Neurotrauma: Traumatic Brain Injury

Neurotrauma: Traumatic Brain Injury

Edited by Franklin McDonough

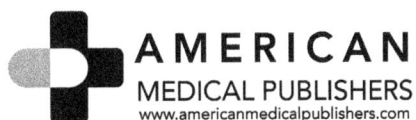

AMERICAN
MEDICAL PUBLISHERS
www.americanmedicalpublishers.com

American Medical Publishers,
41 Flatbush Avenue,
1st Floor, New York,
NY 11217, USA

Visit us on the World Wide Web at:
www.americanmedicalpublishers.com

ISBN: 978-1-63927-321-8

Cataloging-in-Publication Data

Neurotrauma : traumatic brain injury / edited by Franklin McDonough.
     p. cm.
Includes bibliographical references and index.
ISBN 978-1-63927-321-8
1. Nervous system--Wounds and injuries. 2. Brain--Wounds and injuries.
3. Brain--Wounds and injuries--Complications. 4. Brain--Diseases. I. McDonough, Franklin.
RD594 .N48 2022
617.481--dc23

Table of Contents

Preface

Neurotrauma refers to two different types of injuries, namely, acquired brain injury and spinal cord injury. Traumatic brain injury and non-traumatic brain injuries are the two types of acquired brain injuries. Traumatic brain injury occurs when the brain is injured by an external mechanical force. It can cause temporary or permanent impairment in the brain. There are numerous causes which can result in traumatic brain injury such as violence, transportation accidents, sports, etc. Traumatic brain injuries can be classified on the basis of severity into mild, moderate and severe injuries. The signs and symptoms depend on the type of brain injury. A few of the common signs are constant headache, vomiting, nausea, dizziness, blurred vision, ringing in the ears and lack of motor coordination. This book provides comprehensive insights into the field of traumatic brain injury. The extensive content of this book provides the readers with a thorough understanding of the subject. This book is a compilation of chapters that discuss the most vital concepts and emerging trends in this field.

Various studies have approached the subject by analyzing it with a single perspective, but the present book provides diverse methodologies and techniques to address this field. This book contains theories and applications needed for understanding the subject from different perspectives. The aim is to keep the readers informed about the progresses in the field; therefore, the contributions were carefully examined to compile novel researches by specialists from across the globe.

Indeed, the job of the editor is the most crucial and challenging in compiling all chapters into a single book. In the end, I would extend my sincere thanks to the chapter authors for their profound work. I am also thankful for the support provided by my family and colleagues during the compilation of this book.

Editor

Preface

Anti-inflammatory and immunomodulatory mechanisms of mesenchymal stem cell transplantation in experimental traumatic brain injury

Run Zhang[1†], Yi Liu[1†], Ke Yan[1], Lei Chen[2], Xiang-Rong Chen[1], Peng Li[1], Fan-Fan Chen[1] and Xiao-Dan Jiang[1*]

Abstract

Background: Previous studies have shown beneficial effects of mesenchymal stem cell (MSC) transplantation in central nervous system (CNS) injuries, including traumatic brain injury (TBI). Potential repair mechanisms involve transdifferentiation to replace damaged neural cells and production of growth factors by MSCs. However, few studies have simultaneously focused on the effects of MSCs on immune cells and inflammation-associated cytokines in CNS injury, especially in an experimental TBI model. In this study, we investigated the anti-inflammatory and immunomodulatory properties of MSCs in TBI-induced neuroinflammation by systemic transplantation of MSCs into a rat TBI model.

Methods/results: MSCs were transplanted intravenously into rats 2 h after TBI. Modified neurologic severity score (mNSS) tests were performed to measure behavioral outcomes. The effect of MSC treatment on neuroinflammation was analyzed by immunohistochemical analysis of astrocytes, microglia/macrophages, neutrophils and T lymphocytes and by measuring cytokine levels [interleukin (IL)-1α, IL-1β, IL-4, IL-6, IL-10, IL-17, tumor necrosis factor-α, interferon-γ, RANTES, macrophage chemotactic protein-1, macrophage inflammatory protein 2 and transforming growth factor-β1] in brain homogenates. The immunosuppression-related factors TNF-α stimulated gene/protein 6 (TSG-6) and nuclear factor-κB (NF-κB) were examined by reverse transcription-polymerase chain reaction and Western blotting. Intravenous MSC transplantation after TBI was associated with a lower density of microglia/macrophages and peripheral infiltrating leukocytes at the injury site, reduced levels of proinflammatory cytokines and increased anti-inflammatory cytokines, possibly mediated by enhanced expression of TSG-6, which may suppress activation of the NF-κB signaling pathway.

Conclusions: The results of this study suggest that MSCs have the ability to modulate inflammation-associated immune cells and cytokines in TBI-induced cerebral inflammatory responses. This study thus offers a new insight into the mechanisms responsible for the immunomodulatory effect of MSC transplantation, with implications for functional neurological recovery after TBI.

* Correspondence: jiangxiao_dan@163.com
†Equal contributors
[1]The National Key Clinic Specialty, The Neurosurgery Institute of Guangdong Province, Guangdong Provincial Key Laboratory on Brain Function Repair and Regeneration, Department of Neurosurgery, Zhujiang Hospital, Southern Medical University, Guangzhou 510282, China
Full list of author information is available at the end of the article

Background

Traumatic brain injury (TBI) is a major cause of mortality and morbidity among the population worldwide [1]. The inflammatory response is regarded as a key factor in the secondary injury cascade following TBI. Activation of the inflammatory cascade is mediated by the release of pro- and anti-inflammatory cytokines [2,3]. TBI induces a strong inflammatory response characterized by the recruitment of peripheral leukocytes into the cerebral parenchyma and the activation of resident immune cells [4,5]. The infiltration of neutrophils, monocytes and lymphocytes to the injured site directly affects neuronal survival and death [4-7]. Moreover, activated microglia migrate to injured sites and release cytokines, chemotactic cytokines, reactive oxygen species, nitric oxide, proteases and other factors with cytotoxic effects, which may in turn exacerbate neuronal death [6,8].

However, these immune cells and inflammatory mediators can also have neuroprotective effects in TBI [3,9]. For example, T lymphocytes may contribute to later repair processes in brain injury [10,11]; proinflammatory cytokines such as interleukin (IL)-1, IL-6 and tumor necrosis factor (TNF)-α have both deleterious and beneficial effects on neural cells [7,12,13]; and microglia can remove cell debris, promote tissue remodeling and exert numerous neuroprotective effects under certain conditions [4,14,15]. Of these, TBI-induced inflammation appears to be a key factor in secondary brain damage, which suggests that anti-inflammatory or immunoregulatory strategies could provide effective treatments for the management of TBI-induced pathology.

Previous studies have shown beneficial effects of mesenchymal stem cell (MSC) transplantation in central nervous system (CNS) injuries, including TBI, stroke and spinal cord injury animal models. The main findings of these studies suggested that MSCs improved neurological functional recovery, decreased apoptosis, increased endogenous cell proliferation, promoted angiogenesis and reduced lesion size [16]. The potential mechanisms whereby transplanted MSCs might exert beneficial effects in CNS injury include their ability to migrate to injured tissues, transdifferentiation to replace damaged neural cells and the production of growth factors by MSCs [16-18]. However, recent evidence indicates that the therapeutic effect of MSC transplantation may not be through direct cell replacement, but via modulating the host microenvironment [19]. MSCs can secrete a variety of bioactive molecules such as trophic factors and anti-apoptotic molecules, which may provide the main mechanism responsible for their therapeutic effect [20].

More recently, many studies have demonstrated that MSCs possess immunomodulatory properties [21,22]. MSCs can directly inhibit the proliferation of T lymphocytes and microglial cells, and can modulate the cytokine-secretion profile of dendritic cells and monocytes and/or macrophages [20,23-25]. MSCs are also known to inhibit basal and formyl-methionyl-leucyl-phenylalanine-stimulated production of reactive oxygen species by neutrophils [26]. In experimental autoimmune encephalomyelitis models, MSCs inhibited myelin-specific T cells and induced peripheral tolerance [27,28]. The immunosuppressive effect of transplanted MSCs has also been demonstrated in acute, severe graft-versus-host disease [29] and in multiple system atrophy [30]. In addition, MSCs can induce peripheral tolerance and migrate to injured tissues, where they can inhibit the release of proinflammatory cytokines and promote the survival of damaged cells [21]. For example, the therapeutic benefit of MSC transplantation has been observed in acute lung injury [31,32], myocardial infarction [33], acute renal failure [34], cerebral ischemia [35] and Alzheimer's disease [36]. Furthermore, some studies have found an inflammation-modulatory function for transplanted stem cells. One study demonstrated anti-inflammatory effects of human cord blood cells in a rat model of stroke [37]. Another study reported that intravenous NSCs, administered during the hyperacute stage in stroke, could modulate innate cerebral inflammatory responses by interacting with peripheral inflammatory systems [38].

These studies indicate the feasibility of using MSCs to reduce cerebral inflammation and modulate the immune response after TBI. However, few studies have focused simultaneously on the effects of MSCs on inflammation-associated cytokines and immune cells in CNS injury, especially in an experimental TBI model. In this study, we therefore investigated the anti-inflammatory and immunomodulatory properties of MSCs in TBI-induced neuroinflammation using systemic MSC transplantation in a rat TBI model.

Materials and methods

Sprague–Dawley (SD) rats were purchased from the Animal Experiment Center of Southern Medical University (Guangzhou, China). Animals were housed under a 12-h light/dark cycle, with food and water freely available. Animal experimental procedures were approved by the Southern Medical University Ethics Committee. All surgery was performed under sodium pentobarbital anesthesia, and all efforts were made to minimize animal suffering.

Isolation, expansion and characterization of MSCs

MSCs were generated from the bone marrow of SD rats. Mononuclear cells were isolated by gradient centrifugation at 900 g for 30 min on Percoll (Invitrogen, Carlsbad, CA, USA) at a density of 1.073 g/ml. The cells were then washed twice with phosphate-buffered saline (PBS) and plated at 1×10^6 cells/25 cm^2 in culture flasks in 5 ml DMEM/F12 (1:1) with 10% fetal bovine serum. After 72 h of incubation, non-adherent cells were removed from the cultures, and fresh culture medium was added to the flasks. When the cells reached 90% confluence, adherent cells were trypsinized, harvested and expanded [39]. Expanded cells from passages three–eight were used for further testing or transplantation.

MSCs were assessed by flow cytometry analysis of CD44, CD90 and CD105, and the hematopoietic markers CD14, CD34, CD45 and HLA-DR [40]. The primary antibodies used were fluorescein isothiocyanate-conjugated anti-CD44, -CD45 and -CD105, and phycoerythrin-conjugated anti-CD14, -CD34, -CD90 and -HLA-DR. All antibodies were purchased from AbD Serotec (1:10, Kidlington, UK).

Experimental groups
SD rats were divided into three groups: (1) sham group (21 rats); (2) TBI + saline group (52 rats); (3) TBI + MSCs group (52 rats).

Traumatic brain injury animal models
TBI animal models were produced as previously described [41]. Adult male SD rats (220–250 g) were anesthetized with 2% pentobarbital (30 mg/kg) intraperitoneally and maintained at 37°C throughout the surgical procedure using a water-heating pad. The rats were placed in a stereotactic frame. A 6-mm-diameter craniotomy was performed over the right cortex midway between the lambda and the bregma. Injury was induced using a weight-drop hitting device (ZH-ZYQ, Electronic Technology Development Co., Xuzhou, China) with a 4.5-mm-diameter cylinder bar weighing 40 g from a height of 20 cm. Rats in the sham group were subjected to the same craniotomy procedure without cortical impact.

MSC transplantation
Two hours after TBI, the rats were neurologically evaluated using a modified neurological severity score (mNSS) test. Rats with similar neurological severity scores (13–15 points) were randomly divided into two groups that received 4×10^6 MSCs in 100 μl PBS or PBS alone, respectively, via the jugular vein.

Behavioral testing
Behavioral testing was conducted on days 1, 3, 7, 14, 21 and 28 after TBI using mNSS tests. The mNSS test includes motor, sensory, reflex and balance tests, as described previously [42]. The mNSS test is graded on a scale of 0–18, where a total score of 18 points indicates severe neurological deficit and a score of 0 indicates normal performance; 13–18 points indicates severe injury, 7–12 indicates mean-moderate injury, and 1–6 indicates mild injury.

Measurements of brain water content
Brain water content was measured at 72 h after TBI. Following anesthesia and decapitation, the brains were removed immediately and divided into two hemispheres along the midline, and the cerebella were removed. Ipsilateral hemispheres were placed on a pre-weighed piece of aluminum foil to give the wet weight and then dried in an electric oven at 100°C for 24 h [38]. The brain water percentage was calculated as follows: (wet weight - dry weight)/(wet weight).

Immunohistochemistry and terminal deoxynucleotidyl transferase dUTP nick end labeling staining
At 72 h after TBI, rats were anesthetized and transcardially perfused with 100 ml cold PBS and 100 ml of 4% paraformaldehyde in 0.1 M PBS. The brains were then removed, post-fixed and paraffin-embedded, and consecutive coronal sections were cut at 5-μm intervals from bregma –2.0 mm to bregma –7.0 mm to collect the entire lesioned cortex. For immunohistochemistry, slides with brain sections were deparaffinized and boiled in 10 mM citrate buffer (pH 6.0) in a microwave to expose the antigens and then blocked with 10% normal goat serum. Slides were incubated with primary antibody against glial fibrillary acidic protein (GFAP) (rabbit polyclonal to GFAP, 1:200), microglia/macrophage-specific calcium-binding protein (goat polyclonal to Iba1, 1:100, Abcam, New Territories, HK), myeloperoxidase (MPO) (rabbit polyclonal to MPO, 1:100, Abcam) and CD3 (rabbit polyclonal to CD3, 1:100, Abcam) at 4°C overnight. Following primary antibody incubation, slides were incubated in biotin-conjugated anti-rabbit IgG or anti-goat IgG (1:100, Boster, Wuhan, China), then treated with an avidin-biotin-peroxidase system (Boster) (negative controls for immunostaining was secondary antibody only). Finally, slides were stained with diaminobenzidine, and the nucleus was counterstained with hematoxylin. Terminal deoxynucleotidyl transferase-mediated dUTP nick 3′-end labeling was performed to detect dying cells using an In Situ Cell Detection Kit (Roche, South San Francisco, CA, USA) according to the manufacturer's instructions. The number of positive cells near the injured areas was counted (8 to10 sections per brain, 500 μm apart) in a blinded manner.

Cytokine analysis
To measure cytokine levels, rats were killed at 12, 24 and 72 h after TBI or sham operation. Brains were immediately collected, and punch biopsies (5 mm diameter) of the injured cortex were isolated and stored at –80°C. The tissue was homogenized in chilled extraction buffer containing Tris–HCl (50 mmol/l, pH 7.2), NaCl (150 mmol/l), 1% Triton X-100 and 1 mg/ml protease inhibitor cocktail (Biovision, Mountain View, CA, USA) at a ratio of 1:10 (tissue: buffer), shaken for 90 min on ice, centrifuged at

12,000 g for 15 min at 4°C and frozen at −80°C [43]. Total protein concentrations were measured using a BCA Protein Assay Kit (Thermo, Rockford, IL, USA). The levels of 12 cytokines [IL-1α, IL-1β, IL-4, IL-6, IL-10, IL-17, tumor necrosis factor (TNF)-α, interferon (IFN)-γ, RANTES, macrophage chemotactic protein (MCP)-1, macrophage inflammatory protein (MIP)-2 and transforming growth factor (TGF)-β1] were determined in 1 mg of total protein using the Rat Bio-Plex Pro Assays (Bio- Rad, Hercules, CA, USA), according to the manufacturer's instructions.

Quantitative real-time polymerase chain reaction

Total RNA was extracted from injured brain tissues at 12, 24 and 72 h after TBI using TRIzol Reagent (Invitrogen), according to the manufacturer's instructions. Levels of TNF-α stimulated gene/protein 6 (TSG-6) and nuclear factor (NF)-κB mRNA were quantitated using an ABI 7500HT Fast Real-Time PCR System (Applied Biosystems, Grand Island, NY, USA). Glyceraldehyde-3-phosphate dehydrogenase (GAPDH) was used as an endogenous control. Sequence-specific primers for the above genes were designed using Premier 5 software as follows:

TSG-6-up: GCAGCTAGAAGCAGCCAGAAAG,
TSG-6-dn: TTGTAGCAATAGGCGTCCCACC;
NF-κB-up: CTACACTTAGCCATCATCCACCTT,
NF-κB-dn: AGTCCTCCACCACATCTTCCTG;
GAPDH-up: AAGGTGAAGGTCGGAGTCAA,
GAPDH-dn: AATGAAGGGGTCATTGATGG.

The $2^{-\Delta\Delta Ct}$ method was used to calculate the relative expression levels.

Western blot analysis

Total protein was isolated from rat injured brain tissues using ice-cold RIPA buffer. Total protein concentrations were measured with the BCA Protein Assay Kit (Thermo). Protein samples (30 μg per lane) were separated using sodium dodecyl sulfate-polyacrylamide gel electrophoresis and transferred to polyvinylidene difluoride membranes. Proteins were detected by incubation with primary antibodies (mouse polyclonal to TSG-6 and mouse anti-NF-κB p65 1:250, BD Biosciences, San Jose, CA, USA) followed by secondary antibodies (goat anti- mouse IgG, horseradish-peroxidase conjugate, 1:1,000, Sigma Aldrich, St. Louis, MO, USA). Immunoblots were visualized using a Millipore ECL Western Blotting Detection System (Millipore, Billerica, MA, USA). GAPDH (1:3,000, Santa Cruz Biotechnology, Santa Cruz, CA, USA.) was employed as the loading control.

Statistical analysis

Statistical analyses were performed using SPSS version 13.0 (SPSS, Chicago, IL, USA), and all data are presented as mean ± S.D. Statistical differences among the groups were assessed by one-way ANOVA and post hoc multiple comparisons were performed using Student-Newman-Keuls tests. The significance level was set at $p < 0.05$.

Results

Isolation and characterization of MSCs

MSCs were isolated from SD rats' bone marrow and maintained in culture for several passages. Before intravenous transplantation, third- and eighth-passage cells were characterized, and flow cytometry analysis confirmed that the cells at transplantation were positive for CD44 (99.01%), CD90 (99.28%) and CD105 (97.71%), and had low expression of CD14 (0.79%), CD34 (0.78%), CD45 (0.67%) and HLA-DR (1.11%) (Figure 1).

Treatment with MSCs improved neurological recovery after TBI

In order to assess the effects of systemic administration of MSCs after TBI, mNSS was performed on days 1, 3, 7, 14, 21 and 28 after TBI. There was a significant improvement in neurological function in the MSC-treated group compared with the PBS group from days 3–28 post-TBI ($p < 0.05$). There was no significant difference between the scores in the two groups only at 24 h post-TBI (Figure 2A).

MSC treatment reduced brain water content after TBI

To investigate whether treatment with MSCs could reduce brain edema, we measured brain water contents in the two experimental groups. Increased water content directly causes brain edema, which is one of the most important surrogate markers of brain damage, and it peaks at 72 h after brain injury [44]. The PBS group had a significantly higher brain water content than the sham-injured control group. However, treatment with MSCs significantly reduced the brain water contents compared with the PBS group ($p < 0.05$). The brain water contents in the sham, PBS and MSC groups were 78.62 ± 0.32, 82.48 ± 0.74% and 79.87 ± 0.70%, respectively (Figure 2B).

MSC treatment reduced brain inflammatory cell infiltration, microglia and apoptotic cell numbers

To test the effects of MSC treatment on the number of peripheral infiltrating and resident immune cells in the injured brain, we identified GFAP+ astrocytes, Iba-1+ microglia cells/macrophages, MPO+ neutrophils and CD3+ lymphocytes by immunohistochemistry. The densities of astrocytes were not significantly different after MSC treatment (Figure 3B,D). The number of microglia/macrophages (sham: 142. 7 ± 45. 4 cells/mm²; PBS: 1,524. 7 ± 60.1 cells/mm²; MSCs: 1,124.3 ± 104.5 cells/mm²) (Figure 3C,E) was significantly reduced after MSC

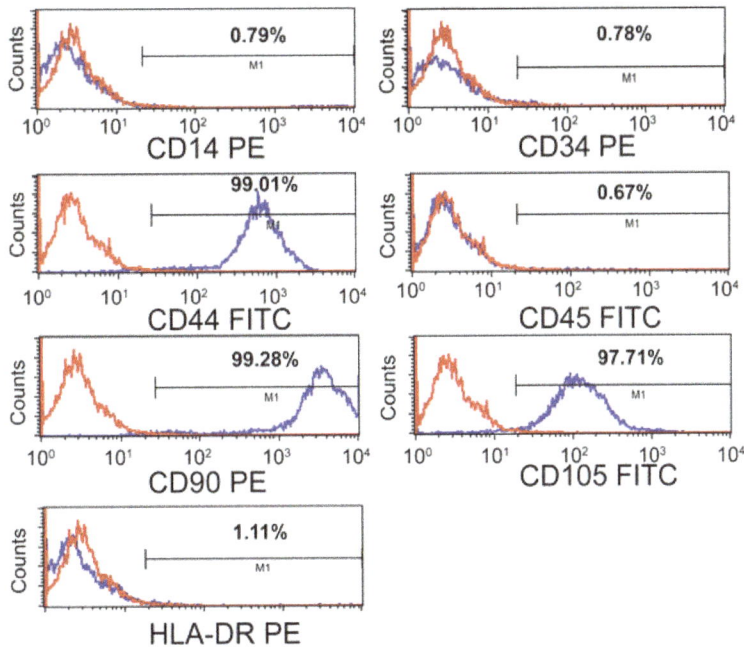

Figure 1 Surface marker expression in MSCs. MSCs were confirmed by flow cytometry analysis after three passages as positive for CD44 (99.01%), CD90 (99.28%) and CD105 (97.71%), with low positivity for CD14 (0.79%), CD34 (0.78%), CD45 (0.67%) and HLA-DR (1.11%).

administration at 72 h post-TBI compared with the PBS treatment group ($p < 0.05$). Meanwhile, MSCs decreased the densities of infiltrated MPO^+ neutrophils (PBS: 775.0 ± 55.34 cells/mm^2; MSCs: 638.67 ± 72.15 cells/mm^2) (Figure 4A,C) and $CD3^+$ lymphocytes (PBS: 421.67 ± 28.15 cells/mm^2; MSCs: 367.67 ± 17.5 cells/mm^2) (Figure 4B,D) and apoptotic cells (sham: 18. 7 ± 8.1 cells/mm^2; PBS: 295 ± 15 cells/mm^2; MSCs: 179.3 ± 25.8 cells/mm^2) (Figure 5) in the injured cortex at 72 h post-TBI ($p < 0.05$).

MSCs influenced cytokine levels in injured cortex

To investigate the anti-inflammatory functions of MSCs, we assessed an array of inflammatory cytokines in injured

cortex homogenates at 12, 24 and 72 h after TBI (Figure 6). Levels of the proinflammatory cytokines IL-1β at 12 h ($p < 0.01$), 24 h ($p < 0.05$) and 72 h ($p < 0.05$), IL-6 at 24 h ($p < 0.05$) and 72 h ($p < 0.05$), IL-17 at 24 h ($p < 0.05$) and 72 h ($p < 0.01$), TNF-α at 24 h ($p < 0.05$) and 72 h ($p < 0.01$), and IFN-γ at 72 h ($p < 0.05$) were all significantly decreased in the MSC-treatment group compared with the PBS group (Figure 6A-E). In contrast, production of the anti-inflammatory cytokines IL-10 at 24 h ($p < 0.01$) and 72 h ($p < 0.05$) and TGF-β1 at 24 h ($p < 0.01$) and 72 h ($p < 0.01$) (Figure 6F,G) after TBI were increased in the MSC-treatment group compared with the PBS group. The chemokines MCP-1,

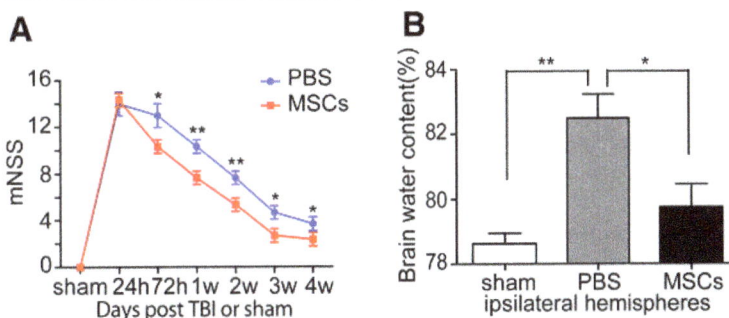

Figure 2 Modified neurologic severity score (mNSS) and brain water content. (A) Neurological function was analyzed by mNSS on days 1, 3, 7, 14, 21 and 28 after TBI. Treatment with MSCs significantly lowered mNSS from days 3–28 compared with the PBS group. There was no significant difference in scores between the MSC- and PBS-treated groups only at 24 h post-TBI ($n = 6$ per group). **(B)** Brain water content of ipsilateral hemispheres was measured at 72 h after injury. The PBS group had a significantly higher brain water content than the sham-injured control group. MSC treatment significantly reduced brain water content compared with the PBS group ($n = 6$ per group). Data are presented as the mean ± SD. *$p < 0.05$, **$p < 0.01$.

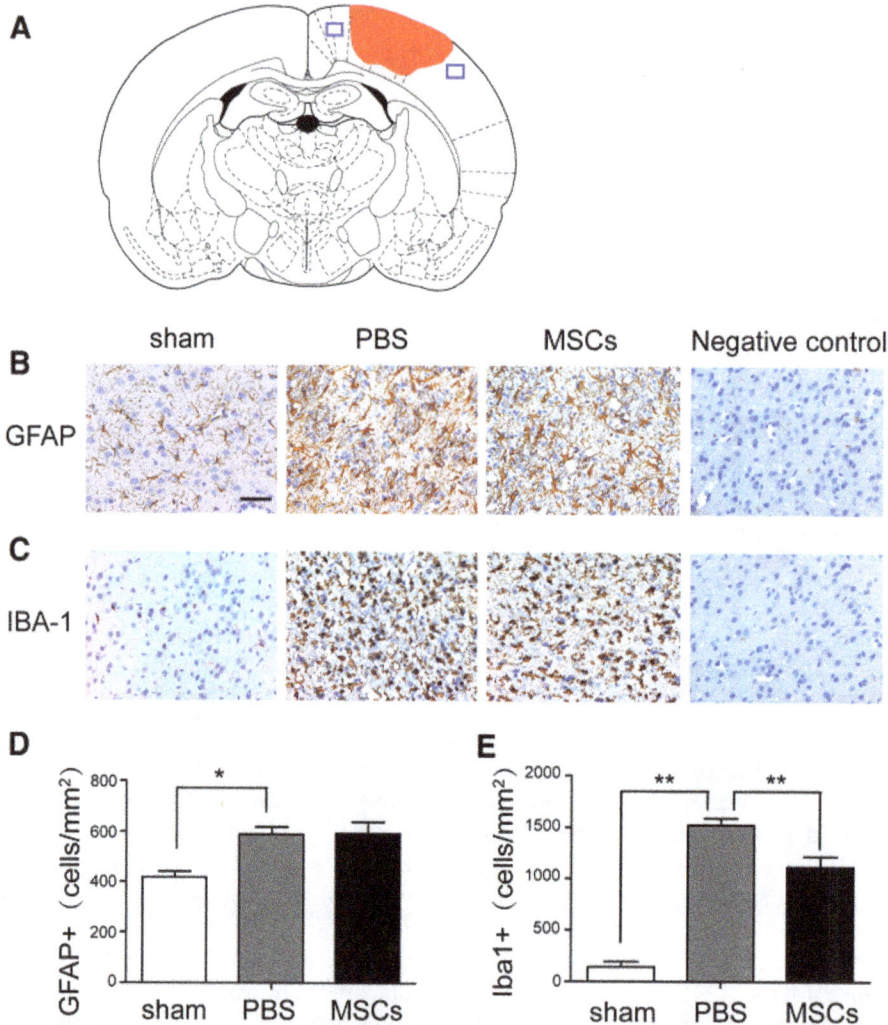

Figure 3 Effect of MSC treatment on GFAP⁺ astrocytes and Iba-1⁺ microglia/macrophages. (A) Diagram of a coronal rat brain section showing the relationship of the lesion cavity (*red*) to the regions photographed (*blue squares*). The density of astrocytes was not significantly different after MSC treatment (**B, D**) ($n = 6$ per group). The number of microglia/macrophages (**C, E**) (sham: 142.7 ± 45.4 cells/mm^2; PBS: $1,524.7 \pm 60.1$ cells/mm^2; MSCs: $1,124.3 \pm 104.5$ cells/mm^2) was significantly decreased after MSC administration at 72 h post-TBI compared with the PBS-treatment group ($n = 6$ per group). Data are presented as mean $\pm$ SD. *Bar* = 50 µm. *$p < 0.05$.

MIP-2 and RANTES were reduced at 12, 24 and 72 h after TBI in the MSC group compared with the PBS group (Figure 6H-J). There were no significant differences in levels of the cytokines IL-1α and IL-4 (Figure 6K,L) between the two groups.

MSC treatment upregulated TSG-6 expression

To elucidate the potential mechanisms responsible for the effects of MSCs on anti-inflammatory and immuno-modulatory properties, we analyzed the expression of the inhibitory factors TSG-6 and transcription factor NF-κB at the mRNA and protein levels. TSG-6 was upregulated from 12–72 h in the injured cortex after TBI in the MSC-treatment group ($p < 0.01$) (Figure 7A). mRNA levels of NF-κB (Figure 7B) were decreased from

12–48 h after MSC transplantation ($p < 0.01$). Similar results were obtained by Western blotting for TSG-6 and NF-κB p65 (Figure 7C).

Discussion

In this study, we investigated the anti-inflammatory and immunomodulatory properties of MSCs by systemic transplantation into TBI model rats. The main observations were that MSC treatment reduced the presence of microglia/macrophages in the damaged brain parenchyma and decreased the density of peripheral infiltrating leukocytes at the injured site, as well as reducing proinflammatory cytokines and increasing anti-inflammatory cytokines, possibly through enhanced expression of TSG-6. TSG-6 may, in turn, act by suppressing activation of the NF-κB signaling

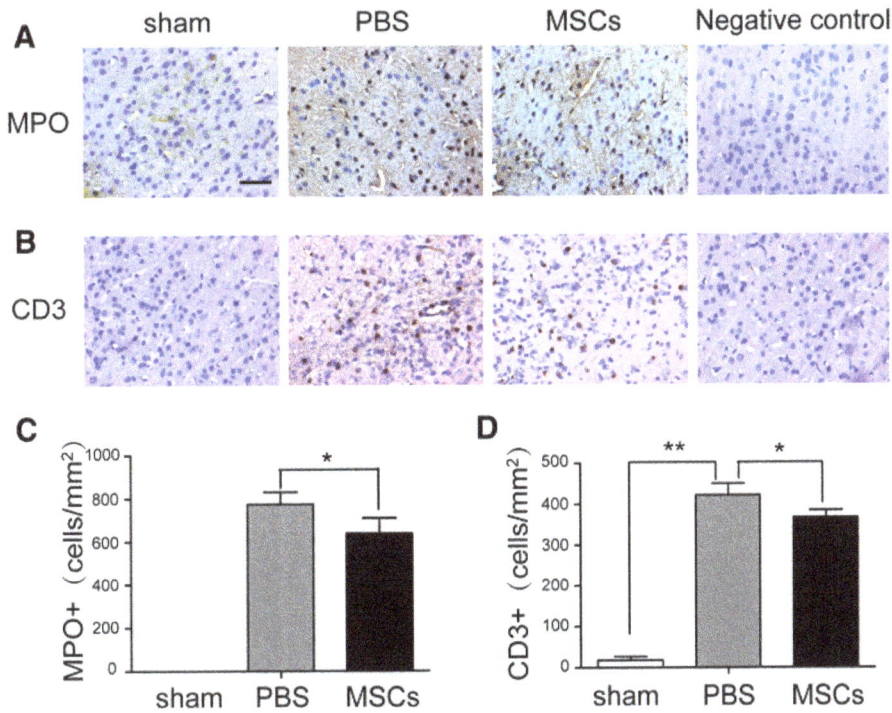

Figure 4 Influence of MSC administration on MPO+ neutrophils and CD3+ lymphocytes. MSCs reduced the numbers of infiltrating MPO+ neutrophils **(A, C)** (PBS: 775.0 ± 55.34 cells/mm²; MSCs: 638.67 ± 72.15 cells/mm²), CD3+ lymphocytes **(B, D)** (PBS: 421.67 ± 28.15 cells/mm²; MSCs: 367.67 ± 17.5 cells/mm²). Data are presented as the mean ± SD. Bar = 50 μm; n = 6 per group, *p < 0.05.

pathway and decreasing the production of proinflammatory cytokines to initiate a proinflammatory cytokine cascade.

Proinflammatory cytokines such as TNF-α, IL-1 and IL-6 are produced mainly by microglia, with some also produced by astrocytes, neurons and endothelial cells, which in turn activate glial cells, inducing further cytokine production and astrogliosis [4,45,46]. Reduced activation of microglia can thus reduce inflammation and improve histological and functional outcomes after TBI [8]. Anti-inflammatory cytokines such as IL-4, IL-10 and TGF-β1 have the ability to counteract and downregulate inflammatory and cytotoxic reactions [4,47]. For instance, IL-10 is produced by microglia and astrocytes and by lymphocytes in the periphery, and can suppress microglia and astroglia activation, as

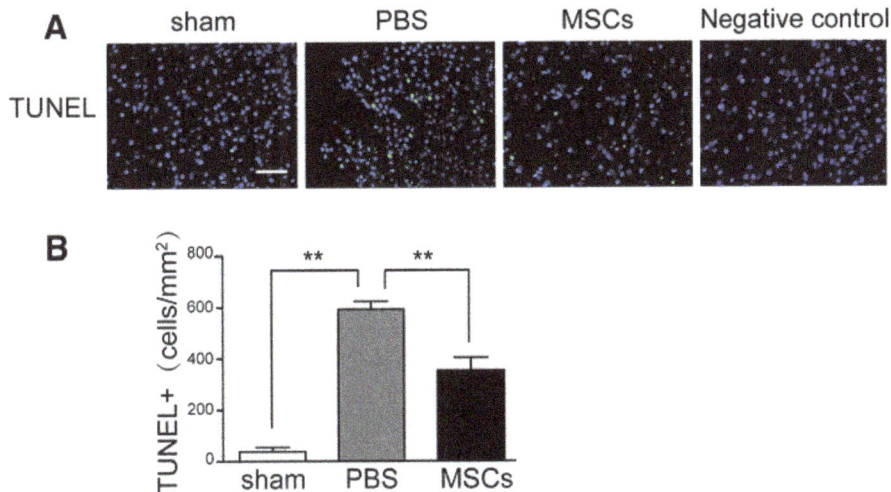

Figure 5 Effect of MSC transplantation on apoptosis. Apoptotic cells (sham: 18.7 ± 8.1 cells/mm²; PBS: 295 ± 15 cells/mm²; MSCs: 179.3 ± 25.8 cells/mm²) in the injured cortex at 72 h after TBI were reduced in the MSC treatment group compared with the PBS group **(A, B)** (n = 6 per group). Number of apoptotic cells is presented as the mean ± SD. Bar = 50 μm. **p < 0.01.

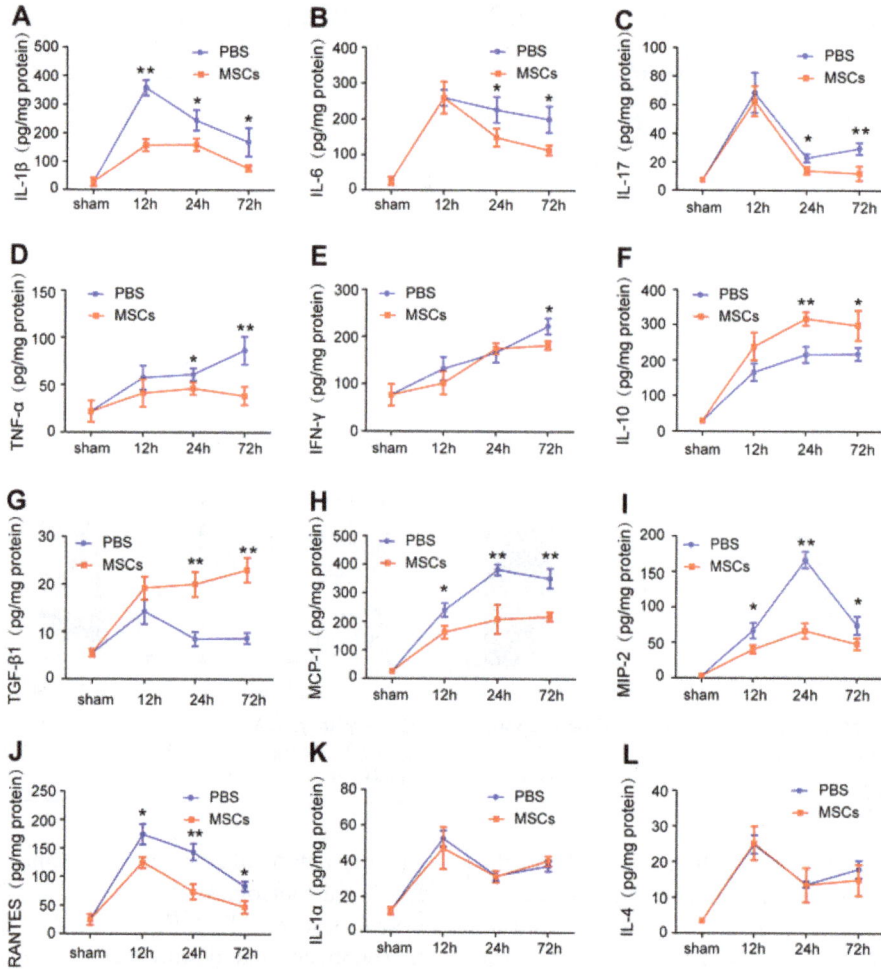

Figure 6 Influence of MSC treatment on cytokine concentrations. Levels of the proinflammatory cytokines IL-1β (at 12, 24 and 72 h), IL-6 (at 24 and 72 h), IL-17 (at 24 and 72 h), TNF-α (at 24 and 72 h) and IFN-γ (at 72 h) were significantly decreased in the MSC-treatment group compared with the PBS group **(A–E)**. Levels of the anti-inflammatory cytokines IL-10 and TGF-β1 (at 24 and 72 h after TBI) **(F, G)** were increased in the MSC-treatment group compared with the PBS group. The chemokines MCP-1, MIP-2 and RANTES were reduced at 12, 24 and 72 h after TBI in the MSC group compared with the PBS group **(H–J)**. There were no significant differences in levels of the cytokines IL-1α and IL-4 **(K, L)** between the two groups. $n = 6$ in each time point of per group. Data are presented as the mean ± SD. *$p < 0.05$, **$p < 0.01$.

well as decreasing production of proinflammatory cytokines [48,49]. MSCs have been shown to decrease proinflammatory cytokine gene expression in experimental acute lung injury [31,32], myocardial infarction [33] and acute renal failure [34] and to upregulate IL-10 expression in rat models of myocardial infarction and cerebral infarction [50,51]. Although astrocytes are not directly immune-related cells, activated astrocytes are a major source of inflammatory-related molecules such as pro- and anti-inflammatory cytokines and chemokines. In addition, astrocyte activation and proliferation after TBI seem to impair axonal regrowth, but these cells also release neurotrophic factors promoting tissue repair and neurogenesis [52]. However, the immuno-modulatory effects of MSCs on astrocytes are still limited. One study has shown that MSCs can inhibit

the production of cytokines in LPS-activated astrocyte cultures, reducing not only the proinflammatory cytokines, but also the expression of the anti-inflammatory IL-10 [53].

In the CNS, chemokines secreted by glia and neurons are considered to be essential mediators in the recruitment of leukocytes into damaged parenchyma in post-traumatic neuroinflammation [43]. MIP-2, also known as CXCL2, contributes to neutrophil infiltration and subsequent secondary neurodegeneration following TBI [54], and it has been shown to increase rapidly following TBI in experimental TBI models [55,56]. MCP-1, also known as CCL2, is the most potent chemoattractant for monocytes, macrophages and microglia, which play significant roles in mediating post-traumatic secondary brain damage [43]. CCL2 expression is elevated rapidly after diffuse axonal injury, and its overexpression exacerbated ischemic brain injury in

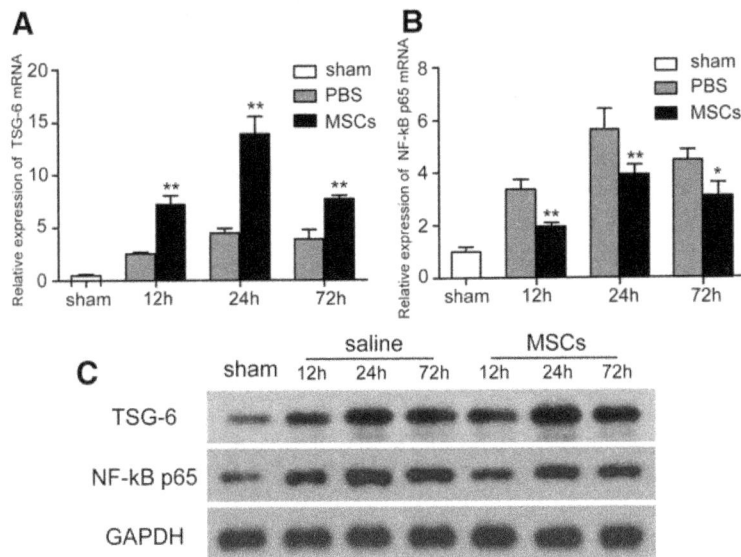

Figure 7 MSC treatment upregulates TSG-6 and downregulates NF-κB expression. Upregulation of TSG-6 **(A)** was observed from 12 to 72 h in the injured cortex after TBI in the MSC-treatment group. mRNA levels of NF-κB **(B)** decreased from 12 to 48 h after MSC transplantation. Similar results were observed at the protein level **(C)** for TSG-6 and NF-κB p65. $n = 6$ in each time point of per group. Data are presented as the mean ± SD. $*p < 0.05$, $**p < 0.01$ versus PBS group.

mice [57,58]. Expression of the chemokine RANTES (regulated upon activation, normal T cell expressed and secreted) increased after brain injury in rats and has the ability to activate T cells [59]. The role of T lymphocytes in TBI is largely unknown, although in ischemic stroke, these cells infiltrate into the brain and release proinflammatory cytokines and cytotoxic substances, which contribute to early inflammation and brain injury [10]. One study has shown that reduction of T-lymphocyte recruitment significantly enhances tissue preservation and functional outcome after spinal cord injury [60]. Therefore, reduction of neutrophil and T lymphocyte infiltrations at an early stage is a key feature in improving TBI outcome [61]. In contrast, T lymphocytes can also have beneficial effects on the repair and regeneration of the brain at later stages following injury [10]. Our results indicated that MSCs reduce production of the chemokines MIP-2, MCP-1 and RANTES, suggesting that they could act through reducing chemokine production, thus decreasing the recruitment of peripheral leukocytes.

The anti-inflammatory and immunosuppressive effects of MSCs were related to several inhibitory factors such as inducible nitric oxide synthase, indoleamine 2,3-dioxygenase, prostaglandin E2 and TSG-6, which are produced by MSCs or released following cross-talk with target cells, and which have been reported to be involved in MSC-mediated immune regulation [22]. The current study did not investigate inhibitory factors produced by MSCs, such as inducible nitric oxide synthase,

indoleamine 2,3-dioxygenase or prostaglandin E2, because their short half-lives mean that their immunosuppressive effects can only be observed *in vitro* or because they have adverse effects when administered systemically [62]. TSG-6 is an anti-inflammatory protein with multiple anti-inflammatory effects that is induced by the inflammatory cytokines TNF-α and IL-1 [63]. Transplanted MSCs played a crucial role in the suppression of inflammation in models of myocardial infarction and corneal injury, and these anti-inflammatory effects may be attributable to the secretion of TSG-6 by MSCs [33,64]. NF-κB is an important transcription factor that regulates many genes with key roles in immune and inflammatory responses. It is activated in the brain after TBI and contributes to neuronal death [65,66]. Inhibition of NF-κB activation may thus reduce adverse inflammatory response events and reduce the loss of neuronal cells after TBI. TSG-6 can reduce the production of proinflammatory cytokines through suppressed activation of the NF-κB signaling pathway, thus initiating the cascade of proinflammatory cytokines [67]. Our results suggest that the beneficial effects of MSCs may be partially explained by the effect of TSG-6 on the NF-κB pathway.

The results of this study raise several issues regarding the clinical use of MSCs. First, the schedule of MSC administration is important. MSCs are not spontaneously immunosuppressive and only exhibit this property under special conditions [22]; stimulation with certain inflammatory cytokines such as IFN-γ is essential for MSC-mediated immunosuppression [68]. If the levels of inflammatory cytokines are too low, the immunosuppressive effect of

MSCs will not be triggered. Inflammatory cytokines are rapidly upregulated following brain injury, and some peak at as little as 2 h after TBI [7]. In addition, neutrophil and T lymphocyte infiltrations peak at 24 h after TBI [61], and microglia activation is induced immediately after injury [69,70]. Later MSC treatment may therefore not be effective in terms of anti-inflammatory or immunosuppressive activity, while MSC administration at the onset of the inflammatory response after TBI is more likely to be effective. In this study, we therefore transplanted MSCs at 2 h after TBI. Second, the route taken by the cells is also important. Previous studies showed that in the case of intravenously injected MSCs, few cells reached the brain parenchyma after the pulmonary first-pass effect [16]. The ideal treatment combined intravenous injection with direct injection to provide both systemic and local therapeutic effects [21]. Finally, multiple administrations of MSCs may be needed to sustain and prolong their inhibitory effects, as demonstrated in a mouse graft-versus-host disease model [71].

MSCs are known to modulate both systemic and local inflammation systems in neuroinflammation [72]. We did not investigate the effect of MSCs on systemic inflammation, but the possibility that the neuroprotective effects of MSCs are caused by modulation of the systemic inflammatory system cannot be ruled out. Recent evidence suggests a link between brain injury and the autonomic release of proinflammatory cytokines by resident macrophages in the spleen [73]. Inhibiting this release by splenectomy was shown to improve outcomes in animal models of TBI [44], implying that transplanted MSCs acting directly on resident macrophages in the spleen could contribute to the neuroprotective effect. Overall, these results suggest that novel MSC-mediated immunosuppression mechanisms may be developed for the therapy of TBI.

Conclusions

These results suggest that MSCs have the ability to modulate inflammation-associated cytokine release and immune cells in TBI-induced cerebral inflammatory responses. This study serves as the basis for future studies and offers new insights into the mechanisms responsible for the beneficial immunomodulatory effect of MSC transplantation in terms of functional neurological recovery after TBI. However, further studies are needed to resolve outstanding issues regarding the clinical use of MSCs in TBI.

Abbreviations

MSC: Mesenchymal stem cell; TBI: Traumatic brain injury; CNS: Central nervous system; mNSS: Modified neurologic severity score; TSG-6: Stimulated gene/protein 6; NF-κB: Nuclear factor-κB.

Competing interests

The authors declare that they have no competing interests.

Authors' contributions

Conceived and designed the experiments: RZ, XDJ. Performed the experiments: RZ, YL, KY, XRC, LC. Analyzed the data: FFC, PL. Wrote the paper: RZ, XDJ. Paper revision: XDJ. All authors read and approved the final manuscript.

Acknowledgments

This work was supported by grants from the funds for National Key Clinic Department, the Natural Science Fund of China (nos. 81171179, 81272439), the Funds for Key Sci-Tech Research Projects of Guangdong (no. 2008A030201019) and Guangzhou (no. 09B52120112-2009J1-C418-2, no. 2008A1-E4011-6) to Prof. Xiaodan Jiang.

Author details

[1]The National Key Clinic Specialty, The Neurosurgery Institute of Guangdong Province, Guangdong Provincial Key Laboratory on Brain Function Repair and Regeneration, Department of Neurosurgery, Zhujiang Hospital, Southern Medical University, Guangzhou 510282, China. [2]Department of Neurosurgery, Shenzhen Second People's Hospital, the First Affiliated Hospital of Shenzhen University, Shenzhen 518000, China.

References

1. Xiong Y, Mahmood A, Chopp M: Neurorestorative treatments for traumatic brain injury. *Discov Med* 2010, 10:434–442.
2. Helmy A, Carpenter KL, Menon DK, Pickard JD, Hutchinson PJ: The cytokine response to human traumatic brain injury: temporal profiles and evidence for cerebral parenchymal production. *J Cereb Blood Flow Metab* 2011, 31:658–670.
3. Correale J, Villa A: The neuroprotective role of inflammation in nervous system injuries. *J Neurol* 2004, 251:1304–1316.
4. Ziebell JM, Morganti-Kossmann MC: Involvement of pro- and anti-inflammatory cytokines and chemokines in the pathophysiology of traumatic brain injury. *Neurotherapeutics* 2010, 7:22–30.
5. Rhodes J: Peripheral immune cells in the pathology of traumatic brain injury? *Curr Opin Crit Care* 2011, 17:122–130.
6. Lucas SM, Rothwell NJ, Gibson RM: The role of inflammation in CNS injury and disease. *Br J Pharmacol* 2006, 147(Suppl 1):S232–S240.
7. Helmy A, De Simoni MG, Guilfoyle MR, Carpenter KL, Hutchinson PJ: Cytokines and innate inflammation in the pathogenesis of human traumatic brain injury. *Prog Neurobiol* 2011, 95:352–372.
8. d'Avila JC, Lam TI, Bingham D, Shi J, Won SJ, Kauppinen TM, Massa S, Liu J, Swanson RA: Microglial activation induced by brain trauma is suppressed by post-injury treatment with a PARP inhibitor. *J Neuroinflammation* 2012, 9:31.
9. Morganti-Kossmann MC, Satgunaseelan L, Bye N, Kossmann T: Modulation of immune response by head injury. *Injury* 2007, 38:1392–1400.
10. Brait VH, Arumugam TV, Drummond GR, Sobey CG: Importance of T lymphocytes in brain injury, immunodeficiency, and recovery after cerebral ischemia. *J Cereb Blood Flow Metab* 2012, 32:598–611.
11. Arneth BM: Protective autoimmunity and protein localization. *J Neuroimmunol* 2010, 219:123–125.
12. Winter CD, Pringle AK, Clough GF, Church MK: Raised parenchymal interleukin-6 levels correlate with improved outcome after traumatic brain injury. *Brain* 2004, 127:315–320.
13. Turrin NP, Rivest S: Tumor necrosis factor alpha but not interleukin 1 beta mediates neuroprotection in response to acute nitric oxide excitotoxicity. *J Neurosci* 2006, 26:143–151.
14. Biber K, Neumann H, Inoue K, Boddeke HW: Neuronal 'on' and 'off' signals control microglia. *Trends Neurosci* 2007, 30:596–602.
15. Aloisi F: Immune function of microglia. *Glia* 2001, 36:165–179.
16. Parr AM, Tator CH, Keating A: Bone marrow-derived mesenchymal stromal cells for the repair of central nervous system injury. *Bone Marrow Transplant* 2007, 40:609–619.
17. Chopp M, Li Y: Treatment of neural injury with marrow stromal cells. *Lancet Neurol* 2002, 1:92–100.
18. Si YL, Zhao YL, Hao HJ, Fu XB, Han WD: MSCs: Biological characteristics, clinical applications and their outstanding concerns. *Ageing Res Rev* 2011, 10:93–103.

19. Scuteri A, Miloso M, Foudah D, Orciani M, Cavaletti G, Tredici G: Mesenchymal stem cells neuronal differentiation ability: a real perspective for nervous system repair? *Curr Stem Cell Res Ther* 2011, 6:82–92.

20. Meirelles Lda S, Fontes AM, Covas DT, Caplan AI: Mechanisms involved in the therapeutic properties of mesenchymal stem cells. *Cytokine Growth Factor Rev* 2009, 20:419–427.

21. Uccelli A, Moretta L, Pistoia V: Mesenchymal stem cells in health and disease. *Nat Rev Immunol* 2008, 8:726–736.

22. Shi Y, Su J, Roberts AI, Shou P, Rabson AB, Ren G: How mesenchymal stem cells interact with tissue immune responses. *Trends Immunol* 2012, 33:136–143.

23. Di Nicola M, Carlo-Stella C, Magni M, Milanesi M, Longoni PD, Matteucci P, Grisanti S, Gianni AM: Human bone marrow stromal cells suppress T-lymphocyte proliferation induced by cellular or nonspecific mitogenic stimuli. *Blood* 2002, 99:3838–3843.

24. Ooi YY, Ramasamy R, Rahmat Z, Subramaiam H, Tan SW, Abdullah M, Israf DA, Vidyadaran S: Bone marrow-derived mesenchymal stem cells modulate BV2 microglia responses to lipopolysaccharide. *Int Immunopharmacol* 2010, 10:1532–1540.

25. Nemeth K, Leelahavanichkul A, Yuen PS, Mayer B, Parmelee A, Doi K, Robey PG, Leelahavanichkul K, Koller BH, Brown JM, et al: Bone marrow stromal cells attenuate sepsis via prostaglandin E(2)-dependent reprogramming of host macrophages to increase their interleukin-10 production. *Nat Med* 2009, 15:42–49.

26. Raffaghello L, Bianchi G, Bertolotto M, Montecucco F, Busca A, Dallegri F, Ottonello L, Pistoia V: Human mesenchymal stem cells inhibit neutrophil apoptosis: a model for neutrophil preservation in the bone marrow niche. *Stem Cells* 2008, 26:151–162.

27. Zappia E, Casazza S, Pedemonte E, Benvenuto F, Bonanni I, Gerdoni E, Giunti D, Ceravolo A, Cazzanti F, Frassoni F, et al: Mesenchymal stem cells ameliorate experimental autoimmune encephalomyelitis inducing T-cell anergy. *Blood* 2005, 106:1755–1761.

28. Gerdoni E, Gallo B, Casazza S, Musio S, Bonanni I, Pedemonte E, Mantegazza R, Frassoni F, Mancardi G, Pedotti R, Uccelli A: Mesenchymal stem cells effectively modulate pathogenic immune response in experimental autoimmune encephalomyelitis. *Ann Neurol* 2007, 61:219–227.

29. Le Blanc K, Rasmusson I, Sundberg B, Gotherstrom C, Hassan M, Uzunel M, Ringden O: Treatment of severe acute graft-versus-host disease with third party haploidentical mesenchymal stem cells. *Lancet* 2004, 363:1439–1441.

30. Stemberger S, Jamnig A, Stefanova N, Lepperdinger G, Reindl M, Wenning GK: Mesenchymal stem cells in a transgenic mouse model of multiple system atrophy: immunomodulation and neuroprotection. *PLoS One* 2011, 6:e19808.

31. Ortiz LA, Dutreil M, Fattman C, Pandey AC, Torres G, Go K, Phinney DG: Interleukin 1 receptor antagonist mediates the antiinflammatory and antifibrotic effect of mesenchymal stem cells during lung injury. *Proc Natl Acad Sci U S A* 2007, 104:11002–11007.

32. Gupta N, Su X, Popov B, Lee JW, Serikov V, Matthay MA: Intrapulmonary delivery of bone marrow-derived mesenchymal stem cells improves survival and attenuates endotoxin-induced acute lung injury in mice. *J Immunol* 2007, 179:1855–1863.

33. Lee RH, Pulin AA, Seo MJ, Kota DJ, Ylostalo J, Larson BL, Semprun-Prieto L, Delafontaine P, Prockop DJ: Intravenous hMSCs improve myocardial infarction in mice because cells embolized in lung are activated to secrete the anti-inflammatory protein TSG-6. *Cell Stem Cell* 2009, 5:54–63.

34. Togel F, Hu Z, Weiss K, Isaac J, Lange C, Westenfelder C: Administered mesenchymal stem cells protect against ischemic acute renal failure through differentiation-independent mechanisms. *Am J Physiol Renal Physiol* 2005, 289:F31–F42.

35. Sheikh AM, Nagai A, Wakabayashi K, Narantuya D, Kobayashi S, Yamaguchi S, Kim SU: Mesenchymal stem cell transplantation modulates neuroinflammation in focal cerebral ischemia: contribution of fractalkine and IL-5. *Neurobiol Dis* 2011, 41:717–724.

36. Lee JK, Jin HK, Endo S, Schuchman EH, Carter JE, Bae JS: Intracerebral transplantation of bone marrow-derived mesenchymal stem cells reduces amyloid-beta deposition and rescues memory deficits in Alzheimer's disease mice by modulation of immune responses. *Stem Cells* 2010, 28:329–343.

37. Vendrame M, Gemma C, de Mesquita D, Collier L, Bickford PC, Sanberg CD, Sanberg PR, Pennypacker KR, Willing AE: Anti-inflammatory effects of human cord blood cells in a rat model of stroke. *Stem Cells Dev* 2005, 14:595–604.

38. Lee ST, Chu K, Jung KH, Kim SJ, Kim DH, Kang KM, Hong NH, Kim JH, Ban JJ, Park HK et al: Anti-inflammatory mechanism of intravascular neural stem cell transplantation in haemorrhagic stroke. *Brain* 2008, 131:616–629.

39. Aggarwal S, Pittenger MF: Human mesenchymal stem cells modulate allogeneic immune cell responses. *Blood* 2005, 105:1815–1822.

40. Dominici M, Le Blanc K, Mueller I, Slaper-Cortenbach I, Marini F, Krause D, Deans R, Keating A, Prockop D, Horwitz E: Minimal criteria for defining multipotent mesenchymal stromal cells. The International Society for Cellular Therapy position statement. *Cytotherapy* 2006, 8:315–317.

41. Feeney DM, Boyeson MG, Linn RT, Murray HM, Dail WG: Responses to cortical injury: I. Methodology and local effects of contusions in the rat. *Brain Res* 1981, 211:67–77.

42. Lu M, Chen J, Lu D, Yi L, Mahmood A, Chopp M: Global test statistics for treatment effect of stroke and traumatic brain injury in rats with administration of bone marrow stromal cells. *J Neurosci Methods* 2003, 128:183–190.

43. Semple BD, Bye N, Rancan M, Ziebell JM, Morganti-Kossmann MC: Role of CCL2 (MCP-1) in traumatic brain injury (TBI): evidence from severe TBI patients and CCL2–/– mice. *J Cereb Blood Flow Metab* 2010, 30:769–782.

44. Li M, Li F, Luo C, Shan Y, Zhang L, Qian Z, Zhu G, Lin J, Feng H: Immediate splenectomy decreases mortality and improves cognitive function of rats after severe traumatic brain injury. *J Trauma* 2011, 71:141–147.

45. Lau LT, Yu AC: Astrocytes produce and release interleukin-1, interleukin-6, tumor necrosis factor alpha and interferon-gamma following traumatic and metabolic injury. *J Neurotrauma* 2001, 18:351–359.

46. Konsman JP, Drukarch B, Van Dam AM: (Peri)vascular production and action of pro-inflammatory cytokines in brain pathology. *Clin Sci (Lond)* 2007, 112:1–25.

47. Cederberg D, Siesjo P: What has inflammation to do with traumatic brain injury? *Childs Nerv Syst* 2010, 26:221–226.

48. Kremlev SG, Palmer C: Interleukin-10 inhibits endotoxin-induced pro-inflammatory cytokines in microglial cell cultures. *J Neuroimmunol* 2005, 162:71–80.

49. Knoblach SM, Faden AI: Interleukin-10 improves outcome and alters proinflammatory cytokine expression after experimental traumatic brain injury. *Exp Neurol* 1998, 153:143–151.

50. Liu N, Chen R, Du H, Wang J, Zhang Y, Wen J: Expression of IL-10 and TNF-alpha in rats with cerebral infarction after transplantation with mesenchymal stem cells. *Cell Mol Immunol* 2009, 6:207–213.

51. Du YY, Zhou SH, Zhou T, Su H, Pan HW, Du WH, Liu B, Liu QM: Immuno-inflammatory regulation effect of mesenchymal stem cell transplantation in a rat model of myocardial infarction. *Cytotherapy* 2008, 10:469–478.

52. Bush TG, Puvanachandra N, Horner CH, Polito A, Ostenfeld T, Svendsen CN, Mucke L, Johnson MH, Sofroniew MV: Leukocyte infiltration, neuronal degeneration, and neurite outgrowth after ablation of scar-forming, reactive astrocytes in adult transgenic mice. *Neuron* 1999, 23:297–308.

53. Schafer S, Calas AG, Vergouts M, Hermans E: Immunomodulatory influence of bone marrow-derived mesenchymal stem cells on neuroinflammation in astrocyte cultures. *J Neuroimmunol* 2012, 249:40–48.

54. Semple BD, Bye N, Ziebell JM, Morganti-Kossmann MC: Deficiency of the chemokine receptor CXCR2 attenuates neutrophil infiltration and cortical damage following closed head injury. *Neurobiol Dis* 2010, 40:394–403.

55. Bye N, Habgood MD, Callaway JK, Malakooti N, Potter A, Kossmann T, Morganti-Kossmann MC: Transient neuroprotection by minocycline following traumatic brain injury is associated with attenuated microglial activation but no changes in cell apoptosis or neutrophil infiltration. *Exp Neurol* 2007, 204:220–233.

56. Rhodes JK, Sharkey J, Andrews PJ: The temporal expression, cellular localization, and inhibition of the chemokines MIP-2 and MCP-1 after traumatic brain injury in the rat. *J Neurotrauma* 2009, 26:507–525.

57. Rancan M, Otto VI, Hans VH, Gerlach I, Jork R, Trentz O, Kossmann T, Morganti-Kossmann MC: Upregulation of ICAM-1 and MCP-1 but not of MIP-2 and sensorimotor deficit in response to traumatic axonal injury in rats. *J Neurosci Res* 2001, 63:438–446.

58. Chen Y, Hallenbeck JM, Ruetzler C, Bol D, Thomas K, Berman NE, Vogel SN: Overexpression of monocyte chemoattractant protein 1 in the brain exacerbates ischemic brain injury and is associated with recruitment of inflammatory cells. *J Cereb Blood Flow Metab* 2003, 23:748–755.

59. Lumpkins K, Bochicchio GV, Zagol B, Ulloa K, Simard JM, Schaub S, Meyer W, Scalea T: Plasma levels of the beta chemokine regulated upon activation,

normal T cell expressed, and secreted (RANTES) correlate with severe brain injury. *J Trauma* 2008, **64**:358–361.

60. Gonzalez R, Glaser J, Liu MT, Lane TE, Keirstead HS: **Reducing inflammation decreases secondary degeneration and functional deficit after spinal cord injury.** *Exp Neurol* 2003, **184**:456–463.

61. Clausen F, Lorant T, Lewen A, Hillered L: **T lymphocyte trafficking: a novel target for neuroprotection in traumatic brain injury.** *J Neurotrauma* 2007, **24**:1295–1307.

62. Prockop DJ, Oh JY: **Mesenchymal stem/stromal cells (MSCs): role as guardians of inflammation.** *Mol Ther* 2012, **20**:14–20.

63. Wisniewski HG, Vilcek J: **TSG-6: an IL-1/TNF-inducible protein with anti-inflammatory activity.** *Cytokine Growth Factor Rev* 1997, **8**:143–156.

64. Roddy GW, Oh JY, Lee RH, Bartosh TJ, Ylostalo J, Coble K, Rosa RH Jr, Prockop DJ: **Action at a distance: systemically administered adult stem/progenitor cells (MSCs) reduce inflammatory damage to the cornea without engraftment and primarily by secretion of TNF-alpha stimulated gene/protein 6.** *Stem Cells* 2011, **29**:1572–1579.

65. Chen G, Shi J, Ding Y, Yin H, Hang C: **Progesterone prevents traumatic brain injury-induced intestinal nuclear factor kappa B activation and proinflammatory cytokines expression in male rats.** *Mediators Inflamm* 2007, **2007**:93431.

66. Qu C, Mahmood A, Ning R, Xiong Y, Zhang L, Chen J, Jiang H, Chopp M: **The treatment of traumatic brain injury with velcade.** *J Neurotrauma* 2010, **27**:1625–1634.

67. Choi H, Lee RH, Bazhanov N, Oh JY, Prockop DJ: **Anti-inflammatory protein TSG-6 secreted by activated MSCs attenuates zymosan-induced mouse peritonitis by decreasing TLR2/NF-kappaB signaling in resident macrophages.** *Blood* 2011, **118**:330–338.

68. Ren G, Zhang L, Zhao X, Xu G, Zhang Y, Roberts AI, Zhao RC, Shi Y: **Mesenchymal stem cell-mediated immunosuppression occurs via concerted action of chemokines and nitric oxide.** *Cell Stem Cell* 2008, **2**:141–150.

69. Koshinaga M, Katayama Y, Fukushima M, Oshima H, Suma T, Takahata T: **Rapid and widespread microglial activation induced by traumatic brain injury in rat brain slices.** *J Neurotrauma* 2000, **17**:185–192.

70. Koshinaga M, Suma T, Fukushima M, Tsuboi I, Aizawa S, Katayama Y: **Rapid microglial activation induced by traumatic brain injury is independent of blood brain barrier disruption.** *Histol Histopathol* 2007, **22**:129–135.

71. Yanez R, Lamana ML, Garcia-Castro J, Colmenero I, Ramirez M, Bueren JA: **Adipose tissue-derived mesenchymal stem cells have in vivo immunosuppressive properties applicable for the control of the graft-versus-host disease.** *Stem Cells* 2006, **24**:2582–2591.

72. Kassis I, Grigoriadis N, Gowda-Kurkalli B, Mizrachi-Kol R, Ben-Hur T, Slavin S, Abramsky O, Karussis D: **Neuroprotection and immunomodulation with mesenchymal stem cells in chronic experimental autoimmune encephalomyelitis.** *Arch Neurol* 2008, **65**:753–761.

73. Rasouli J, Lekhraj R, Ozbalik M, Lalezari P, Casper D: **Brain-spleen inflammatory coupling: a literature review.** *Einstein J Biol Med* 2011, **27**:74–77.

2

Inflammation in epileptogenesis after traumatic brain injury

Kyria M. Webster[1], Mujun Sun[1], Peter Crack[2], Terence J. O'Brien[1], Sandy R. Shultz[1] and Bridgette D. Semple[1*]

Abstract

Background: Epilepsy is a common and debilitating consequence of traumatic brain injury (TBI). Seizures contribute to progressive neurodegeneration and poor functional and psychosocial outcomes for TBI survivors, and epilepsy after TBI is often resistant to existing anti-epileptic drugs. The development of post-traumatic epilepsy (PTE) occurs in a complex neurobiological environment characterized by ongoing TBI-induced secondary injury processes. Neuroinflammation is an important secondary injury process, though how it contributes to epileptogenesis, and the development of chronic, spontaneous seizure activity, remains poorly understood. A mechanistic understanding of how inflammation contributes to the development of epilepsy (epileptogenesis) after TBI is important to facilitate the identification of novel therapeutic strategies to reduce or prevent seizures.

Body: We reviewed previous clinical and pre-clinical data to evaluate the hypothesis that inflammation contributes to seizures and epilepsy after TBI. Increasing evidence indicates that neuroinflammation is a common consequence of epileptic seizure activity, and also contributes to epileptogenesis as well as seizure initiation (ictogenesis) and perpetuation. Three key signaling factors implicated in both seizure activity and TBI-induced secondary pathogenesis are highlighted in this review: high-mobility group box protein-1 interacting with toll-like receptors, interleukin-1β interacting with its receptors, and transforming growth factor-β signaling from extravascular albumin. Lastly, we consider age-dependent differences in seizure susceptibility and neuroinflammation as mechanisms which may contribute to a heightened vulnerability to epileptogenesis in young brain-injured patients.

Conclusion: Several inflammatory mediators exhibit epileptogenic and ictogenic properties, acting on glia and neurons both directly and indirectly influence neuronal excitability. Further research is required to establish causality between inflammatory signaling cascades and the development of epilepsy post-TBI, and to evaluate the therapeutic potential of pharmaceuticals targeting inflammatory pathways to prevent or mitigate the development of PTE.

Keywords: Inflammation, Traumatic brain injury, Epilepsy, Post-traumatic epilepsy, Seizures, Cytokine, Interleukin, Astrocytes

Background

Epilepsy is a common and debilitating consequence of traumatic brain injuries (TBI), with recurrent spontaneous seizures contributing to progressive neurodegeneration and greatly interfering with quality of life as well as increasing the risk of injury and death. Epileptogenesis, the neurobiological process by which epilepsy develops, occurs as part of the ongoing secondary injury events triggered by a brain insult, including neuroinflammation. Previous evidence from clinical and pre-clinical studies has suggested that aspects of the inflammatory response may also promote seizure activity itself (ictogenesis).

The aim of this review was to evaluate the published evidence regarding the role of inflammation in the development of post-traumatic epilepsy (PTE), drawing upon data from both clinical studies and experimental models. In particular, we summarize the current understanding of mechanisms by which neuroinflammatory mediators can influence neuronal excitability, either directly or indirectly. We focused in particular on three

* Correspondence: Bridgette.Semple@unimelb.edu.au
[1]Department of Medicine (The Royal Melbourne Hospital), The University of Melbourne, Kenneth Myer Building, Melbourne Brain Centre, Royal Parade, Parkville, VIC 3050, Australia
Full list of author information is available at the end of the article

key signaling pathways which are known to be involved in TBI-induced secondary pathogenesis, and more recently, have been implicated in seizure activity and the process of epileptogenesis. Lastly, potential mechanisms underlying age-specific vulnerability to hyperexcitability and epileptogenesis are discussed. This review also acts to highlight knowledge gaps in the field, identifying key areas for future research. Ultimately, a mechanistic understanding of how neuroinflammation contributes to the development of epilepsy after brain injury may identify novel therapeutic targets, to reduce or prevent PTE for survivors of brain injuries.

Traumatic brain injury and epilepsy

TBI is a major global public health problem and a leading cause of mortality and morbidity [1, 2]. It is particularly prevalent in childhood and adolescence, as a result of falls, inflicted trauma, sports-related injuries, and motor vehicle accidents. An earlier review of 11 studies examining TBI incidence in Australia, North America, and Europe estimated a median of 691 injuries per 100,000 population under 20 years of age [2]. Of note, children under the age of 5 had the highest incidence of Emergency Department admissions for TBI [2].

TBI is any insult to the brain from an external mechanical force, including penetrative or blunt trauma [1, 3]. These can include focal injuries, such as lesions caused by contusions or hemorrhages, or diffuse injuries, such as with traumatic axonal injury [4]. TBI involves a

primary insult, defined as the immediate structural damage caused by the external mechanical force. This is followed by a secondary injury, which includes a myriad of neuropathological processes including excitotoxicity, neuroinflammation, oxidative stress, and apoptosis [1, 3, 5]. These secondary processes commence within minutes after TBI, can persist for months to years, and are thought to contribute to the expansion of tissue damage [6, 7]. The manifestation and severity of secondary injury processes can differ depending on injury type, severity, and individual factors [8]. The biomechanics and biochemical components of the physiological response to TBI have been reviewed in detail elsewhere [7, 9].

PTE is a common consequence of TBI, defined as spontaneous, recurrent, and chronic seizures following a head injury [10, 11]. Clinical diagnosis is often based upon one or more unprovoked seizures occurring later than 1 week after a TBI, as an indicator that epileptogenesis is occurring [12]. Epileptogenesis is the process by which epilepsy develops; that is, when an otherwise normally functioning brain becomes biased towards abnormal recurrent electrical activity, increasing the propensity to develop spontaneous recurrent seizures [13, 14]. It is thought to develop through three phases: (1) the initial trigger; (2) the latency period, during which the changes initiated in phase one cause a transformational bias in the brain towards epileptic activity; and (3) the onset of spontaneous seizures and the establishment of chronic epilepsy (Fig. 1) [15–18]. After TBI, the

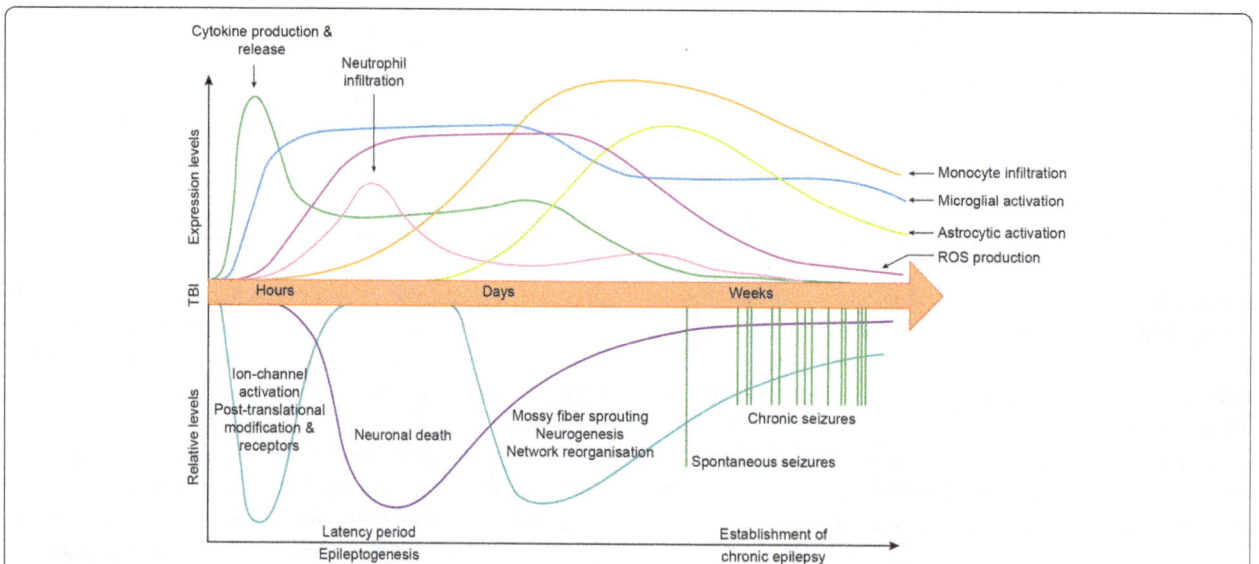

Fig. 1 Summary of the progression of inflammatory factors and epileptogenesis after TBI. After TBI, epileptogenesis occurs after a latent period of months to years. Within hours after the injury, a myriad of cytokines are released at high levels which can continue for days. This is concurrent with activation of ion-channels and post-translational modifications of various receptors associated with neuronal excitation and inhibition, which can occur as early as minutes after the injury. Local immune cells are activated, and peripheral immune cells are also recruited to the area within hours to days. Neuroinflammation can persist for weeks after the injury, coincidental with widespread neuronal loss. In the later phase of epileptogenesis, processes such as neurogenesis and mossy fiber sprouting in the hippocampus contribute to an increasingly excitable neuronal environment. It may be weeks, months, or years before spontaneous seizures and the establishment of chronic and persistent epilepsy manifests

latency period may be many years in duration, and epileptogenesis is associated with ongoing secondary injury processes which can bias towards hyperexcitability [14].

The reported incidence of developing epilepsy after TBI ranges from 4.4 to 53%, depending on the population studied [12]. There are several factors that have been associated with a greater risk of developing PTE, including higher injury severity and a lower age-at-insult [10, 19, 20]. It has been estimated that 10–20% of children with severe TBI develop PTE, although the risk after injury has been reported at up to 60%, with the wide range of estimates most likely due to the large variation in severity, heterogeneity of the initial insult, and difficulties in diagnosis and follow-up [10, 20]. Children under the age of 5 may be at highest risk for early post-traumatic seizure development [10, 12, 21], with one study finding that this age group were more likely to have a seizure within the first week after injury (17%), compared to patients over 5 years of age with similar injuries (2%) [22]. In adults, the presence of acute intracerebral hematoma has been consistently associated with a higher risk of developing PTE, as are penetrative insults and depressed skull fractures [12, 22, 23].

Several neuropathological hallmarks have been associated with the development of PTE. An early and persistent increase in hippocampal excitability has been observed in both patients and animal models [24]. This net increase in excitability is thought to result from the selective loss of vulnerable inhibitory interneurons concurrent with the reorganization of excitatory circuitry [25, 26]. Recurrent excitatory circuitry in the hippocampal dentate gyrus may manifest as mossy fiber sprouting, where the axons of dentate granule cells form abnormal connections with neighboring neurons in response to a loss of CA3 pyramidal cell targets and hilar interneurons [27, 28].

The onset of PTE is also commonly associated with hippocampal sclerosis, involving the loss of pyramidal neurons, and concurrent reactive gliosis, consistent with temporal lobe epilepsy (TLE) [29]. An estimated 35–62% of patients with PTE have seizures originating from the temporal lobe [30, 31]. However, overlaying cortical regions have also been implicated in post-TBI epileptogenesis, as these regions may also exhibit neuronal loss, chronic neuroinflammation, and network reorganization resulting in spontaneous epileptiform activity [26, 32].

Clinical management and treatment of PTE is challenging, as seizures are commonly resistant to existing anti-seizure drugs (ASDs) [10, 20, 33, 34]. Classical ASDs, such as phenytoin, carbamazepine, valproate benzodiazepines, are ineffective in reducing or preventing PTE [34–36]. While early post-injury prophylaxis with ASDs may reduce or prevent early post-injury seizures [37], there is little evidence to indicate that these treatments can be disease-modifying and prevent the development of PTE or spontaneous unprovoked seizures long-term [38]. Once a patient has developed seizures, polypharmacy is often employed in an attempt to control the seizures, yet a significant proportion of TBI patients who develop epilepsy will develop drug-resistance, defined as a failure to achieve seizure cessation after trialling more than two tolerated and appropriate ASD treatments [33, 34]. However, the use of multiple ASDs simultaneously could have unpredictable consequences due to potential interactions with various secondary processes and the reduced cerebral perfusion commonly present after TBI [20]. Seizures are particularly detrimental during periods of brain development as they can cause permanent adverse effects, including cognitive deficits [39, 40]. Due to increased susceptibility to post-traumatic seizures after an early age-of-insult, as well as inherent difficulties in controlling or treating PTE, further research is needed to understand the mechanisms that contribute to the generation of post-traumatic seizures, particularly in pediatric age groups.

Neuroinflammation after TBI

Inflammation is a central component of the secondary injury after TBI, and the subject of intense research as a promising target for treatment. In healthy tissue, inflammation typically acts to combat invading pathogens and preserve the health of the tissue [41]. However, in pathological conditions such as trauma, inflammation can also function as a reactionary system to either aggravate or ameliorate tissue damage [42, 43]. Increased neuroinflammation after TBI has been associated with poor outcomes and progression to various sequelae including neurodegenerative diseases [43–47].

The main hallmarks of the cerebral inflammatory response after TBI include blood-brain barrier (BBB) dysfunction, edema, microglial, and astrocytic activation and migration, the release of inflammatory factors such as cytokines and the recruitment of blood-derived leukocytes into brain parenchyma [48]. Neutrophils, recruited from the peripheral circulation within hours after TBI, mediate early pathogenesis by promoting edema and oxidative stress, and the production of inflammatory cytokines and neurotoxic proteases [49, 50]. Cytokines can be released rapidly after injury as they are synthesized and stored locally by neurons and glia [48].

Under physiological conditions, the BBB is a highly stringent barrier between vessels and brain tissue, which mediates the transport of blood components such as immune cells into the brain [51]. After TBI, this barrier can be compromised, allowing peripheral inflammatory cells into the brain and the injured area [52]. Chemoattractant cytokines, called chemokines, further facilitate the recruitment and transmigration of inflammatory leukocytes [53]. By their actions at the BBB as well as direct chemoattraction, chemokines including CXCL8 and CCL2 (also known as monocyte chemoattractant protein-1) are key mediators in the migration of neutrophils and monocytes, respectively, to the site of injury [54].

Once in the brain, these cells release a plethora of inflammatory cytokines, chemokines, and reactive oxygen species (ROS) to perpetuate inflammation and oxidative stress in the injured brain. Both clinical and experimental studies have demonstrated a pronounced elevation of many cytokines after TBI, including tumor necrosis factor (TNF-α), transforming growth factor-β (TGF-β), and interleukin-1β (IL-1β), -6, and -10, with downstream activation of intracellular signaling cascades involving nuclear factor Kappa-light-chain-enhancer of activated B cells (NF-κB) [1, 44, 48, 55–57]. Released cytokines in turn can recruit additional blood-borne neutrophils and monocytes into the injured tissue, propagating the inflammatory cascade.

Inflammation in the brain has a duality in function after injury, which manifests through the actions of many different cell types. For example, microglial activation is integral in tissue repair, surveillance of pathogenic factors and host defense [58]. However, activated microglia can also release cytotoxic factors such as ROS to induce oxidative stress [59–61]. Astrocytes can promote tissue repair in the central nervous system (CNS) through the release of insulin-like growth factor [47], but are also implicated in the perpetuation of inflammation by an over-production of cytokines such as IL-6 [62, 63], as well as modulation of the BBB and neuronal function to promote excitability and seizure production [64].

Cytokines themselves also have a complex role after TBI, as experimental studies have yielded conflicting findings of both deleterious contributions and participation in repair processes after CNS insult [48]. One cytokine that displays such paradox is TNF-α, which has been associated with increased neurological damage, including demyelination and BBB breakdown, in several experimental models of TBI [65, 66]. However, increased levels of TNF-α may conversely have a neuroprotective function in the late stages of inflammation post-TBI, at 2–4 weeks after the injury, as suggested from a mouse model of TBI [56]. The varied roles of inflammatory mediators in the pathological environment after TBI is likely dependent on many different factors, including timing of release, the location and cell types involved, the differing physics of protein-protein interactions of cytokines, and their relative amounts. The multifarious dynamics of this response may contribute to the progression of a chronic state of damage, leading to the myriad of secondary consequences of TBI, including PTE.

Inflammation in epileptogenesis

The long-standing concept that seizures result from an imbalance between reduced γ-aminobutyric acid (GABA)-ergic inhibition and enhanced glutamatergic excitation [67, 68], based upon the presence of large amplitude EEG discharges during the seizure event itself, is an over-simplified of a very complex network response. While excessive glutamatergic excitation has historically been considered of as the precipitating factor for a focal seizure, there is a lack of strong data to support this hypothesis. Instead, paradoxically, accumulating evidence indicates that increased synchronised GABAergic interneuronal activity is sufficient to disrupt neuronal networks and initiate the transition from interictal to ictal activity resulting in focal seizures [69]. The recruitment of neighboring neurons and subsequent seizure progression is then hypothesized to be mediated by an elevation in extracellular potassium [70]. Adding to the complexity of network-based activity, both excitatory and inhibitory roles of GABA and glutamatergic neurons have been reported, and a range of extrasynaptic as well as synaptic neurotransmitter receptors and ion channels have been implicated in seizures, in addition to those traditionally implicated, such as NMDA and GABA$_A$ receptors [71].

However, strong evidence also implicates a role for inflammation in seizure pathologies [45]. Seizure activity readily induces an inflammatory response, including the activation of microglia and production of pro-inflammatory cytokines [47, 63]. More importantly, experimental data has suggested that inflammatory mediators may initiate or trigger early seizures, preceding the onset of diagnosed epilepsy. For example, systemic inflammation by injection of bacterial lipopolysaccharide results in a lowered seizure threshold [72]. In the next sections, we will review clinical and experimental evidence suggesting an inherent link between inflammatory signaling, neuropathology, and seizure activity in the injured brain, as a likely mechanism of importance in the development and progression of PTE.

Seizures increase inflammation

Experimentally, induction of a seizure induces the rapid activation of glial cells in surrounding parenchyma, which respond by the production and release of inflammatory molecules [73]. Much of the research that has shown an increase in inflammation after seizures have used experimental models of status epilepticus. This involves the administration of a chemical or electrical pro-convulsant stimulus to create a sustained seizure event (the initial insult) followed by a latency period before the onset of spontaneous recurrent seizures to model epilepsy [74, 75]. In these experimental models, the inflammatory response displays a distinct temporal profile after induction, characterized by the early activation of astrocytes and microglia followed by BBB breakdown and neuronal activation [63, 76, 77]. In addition to the investigation of protein release, microarray analysis of gene transcripts have also demonstrated an upregulation of inflammatory genes [78]. Specific cell surface toll-like receptors (TLR's), which respond to a range of inflammatory cytokines and other stress-related factors, are highly upregulated after pilocarpine-induced seizures on forebrain microglia of adult mice [77]. Simultaneously, a robust increase in cytokine levels has been observed in both chemically and electrically induced experimental models of epilepsy in adult rodents [77, 79, 80]. For example, IL-1β is expressed at low levels in a healthy brain, but is robustly upregulated for up to 60 days after the induction of self-sustaining limbic status epilepticus in rodents, a model using hippocampal electrical stimulation [76]. TNF-α and IL-6 are also rapidly upregulated after status epilepticus, peaking within 30 min of seizure onset and remaining elevated for up to 72 h in rats that progressed to spontaneous seizures [76].

These experimental findings that seizures result in inflammation are confirmed by evidence in the clinical setting. Analysis of cerebrospinal fluid (CSF) from newly diagnosed adult patients with tonic-clonic seizures detected an upregulation of IL-6 and IL-1 receptors (IL-1Rs) [81, 82]. Matched serum samples revealed a higher levels of IL-6 compared to in the CSF, suggesting that these cytokines likely originated in the brain [82]. High levels of cytokines including IL-1β and high-mobility group box protein-1 (HMGB1) have also been identified in neurons and glia of surgically resected epileptic tissue [83]. Together, these findings indicate that neuroinflammation is a common consequence of seizure activity.

Inflammation contributing to seizures

Accumulating evidence suggests that neuroinflammation is also a contributor to epileptogenic pathology after TBI [45, 63, 84]. In particular, experimental models have demonstrated that glial cell activation and recruitment and the synthesis of inflammatory factors, may precede and/or occur concurrently with epileptogenic events [85, 86]. For example, in a rodent model of experimental TBI, a reduced threshold to electroconvulsive shock-induced seizures was reversed when minocycline, a tetracycline antibiotic known to inhibit brain infiltration of monocytes and microglia, was applied [87, 88], implicating both microglial activity and pro-inflammatory cytokines in post-traumatic seizure activity.

Much of the evidence for a role of inflammation in epileptogenesis has focused on the effect of cytokines in seizure susceptibility. Cytokines can act as classical neurotransmitters through receptor modulation and phosphorylation at the neuronal membrane [89]. Models of chronic inflammation, such as transgenic mice systemically overexpressing IL-6 or TNF-α, can reduce seizure threshold and predispose the brain to seizure induced-neuronal loss [90, 91]. Indeed, inflammatory signaling may promote the loss of GABAergic neurons in the hippocampus, resulting in an increased propensity for seizures due to a reduction in synaptic inhibition [92].

N-methyl-D-aspartate (NMDA) receptors play a critical role in the glutamatergic system to contribute to neuronal excitability, and previous evidence suggests both direct and indirect interactions between these receptors and cyokines [93]. Cytokines have been found to inhibit the uptake of glutamate by astrocytes in culture [94] and modulate excitatory neurotransmission in the brain through NMDA and alpha-amino-3-hydroxyl-5-methyl-4-isoxazole-propoinate (AMPA) receptors [95, 96]. For example, IL-1β produced by microglia can enhance NMDA-mediated Ca^{2+} currents through cell surface type 1 IL-1R (IL-1R1) co-localized on pyramidal cell dendrites [89]. Pre-synaptic NMDA receptors are agonists for Ca^{2+}-mediated glutamate release, and when activated by inflammatory factors such as IL-1β and HMGB1 can cause an excess of intracellular Ca^{2+} leading to an extracellular hyperexcitability and excitotoxicity [95]. Several other cytokines including TNF-α and IL-10 have also been associated with the regulation of seizure duration in experimental kindling models [97, 98]. Though these correlations have been seen in multiple studies with different models, the mechanisms underlying the relationship between the inflammatory environment and epileptogenesis, particularly in the context of brain injury, remain still poorly understood.

There is limited clinical data to confirm a cause-and-effect link between inflammation and the pathophysiology of epilepsy, however increasing evidence supports this hypothesis. Many studies have now demonstrated that early exposure of the brain to immune responses can have varied and persistent consequences on adult physiology [99–102]. Febrile seizures (FS) and febrile status epilepticus in children is a risk factor for developing epilepsy later in life [103], which may be induced by fever often associated with inflammation and infection [47]. Although the mechanisms underlying FS remains unclear, it is thought that cytokines play a key role in its development [104]. One study has reported specific polymorphisms in the promoter region of cytokine genes, including IL-1β, in children with FS compared to controls [105]. Such genetic variation may influence the production of IL-1β in both healthy tissue and after injury or stimulus [106], and similar polymorphisms have also been observed at a high frequency in patients with TLE [107].

Recently, the hypothesis of glial functions playing a pivotal role in biasing the neuronal network towards an epileptogenic environment has been gaining traction [108, 109]. In particular, interactions between neurons, glia, and the inflammatory mediators IL-1β, HMGB-1, and TGF-β, have been implicated in promoting seizure susceptibility, as described below. The main signaling pathways implicated in the proposed link between inflammation and epileptogenesis of these three mediators is summarized in Fig. 2.

IL-1β/IL-1R signaling in TBI and PTE

IL-1 is a family of pro-inflammatory cytokines that act as key mediators of the innate immune response [110]. The IL-1 family consists of 7 agonists (e.g., IL-1α and β) and 3 receptor antagonists [110], and amongst these the IL-1β isoform has been the most commonly studied in the brain injury and epilepsy settings. In the CNS, IL-1β can be produced by a range of cells including microglia, astrocytes, endothelial cells (EC), neurons, and peripheral leukocytes upon infiltrating into the brain [111–113]. IL-1β exerts its action on multiple cell types primarily via IL-1R1 [114–119]. This initiates intracellular signaling via NF-κB transcription factor, p38 mitogen-activated protein kinase (MAPK), or other factors [118, 120]. Several studies have demonstrated that IL-1β binding to IL-1R stimulates immune cell activation and induces the production of neurotoxic molecules [114, 115, 117–119].

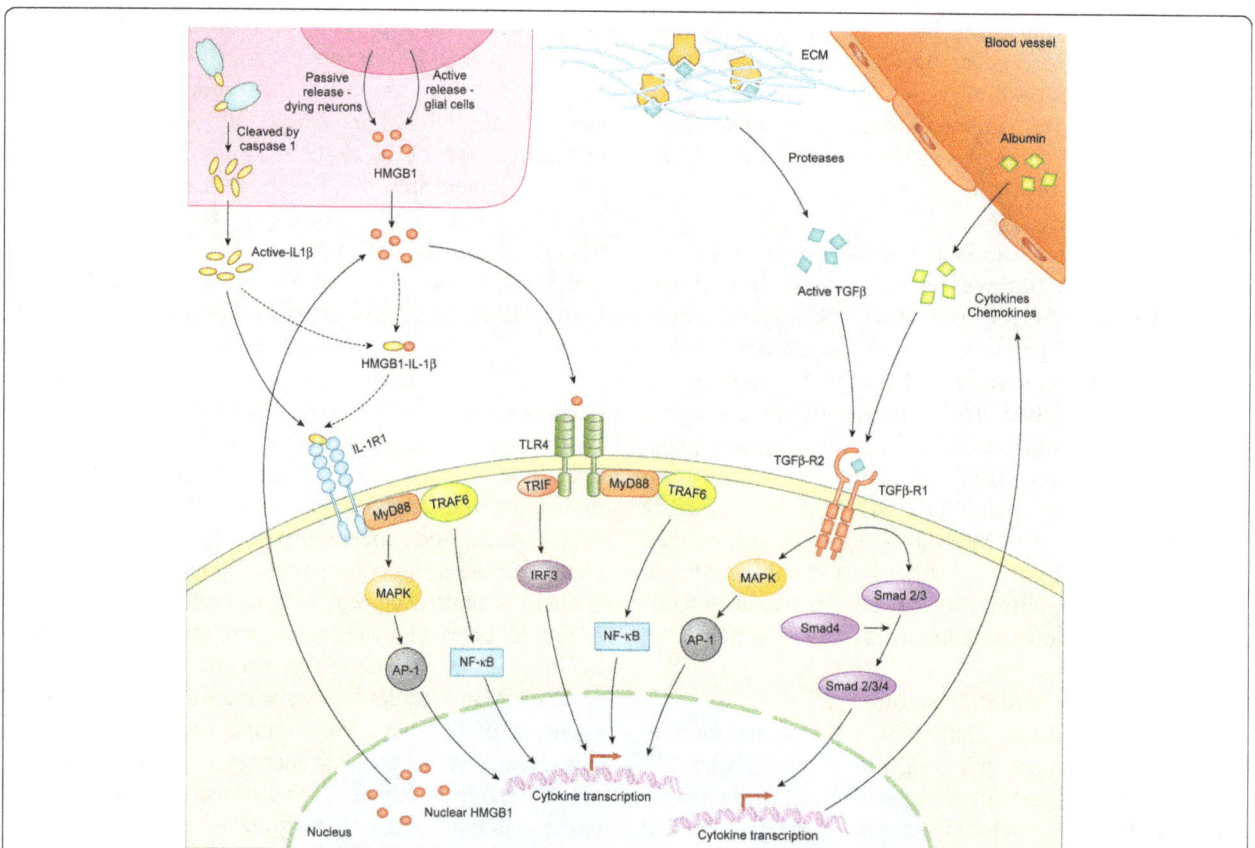

Fig. 2 Summary of three key signaling cascades that may mediate the link between inflammation and epileptogenesis. HMGB1, IL-1β, TGF-β, and serum albumin have varied release mechanisms from multiple cell types in order to activate their signaling pathways. After injury, HMGB1 may be passively released from necrotic neurons to the extracellular space, or released actively from activated microglia and astrocytes. HMGB1 can bind to multiple receptors on many different cell types, such as TLR4, which can activate MyD88 independent pathways such as the phosphorylation of interferon regulatory transcription factor 3 (IRF3) leading to the transcription and release of interferons-α and -β, as well as other interferon-induced genes. HMGB1-TLR4 can also activate NF-κB signaling both directly or via TNF receptor-associated factor 6 (TRAF6). This can lead to a rapid nuclear transcription of various immune-related processes, as reviewed elsewhere [250]. Caspase-1 mediates cleavage of inactive pro-IL-1β to active IL-1β, allowing for its relocation into the extracellular space, where IL-1β can bind to IL-1R1 either directly or in complex with HMGB1. The IL-1β/IL-1R1 complex can then induce NF-κB signaling via TRAF6 or activate MyD88-dependent MAPK signaling, which has been linked to the production of various neurotoxic molecules. TGF-β is released in an inactive form from cells and binds to the extracellular matrix. Proteases, released after injury, cleave the inactive protein to active TGF-β, which is able to bind to the two TGF-β receptors. Mechanical breakdown of the BBB allows serum albumin into the extracellular space, where it can also bind to TGF-β receptor1 and receptor2, which signal via Smad complex proteins or MAPK signaling pathways, respectively, to regulate the immune response. This pathway has also been implicated in post-translational changes to a variety of voltage-dependent ion channels implicated in changes to neuronal excitability [94]

There are several lines of evidence implicating IL-1β in the development of PTE. Firstly, IL-1β is rapidly and highly upregulated following experimental and clinical TBI. In rodent models, Il-1β expression is upregulated as early as 1 h post-TBI [121, 122] and peaks between 12 and 24 h [54, 123, 124]. This response may then persist for several months post-injury [125]. Consistent with experimental findings, analysis of protein, and gene expression in post-mortem brain tissue from TBI patients found that IL-1β was upregulated in individuals who died 6–122 h post-injury [126]. This is consistent with reports of elevated IL-1β in the CSF and serum of severe TBI patients [127, 128], correlated with poor outcomes in both children and adults [19, 129]. Thus IL-1β levels are elevated during the period of secondary injury after TBI, which has been postulated to also be an important time period for the epileptogenic process [130]. Notably, numerous studies indicate that modulating IL-1β signaling is broadly beneficial in experimental TBI models. Treatment with an IL-1β neutralizing antibody alleviated TBI-induced microglial activation, neutrophil infiltration, cerebral edema, and cognitive deficits in mouse models of TBI [131, 132]. In line with this finding, IL-1R1 deficient mice also showed decreased cerebral edema and leukocyte infiltration following TBI [133], and post-injury administration of an IL-1R1 antagonist attenuated neuronal cell death and cognitive dysfunction in rats [134]. A phase II clinical trial employing an IL-1R antagonist treatment (100 mg/day subcutaneously administered for 5 days) was recently conducted in patients with severe diffuse TBI, demonstrating safety penetration into the plasma and brain extracellular fluid, and an alteration of the immune profile [135].

One of the key clinical studies linking IL-1β with PTE was conducted by Diamond and colleagues, who examined whether genetic variation in the IL-1β gene and CSF/serum IL-1β ratios correlated with PTE development in a cohort of 256 patients with moderate to severe TBI [136]. Serum and CSF were collected from a portion of subjects within the first week post-injury, and IL-1β levels were assessed in relation to the later incidence of PTE. Further, IL-1β tagging and functional single nucleotide polymorphisms (SNPs) were genotyped to evaluate its association to PTE. Elevated CSF/serum IL-1β ratios were found to be associated with increased risk of PTE, and one of IL-1β SNPs, rs1143634, showed an association between the heterozygote genotype and increased PTE risk [136]. Further research is required to determine the contribution of genetic variability to IL-1β function and how this may influence the inflammatory response after TBI.

IL-1β has also been linked to other epilepsies in addition to PTE. For example, IL-1β may play a role in epileptogenesis that follows FS. Specifically, IL-1β levels were found to be acutely upregulated in rats after prolonged FS, and IL-1β levels remained elevated only in rats that developed spontaneous limbic seizures after prolonged FS [137]. In another study, IL-1R1 deficient mice were found to be resistant to experimental FS [138].

There are a number of possible mechanisms by which IL-1β may contribute to PTE. IL-1β can modulate neuronal hyperexcitability through Ca^{2+}, glutamatergic, and GABAergic pathways [139]. By acting on glia cells, IL-1β mediates astrocytes and microglia activation, formation of a glial scar, and the release of neurotoxic mediators to promote cell loss, features which are associated with epileptic foci in the brain [140]. Furthermore, IL-1β signaling may promote epileptogenesis by enhancing BBB permeability and enhancing the recruitment of peripheral leukocytes into the brain [141–144]. There are many proposed mechanisms of IL-1β signaling in areas that are still poorly understood, and future research into these may reveal the way in which they interact to increase the risk of epileptogenesis.

Although less commonly studied, other members of the IL-1 family have also been investigated in the context of TBI and epilepsy. For example, an upregulation of IL-1α has been reported in brain tissue following experimental TBI [145, 146]. In the clinical setting, peripheral blood mononuclear cells collected from epilepsy patients exhibited greater production of IL-1α in response to stimulation in vitro compared to cells from non-epileptic controls [147]. However, no association has been found between gene polymorphisms of IL-1α and TBI outcomes [148], nor IL-1α and seizure pathogenesis [149]. Taken together, there is much accumulating experimental and clinical evidence implicating IL-1 cytokines in epileptogenesis, however further studies are needed to delineate their precise roles and whether therapeutically targeting them can mitigate PTE.

HMGB1/TLR4 signaling in PTE

HMGB1 was originally identified as a ubiquitous, highly evolutionarily conserved, chromatin-binding protein, most often found in the cell nucleus of healthy tissues [150–152]. Discovered in 1973, and named due to its ability to migrate quickly during gel electrophoresis [153], HMGB1 participates in the formation of nucleosomes and is important in the regulation of gene transcription [151, 154, 155]. More recently, HMGB1 has been identified as a damage-associated molecular pattern (DAMP) [150], which are molecules that are able to initiate or perpetuate inflammation. Complete gene deficiency of HMGB1 is lethal during early postnatal life, indicating its essential role in transcriptional control [156]. A 98% homology between human HMGB1 and mouse HMGB1 enables clinically relevant experimental investigation through animal models [157].

HMGB1 has two modes of cellular release in injured tissue. Immediately after injury, necrosis allows a passive release of significant amounts of HMGB1 from the nucleus into the extracellular space [158]. HMGB1 may undergo post-translational oxidation and acetylation, resulting in its active release by immune cells in response to various cytokines including itself, allowing a powerful positive feedback loop during inflammation [157, 159–161]. In addition, HMGB1 may be released upon activation by a wide range of cells in the CNS including neurons, microglia, macrophages, monocytes, natural killer cells, dendritic cells, ECs, and platelets [162].

High levels of HMGB1 have been found in epileptogenic tissue resected during surgery [83, 163], implicating a role for this DAMP in neuronal hyperexcitability. Experimental evidence from an animal model of temporal lobe epilepsy suggests that HMGB1 contributes to seizure activity and epilepsy [164]. One previous study by Maroso and colleagues demonstrated that intracerebral injection of HMGB1 in wild type mice increased seizure activity in response to a stimulus [165]. This pro-convulsant effect of HMGB1 is most likely mediated through one of its key signaling receptors, TLR4, as a comparable increase in seizure susceptibility was not seen in non-functional TLR4 mutant mice [165]. TLR4 mutant mice were also found to be intrinsically resistant to seizures as compared to wild type mice [165]. Interfering with the binding of HMGB1 to TLR4 has been shown to reduce both seizure frequency and onset. For example, TLR4 antagonists and BoxA, a competitive antagonist to HMGB1 comprising of the BoxA domain of the protein, have been reported to reduce and even inhibit epileptic activity that is resistant to standard ASDs in an animal model of temporal lobe epilepsy [166].

In another recent study, the mechanism by which HMGB1 signaling promotes neuronal hyperexcitability and seizure activity was found to be through an increase in NMDA receptor function in TLR4-expressing hippocampal neurons [167]. This effect was dependent on the oxidation of HMGB1 characteristic of its active release from immune cells, and was associated with high levels of NMDA-induced excitotoxic cell death [167]. Because the inflammatory environment after TBI involves the rapid production of ROS and free radicals [168, 169], there is a physiological preference towards the extracellular oxidation of HMGB1, thus increasing TLR4-mediated augmentation of NMDA functionality and promoting seizure susceptibility [167].

Downstream of HMGB1, TLR4 mRNA expression is upregulated in response to brain insult [170], consistent with upregulation of this receptor during seizure activity in experimental models of epilepsy [165]. TLR4 is able to transmit signals via both myeloid differentiation primary response gene 88 (MyD88) dependent and

independent pathways [171]. It is through the MyD88 dependent pathway that TLR4 is able to activate NF-κB, which may be responsible for increasing pro-inflammatory cytokine expression to augment the inflammatory response [172, 173]. This pathway has generated great interest recently, and with the potential to modulate epileptic activity, even in drug-resistant epilepsy, further research is needed to confirm the potential of this pathway as a target for therapeutic intervention in the development of PTE.

Previous research has also suggested that HMGB1 is able to enhance inflammation through forming a complex with different cytokines, including IL-1β [174]. HMGB1 bound to IL-1β has been isolated from cell cultures when co-incubated [174]. Studies of joint inflammation in animals have also shown that when HMGB1 is present with IL-1β there is an enhanced inflammatory response, most likely through action on with IL-1 receptor 1[175], Whilst this complex has yet to be identified in brain tissue, further research is needed into this pathway as it may play a vital role in extending a bias towards epileptogenesis.

By contributing to acute and chronic seizures, both directly and indirectly, the HMGB1-TLR4 axis is therefore a promising target for TLEs that are resistant to ASDs [165, 167]. This is important in the context of TBI, as seizure pathology can begin as early as the day of a brain injury [176]. Together, these data support a key role for HMGB1 in neuronal hyperexcitability and implicate the HMGB1-TLR4 signaling pathway as a potential therapeutic target to modulate post-traumatic epileptogenesis.

TGF-β/albumin involvement in PTE

Vascular dysfunction has been associated with many types of focal and acquired epilepsies, including PTE [177]. BBB dysfunction is also a common feature of TBI in both patients and experimental models [6, 178]. Vascular dysfunction after TBI, in particular the localized breakdown of the BBB surrounding focal regions of tissue damage, is hypothesized to trigger a series of epileptogenic processes [179]. For example, increased permeability of the BBB is evident by magnetic resonance imaging with gadolinium and co-localized with the focal epileptogenic region in patients with PTE [180, 181].

A proposed mechanism of BBB breakdown in this context is through the TGF-β/albumin-mediated signaling pathway. In the laboratory, experimental opening of the BBB in the rodent neocortex was found to trigger epileptogenesis, which was recapitulated by exposure of the brain to serum albumin [182]. Albumin has been shown to induce the production of excitatory synapses experimentally both in vitro and in vivo [183]. Serum albumin in the rodent brain has been shown to result in hypersynchronized responses to electrical stimulation [184], analogous to those observed in animal models of epilepsy [185, 186]. The formation of epileptiform activity after albumin exposure is delayed, suggesting that the mechanism of action is complex rather than a direct effect by albumin [184]. One possible mechanism which has been receiving scrutiny is the activation of astrocytes by serum albumin [109, 187], activating a TGF-β receptor-mediated signaling cascade [64, 182, 184].

TGF-β is a pleiotropic cytokine involved in various cellular processes, including cell growth, differentiation, morphogenesis, apoptosis, and immune responses through intercellular communication in many different cell types [188–190]. Signaling is mediated by binding of TGF-β to two serine threonine kinase receptors, which when activated cause the phosphorylation of the Smad protein complex and the p38 MAPK pathway [191]. A role for TGF-β has been implicated in many different CNS diseases, related to its upregulation in Alzheimer's disease, multiple sclerosis, ischemic brain injury, and TBI [192]. TGF-β is thought to have neuroprotective properties, and is associated with both microglial activation and the wound healing response [193]. Paradoxically, TGF-β also appears to contribute to excitotoxicity, adding to the dual role of inflammation which is dependent on the context and cell types involved [194]. Further research into the variation in response from this pathway is needed, as this may reveal insights into the dual role of inflammation and how to bias the brain towards neuroprotection rather than neurodegeneration.

The binding of albumin to TGF-β receptor has been characterized experimentally in rodent models of BBB disruption, resulting in the activation of TGF-β signaling [184]. The induction of experimental BBB dysfunction to induce epileptiform activity can be prevented through blockage of albumin binding to TGF-β receptors [184]. Much of the published literature has focused on albumin's interaction with the TGF-β signaling pathway in disease models, but there is some suggestion that TGF-β may also play a role in PTE from animal models with similar pathologies. In rodent models of epilepsy, TGF-β is reportedly upregulated in both neurons [195] and hippocampal astrocytes [196]. The action of TGF-β in astrocytes following exposure to albumin has also been shown to induce pro-ictogenic cytokine production, resulting in increased neuronal excitability in experimental models [197]. TGF-β has also been implicated experimentally in excitatory synaptogenesis in a post-injury epilepsy model [183]. As neuronal reorganization and synaptogenesis are hypothesized to be a potential mechanism underlying chronic seizures and are well-documented consequences of CNS trauma, this action of TGF-β may be critical for the progression of brain injury to epilepsy [183, 198, 199]. In summary,

the actions of TGF-β in the injured and epileptic brain remain poorly understood, but the potentially paradoxical behavior of this cytokine warrants further investigation.

Age-specific vulnerability to PTE

Neuroinflammation is a key aspect of secondary injury that can vary according to the stage of brain development, which may underlie differences in clinical outcomes between patients who suffer a TBI during childhood and patients who suffer a TBI during adulthood [200]. Many studies now suggest that the early postnatal brain has an enhanced propensity for inflammation, described as a 'window of susceptibility' [200–202]. Early support for this hypothesis came from experimental evidence that 3-week old (juvenile) rats showed a higher susceptibility to IL-1β-induced BBB breakdown compared to adult rats [203, 204]. These observations are most likely not due to an immaturity of the BBB integrity at a younger age, as the tight junctions that maintain the BBB are fully developed from prenatal stages [205], but rather to a unique global chemokine expression profile that is distinctly different to the adult CNS [200]. In experimental autoimmune encephalomyelitis, a model of multiple sclerosis that shares some of the inflammatory processes of PTE, many chemokines involved in the recruitment of T cells and monocytes into the brain are robustly upregulated to 2–6-fold higher in juveniles compared to adults, including CCL2, CCL3, and CCL6 [200, 206–208]. There is also some evidence in the clinical context that the response of the immune system in the brain after a pathogenic challenge also differs between adults and children, with children presenting with higher production of IL-1 and IL-10 from peripheral blood monocytes after pathogenic stimulation [209]. Several cytokines have been detected at elevated levels in both CSF and serum of children after TBI, including IL-1α, IL-6, IL-12, and TNF-α, though how this response may correspond to the clinical differences at different ages after TBI are still relatively underinvestigated [210–212].

Microglia present differently within the immature brain compared to adults. During early postnatal development, their morphology is distinct, with fewer processes than those in the adult brain [213], and in an experimental pathogenic model, neonatal brain injury induced a markedly reduced activation compared to the robust activation seen in adult brain tissue [214]. Activated microglia typically adopt a phagocytic morphology and are associated with neuronal death, which is thought to be a critical aspect of normal brain development [201, 215]. There are also more circulating macrophages in the developing brain compared to adults under basal conditions associated with dying neurons and glia, particularly in the corpus callosum [213, 216]. Neutrophil infiltration into brain parenchyma after injury differs across ages, with a much higher level of infiltration detected experimentally in postnatal day 7 (p7) rats than in adults [214]. This neutrophil infiltration can persist 2–3 days after a pathogenic challenge and was found to be concurrent with damage to vasculature [203, 204, 214].

Increased seizure susceptibility in the immature brain may result from several contributing factors. Glutamate is the primary neurotransmitter in both the adult and developing brain [217], yet there is low expression of the glutamate type 1 transporter, therefore, clearance from the synaptic cleft is markedly slower compared that in the adult brain [218]. GABA receptor action is normally inhibitory in the adult brain, but is predominantly excitatory during early brain development due to high intracellular concentrations of chloride as a result of differential developmental expression of specific chloride ion transporters [219–221]. During early cortical development, experimental models have shown that GABA is predominantly depolarizing, progressing through childhood to the hyperpolarizing state found in the healthy adult brain [222, 223]. A recent study of experimental mesial temporal lobe epilepsy found a depolarizing role of GABA receptor, which was highly upregulated in surviving epileptic neurons [224], suggesting that the early neurodevelopmental environment may be more vulnerable to hyperexcitability after an insult. NMDA receptors are also more permeable to Ca^{2+} during development and desensitize more slowly [225]. In addition to a shorter post-ictal refractory period compared to the adult brain [226, 227], this inherently increased excitability of the pediatric brain may underlie an increased propensity for PTE after TBI during early childhood.

However, other studies have noted that the immature brain may conversely show resistance to seizure-related pathology; for example, chemical stimulation to experimentally induce sustained hyperexcitability is more difficult in the immature brain [39]. Infant brains may also be more resistant to excitotoxic-induced cell death than the adult brain [228]. Due to the apparent paradox of age-related differences, further study pertaining to the specific excitability of the developing environment is needed, particularly in the context of brain injury.

Inflammation in pediatric PTE
As a result of the abovementioned evidence of age-specific responses to both inflammatory stimuli and seizures, a potential link between neuroinflammation and seizure susceptibility particularly during early childhood is under intense scrutiny. Experimental studies have implicated a role for neuroinflammation in increased seizure susceptibility in the immature brain; for

example, exposure to several chemoconvulsant challenges revealed a lower seizure threshold in immature rats compared to adults [102]. The authors attribute this response to increased TNF-α or IL-1β production by activated microglia in the hippocampus in immature rats, which was associated with cognitive deficits and widespread neuronal loss [102, 229]. Changes in seizure threshold caused by neuroinflammation in the pediatric brain are associated with long-term alterations in glutamate receptors in the hippocampus, and a resultant increase in neuronal network excitability [229, 230].

In addition to the younger brain having an increased propensity for an enhanced neuroinflammatory response, age-specific differences in important epileptogenic factors have been identified. One such difference is NMDA receptor density, which has been shown experimentally to peak at p28 at approximately 160% of adult levels [231]. NMDA receptors also have a different subunit composition in the developing brain compared to the adult brain, resulting in different functional properties [232, 233]. Due to these changes, NMDA receptors are able to depolarize more easily in the presence of glutamate, resulting in a longer duration of excitatory postsynaptic currents [218, 234].

Therapeutic targeting of post-traumatic inflammation to prevent PTE
TBI induces a neuroinflammatory cascade in the brain, leading to persistent and perpetuating neurodegeneration and likely contributing to an increased risk of initiating epileptogenesis, resulting in the development of PTE. In the context of the ongoing pursuit of novel therapeutic targets to prevent PTE, both clinical and experimental studies provide compelling evidence implicating IL-1β and HMGB1 as pivotal players in the cascade. Due to their early and varied role in the neuroinflammatory cascade after injury and emerging roles in the regulation of neuronal excitability, pharmacological targeting of these mechanisms may prove beneficial at reducing PTE. Further pre-clinical studies are needed to elucidate the exact mechanisms by which these and other inflammatory mediators initiate or perpetuate the process of epileptogenesis.

Several different animal models of PTE have been well studied over the past decade [235]. These experimental models have demonstrated that TBI results in both acute and chronic changes to the neuronal environment that likely contribute to epileptogenesis, such as hyperexcitable recurrent circuitry in the dentate gyrus of the hippocampus [235–237]. Whilst these models allow for the investigation of various mechanisms and testing of potential therapeutics, rodent models of PTE are not without limitations. Some models can produce a high level of epileptiform activity when measured with electroencephalogram, but most models are limited in the amount of spontaneous seizure activity they induce, leading to the need for higher animal numbers [11, 238]. One study that used a controlled cortical impact model of PTE, found that only 20–36% of animals given a severe TBI developed spontaneous behavioral seizures [239]. Though this presents logistical challenges, this incidence is only slightly higher than the estimated incidence in the clinical setting, which one study found to be 16.7% for severe TBI [240]. Animal models are also notoriously time-consuming as the latency to spontaneous seizure onset can be weeks to months after the initial injury [238, 241]. To increase the number of animals that can be investigated in relation to epileptogenesis and combat time restraints, some studies incorporate the administration of a pro-convulsant agent, such as pentylenetetrazol (PTZ), to unveil changes to seizure threshold as a surrogate marker of seizure susceptibility [235, 238, 241]. Many neuropathological processes that occur following TBI, including the neuroinflammatory response, can also differ greatly due to the developmental state of the brain at the time of impact [1]. This confound should be taken into account when investigating both the underlying mechanisms of epileptogenesis and piloting novel therapeutic interventions. Despite these limitations, these models show high clinical relevance and are useful tools with which to study PTE, and they are continually being improved upon.

Much investigation of neuroinflammatory intervention as a therapeutic option after TBI has focused on broad-target agents, such as minocycline, erythropoietin, and progesterone. All of these treatments were proposed to reduce neuroinflammation after TBI, generating promising results in pre-clinical research but failing to produce short-term improvement after TBI during clinical trials, as reviewed elsewhere [242]. However, these treatments, which are both pleiotropic in nature and relatively safe for long-term use, may have more success in relation to the chronic outcomes such as PTE as many of the effects of neuroinflammation persist long after the offending insult, yet few studies have considered the potential effects of anti-inflammatory treatments on long-term epileptogenesis after injury. Hypothermia is another broad-target treatment for neuroinflammation that has had some success in providing neuroprotection in the context of TBI and spinal cord injuries, with some evidence suggesting that it may also prevent epileptogenesis [243–245]. The potential to prevent or reduce PTE by targeting other inflammatory mediators in the post-injury neural environment, such as serum albumin and TGF-β, have not yet been explored. Additional potential targets include TNF-α, which has been shown to influence neurotransmission by altering excitatory post-synaptic currents and decreasing GABA-mediated inhibitory synaptic strength in hippocampal neurons [246]; the prostaglandin receptor EP2, which mediates COX-2 inflammatory signaling and appears to promote seizures by aggravating neuronal injury [247]; as well as factors involved in regeneration and regrowth such as fibroblast growth factor, tropomyosin receptor kinase B, and insulin-like growth factor-1. [248, 249]

Conclusion

This review of the published literature has found that several inflammatory mediators, including IL-1β and HMGB1, exhibit epileptogenic and ictogenic properties, acting on glia and neurons both directly and indirectly to influence neuronal excitability. As neuroinflammation is a central component of the neuropathology after TBI, comparable mechanisms are likely to be involved in the process of epileptogenesis leading to PTE. An increased understanding of how inflammation influences epileptogenesis may reveal novel therapeutic targets and strategies to prevent or reduce seizures after TBI. As PTE is often resistant to existing pharmaceutical treatments [33, 34, 36], there is an urgent need for further research to develop preventative treatments to improve both the quality and longevity of life for TBI survivors.

Abbreviations

ASDs: Anti-seizure drugs; AMPA: Alpha-amino-3-hydroxy-5-methyl-4-isoxazole-propoinate; BBB: Blood-brain barrier; CA3: Region III of hippocampus proper; CCL2: Chemokine (C-C Motif) ligand 2; CCL3: Chemokine (C-C Motif) ligand 3; CCL6: Chemokine (C-C Motif) ligand 6; CNS: Central nervous system; COX-2: Cyclooxygenase-2; CSF: Cerebrospinal fluid; CXCL8: Chemokine (C-X-C motif) ligand 8; DAMP: Damage associated molecular pattern; EC: Endothelial cells; EP2: Receptor for prostaglandin E2; FS: Febrile seizures; GABA: γ-aminobutyric acid; HMGB1: High mobility group box 1 protein; IL-1R: IL-1 receptor; IL-1R1: Cell surface type 1 IL-1 receptor; IL-1α: Interleukin-1α; IL-1β: Interleukin-1β; IL-6: Interleukin-6; IL-10: Interleukin-10; IL-12: Interleukin-12; IRF3: Interferon regulatory transcription factor 3; MAPK: Mitogen-activated protein kinase; MyD88: Myeloid differentiation primary response gene 88; NF-κB: Nuclear factor Kappa-light-chain-enhancer of activated B cells; NMDA: N-methyl-d-aspartate; p7: Postnatal day 7; p28: Postnatal day 28; PTE: Post-traumatic epilepsy; PTZ: Pentylenetetrazol; ROS: Reactive oxygen species; SNPs: Single nucleotide polymorphisms; TBI: Traumatic brain injury; TGF-β: Transforming growth factor-β; TLE: Temporal lobe epilepsy; TLR: Toll-like receptor; TNF-α: Tumor necrosis factor- α; TRAF6: TNF receptor associated factor 6

Acknowledgements
Figures were prepared by Elsevier Illustration Services.

Funding
BDS and SRS are supported by fellowships from the National Health and Medical Research Council of Australia. This manuscript was written with support from the Rebecca L Cooper Medical Research Foundation.

Authors' contributions
KMW and BDS conceptualized and designed the manuscript; KMW, MS, and BDS drafted the manuscript; PC, TJO'B, and SRS provided critical revisions and intellectual input. All authors read and approved the final manuscript.

Competing interests

The authors declare that they have no competing interests.

Consent for publication

Not Applicable.

Author details

[1]Department of Medicine (The Royal Melbourne Hospital), The University of Melbourne, Kenneth Myer Building, Melbourne Brain Centre, Royal Parade, Parkville, VIC 3050, Australia. [2]Department of Pharmacology and Therapeutics, The University of Melbourne, Parkville, VIC 3050, Australia.

References

1. Potts MB, Koh S-E, Whetstone WD, Walker BA, Yoneyama T, Claus CP, et al. Traumatic injury to the immature brain: inflammation, oxidative injury, and iron-mediated damage as potential therapeutic targets. NeuroRx. 2006;3(2): 143–53.
2. Thurman DJ. The epidemiology of traumatic brain injury in children and youths: a review of research since 1990. J Child Neurol. 2016;31(1):20–7.
3. Maas AIR, Stocchetti N, Bullock R. Moderate and severe traumatic brain injury in adults. Lancet Neurol. 2008;7(8):728–41.
4. Khoshyomn S, Tranmer BI. Diagnosis and management of pediatric closed head injury. Semin Pediatr Surg. 2004;13(2):80–6.
5. Schouten JW. Neuroprotection in traumatic brain injury: a complex struggle against the biology of nature. Curr Opin Crit Care. 2007;13(2):134–42.
6. Hinson HE, Rowell S, Schreiber M. Clinical evidence of inflammation driving secondary brain injury: a systematic review. J Trauma Acute Care Surg. 2015;78(1):184–91.
7. Dashnaw ML, Petraglia AL, Bailes JE. An overview of the basic science of concussion and subconcussion: where we are and where we are going. Neurosurg Focus. 2012;33(6):1–9.
8. Prins ML, Hovda DA. Developing experimental models to address traumatic brain injury in children. J Neurotrauma. 2003;20(2):123–37.
9. Blennow K, Hardy J, Zetterberg H. The neuropathology and neurobiology of traumatic brain injury. Neuron. 2012;76(5):886–99.
10. Appleton RE, Demellweek C. Post-traumatic epilepsy in children requiring inpatient rehabilitation following head injury. J Neurol Neurosurg Psychiatry. 2002;72(5):669–72.
11. Statler KD, Scheerlinck P, Pouliot W, Hamilton M, White HS, Dudek FE. A potential model of pediatric posttraumatic epilepsy. Epilepsy Res. 2009;86(2-3):221–3.
12. Frey LC. Epidemiology of posttraumatic epilepsy: a critical review. Epilepsia. 2003;44:11–7.
13. Fisher RS, Boas WV, Blume W, Elger C, Genton P, Lee P, et al. Epileptic seizures and epilepsy: definitions proposed by the International League against Epilepsy (ILAE) and the International Bureau for Epilepsy (IBE). Epilepsia. 2005;46(4):470–2.
14. Pitkanen A, Immonen R. Epilepsy related to traumatic brain injury. Neurotherapeutics. 2014;11(2):286–96.
15. DeLorenzo RJ, Sun DA, Deshpande LS. Cellular mechanisms underlying acquired epilepsy: the calcium hypothesis of the induction and maintenance of epilepsy (vol 105, pg 229, 2005). Pharmacol Ther. 2006;111(1):287–325.
16. Goldberg EM, Coulter DA. Mechanisms of epileptogenesis: a convergence on neural circuit dysfunction. Nat Rev Neurosci. 2013;14(5):337–49.
17. Temkin NR. Preventing and treating posttraumatic seizures: the human experience. Epilepsia. 2009;50:10–3.
18. Walker MC, White HS, Sander J. Disease modification in partial epilepsy. Brain. 2002;125:1937–50.
19. Chiaretti A, De Benedictis R, Polidori G, Piastra M, Iannelli A, Di Rocco C. Early post-traumatic seizures in children with head injury. Childs Nerv Syst. 2000;16(12):862–6.
20. Barlow KM, Spowart JJ, Minns RA. Early posttraumatic seizures in non-accidental head injury: relation to outcome. Dev Med Child Neurol. 2000;42(9):591–4.
21. Hahn YS, Fuchs S, Flannery AM, Barthel MJ, McLone DG. Factors influencing posttraumatic seizures in children. Neurosurgery. 1988;22(5):864–7.
22. Jennett B. Trauma as a cause of epilepsy in childhood. Dev Med Child Neurol. 1973;15(1):56–62.
23. Desai BT, Whitman S, Coonleyhoganson R, Coleman TE, Gabriel G, Dell J. Seizures and civilian head-injuries. Epilepsia. 1983;24(3):289–96.
24. Li H, McDonald W, Parada I, Faria L, Graber K, Takahashi DK, et al. Targets for preventing epilepsy following cortical injury. Neurosci Lett. 2011;497(3):172–6.
25. Santhakumar V, Ratzliff ADH, Jeng J, Toth Z, Soltesz I. Long-term hyperexcitability in the hippocampus after experimental head trauma. Ann Neurol. 2001;50(6):708–17.
26. Cantu D, Walker K, Andresen L, Taylor-Weiner A, Hampton D, Tesco G, et al. Traumatic brain injury increases cortical glutamate network activity by compromising GABAergic control. Cereb Cortex. 2015;25(8):2306–20.
27. Santhakumar V, Bender R, Frotscher M, Ross ST, Hollrigel GS, Toth Z, et al. Granule cell hyperexcitability in the early post-traumatic rat dentate gyrus: the 'irritable mossy cell' hypothesis. J Physiol London. 2000;524(1):117–34.
28. Santhakumar V, Aradi I, Soltesz I. Role of mossy fiber sprouting and mossy cell loss in hyperexcitability: a network model of the dentate gyrus incorporating cell types and axonal topography. J Neurophysiol. 2005;93(1):437–53.
29. Lowenstein DH, Thomas MJ, Smith DH, McIntosh TK. Selective vulnerability of dentate hilar neurons following traumatic brain injury - a potential mechanistic link between head trauma and disorders of the hippocampus. Neurology. 1992;42(7):1427.
30. Diaz-Arrastia R, Agostini MA, Frol AB, Mickey B, Fleckenstein J, Van Ness PC. Neurophysiologic and neuroradiologic features of intractable epilepsy after traumatic brain injury in adults. Arch Neurol. 2000;57(11):1611–6.
31. Hudak AM, Trivedi K, Harper CR, Booker K, Caesar RR, Agostini M, et al. Evaluation of seizure-like episodes in survivors of moderate and severe traumatic brain injury. J Head Trauma Rehab. 2004;19(4):290–5.
32. Yang L, Afroz S, Michelson HB, Goodman JH, Valsamis HA, Ling DSF. Spontaneous epileptiform activity in rat neocortex after controlled cortical impact injury. J Neurotrauma. 2010;27(8):1541–8.
33. Semah F, Picot MC, Adam C, Broglin D, Arzimanoglou A, Bazin B, et al. Is the underlying cause of epilepsy a major prognostic factor for recurrence? Neurology. 1998;51(5):1256–62.
34. Larkin M, Meyer RM, Szuflita NS, Severson MA, Levine ZT. Post-traumatic, drug-resistant epilepsy and review of seizure control outcomes from blinded, randomized controlled trials of brain stimulation treatments for drug-resistant epilepsy. Cureus. 2016;8(8):e744.
35. Temkin NR. Antiepileptogenesis and seizure prevention trials with antiepileptic drugs: meta-analysis of controlled trials. Epilepsia. 2001;42(4):515–24.
36. Beghi E. Overview of studies to prevent posttraumatic epilepsy. Epilepsia. 2003;44:21–6.
37. Torbic H, Forni AA, Anger KE, Degrado JR, Greenwood BC. Use of antiepileptics for seizure prophylaxis after traumatic brain injury. Am J Health Syst Pharm. 2013;70(9):759–66.
38. Kirmani BF, Robinson DM, Fonkem E, Graf K, Huang JH. Role of anticonvulsants in the management of posttraumatic epilepsy. Front Neurol. 2016;7:32.
39. Kubova H, Mares P, Suchomelova L, Brozek G, Druga R, Pitkanen A. Status epilepticus in immature rats leads to behavioural and cognitive impairment and epileptogenesis. Eur J Neurosci. 2004;19(12):3255–65.
40. Statler KD. Pediatric posttraumatic seizures: epidemiology, putative mechanisms of epileptogenesis and promising investigational progress. Dev Neurosci. 2006;28(4-5):354–63.
41. Hickey WF. Basic principles of immunological surveillance of the normal central nervous system. Glia. 2001;36(2):118–24.
42. Auffray C, Sieweke MH, Geissmann F. Blood monocytes: development, heterogeneity, and relationship with dendritic cells. Annu Rev Immunol. 2009;27:669–92.
43. Cederberg D, Siesjo P. What has inflammation to do with traumatic brain injury? Childs Nerv Syst. 2010;26(2):221–6.
44. DeKosky ST, Blennow K, Ikonomovic MD, Gandy S. Acute and chronic traumatic encephalopathies: pathogenesis and biomarkers. Nat Rev Neurol. 2013;9(4):192–200.
45. Riazi K, Galic MA, Pittman QJ. Contributions of peripheral inflammation to seizure susceptibility: cytokines and brain excitability. Epilepsy Res. 2010;89(1):34–42.
46. Utagawa A, Truettner JS, Dietrich WD, Bramlett HM. Systemic inflammation exacerbates behavioral and histopathological consequences of isolated traumatic brain injury in rats. Exp Neurol. 2008;211(1):283–91.

47. Vezzani A, Granata T. Brain inflammation in epilepsy: experimental and clinical evidence. Epilepsia. 2005;46(11):1724–43.

48. Morganti-Kossmann MC, Rancan M, Stahel PF, Kossmann T. Inflammatory response in acute traumatic brain injury: a double-edged sword. Curr Opin Crit Care. 2002;8(2):101–5.

49. Hudome S, Palmer C, Roberts RL, Mauger D, Housman C, Towfighi J. The role of neutrophils in the production of hypoxic-ischemic brain injury in the neonatal rat. Pediatr Res. 1997;41(5):607–16.

50. Owen CA, Campbell EJ. The cell biology of leukocyte-mediated proteolysis. J Leukoc Biol. 1999;65(2):137–50.

51. Chodobski A, Zink BJ, Szmydynger-Chodobska J. Blood-brain barrier pathophysiology in traumatic brain injury. Transl Stroke Res. 2011;2(4):492–516.

52. Dempsey RJ, Baskaya MK, Dogan A. Attenuation of brain edema, blood-brain barrier breakdown, and injury volume by ifenprodil, a polyamine-site N-methyl-D-aspartate receptor antagonist, after experimental traumatic brain injury in rats. Neurosurgery. 2000;47(2):399–404.

53. Ransohoff RM, Tani M. Do chemokines mediate leukocyte recruitment in post-traumatic CNS inflammation? Trends Neurosci. 1998;21(4):154–9.

54. Semple BD, Bye N, Rancan M, Ziebell JM, Morganti-Kossmann MC. Role of CCL2 (MCP-1) in traumatic brain injury (TBI): evidence from severe TBI patients and CCL2-/- mice. J Cereb Blood Flow Metab. 2010;30(4):769–82.

55. Nonaka M, Chen XH, Pierce JES, Leoni MJ, McIntosh TK, Wolf JA, et al. Prolonged activation of NF-kappa B following traumatic brain injury in rats. J Neurotrauma. 1999;16(11):1023–34.

56. Scherbel U, Raghupathi R, Nakamura M, Saatman KE, Trojanowski JQ, Neugebauer E, et al. Differential acute and chronic responses of tumor necrosis factor-deficient mice to experimental brain injury. Proc Natl Acad Sci U S A. 1999;96(15):8721–6.

57. Sherwood ER, Prough DS. Interleukin-8, neuroinflammation, and secondary brain injury. Crit Care Med. 2000;28(4):1221–3.

58. Kreutzberg GW. Microglia: a sensor for pathological events in the CNS. Trends Neurosci. 1996;19(8):312–8.

59. Braughler JM, Hall ED. Central nervous system trauma and stroke. I. Biochemical considerations for oxygen radical formation and lipid peroxidation. Free Radic Biol Med. 1989;6(3):289–301.

60. Hall ED, Braughler JM. Central nervous system trauma and stroke. II. Physiological and pharmacological evidence for involvement of oxygen radicals and lipid peroxidation. Free Radic Biol Med. 1989;6(3):303–13.

61. Smith SL, Andrus PK, Zhang JR, Hall ED. Direct measurement of hydroxyl radicals, lipid peroxidation, and blood-brain barrier disruption following unilateral cortical impact head injury in the rat. J Neurotrauma. 1994;11(4):393–404.

62. Campbell IL, Abraham CR, Masliah E, Kemper P, Inglis JD, Oldstone MB, et al. Neurologic disease induced in transgenic mice by cerebral overexpression of interleukin 6. Proc Natl Acad Sci U S A. 1993;90(21):10061–5.

63. Ravizza T, Balosso S, Vezzani A. Inflammation and prevention of epileptogenesis. Neurosci Lett. 2011;497(3):223–30.

64. David Y, Cacheaux LP, Ivens S, Lapilover E, Heinemann U, Kaufer D, et al. Astrocytic dysfunction in epileptogenesis: consequence of altered potassium and glutamate homeostasis? J Neurosci. 2009;29(34):10588–99.

65. Tchelingerian JL, Monge M, Lesaux F, Zalc B, Jacque C. Differential oligodendroglial expression of the tumor-necrosis-factor receptors in-vivo and in-vitro. J Neurochem. 1995;65(5):2377–80.

66. Shohami E, Ginis I, Hallenbeck JM. Dual role of tumor necrosis factor alpha in brain injury. Cytokine Growth Factor Rev. 1999;10(2):119–30.

67. Matsumoto H, Marsan CA. Cortical cellular phenomena in experimental epilepsy: ictal manifestations. Exp Neurol. 1964;9:305–26.

68. Cobb SR, Buhl EH, Halasy K, Paulsen O, Somogyi P. Synchronization of neuronal activity in hippocampus by individual GABAergic interneurons. Nature. 1995;378(6552):75–8.

69. Avoli M, de Curtis M, Gnatkovsky V, Gotman J, Kohling R, Levesque M, et al. Specific imbalance of excitatory/inhibitory signaling establishes seizure onset pattern in temporal lobe epilepsy. J Neurophysiol. 2016;115(6):3229–37.

70. de Curtis M, Avoli M. GABAergic networks jump-start focal seizures. Epilepsia. 2016;57(5):679–87.

71. Lason W, Chlebicka M, Rejdak K. Research advances in basic mechanisms of seizures and antiepileptic drug action. Pharmacol Rep. 2013;65(4):787–801.

72. Sayyah M, Javad-Pour M, Ghazi-Khansari M. The bacterial endotoxin lipopolysaccharide enhances seizure susceptibility in mice: involvement of proinflammatory factors: nitric oxide and prostaglandins. Neuroscience. 2003;122(4):1073–80.

73. Dhote F, Peinnequin A, Carpentier P, Baille V, Delacour C, Foquin A, et al. Prolonged inflammatory gene response following soman-induced seizures in mice. Toxicology. 2007;238(2-3):166–76.

74. Levesque M, Avoli M, Bernard C. Animal models of temporal lobe epilepsy following systemic chemoconvulsant administration. J Neurosci Methods. 2016;260:45–52.

75. Gorter JA, van Vliet EA, da Silva FH L. Which insights have we gained from the kindling and post-status epilepticus models? J Neurosci Methods. 2016;260:96–108.

76. De Simoni MG, Perego C, Ravizza T, Moneta D, Conti M, Marchesi F, et al. Inflammatory cytokines and related genes are induced in the rat hippocampus by limbic status epilepticus. Eur J Neurosci. 2000;12(7):2623–33.

77. Turrin NP, Rivest S. Innate immune reaction in response to seizures: implications for the neuropathology associated with epilepsy. Neurobiol Dis. 2004;16(2):321–34.

78. Gorter JA, van Vliet EA, Aronica E, Breit T, Rauwerda H, da Silva FHL, et al. Potential new antiepileptogenic targets indicated by microarray analysis in a rat model for temporal lobe epilepsy. J Neurosci. 2006;26(43):11083–110.

79. Oprica M, Eriksson C, Schultzberg M. Inflammatory mechanisms associated with brain damage induced by kainic acid with special reference to the interleukin-1 system. J Cell Mol Med. 2003;7(2):127–40.

80. Vezzani A, Conti N, De Luigi A, Ravizza T, Moneta D, Marchesi F, et al. Interleukin-l beta immunoreactivity and microglia are enhanced in the rat hippocampus by focal kainate application: functional evidence for enhancement of electrographic seizures. J Neurosci. 1999;19(12):5054–65.

81. Peltola J, Laaksonen J, Haapala AM, Hurme M, Rainesalo S, Keranen T. Indicators of inflammation after recent tonic-clonic epileptic seizures correlate with plasma interleukin-6 levels. Seizure Eur J Epilepsy. 2002;11(1):44–6.

82. Peltola J, Palmio J, Korhonen L, Suhonen J, Miettinen A, Hurme M, et al. Interleukin-6 and Interleukin-1 receptor antagonist in cerebrospinal fluid from patients with recent tonic-clonic seizures. Epilepsy Res. 2000;41(3):205–11.

83. Crespel A, Coubes P, Rousset M-C, Brana C, Rougier A, Rondouin G, et al. Inflammatory reactions in human medial temporal lobe epilepsy with hippocampal sclerosis. Brain Res. 2002;952(2):159–69.

84. Kharatishvili I, Pitkanen A. Association of the severity of cortical damage with the occurrence of spontaneous seizures and hyperexcitability in an animal model of posttraumatic epilepsy. Epilepsy Res. 2010;90(1-2):47–59.

85. Kirkman NJ, Libbey JE, Wilcox KS, White HS, Fujinami RS. Innate but not adaptive immune responses contribute to behavioral seizures following viral infection. Epilepsia. 2010;51(3):454–64.

86. Vezzani A, Balosso S, Ravizza T. The role of cytokines in the pathophysiology of epilepsy. Brain Behav Immun. 2008;22(6):797–803.

87. Lloyd E, Somera-Molina K, Van Eldik LJ, Watterson DM, Wainwright MS. Suppression of acute proinflammatory cytokine and chemokine upregulation by post-injury administration of a novel small molecule improves long-term neurologic outcome in a mouse model of traumatic brain injury. J Neuroinflammation. 2008;5:28.

88. Somera-Molina KC, Robin B, Somera CA, Anderson C, Stine C, Koh S, et al. Glial activation links early-life seizures and long-term neurologic dysfunction: evidence using a small molecule inhibitor of proinflammatory cytokine upregulation. Epilepsia. 2007;48(9):1785–800.

89. Viviani B, Gardoni F, Marinovich M. Cytokines and neuronal ion channels in health and disease. Int Rev Neurobiol. 2007;82:247–63.

90. Cunningham AJ, Murray CA, O'Neill LA, Lynch MA, O'Connor JJ. Interleukin-1 beta (IL-1 beta) and tumour necrosis factor (TNF) inhibit long-term potentiation in the rat dentate gyrus in vitro. Neurosci Lett. 1996;203(1):17–20.

91. Probert L, Akassoglou K, Pasparakis M, Kontogeorgos G, Kollias G. Spontaneous inflammatory demyelinating disease in transgenic mice showing central nervous system-specific expression of tumor necrosis factor alpha. Proc Natl Acad Sci U S A. 1995;92(24):11294–8.

92. Samland H, Huitron-Resendiz S, Masliah E, Criado J, Henriksen SJ, Campbell IL. Profound increase in sensitivity to glutamatergic- but not cholinergic agonist-induced seizures in transgenic mice with astrocyte production of IL-6. J Neurosci Res. 2003;73(2):176–87.

93. Bradford HF. Glutamate, GABA and epilepsy. Prog Neurobiol. 1995;47(6):477–511.

94. Hu S, Sheng WS, Ehrlich LC, Peterson PK, Chao CC. Cytokine effects on glutamate uptake by human astrocytes. Neuroimmunomodulation. 2000;7(3):153–9.

95. Balosso S, Ravizza T, Pierucci M, Calcagno E, Invernizzi R, Di Giovanni G, et al. Molecular and functional interactions between tumor necrosis factor-alpha receptors and the glutamatergic system in the mouse hippocampus: implications for seizure susceptibility. Neuroscience. 2009;161(1):293–300.

96. Pickering M, Cumiskey D, O'Connor JJ. Actions of TNF-alpha on glutamatergic synaptic transmission in the central nervous system. Exp Physiol. 2005;90(5):663–70.

97. Godukhin OV, Levin SG, Parnyshkova EY. The effects of interleukin-10 on the development of epileptiform activity in the hippocampus induced by transient hypoxia, bicuculline, and electrical kindling. Neurosci Behav Physiol. 2009;39(7):625–31.

98. Shandra AA, Godlevsky LS, Vastyanov RS, Oleinik AA, Konovalenko VL, Rapoport EN, et al. The role of TNF-alpha in amygdala kindled rats. Neurosci Res. 2002;42(2):147–53.

99. Bilbo SD, Rudy JW, Watkins LR, Maier SF. A behavioural characterization of neonatal infection-facilitated memory impairment in adult rats. Behav Brain Res. 2006;169(1):39–47.

100. Boisse L, Mouihate A, Ellis S, Pittman QJ. Long-term alterations in neuroimmune responses after neonatal exposure to lipopolysaccharide. J Neurosci. 2004;24(21):4928–34.

101. Ellis S, Mouihate A, Pittman QJ. Neonatal programming of the rat neuroimmune response: stimulus specific changes elicited by bacterial and viral mimetics. J Physiol. 2006;571(Pt 3):695–701.

102. Galic MA, Riazi K, Henderson AK, Tsutsui S, Pittman QJ. Viral-like brain inflammation during development causes increased seizure susceptibility in adult rats. Neurobiol Dis. 2009;36(2):343–51.

103. Hesdorffer DC, Shinnar S, Lax DN, Pellock JM, Nordli Jr DR, Seinfeld S, et al. Risk factors for subsequent febrile seizures in the FEBSTAT study. Epilepsia. 2016;57(7):1042–7.

104. Baulac S, Gourfinkel-An I, Nabbout R, Huberfeld G, Serratosa J, Leguern E, et al. Fever, genes, and epilepsy. Lancet Neurol. 2004;3(7):421–30.

105. Virta M, Hurme M, Helminen M. Increased frequency of interleukin-1beta (-511) allele 2 in febrile seizures. Pediatr Neurol. 2002;26(3):192–5.

106. Hulkkonen J, Laippala P, Hurme M. A rare allele combination of the interleukin-1 gene complex is associated with high interleukin-1 beta plasma levels in healthy individuals. Eur Cytokine Netw. 2000;11(2):251–5.

107. Kanemoto K, Kawasaki J, Miyamoto T, Obayashi H, Nishimura M. Interleukin (IL)1beta, IL-1alpha, and IL-1 receptor antagonist gene polymorphisms in patients with temporal lobe epilepsy. Ann Neurol. 2000;47(5):571–4.

108. Binder DK, Steinhauser C. Functional changes in astroglial cells in epilepsy. Glia. 2006;54(5):358–68.

109. Heinemann U, Kaufer D, Friedman A. Blood-brain barrier dysfunction, TGFbeta signaling, and astrocyte dysfunction in epilepsy. Glia. 2012;60(8):1251–7.

110. Garlanda C, Dinarello CA, Mantovani A. The interleukin-1 family: back to the future. Immunity. 2013;39(6):1003–18.

111. Kim Y-J, Hwang S-Y, Oh E-S, Oh S, Han I-O. IL-1beta, an immediate early protein secreted by activated microglia, induces iNOS/NO in C6 astrocytoma cells through p38 MAPK and NF-kappaB pathways. J Neurosci Res. 2006;84(5):1037–46.

112. Lau LT, Yu AC. Astrocytes produce and release interleukin-1, interleukin-6, tumor necrosis factor alpha and interferon-gamma following traumatic and metabolic injury. J Neurotrauma. 2001;18(3):351–9.

113. Miossec P, Cavender D, Ziff M. Production of interleukin 1 by human endothelial cells. J Immunol. 1986;136(7):2486–91.

114. John GR, Lee SC, Song X, Rivieccio M, Brosnan CF. IL-1-regulated responses in astrocytes: relevance to injury and recovery. Glia. 2005;49(2):161–76.

115. Konsman JP, Vigues S, Mackerlova L, Bristow A, Blomqvist A. Rat brain vascular distribution of interleukin-1 type-1 receptor immunoreactivity: relationship to patterns of inducible cyclooxygenase expression by peripheral inflammatory stimuli. J Comp Neurol. 2004;472(1):113–29.

116. Pinteaux E, Parker LC, Rothwell NJ, Luheshi GN. Expression of interleukin-1 receptors and their role in interleukin-1 actions in murine microglial cells. J Neurochem. 2002;83(4):754–63.

117. Sato A, Ohtaki H, Tsumuraya T, Song D, Ohara K, Asano M, et al. Interleukin-1 participates in the classical and alternative activation of microglia/macrophages after spinal cord injury. J Neuroinflammation. 2012;9:65.

118. Srinivasan D, Yen J-H, Joseph DJ, Friedman W. Cell type-specific interleukin-1beta signaling in the CNS. J Neurosci. 2004;24(29):6482–8.

119. Vela JM, Molina-Holgado E, Arevalo-Martin A, Almazan G, Guaza C. Interleukin-1 regulates proliferation and differentiation of oligodendrocyte progenitor cells. Mol Cell Neurosci. 2002;20(3):489–502.

120. Moynagh PN. The interleukin-1 signalling pathway in astrocytes: a key contributor to inflammation in the brain. J Anat. 2005;207(3):265–9.

121. Fan L, Young PR, Barone FC, Feuerstein GZ, Smith DH, McIntosh TK. Experimental brain injury induces expression of interleukin-1 beta mRNA in the rat brain. Brain Res Mol Brain Res. 1995;30(1):125–30.

122. Kinoshita K, Chatzipanteli IK, Vitarbo E, Truettner JS, Alonso OF, Dietrich WD. Interleukin-1beta messenger ribonucleic acid and protein levels after fluid-percussion brain injury in rats: importance of injury severity and brain temperature. Neurosurgery. 2002;51(1):195–203. discussion.

123. Ciallella JR, Ikonomovic MD, Paljug WR, Wilbur YI, Dixon CE, Kochanek PM, et al. Changes in expression of amyloid precursor protein and interleukin-1beta after experimental traumatic brain injury in rats. J Neurotrauma. 2002;19(12):1555–67.

124. Kamm K, Vanderkolk W, Lawrence C, Jonker M, Davis AT. The effect of traumatic brain injury upon the concentration and expression of interleukin-1beta and interleukin-10 in the rat. J Trauma. 2006;60(1):152–7.

125. Acosta SA, Tajiri N, Shinozuka K, Ishikawa H, Grimmig B, Diamond DM, et al. Long-term upregulation of inflammation and suppression of cell proliferation in the brain of adult rats exposed to traumatic brain injury using the controlled cortical impact model. PLoS One. 2013;8(1):e53376.

126. Frugier T, Morganti-Kossmann MC, O'Reilly D, McLean CA. In situ detection of inflammatory mediators in post mortem human brain tissue after traumatic injury. J Neurotrauma. 2010;27(3):497–507.

127. Holmin S, Soderlund J, Biberfeld P, Mathiesen T. Intracerebral inflammation after human brain contusion. Neurosurgery. 1998;42(2):291–8.

128. Winter CD, Iannotti F, Pringle AK, Trikkas C, Clough GF, Church MK. A microdialysis method for the recovery of IL-1 beta, IL-6 and nerve growth factor from human brain in vivo. J Neurosci Methods. 2002;119(1):45–50.

129. Shiozaki T, Hayakata T, Tasaki O, Hosotubo H, Fuijita K, Mouri T, et al. Cerebrospinal fluid concentrations of anti-inflammatory mediators in early-phase severe traumatic brain injury. Shock. 2005;23(5):406–10.

130. Hunt RF, Boychuk JA, Smith BN. Neural circuit mechanisms of post-traumatic epilepsy. Front Cell Neurosci. 2013;7:89. doi:10.3389/fncel.2013.00089.

131. Clausen F, Hanell A, Bjork M, Hillered L, Mir AK, Gram H, et al. Neutralization of interleukin-1beta modifies the inflammatory response and improves histological and cognitive outcome following traumatic brain injury in mice. Eur J Neurosci. 2009;30(3):385–96.

132. Clausen F, Hanell A, Israelsson C, Hedin J, Ebendal T, Mir AK, et al. Neutralization of interleukin-1beta reduces cerebral edema and tissue loss and improves late cognitive outcome following traumatic brain injury in mice. Eur J Neurosci. 2011;34(1):110–23.

133. Lazovic J, Basu A, Lin H-W, Rothstein RP, Krady JK, Smith MB, et al. Neuroinflammation and both cytotoxic and vasogenic edema are reduced in interleukin-1 type 1 receptor-deficient mice conferring neuroprotection. Stroke. 2005;36(10):2226–31.

134. Sanderson KL, Raghupathi R, Saatman KE, Martin D, Miller G, McIntosh TK. Interleukin-1 receptor antagonist attenuates regional neuronal cell death and cognitive dysfunction after experimental brain injury. J Cereb Blood Flow Metab. 1999;19(10):1118–25.

135. Helmy A, Guilfoyle MR, Carpenter KLH, Pickard JD, Menon DK, Hutchinson PJ. Recombinant human interleukin-1 receptor antagonist in severe traumatic brain injury: a phase II randomized control trial. J Cereb Blood Flow Metab. 2014;34(5):845–51.

136. Diamond ML, Ritter AC, Failla MD, Boles JA, Conley YP, Kochanek PM, et al. IL-1beta associations with posttraumatic epilepsy development: a genetics and biomarker cohort study. Epilepsia. 2015;56(7):991–1001.

137. Dube CM, Ravizza T, Hamamura M, Zha Q, Keebaugh A, Fok K, et al. Epileptogenesis provoked by prolonged experimental febrile seizures: mechanisms and biomarkers. J Neurosci. 2010;30(22):7484–94.

138. Dube C, Vezzani A, Behrens M, Bartfai T, Baram TZ. Interleukin-1beta contributes to the generation of experimental febrile seizures. Ann Neurol. 2005;57(1):152–5.

139. Zhu G, Okada M, Yoshida S, Mori F, Ueno S, Wakabayashi K, et al. Effects of interleukin-1beta on hippocampal glutamate and GABA releases associated with Ca2 + -induced Ca2+ releasing systems. Epilepsy Res. 2006;71(2-3):107–16.

140. Wetherington J, Serrano G, Dingledine R. Astrocytes in the epileptic brain. Neuron. 2008;58(2):168–78.

141. Ferrari CC, Depino AM, Prada F, Muraro N, Campbell S, Podhajcer O, et al. Reversible demyelination, blood-brain barrier breakdown, and pronounced neutrophil recruitment induced by chronic IL-1 expression in the brain. Am J Pathol. 2004;165(5):1827–37.

142. Proescholdt MG, Chakravarty S, Foster JA, Foti SB, Briley EM, Herkenham M. Intracerebroventricular but not intravenous interleukin-1beta induces widespread vascular-mediated leukocyte infiltration and immune signal mRNA expression followed by brain-wide glial activation. Neuroscience. 2002;112(3):731–49.

143. Quagliarello VJ, Wispelwey B, Long Jr WJ, Scheld WM. Recombinant human interleukin-1 induces meningitis and blood-brain barrier injury in the rat. Characterization and comparison with tumor necrosis factor. J Clin Invest. 1991;87(4):1360–6.

144. Shaftel SS, Carlson TJ, Olschowka JA, Kyrkanides S, Matousek SB, O'Banion MK. Chronic interleukin-1beta expression in mouse brain leads to leukocyte infiltration and neutrophil-independent blood brain barrier permeability without overt neurodegeneration. J Neurosci. 2007;27(35):9301–9.

145. Harting MT, Jimenez F, Adams SD, Mercer DW, Cox Jr CS. Acute, regional inflammatory response after traumatic brain injury: implications for cellular therapy. Surgery. 2008;144(5):803–13.

146. Lu K-T, Wang Y-W, Yang J-T, Yang Y-L, Chen H-I. Effect of interleukin-1 on traumatic brain injury-induced damage to hippocampal neurons. J Neurotrauma. 2005;22(8):885–95.

147. Pacifici R, Paris L, Di Carlo S, Bacosi A, Pichini S, Zuccaro P. Cytokine production in blood mononuclear cells from epileptic patients. Epilepsia. 1995;36(4):384–7.

148. Tanriverdi T, Uzan M, Sanus GZ, Baykara O, Is M, Ozkara C, et al. Lack of association between the IL1A gene (-889) polymorphism and outcome after head injury. Surg Neurol. 2006;65(1):7–10. discussion.

149. Haspolat S, Baysal Y, Duman O, Coskun M, Tosun O, Yegin O. Interleukin-1alpha, interleukin-1beta, and interleukin-1Ra polymorphisms in febrile seizures. J Child Neurol. 2005;20(7):565–8.

150. Bianchi ME, Manfredi AA. High-mobility group box 1 (HMGB1) protein at the crossroads between innate and adaptive immunity. Immunol Rev. 2007;220:35–46.

151. Stros M. HMGB proteins: interactions with DNA and chromatin. Biochim Biophys Acta. 2010;1799(1-2):101–13.

152. Yanai H, Ban T, Taniguchi T. Essential role of high-mobility group box proteins in nucleic acid-mediated innate immune responses. J Intern Med. 2011;270(4):301–8.

153. Goodwin GH, Sanders C, Johns EW. A new group of chromatin-associated proteins with a high content of acidic and basic amino acids. Eur J Biochem. 1973;38(1):14–9.

154. Gerlitz G, Hock R, Ueda T, Bustin M. The dynamics of HMG protein-chromatin interactions in living cells. Biochem Cell Biol. 2009;87(1):127–37.

155. Venters BJ, Pugh BF. How eukaryotic genes are transcribed. Crit Rev Biochem Mol Biol. 2009;44(2-3):117–41.

156. Calogero S, Grassi F, Aguzzi A, Voigtlander T, Ferrier P, Ferrari S, et al. The lack of chromosomal protein Hmg1 does not disrupt cell growth but causes lethal hypoglycaemia in newborn mice. Nat Genet. 1999;22(3):276–80.

157. Yang H, Antoine DJ, Andersson U, Tracey KJ. The many faces of HMGB1: molecular structure-functional activity in inflammation, apoptosis, and chemotaxis. J Leukoc Biol. 2013;93(6):865–73.

158. Scaffidi P, Misteli T, Bianchi ME. Release of chromatin protein HMGB1 by necrotic cells triggers inflammation. Nature. 2002;418(6894):191–5.

159. Bonaldi T, Talamo F, Scaffidi P, Ferrera D, Porto A, Bachi A, et al. Monocytic cells hyperacetylate chromatin protein HMGB1 to redirect it towards secretion. EMBO J. 2003;22(20):5551–60.

160. Lu B, Nakamura T, Inouye K, Li J, Tang Y, Lundback P, et al. Novel role of PKR in inflammasome activation and HMGB1 release. Nature. 2012;488(7413):670–4.

161. Wang H, Bloom O, Zhang M, Vishnubhakat JM, Ombrellino M, Che J, et al. HMG-1 as a late mediator of endotoxin lethality in mice. Science (New York, NY). 1999;285(5425):248–51.

162. Harris HE, Andersson U, Pisetsky DS. HMGB1: a multifunctional alarmin driving autoimmune and inflammatory disease. Nat Rev Rheumatol. 2012;8(4):195–202.

163. Aronica E, Crino PB. Inflammation in epilepsy: clinical observations. Epilepsia. 2011;52 Suppl 3:26–32.

164. Chiavegato A, Zurolo E, Losi G, Aronica E, Carmignoto G. The inflammatory molecules IL-1 beta and HMGB1 can rapidly enhance focal seizure generation in a brain slice model of temporal lobe epilepsy. Front Cell Neurosci. 2014;8:155.

165. Maroso M, Balosso S, Ravizza T, Liu J, Aronica E, Iyer AM, et al. Toll-like receptor 4 and high-mobility group box-1 are involved in ictogenesis and can be targeted to reduce seizures. Nat Med. 2010;16(4):413–U91.

166. Iori V, Maroso M, Rizzi M, Iyer AM, Vertemara R, Carli M, et al. Receptor for advanced glycation endproducts is upregulated in temporal lobe epilepsy and contributes to experimental seizures. Neurobiol Dis. 2013;58:102–14.

167. Balosso S, Liu J, Bianchi ME, Vezzani A. Disulfide-containing high mobility group box-1 promotes n-methyl-d-aspartate receptor function and excitotoxicity by activating toll-like receptor 4-dependent signaling in hippocampal neurons. Antioxid Redox Signal. 2014;21(12):1726–40.

168. Tang D, Kang R, Zeh 3rd HJ, Lotze MT. High-mobility group box 1, oxidative stress, and disease. Antioxid Redox Signal. 2011;14(7):1315–35.

169. Waldbaum S, Patel M. Mitochondria, oxidative stress, and temporal lobe epilepsy. Epilepsy Res. 2010;88(1):23–45.

170. Chen G, Shi J, Jin W, Wang L, Xie W, Sun J, et al. Progesterone administration modulates TLRs/NF-kappa B signaling pathway in rat brain after cortical contusion. Ann Clin Lab Sci. 2008;38(1):65–74.

171. Okun E, Griffioen KJ, Lathia JD, Tang S-C, Mattson MP, Arumugam TV. Toll-like receptors in neurodegeneration. Brain Res Rev. 2009;59(2):278–92.

172. Chang ZL. Important aspects of toll-like receptors, ligands and their signaling pathways. Inflamm Res. 2010;59(10):791–808.

173. Lu Y-C, Yeh W-C, Ohashi PS. LPS/TLR4 signal transduction pathway. Cytokine. 2008;42(2):145–51.

174. Sha YG, Zmijewski J, Xu ZW, Abraham E. HMGB1 develops enhanced binding to cytokines. J Immunol. 2008;180(4):2531–7.

175. Garcia-Arnandis I, Guillen MI, Gomar F, Pelletier JP, Martel-Pelletier J, Alcaraz MJ. High mobility group box 1 potentiates the pro-inflammatory effects of interleukin-1 beta in osteoarthritic synoviocytes. Arthr Res Ther. 2010;12(4):R165.

176. Annegers JF, Grabow JD, Groover RV, Laws Jr ER, Elveback LR, Kurland LT. Seizures after head trauma: a population study. Neurology. 1980;30(7 Pt 1):683–9.

177. Shlosberg D, Benifla M, Kaufer D, Friedman A. Blood-brain barrier breakdown as a therapeutic target in traumatic brain injury. Nat Rev Neurol. 2010;6(7):393–403.

178. Kelley BJ, Lifshitz J, Povlishock JT. Neuroinflammatory responses after experimental diffuse traumatic brain injury. J Neuropathol Exp Neurol. 2007;66(11):989–1001.

179. Friedman A, Kaufer D, Heinemann U. Blood-brain barrier breakdown-inducing astrocytic transformation: novel targets for the prevention of epilepsy. Epilepsy Res. 2009;85(2-3):142–9.

180. Tomkins O, Feintuch A, Benifla M, Cohen A, Friedman A, Shelef I. Blood-brain barrier breakdown following traumatic brain injury: a possible role in posttraumatic epilepsy. Cardiovasc Psychiatr Neurol. 2011;2011:765923.

181. Tomkins O, Shelef I, Kaizerman I, Eliushin A, Afawi Z, Misk A, et al. Blood-brain barrier disruption in post-traumatic epilepsy. J Neurol Neurosurg Psychiatry. 2008;79(7):774–7.

182. Cacheaux LP, Ivens S, David Y, Lakhter AJ, Bar-Klein G, Shapira M, et al. Transcriptome profiling reveals TGF-beta signaling involvement in epileptogenesis. J Neurosci. 2009;29(28):8927–35.

183. Weissberg I, Wood L, Kamintsky L, Vazquez O, Milikovsky DZ, Alexander A, et al. Albumin induces excitatory synaptogenesis through astrocytic TGF-beta/ALK5 signaling in a model of acquired epilepsy following blood-brain barrier dysfunction. Neurobiol Dis. 2015;78:115–25.

184. Ivens S, Kaufer D, Flores LP, Bechmann I, Zumsteg D, Tomkins O, et al. TGF-beta receptor-mediated albumin uptake into astrocytes is involved in neocortical epileptogenesis. Brain. 2007;130(Pt 2):535–47.

185. Barkai E, Grossman Y, Gutnick MJ. Long-term changes in neocortical activity after chemical kindling with systemic pentylenetetrazole: an in vitro study. J Neurophysiol. 1994;72(1):72–83.

186. Sanabria ERG, Silva AV, Spreafico R, Cavalheiro EA. Damage, reorganization, and abnormal neocortical hyperexcitability in the pilocarpine model of temporal lobe epilepsy. Epilepsia. 2002;43 Suppl 5:96–106.

187. Tigyi G, Hong L, Yakubu M, Parfenova H, Shibata M, Leffler CW. Lysophosphatidic acid alters cerebrovascular reactivity in piglets. Am J Phys. 1995;268(5 Pt 2):H2048–55.

188. Blobe GC, Schiemann WP, Lodish HF. Role of transforming growth factor beta in human disease. N Engl J Med. 2000;342(18):1350–8.

189. Gold LI, Parekh TV. Loss of growth regulation by transforming growth factor-beta (TGF-beta) in human cancers: studies on endometrial carcinoma. Semin Reprod Endocrinol. 1999;17(1):73–92.

190. Shi Y, Massague J. Mechanisms of TGF-beta signaling from cell membrane to the nucleus. Cell. 2003;113(6):685–700.

191. Szelenyi J. Cytokines and the central nervous system. Brain Res Bull. 2001;54(4):329–38.

192. Phillips DJ, Nguyen P, Adamides AA, Bye N, Rosenfeld JV, Kossmann T, et al. Activin a release into cerebrospinal fluid in a subset of patients with severe traumatic brain injury. J Neurotrauma. 2006;23(9):1283–94.

193. Brionne TC, Tesseur I, Masliah E, Wyss-Coray T. Loss of TGF-beta 1 leads to increased neuronal cell death and microgliosis in mouse brain. Neuron. 2003;40(6):1133–45.

194. Prehn JH, Bindokas VP, Marcuccilli CJ, Krajewski S, Reed JC, Miller RJ. Regulation of neuronal Bcl2 protein expression and calcium homeostasis by transforming growth factor type beta confers wide-ranging protection on rat hippocampal neurons. Proc Natl Acad Sci U S A. 1994;91(26):12599–603.

195. Plata-Salaman CR, Ilyin SE, Turrin NP, Gayle D, Flynn MC, Romanovitch AE, et al. Kindling modulates the IL-1beta system, TNF-alpha, TGF-beta1, and neuropeptide mRNAs in specific brain regions. Brain Res Mol Brain Res. 2000;75(2):248–58.

196. Aronica E, van Vliet EA, Mayboroda OA, Troost D, da Silva FH, Gorter JA. Upregulation of metabotropic glutamate receptor subtype mGluR3 and mGluR5 in reactive astrocytes in a rat model of mesial temporal lobe epilepsy. Eur J Neurosci. 2000;12(7):2333–44.

197. Frigerio F, Frasca A, Weissberg I, Parrella S, Friedman A, Vezzani A, et al. Long-lasting pro-ictogenic effects induced in vivo by rat brain exposure to serum albumin in the absence of concomitant pathology. Epilepsia. 2012;53(11):1887–97.

198. Jin X, Prince DA, Huguenard JR. Enhanced excitatory synaptic connectivity in layer v pyramidal neurons of chronically injured epileptogenic neocortex in rats. J Neurosci. 2006;26(18):4891–900.

199. Scheff SW, Price DA, Hicks RR, Baldwin SA, Robinson S, Brackney C. Synaptogenesis in the hippocampal CA1 field following traumatic brain injury. J Neurotrauma. 2005;22(7):719–32.

200. Schoderboeck L, Adzemovic M, Nicolussi E-M, Crupinschi C, Hochmeister S, Fischer M-T, et al. The "window of susceptibility" for inflammation in the immature central nervous system is characterized by a leaky blood-brain barrier and the local expression of inflammatory chemokines. Neurobiol Dis. 2009;35(3):368–75.

201. Galea I, Bechmann I, Perry VH. What is immune privilege (not)? Trends Immunol. 2007;28(1):12–8.

202. Umehara F, Qin YF, Goto M, Wekerle H, Meyermann R. Experimental autoimmune encephalomyelitis in the maturing central-nervous-system-transfer of myelin basic protein-specific T-line lymphocytes to neonatal lewis rats. Lab Investig. 1990;62(2):147–55.

203. Anthony D, Dempster R, Fearn S, Clements J, Wells G, Perry VH, et al. CXC chemokines generate age-related increases in neutrophil-mediated brain inflammation and blood-brain barrier breakdown. Curr Biol. 1998;8(16):923–6.

204. Anthony DC, Bolton SJ, Fearn S, Perry VH. Age-related effects of interleukin-1 beta on polymorphonuclear neutrophil-dependent increases in blood-brain barrier permeability in rats. Brain. 1997;120:435–44.

205. Mollgard K, Saunders NR. The development of the human blood-brain and blood-CSF barriers. Neuropathol Appl Neurobiol. 1986;12(4):337–58.

206. Elhofy A, Wang J, Tani M, Fife BT, Kennedy KJ, Bennett J, et al. Transgenic expression of CCL2 in the central nervous system prevents experimental autoimmune encephalomyelitis. J Leukoc Biol. 2005;77(2):229–37.

207. Karpus WJ, Lukacs NW, McRae BL, Strieter RM, Kunkel SL, Miller SD. An important role for the chemokine macrophage inflammatory protein-1 alpha in the pathogenesis of the T cell-mediated autoimmune disease, experimental autoimmune encephalomyelitis. J Immunol. 1995;155(10):5003–10.

208. Luo Y, Fischer FR, Hancock WW, Dorf ME. Macrophage inflammatory protein-2 and KC induce chemokine production by mouse astrocytes. J Immunol. 2000;165(7):4015–23.

209. Levy O. Innate immunity of the newborn: basic mechanisms and clinical correlates. Nat Rev Immunol. 2007;7(5):379–90.

210. Berger RP, Ta'asan S, Rand A, Lokshin A, Kochanek P. Multiplex assessment of serum biomarker concentrations in well-appearing children with inflicted traumatic brain injury. Pediatr Res. 2009;65(1):97–102.

211. Buttram SDW, Wisniewski SR, Jackson EK, Adelson PD, Feldman K, Bayir H, et al. Multiplex assessment of cytokine and chemokine levels in cerebrospinal fluid following severe pediatric traumatic brain injury: effects of moderate hypothermia. J Neurotrauma. 2007;24(11):1707–17.

212. Whalen MJ, Carlos TM, Kochanek PM, Wisniewski SR, Bell MJ, Clark RS, et al. Interleukin-8 is increased in cerebrospinal fluid of children with severe head injury. Crit Care Med. 2000;28(4):929–34.

213. Perry VH, Hume DA, Gordon S. Immunohistochemical localization of macrophages and microglia in the adult and developing mouse brain. Neuroscience. 1985;15(2):313–26.

214. Lawson LJ, Perry VH. The unique characteristics of inflammatory responses in mouse brain are acquired during postnatal development. Eur J Neurosci. 1995;7(7):1584–95.

215. Oppenheim R. Neuronal cell death and some related regressive phenomena during neurogenesis: a selective historical review and progress report. Oxford: Oxford University Press; 1981.

216. Unkeless JC. Characterization of a monoclonal antibody directed against mouse macrophage and lymphocyte Fc receptors. J Exp Med. 1979;150(3):580–96.

217. Johnston MV, Trescher WH, Ishida A, Nakajima W. Neurobiology of hypoxic-ischemic injury in the developing brain. Pediatr Res. 2001;49(6):735–41.

218. Brooks-Kayal AR. Rearranging receptors. Epilepsia. 2005;46 Suppl 7:29–38.

219. Ben-Ari Y. Excitatory actions of gaba during development: the nature of the nurture. Nat Rev Neurosci. 2002;3(9):728–39.

220. Dzhala VI, Staley KJ. Excitatory actions of endogenously released GABA contribute to initiation of ictal epileptiform activity in the developing hippocampus. J Neurosci. 2003;23(5):1840–6.

221. Khazipov R, Khalilov I, Tyzio R, Morozova E, Ben-Ari Y, Holmes GL. Developmental changes in GABAergic actions and seizure susceptibility in the rat hippocampus. Eur J Neurosci. 2004;19(3):590–600.

222. Ruffolo G, Iyer A, Cifelli P, Roseti C, Muhlebner A, van Scheppingen J, et al. Functional aspects of early brain development are preserved in tuberous sclerosis complex (TSC) epileptogenic lesions. Neurobiol Dis. 2016;95:93–101.

223. Hernan AE, Holmes GL. Antiepileptic drug treatment strategies in neonatal epilepsy. Prog Brain Res. 2016;226:179–93.

224. Stamboulian-Platel S, Legendre A, Chabrol T, Platel J-C, Pernot F, Duveau V, et al. Activation of GABA(A) receptors controls mesiotemporal lobe epilepsy despite changes in chloride transporters expression: in vivo and in silico approach. Exp Neurol. 2016;284:11–28.

225. Erecinska M, Cherian S, Silver IA. Energy metabolism in mammalian brain during development. Prog Neurobiol. 2004;73(6):397–445.

226. Holmes GL. Effects of seizures on brain development: lessons from the laboratory. Pediatr Neurol. 2005;33(1):1–11.

227. Szot P, White SS, McCarthy EB, Turella A, Rejniak SX, Schwartzkroin PA. Behavioral and metabolic features of repetitive seizures in immature and mature rats. Epilepsy Res. 2001;46(3):191–203.

228. Liu Z, Stafstrom CE, Sarkisian M, Tandon P, Yang Y, Hori A, et al. Age-dependent effects of glutamate toxicity in the hippocampus. Brain Research. Dev Brain Res. 1996;97(2):178–84.

229. Galic MA, Riazi K, Heida JG, Mouihate A, Fournier NM, Spencer SJ, et al. Postnatal inflammation increases seizure susceptibility in adult rats. J Neurosci. 2008;28(27):6904–13.

230. Harre EM, Galic MA, Mouihate A, Noorbakhsh F, Pittman QJ. Neonatal inflammation produces selective behavioural deficits and alters N-methyl-D-aspartate receptor subunit mRNA in the adult rat brain. Eur J Neurosci. 2008;27(3):644–53.

231. Insel TR, Miller LP, Gelhard RE. The ontogeny of excitatory amino-acid receptors in rat forebrain.1. N-methyl-D-aspartate and quisqualate receptors. Neuroscience. 1990;35(1):31–43.

232. Flint AC, Maisch US, Weishaupt JH, Kriegstein AR, Monyer H. NR2A subunit expression shortens NMDA receptor synaptic currents in developing neocortex. J Neurosci. 1997;17(7):2469–76.

233. Monyer H, Burnashev N, Laurie DJ, Sakmann B, Seeburg PH. Developmental and regional expression in the rat brain and functional-properties of 4 NMDA receptors. Neuron. 1994;12(3):529–40.

234. Hestrin S. Developmental regulation of NMDA receptor-mediated synaptic currents at a central synapse. Nature. 1992;357(6380):686–9.

235. Pitkanen A, McIntosh TK. Animal. models of post-traumatic epilepsy. J Neurotrauma. 2006;23(2):241–61.

236. Golarai G, Greenwood AC, Feeney DM, Connor JA. Physiological and structural evidence for hippocampal involvement in persistent seizure susceptibility after traumatic brain injury. J Neurosci. 2001;21(21):8523–37.

237. Cernak I, Vink R, Zapple DN, Cruz MI, Ahmed F, Chang T, et al. The pathobiology of moderate diffuse traumatic brain injury as identified using a new experimental model of injury in rats. Neurobiol Dis. 2004;17(1):29–43.

238. Pitkanen A, Bolkvadze T, Immonen R. Anti-epileptogenesis in rodent post-traumatic epilepsy models. Neurosci Lett. 2011;497(3):163–71.

239. Hunt RF, Scheff SW, Smith BN. Posttraumatic epilepsy after controlled cortical impact injury in mice. Exp Neurol. 2009;215(2):243–52.

240. Annegers JF, Hauser WA, Coan SP, Rocca WA. A population-based study of seizures after traumatic brain injuries. N Engl J Med. 1998;338(1):20–4.

241. Bolkvadze T, Pitkanen A. Development of post-traumatic epilepsy after controlled cortical impact and lateral fluid-percussion-induced brain injury in the mouse. J Neurotrauma. 2012;29(5):789–812.

242. D'Ambrosio R, Eastman CL, Fattore C, Perucca E. Novel frontiers in epilepsy treatments: preventing epileptogenesis by targeting inflammation. Expert Rev Neurother. 2013;13(6):615–25.

243. Polderman KH. Mechanisms of action, physiological effects, and complications of hypothermia. Crit Care Med. 2009;37(7):S186–202.

244. Atkins CM, Truettner JS, Lotocki G, Sanchez-Molano J, Kang Y, Alonso OF, et al. Post-traumatic seizure susceptibility is attenuated by hypothermia therapy. Eur J Neurosci. 2010;32(11):1912–20.

245. D'Ambrosio R, Eastman CL, Darvas F, Fender JS, Verley DR, Farin FM, et al. Mild passive focal cooling prevents epileptic seizures after head injury in rats. Ann Neurol. 2013;73(2):199–209.

246. Beattie EC, Stellwagen D, Morishita W, Bresnahan JC, Ha BK, Von Zastrow M, et al. Control of synaptic strength by glial TNF alpha. Science. 2002;295(5563):2282–5.

247. Jiang JX, Yang MS, Quan Y, Gueorguieva P, Ganesh T, Dingledine R. Therapeutic window for cyclooxygenase-2 related anti-inflammatory therapy after status epilepticus. Neurobiol Dis. 2015;76:126–36.

248. Song Y, Pimentel C, Walters K, Boller L, Ghiasvand S, Liu J, et al. Neuroprotective levels of IGF-1 exacerbate epileptogenesis after brain injury. Sci Rep. 2016;6:32095.

249. Alyu F, Dikmen M. Inflammatory aspects of epileptogenesis: contribution of molecular inflammatory mechanisms. Acta Neuropsychiatr. 2016:3:1-16. doi: 10.1017/neu.2016.47.

250. Kaltschmidt B, Widera D, Kaltschmidt C. Signaling via NF-kappa B in the nervous system. Biochim Biophys Acta Mol Cell Res. 2005;1745(3):287–99.

3

Cannabinoid receptor type-2 stimulation, blockade, and deletion alter the vascular inflammatory responses to traumatic brain injury

Peter S Amenta[1], Jack I Jallo[1], Ronald F Tuma[3], D. Craig Hooper[2] and Melanie B Elliott[1*]

Abstract

Background: Immunomodulatory therapies have been identified as interventions for secondary injury after traumatic brain injury (TBI). The cannabinoid receptor type-2 (CB$_2$R) is proposed to play an important, endogenous role in regulating inflammation. The effects of CB$_2$R stimulation, blockade, and deletion on the neurovascular inflammatory responses to TBI were assessed.

Methods: Wild-type C57BL/6 or CB$_2$R knockout mice were randomly assigned to controlled cortical impact (CCI) injury or to craniotomy control groups. The effects of treatment with synthetic, selective CB$_2$R agonists (0-1966 and JWH-133), a selective CB$_2$R antagonist, or vehicle solution administered to CCI groups were assessed at 1-day after injury. Changes in TNF-α, intracellular adhesion molecule (ICAM-1), inducible nitric oxide synthase (iNOS), macrophage/microglial ionized calcium-binding adaptor molecule, and blood-brain-barrier (BBB) permeability were assessed using ELISA, quantitative RT-PCR, immunohistochemistry, and fluorometric analysis of sodium fluorescein uptake. CB$_2$R knockouts and wild-type mice with CCI injury were treated with a CB$_2$R agonist or vehicle treatment.

Results: TNF-α mRNA increased at 6 hours and 1 to 3 days after CCI; a CB$_2$R antagonist and genetic knockout of the CB$_2$R exacerbated TNF-α mRNA expression. Treatment with a CB$_2$R agonist attenuated TNF-α protein levels indicating post-transcriptional mechanisms. Intracellular adhesion molecule (ICAM-1) mRNA was increased at 6 hours, and at 1 to 2 days after CCI, reduced in mice treated with a CB$_2$R agonist, and increased in CB$_2$R knockout mice with CCI. Sodium fluorescein uptake was increased in CB$_2$R knockouts after CCI, with and without a CB$_2$R agonist. iNOS mRNA expression peaked early (6 hours) and remained increased from 1 to 3 days after injury. Treatment with a CB$_2$R agonist attenuated increases in iNOS mRNA expression, while genetic deletion of the CB$_2$R resulted in substantial increases in iNOS expression. Double label immunohistochemistry confirmed that iNOS was expressed by macrophage/microglia in the injured cortex.

Conclusion: Findings demonstrate that the endogenous cannabinoid system and CB$_2$R play an important role in regulating inflammation and neurovascular responses in the traumatically injured brain. CB$_2$R stimulation with two agonists (0-1966 and JWH-133) dampened post-traumatic inflammation, while blockade or deletion of the CB$_2$R worsened inflammation. Findings support previous evidence that modulating the CB$_2$R alters infiltrating macrophages and activated resident microglia. Further investigation into the role of the CB$_2$R on specific immune cell populations in the injured brain is warranted.

Keywords: Controlled cortical impact, Traumatic brain injury, Cannabinoid, Inflammation, Intracellular adhesion molecule

* Correspondence: Melanie.elliott@jefferson.edu
[1]Department of Neurological Surgery, Thomas Jefferson University Hospital, 1020 Locust Street, Thomas Jefferson University, Philadelphia, PA 19107, USA
Full list of author information is available at the end of the article

Introduction

Traumatic brain injury (TBI) affects over 1.4 million Americans annually, with many suffering fatal or permanently disabling injuries [1,2]. Blood-brain-barrier (BBB) disruption, a result of the post-traumatic inflammatory response, is a proposed mechanism of secondary injury and contributes to cell death or dysfunction, worsening neurologic function, and ultimately, to poorer clinical outcome [3,4]. It is also well-recognized, however, that this same inflammatory response plays an important role in the processes necessary for repair and recovery [5]. The initial traumatic insult induces the release of pro-inflammatory cytokines and chemokines triggering endothelial cell activation, chemoattractant signaling, and immune cell infiltration [6]. The release of TNF-α up-regulates the expression of intracellular adhesion molecule-1 (ICAM-1), which promotes the adherence of immune cells to the endothelium and subsequent transmigration to sites of inflammation [7]. The result of an inflammatory-driven barrier breakdown is an enhancement of a cytotoxic environment in the setting of already compromised neurons [8-10]. Infiltrating immune cells and resident microglia have been shown to demonstrate opposing pro- and anti-inflammatory phenotypes [11,12]. Pro-inflammatory cell phenotypes release cytokines and express enzymes such as inducible nitric oxide synthase (iNOS) that generate damaging free radicals and further disrupt BBB function. Anti-inflammatory phenotypes produce cytokines and growth factors that down-regulate free radical generating pathways, which can promote healing and regeneration. Optimal modulation of the post-traumatic inflammatory response will limit damage and promote reparative interactions between the immune and nervous systems.

A number of cellular targets have been identified as potential therapeutic interventions for the post-traumatic inflammatory response. The endocannabinoid system, as documented previously, represents a specialized group of endogenous neurotransmitters with a broad range of function [13]. In particular, the cannabinoid receptor type-2 (CB₂R), expressed predominantly by circulating immune cells and resident microglia, plays an important role in the immune response to injury. Upon stimulation with its ligand, the CB₂R possesses potent immunomodulatory and anti-inflammatory properties as reviewed by Cabral *et al.* [14-18]. In a series of studies, stimulation of the CB₂R has been shown to dampen post-TBI inflammation including infiltrating/resident immune cell activation and neurovascular disruption, all of which were accompanied by improved functional outcome following TBI and spinal cord injuries [19-23]. These findings are supported by other laboratories, showing treatment with a CB₂R agonist results in immunomodulation and neuroprotection in models of brain injury and neurodegeneration [18,24].

Acute immunomodulation through CB₂R ligands is associated with improvements in outcome in animal models of brain and spinal cord injury, Huntington's disease, and Parkinson's disease [18-20,22-25]. Emerging evidence points to the modulation of microglia and infiltrating macrophages as a key component in CB₂R-mediated improvements in functional outcome. Furthermore, these same immunomodulatory processes have also been implicated as important moderators underlying the histopathologic changes observed in cases of improved outcome following injury [18,19,22-24,26,27]. Microglial activation and inflammation in the traumatized brain can persist for years after TBI [28,29], and like macrophages, express pro-inflammatory (M1) and anti-inflammatory (M2) phenotypes [11,12,30]. A 'loss of function' in the M2 cell phenotype may underlie chronic inflammation such as occurs with traumatic brain injury [11]. Promoting the healing function of M2 immune cells through CB₂ receptor stimulation may inhibit the detrimental effects of long-term inflammation including synapse loss, neuronal degeneration, and cognitive function [11]. The present study further investigates the role of the CB₂R in regulating acute inflammatory vascular responses to TBI using CB₂ receptor stimulation, blockade and deletion. We also report the evidence linking CB₂R stimulation and alteration of the inflammatory cell phenotype.

Methods

Animal care and housing

Prior to initiating any research, the Thomas Jefferson University Institutional Animal Care and Use Committee (IACUC) reviewed and approved the research protocol and the use of male C57BL/6 mice. Animal care and use was monitored by the University Animal Care and Use Committee to assure compliance with the provisions of Federal Regulations and the NIH 'Guide for the Care and Use of Laboratory Animals'. All mice were housed in the Thomas Jefferson University Laboratory Animal Services Facility which is accredited by the American Association for the Accreditation of Laboratory Animal Care and complies with NIH standards.

Experimental design

Seventy-four (n = 74) adult male mice at approximately 8 weeks of age (weighing 22 to 24 g), including strains of C57BL/6 wild-type mice (Charles River, Wilmington, MA, USA) or CB₂R knockout B6.129P2-*Cnr2^{tm1Dgen}*/J mice (Taconic, Hudson, NY, USA) were randomly assigned to undergo controlled cortical impact injury (n = 66) or serve as craniotomy controls (control) (n = 8). There were three study arms to determine the effects of CB₂R modulation on genes and proteins expression for primary vascular inflammatory markers (TNF-α, ICAM, iNOS, and BBB permeability) which included: (1) CCI injury over time compared to craniotomy, (2) CB_2R agonists and CB_2R antagonist compared to vehicle-treated mice, and (3) CB_2R knockout (CB_2R KO) CCI groups with and without JWH-133 compared to wild-type CCI (Figure 1). Endpoints for CCI time course experiments were at either 6 hours (n = 4) or 1 (n = 10), 2 (n = 7), or 3 (n = 5) days after CCI injury. Two administrations of synthetic selective CB_2R agonists, 0-1966 (n = 8) or JWH-133 (n = 12), a selective CB_2R antagonist, SR144528 (n = 4), or vehicle solution (n = 10) were administered to wild-type CCI mice as described below. To determine the selectivity for the CB_2R, knockout mice lacking the CB_2R were treated with a CB_2R agonist JWH-133 (n = 3) and 0-1966 (n = 4) or vehicle (n = 9) and compared to wild-type CCI mice (n = 8). Controls underwent all surgical procedures including an equal time of isoflurane exposure, buprenorphine injection, incision and craniotomy but were not subjected to CCI injury, did not receive treatment or vehicle, and were euthanized at 3 days post-operatively. All surgeries and experimental *post-mortem* procedures were performed so that, within each cohort of mice, craniotomy or vehicle-treated control groups were run in parallel with their respective experimental groups to insure consistent environmental conditions. On an annual basis, there is a 6 to 8% mortality rate for our CCI injury model due to the formation of fatal hematomas or cerebrovascular blood clots. Controlled cortical impact injury (CCI) injury resulted in a loss of 6 of the original 66experimental CCI mice (9% mortality rate) equally distributed among groups, and final group sizes were reported for each experimental outcome (see figures).

Traumatic brain injury

Traumatic brain injury was induced using CCI injury, a highly reproducible non-penetrating brain injury model [31]. Mice were injured using methods previously described by our laboratory [19,23,32]. Anesthesia was induced with 3% isoflurane and maintained throughout the procedure at a dose of 2.5% isoflurane. Prior to the start of the procedure, all mice were injected with short-acting buprenorphine (0.01 cc subcutaneous) for acute post-operative pain control. A right-sided 4 mm craniotomy was performed at 1 mm posterior to bregma exposing the mouse somatosensory cortex. A rounded aluminum 3 mm diameter stereotaxic impactor tip (MyNeuroLab, St. Louis, MO, USA) was used to produce a cortical injury at a 1.0 mm depth, 3 m/s velocity, and 100 msec contact time. Following injury, the bone flap was sealed with permanent cyanoacrylate-based fast-acting adhesive closures and the skin was closed with 6.0 silk sutures. Post-operative care included warming with indirect heat from a heat lamp until ambulation resumed, and unlimited access to food and water. Brain and core body temperature were maintained at $37 \pm 0.5°C$ throughout the procedure and monitored with temporalis muscle and rectal temperature probes to avoid the neuroprotective effects of anesthesia-induced hypothermia.

Treatment administration

Stimulation of the CB_2 receptor was performed using agonists 0-1966 (Organix Inc., Woburn, MA, USA) or JWH-133 (Tocris Bioscience, Minneapolis, MN, USA). 0-1966 was used for the TNF and ICAM PCR experiments, while

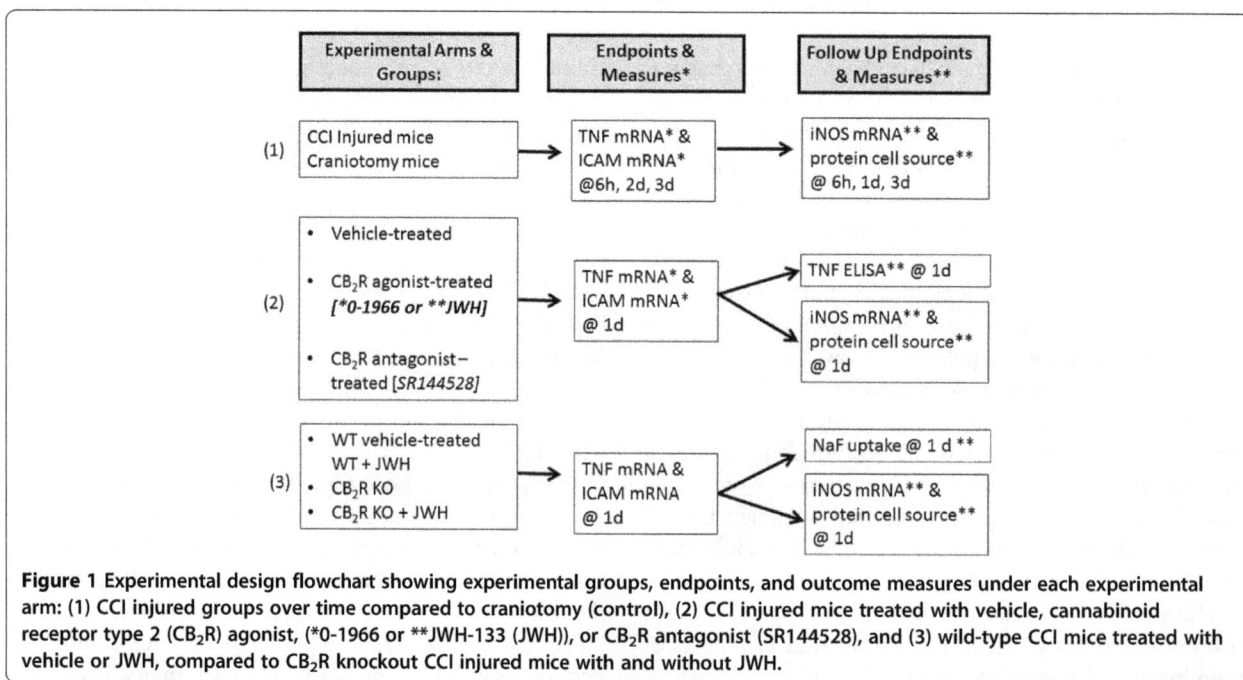

Figure 1 Experimental design flowchart showing experimental groups, endpoints, and outcome measures under each experimental arm: (1) CCI injured groups over time compared to craniotomy (control), (2) CCI injured mice treated with vehicle, cannabinoid receptor type 2 (CB_2R) agonist, (*0-1966 or **JWH-133 (JWH)), or CB_2R antagonist (SR144528), and (3) wild-type CCI mice treated with vehicle or JWH, compared to CB_2R knockout CCI injured mice with and without JWH.

JWH-133 was used in all other experiments (Figure 1). The CB$_2$R agonist was switched to JWH-133 in the later experiments in this study because it had the same selectivity profile for CB$_2$R as 0-1966 but with better solubility, was easier to administer, and was commercially available as a solution. 0-1966 was dissolved in a pure ethanol:emulphor:normal saline solution (1:1:18) resulting in a final concentration of 0.5 mg/mL. The CB$_2$R agonist, 0-1966, also known as 0-1966A, is an analog of bicyclic resorcinols (dimethoxy-resorcinol-dimethylheptyl) and structurally similar to cannabidiol as described by Wiley *et al.* [33]. 0-1966 demonstrates 225-fold higher selectivity for the CB$_2$R (Ki = 23 ± 2.1 nM) compared to CB$_1$R (Ki = 5,055 ± 984 nM) [33]. JWH-133 selective CB$_2$R agonist (Ki = 3.4 nM), in water-soluble emulsion Tocrisolve TM 100 (Tocris Catalog Number 1684) has appoximately 200-fold selectivity over CB1 receptors. The times for repeated intraperitoneal (ip) injections of 0-1966 (5 mg/kg) and JWH-133 (1 mg/kg) for the one-day endpoint were at either 2 or 18 hours post-CCI. The timing of treatment administrations were based on our previous studies [19]. Dosages were based both on preliminary dosing studies performed by our laboratory for our TBI model as well as on previous studies on models of stroke and spinal cord injury [19-22,34]. Vehicle solution was prepared in an identical manner to include 0.2 mL of pure ethanol: emulphor:normal saline solution (1:1:18) minus the cannabinoid and administered at the same time points as 0-1966. The selective CB$_2$R antagonist, SR144528, (Cayman Chemical, Ann Arbor, MI, USA) was dissolved in DMSO: emulphor:normal saline solution (1:1:18) and injected at 5 mg/kg at 2 and 18 hours post-CCI.

BBB assessment

Fluid-phase BBB permeability was assessed using sodium fluorescein (NaF) at 1 day post-CCI in wild-type, CB$_2$R KO mice with and without a CB$_2$R agonist (JWH-133) or controls as previously described by our laboratories [8]. NaF uptake assay was performed for 20 mice randomly divided into CCI subgroups euthanized at either 1 day (n = 236) or serving as controls (n = 4). CCI subgroups consisted of wild-type treated with vehicle or JWH-133, and CB$_2$R KO receiving vehicle or JWH-133. Brain samples were run in duplicate experiments. We selected NaF to evaluate changes in BBB permeability due to its low molecular weight (376 Da) compared to others probes that bind to albumin such as Evans Blue, horseradish peroxidase (HRP), or IgG (≥67,000 Da). Thus, NaF is a more sensitive probe that allows for detection of smaller leaks in the barrier. Mice were injected ip with 100 µL of 10% NaF in PBS and the NaF was allowed to circulate for 10 minutes. Following administration of a lethal dose of sodium pentobarbital, cardiac blood was collected followed by transcardial perfusion with 15 mL of heparin

(1,000 U/L) in PBS. Brains were sectioned into a left and right hemisphere and micro-dissected to separate the cerebral cortex, and processed immediately. To determine BBB permeability, tissues were weighed, homogenized in 1/10 dilution in PBS and centrifuged at 14,000 × g for 2 minutes. Five-hundred microliters of the clarified supernatant was transferred into 500 µL of 15% trichloroacetic acid and centrifuged at 10,000 × g for 10 minutes while the pellet was retained for RNA isolation. One hundred and twenty-five microliters of 5 N NaOH was added to 500 µL of the supernatant, and the amount of fluorescein for each sample was determined using standards ranging from 125 to 4,000 µg on a Cytofluor II fluorometer (PerSeptive Biosystems, Framingham, MA, USA). Serum levels of sodium fluorescein were assessed as previously described so that signals in CNS tissue samples could be normalized against the amount present in the circulation. NaF uptake into each brain region of interest is expressed as (ug/g NaF in cortex)/(µg NaF in serum).

RT-PCR

The pellet isolated during the BBB assessment outlined above was subsequently used for RNA isolation. Total RNA was extracted with the RNeasy Miniprep Kit (Qiagen, Valencia, CA, USA), reverse transcribed into cDNA with MMLV reverse transcriptase (Promega, Madison, WI, USA) and then measured by quantitative real-time PCR with gene-specific primers and probes [35]. IQ supermix and the iCycler iQ real-time detection system were also used for quantification (Bio-Rad Laboratories, Hercules, CA, USA). All samples were run in duplicate and compared to cDNA gene standards to determine copy numbers, which were normalized to the copy number of each sample's housekeeping gene L13. Levels of mRNA are reported as the fold change in gene expression of normalized to the endogenous reference gene L13 and relative to the untreated, craniotomy controls.

Immunohistochemistry

Mice were administered a lethal dose of sodium pentobarbital (120 mg/kg, ip) and underwent cardiac perfusion with heparinized saline followed by 4% paraformaldehyde. Brains were post-fixed in 4% paraformaldehyde for 24 hours, then transferred to 30% sucrose for storage. Frozen sections were cut coronally with a cryostat at −24°C (20 µm thick), and air dried overnight. Tissues were incubated in 10% NGS in O.3% Triton-100. Coronal brain sections were labeled using the following primary antibodies overnight at room temperature: (1) rabbit anti-mouse iNOS (1:200; Enzo Life Science, Farmingdale, NY, USA) and (2) rabbit anti-mouse ionized calcium-binding adaptor molecule-1 (Iba-1) (1:250; Wako Pure Chemical Industries, Richmond, VA, USA). Fluorescent secondary antibodies DyLight 488- or 549-conjugated AffiniPure

Goat anti-rabbit IgG (Jackson ImmunoResearch, West Grove, PA, USA) were applied for 2 hours at room temperature. Negative control staining was performed by omitting the primary antibodies.

Statistical analyses

All statistical analyses were performed using the GraphPad Prism 5 software program (La Jolla, CA, USA). To determine differences between CCI injury and controls at 6 hour, 2 day and 3 day time points, differences between wild-type and knockout mice, and and differences between vehicle-treated, agonist-treated, and antagonist-treated groups, statistical comparisons were performed using a one-way ANOVA followed by Bonferroni *post hoc* analysis for experimental groups compared to control. Significance levels were set at $P < 0.05$ for all statistical analyses and results are reported as the mean and SEM.

Results

TNF-α

The expression of mRNA specific for the pro-inflammatory cytokine TNF-α was significantly increased by comparison with controls at each time points examined after CCI in wild-type mice including 6 hours ($P < 0.05$), 1 day ($P < 0.001$), 2 and 3 days ($P < 0.001$) (Figure 2A and 2C).

Treatment with a CB$_2$R antagonist, SR144528, significantly increased TNF-α mRNA expression at 1 day post-CCI (ANOVA $P < 0.0001$, F = 23.00), but mRNA levels where not altered after administration of a CB$_2$R agonist, 0-1966 (Figure 2B). The increase in TNF-α mRNA mediated by the antagonist are paralleled by genetic deletion of the CB$_2$R at one day post-CCI compared to control ($P < 0.001$) and wild-type mice, $P < 0.01$ (Figure 2C). As shown in Figure 2D, the elevation in the levels of TNF-α protein at 1 day following CCI were reduced by CB$_2$R agonist treatment (Figure 2D).

ICAM

Increases in intracellular adhesion molecule-1 (ICAM-1) induced by increases in TNF-α were expected to occur in the first few days after injury when macrophage and microglial infiltration to the injured site peaks. ICAM mRNA was found to be significantly increased in the injured cortex at 6 hours, 1 and 2 days compared to controls ANOVA $P < 0.05$ (Figure 3A and 3C). ICAM mRNA expression returned to control levels by 3 days after injury. Administration of a 0-1966 significantly reduced ICAM-1 mRNA at one day post-CCI (ANOVA $P < 0.01$ and F = 9.53), while treatment with a CB$_2$R antagonist, SR144528, did not change mRNA levels (Figure 3B). CCI induction

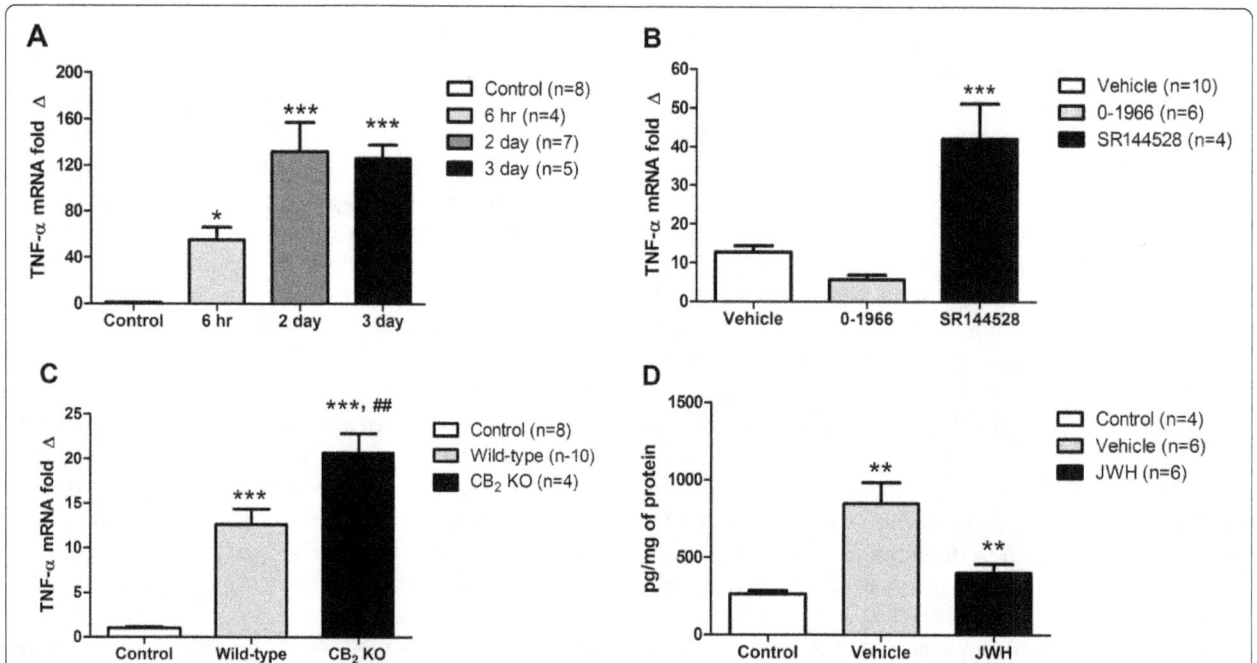

Figure 2 TNF-α mRNA in the injured cortex measured using quantitative real-time PCR (A-C) and TNF-α protein concentration using an enzyme-linked immunosorbent assay (D). (A) TNF-α mRNA at 6 hours, 2 and 3 days after CCI injury compared to craniotomy (control), *$P < 0.05$ and ***$P < 0.001$. **(B)** TNF-α mRNA at 1 day after CCI injury in wild-type mice treated with a vehicle solution (vehicle), cannabinoid receptor type-2 (CB$_2$) agonist (0-1966) or CB$_2$ receptor antagonist (SR144528) compared to vehicle control, ***$P < 0.001$. **(C)** TNF-α mRNA at 1 day after CCI injury in CB$_2$ knockout (CB$_2$ KO) and wild-type mice compared to control, ***$P < 0.001$, and ##$P < 0.01$ compared to wild-type mice. **(D)** TNF-α protein concentration at 1 day post-CCI in vehicle-treated and CB$_2$ agonist-treated (JWH-133) mice compared to control and vehicle, respectively, **$P < 0.01$.

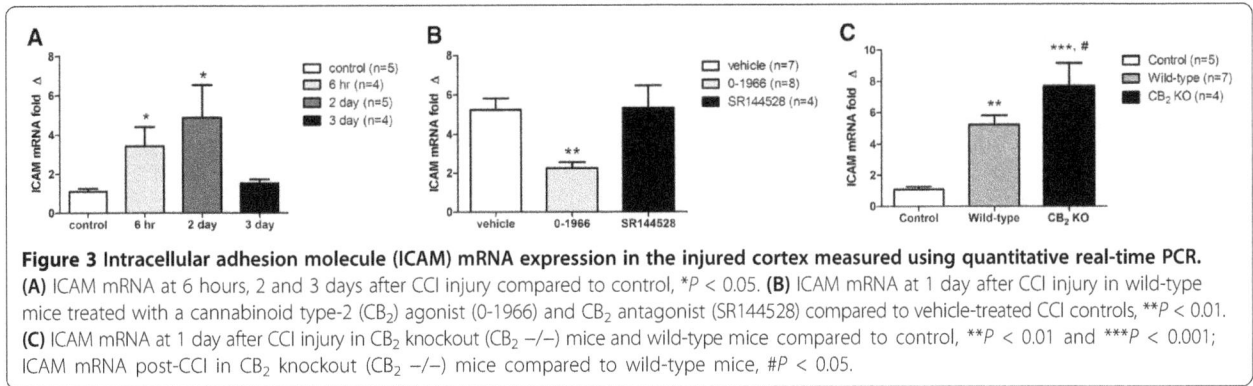

Figure 3 Intracellular adhesion molecule (ICAM) mRNA expression in the injured cortex measured using quantitative real-time PCR.
(A) ICAM mRNA at 6 hours, 2 and 3 days after CCI injury compared to control, $*P < 0.05$. (B) ICAM mRNA at 1 day after CCI injury in wild-type mice treated with a cannabinoid type-2 (CB$_2$) agonist (0-1966) and CB$_2$ antagonist (SR144528) compared to vehicle-treated CCI controls, $**P < 0.01$. (C) ICAM mRNA at 1 day after CCI injury in CB$_2$ knockout (CB$_2$ –/–) mice and wild-type mice compared to control, $**P < 0.01$ and $***P < 0.001$; ICAM mRNA post-CCI in CB$_2$ knockout (CB$_2$ –/–) mice compared to wild-type mice, $\#P < 0.05$.

in genetically modified mice lacking the CB$_2$R KO significantly increased ICAM-1 mRNA expression at 1 day post-CCI compared to wild-type mice with and without CCI (ANOVA $P < 0.001$ F = 16.63) (Figure 3C).

BBB permeability
BBB permeability was assessed by sodium fluorescein (NaF) uptake into the injured cortex (Figure 4). Treatment with JWH-133 reduced the injury-induced increase in NaF uptake, $P < 0.05$. NaF uptake was significantly increased in CCI injured CB$_2$R KO mice treated with the CB$_2$R agonist or vehicle ($P < 0.05$; $P < 0.01$) when compared to CCI-injured wild-type mice. The receptor selectivity of the agonist at the BBB was demonstrated as CB$_2$R KO mice treated with CB$_2$R agonist, JWH-133, were not different from CB$_2$R KO mice treated with vehicle control.

iNOS
iNOS mRNA was significantly increased in the injured cortex at 6 hours, 1 day, 2, and 3 days after injury ($P < 0.001$; F = 10.57) compared to controls (Figure 5A). Increased iNOS mRNA expression in vehicle-treated mice

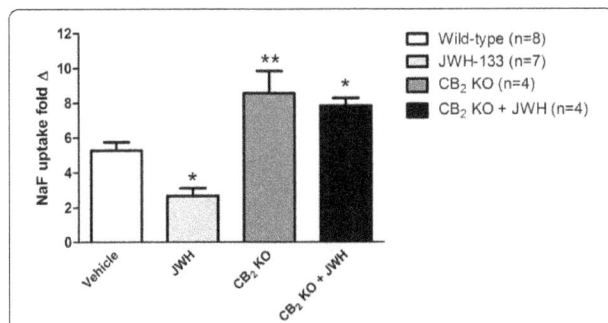

Figure 4 Blood-brain-barrier permeability assessment using sodium fluorescein (NaF) uptake in the injured cortex. NaF uptake for wild-type CCI injured mice treated with vehicle compared to JWH-133 (JWH), $*P < 0.05$ and cannabinoid type-2 knockout CCI mice (CB$_2$R KO) treated with vehicle or JWH, $**P < 0.01$ compared to wild-type vehicle-treated CCI mice (vehicle).

at 1 day post-CCI was attenuated by treatment with a CB$_2$R agonist (JWH-133) ANOVA $P < 0.001$ and F = 38.35 (Figure 5B). Interestingly, CCI injury in knockout mice lacking the CB$_2$R resulted in a considerable increase in iNOS mRNA levels (nearly 10-fold increase) in the injured cortex than in CCI injured wild-type mice (ANOVA $P < 0.0001$ and F = 20.67). Treatment with agonists JWH-133 and 0-1966 reduced the levels of iNOS in CB$_2$R KO mice indicating mechanisms other than the CB$_2$R are involved in the agonist's actions in the injured parenchyma.

Immunohistochemical double labeling for iNOS and a macrophage/microglial specific marker, ionized calcium-binding adaptor molecule (IBA-1) was used to qualitatively evaluate the cellular source of iNOS in the injured cortex (Figure 6). Cells within the cortical tissue surrounding the contusion that were positive for iNOS were co-labeled as macrophage/microglia cells. Some iNOS positive cells were also found distal to the injury in the cingulate cortex and subcortical areas; however, these cells did not co-localize with IBA-1 and showed a neuronal morphology (not shown).

Discussion
Previously, our laboratory found CB$_2$R stimulation reduced BBB permeability and decreased the number of macrophage/microglia in mice with controlled cortical injury [19,23]. We now show that early treatment with a CB$_2$R agonist reduces the post-traumatic increase in intracellular adhesion molecule (ICAM-1) mRNA expression after TBI. This effect is accompanied by reduced levels of TNF-α protein. Conversely, genetic deletion of the CB$_2$R increased the expression of ICAM-1 and TNF-α mRNA and exacerbated the BBB permeability that follows TBI. Pharmacological blockade of the CB$_2$R with an antagonist also increased the levels of TNF-α mRNA. CB$_2$R stimulation improved BBB integrity after TBI, likely secondary to an attenuation of endothelial cell, macrophage, and microglia activation [19,23]. The failure of the CB$_2$R agonist to impact these barrier responses in mice lacking the CB$_2$R

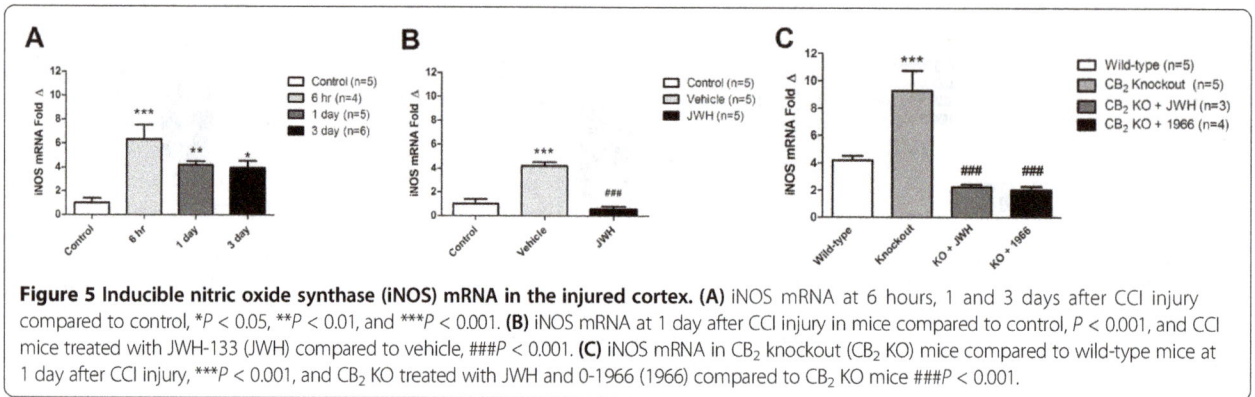

Figure 5 Inducible nitric oxide synthase (iNOS) mRNA in the injured cortex. (A) iNOS mRNA at 6 hours, 1 and 3 days after CCI injury compared to control, $*P < 0.05$, $**P < 0.01$, and $***P < 0.001$. **(B)** iNOS mRNA at 1 day after CCI injury in mice compared to control, $P < 0.001$, and CCI mice treated with JWH-133 (JWH) compared to vehicle, $###P < 0.001$. **(C)** iNOS mRNA in CB_2 knockout (CB_2 KO) mice compared to wild-type mice at 1 day after CCI injury, $***P < 0.001$, and CB_2 KO treated with JWH and 0-1966 (1966) compared to CB_2 KO mice $###P < 0.001$.

demonstrates that the mechanism of action, at least peripherally or at the blood-brain interface, is selective for the CB_2R. Interesting and not entirely surprising findings were that both CB_2R agonists in CB_2R KO mice showed similar effects in reducing iNOS mRNA after injury. This finding indicates the involvement of a non-CB_2 receptor, although due to the low affinity for the CB_1 receptor, activation of the CB_1 receptor is unlikely to be involved but cannot be completely ruled out. JWH-133 improved cerebral infarction but the effect was absent in CB_2R KO mice. [24]. Although there is some overlap between secondary injury mechanisms for stroke and traumatic brain injury, they are in fact distinguishable. CB_2R selective effects on cell infiltration and BBB permeability make a different contribution to the damaged brain in stroke compared to TBI. We conclude that the effects of the drug appear to have CB_2R selectivity peripherally and at the BBB interface; however, once penetrating the brain, there may be non-CB_1 and non- CB_2 receptors involved. Synthetic CB1/CB2 receptor ligands can interact with non-CB_1R, non-CB_2 G protein-coupled receptors, transmitter gated channels, ion channels and/or nuclear receptors and is reviewed by Pertwee et al. [36]. While the G protein-coupled receptor GPR55 and potassium channels have been excluded from the actions of JWH-133, others have not yet been elucidated. These findings provide additional support for the concept that the endogenous cannabinoid system facilitates

protection against secondary injury following TBI [37,38], and that the neuroprotective effects of CB_2R stimulation are due, in part, to the modulation of intracranial microvascular function leading to attenuated immune cell infiltration. Similar effects have been reported in studies of ischemic brain injury, whereby reductions in immune cell trafficking accompanied CB_2R agonist-induced decreases in ICAM-1 expression and BBB damage [20,21,34]. Moreover, following exposure to a variety of inflammatory stimuli, CB_2R stimulation increased endothelial cell tight junction protein expression in the brain microvasculature and reduced vascular permeability and the expression of ICAM-1 and VCAM-1 [39]. Finally, genetic knockout of the CB_2R has been shown to worsen inflammation, injury and behavioral deficits in several models of CNS diseases [18,20,25,39]. These findings indicate the importance of the CB_2R in regulating the immune and vascular response, as well as recovery following injury to the brain.

Early, rapid and robust production of pro-inflammatory cytokines, such as TNF-α after TBI, is responsible for the upregulation of ICAM-1 expression and subsequent immune cell infiltration to the injured brain [7,40]. TNF-α is a key cytokine that has been implicated in the induction of pathological inflammation in a variety of models including TBI. The finding that TNF-α expression following CCI is strongly elevated by administration of a CB_2 antagonist together with its increase in CB_2 knockout mice subject to

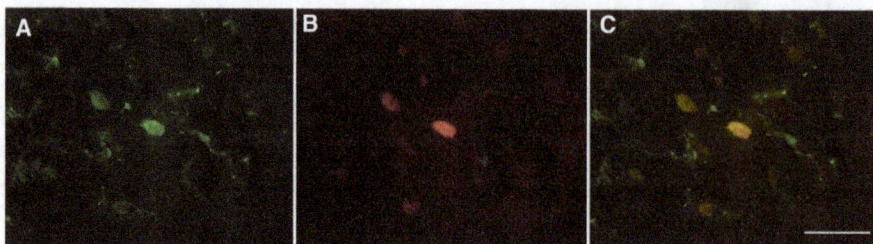

Figure 6 Macrophage/microglial marker, Iba-1, and inducible nitric oxide synthase (iNOS) immunofluorescence in the remaining cortical area adjacent to the contusion. Image shows **(A)** Iba-1 positive cells (green), **(B)** iNOS positive cells (red), and **(C)** merged image showing Iba-1 co-localized with iNOS positive cells with a retracted, amoeboid morphology (yellow).

CCI, confirms the importance of the CB_2 pathway in controlling TNF-α expression after TBI. The lack of changes in TNF message transcription with CB_2R stimulation in this study may be secondary to the post-CCI time point examined. Treatment with a CB_2R agonist reduced TNF-α mRNA at 15 hours after middle cerebral artery occlusion [24]. Fluctuations in TNF-α protein levels have been reported hours to days after CCI injury [41-43]. Cyclical changes in cytokine genes including TNF-α have also been shown after CCI injury in mice [6]. TNF-α mRNA fluctuates over time after injury, in which the levels, albeit increased compared to controls, were at the lowest level at the 1 day time point.

It is important to note that the TNF-α protein levels were reduced by CB_2R agonist treatment. This suggests additional post-transcriptional or post-translational mechanisms may be involved in attenuating the expression of TNF-α protein. Post-transcriptional modification of RNA ultimately determines expression levels by modulating mRNA stability, transport, and translation efficiency. Several key post-transcriptional regulatory elements include RNA-binding proteins, kinases and phosphatases, degradation enzymes, Au-Rich elements (AREs) and microRNA (miRNA). RNA-binding proteins can silence (or facilitate) the translation of TNF mRNA. For example, RNA-binding proteins, T-cell intracellular Ag (TIA-1) and TIA-1-related protein (TIAR), both silence TNF mRNA [44]; kinases and phosphatases change the binding efficiency of RNA-binding proteins and AREs sites. CNS injury alters the mitogen-activated protein kinase (MAPK) pathway enhancing mRNA stability and the efficacy of inflammatory cytokine generation. Interestingly, a CB_2R agonist was shown to reduce spinal MAPKs (p38 and p-ERK-1/2) through increased expression of mitogen-activated protein kinase phosphatases (MKP-1 and MKP-3) in primary microglial cells [45] and may explain the reduction in TNF-α protein expression in this study. Additionally, post-translational processes that interfere with the release of soluble TNF-α from its membrane-anchored pre-cursor or promote degradation of the protein may be involved.

Circulating leukocytes infiltrate the brain after cortical injury, reaching maximal accumulation 2 to 3 days after injury [19,23,46,47], which coincides with increases in barrier permeability [23]. ICAM-integrin interactions, in particular, are important for leukocyte adhesion and transendothelial migration to the injured brain. ICAM-1 (CD54) is a cell surface ligand that binds the integrins lymphocyte function-associated antigen-1 (LFA-1, CD11a/CD18) and macrophage adhesion molecule (Mac-1, CD 11b/CD 18) [7]. After TBI, increased expression of endothelial ICAM-1 helps to precisely guide the migration of leukocytes to the site of injury [43,48,49]. Increased expression of ICAM-1 is tightly coupled with changes in macrophage/microglia activation after CCI injury [49]. Past and present findings by our laboratory support the notion that stimulation of the CB_2R attenuates the inflammatory vascular response to injury. ICAM mRNA levels showed a peak at the 1-day time point that was influenced by the CB_2R deletion but not synthetic blockade. Results indicate a more pronounced effect on the immune-vascular injury response by genetically modifying the endogenous CB receptor system. The process of immune cell infiltration into the damaged parenchyma also enhances the permeability of the BBB. At the site of injury, microglia and accumulating immune cells release pro-inflammatory mediators and free radicals, both of which are known to disrupt the neurovascular unit, compromise the integrity of the BBB, and contribute to excitotoxicity and cell toxicity [8,50,51]. Disruption of the BBB is especially relevant to TBI as it is a proposed secondary injury mechanism creating a cytotoxic environment for neurons [52,53].

Stimulation of the CB_2R suppresses activation, chemotaxis, and migration of peripheral macrophages, monocytes, and T cells, as well as microglial-like cells [15,16,54-58]. These observations suggest that a number of cell types associated with CNS inflammation express the CB_2R. Insults to the CNS and pro-inflammatory conditions have been found to result in significant upregulation of CB_2R mRNA expression [13]. CB_2R mRNA expression is increased 10-fold by activation of microglia and peripheral macrophages in culture [59]. While there is general agreement that circulating immune cells and microglia express the CB_2R, a controversy exists over the expression of the CB_2R on other CNS cell types [14,59-62]. Evidently, this is due to differences in the antibodies used for immunohistochemistry between groups.

Distinctions in the role of infiltrating macrophages and resident microglia in brain injury continues to be a challenge as these cells are both of a monocyte lineage and express many of the same cell-surface markers. Adding to the complexity, is the growing evidence that macrophages and microglia are capable of expressing both pro-inflammatory (M1) and anti-inflammatory (M2) phenotypes [11,12,30]. In addition to pro-inflammatory cytokines and adhesion molecules, iNOS is another marker expressed by a M1 cell phenotype and is useful to study these phenotype differences and injury mechanisms. CB_2R stimulation significantly reduced iNOS mRNA, while genetic deletion substantially exacerbated iNOS expression. Moreover, qualitative analysis of the remaining cortical tissue surrounding the injury showed iNOS expression to be predominantly from a macrophage/microglia cellular source. In a model of TBI, results suggest that the protection offered by a microglial inhibitor, minocycline, may be through cannabinoid receptors as well [63]. Results suggest that selective modulation of the CB_2R transforms the inflammatory phenotype of the infiltrating and/or immune cells after injury.

Conclusion

Modification of the inflammatory vascular responses to TBI through CB$_2$R stimulation, as well as receptor blockade and deletion demonstrate the importance of this receptor in recovery from TBI. The CB$_2$R is an endogenous regulator of the inflammatory response to TBI, working at the interface between the brain and microvasculature. Macrophage/microglial modulation using CB$_2$R agonists has a significant contribution to its protective capabilities [18,24,25]. Interventions that limit prolonged microglial activation and neuroinflammation as occurs after TBI, or facilitate a reparative microglial phenotype are proposed to counteract the development of cognitive and affective disorders [30]. Our results further support that CB$_2$R-dependent pathways regulate the bridge between immune and vascular function following TBI. The development of pharmacological agents to treat TBI may rest in furthering our understanding of the complex immune, vascular, and nervous system interactions that are induced at the time of injury.

Abbreviations

TBI: traumatic brain injury; CCI: controlled cortical impact; CB$_2$R: cannabinoid receptor type-2; TNF-α: tumor necrosis factor-alpha; ICAM-1: intracellular adhesion molecule-1; iNOS: inducible nitric oxide synthase; BBB: blood-brain-barrier; KO: knockout; ELISA: enzyme-linked immunosorbent assay.

Competing interests

The authors declare that they have no competing interests.

Authors' contributions

Dr. MBE is the lead principal investigator and Dr. DCH is the collaborating investigator on this project. Dr. RFT gifted the 0-1966 and made substantial editorial contributions. Dr. JIJ provided translational expertise to the project and made significant editorial contributions. Dr. PSA, contributed surgical contributions, as well as provided substantial editorial input. All authors read and approved the final manuscript.

Acknowledgments

Research support by DOD Award W81XWH-12-1-0326 to Dr. Elliott. We would also like to thank Rhonda Kean (Dr. Hooper's laboratory) for help with RT-PCR and members from Dr. Elliott's laboratory including Brittany Diautolo, Ashley Tyburski, and Christine Macolino for making RT-PCR, immunohistochemistry, and surgical contributions.

Author details

[1]Department of Neurological Surgery, Thomas Jefferson University Hospital, 1020 Locust Street, Thomas Jefferson University, Philadelphia, PA 19107, USA. [2]Department of Cancer Biology, Thomas Jefferson University Hospital, 1020 Locust Street, Thomas Jefferson University, Philadelphia, PA 19107, USA. [3]Department of Physiology, Temple University School of Medicine, 3500 N Broad St, Philadelphia, PA 19140, USA.

References

1. Zaloshnja E, Miller T, Langlois JA, Selassie AW: Prevalence of long-term disability from traumatic brain injury in the civilian population of the United States, 2005. J Head Trauma Rehabil 2008, 23:394–400.
2. Langlois JA, Rutland-Brown W, Wald MM: The epidemiology and impact of traumatic brain injury: a brief overview. J Head Trauma Rehabil 2006, 21:375–378.
3. Erickson MA, Hartvigson PE, Morofuji Y, Owen JB, Butterfield DA, Banks WA: Lipopolysaccharide impairs amyloid beta efflux from brain: altered vascular sequestration, cerebrospinal fluid reabsorption, peripheral clearance and transporter function at the blood-brain barrier. J Neuroinflammation 2012, 9:150.
4. Tomkins O, Feintuch A, Benifla M, Cohen A, Friedman A, Shelef I: Blood-brain barrier breakdown following traumatic brain injury: a possible role in posttraumatic epilepsy. Cardiovasc Psychiatry Neurol 2011, 2011:765923.
5. Lenzlinger PM, Morganti-Kossmann MC, Laurer HL, McIntosh TK: The duality of the inflammatory response to traumatic brain injury. Mol Neurobiol 2001, 24:169–181.
6. Lagraoui M, Latoche JR, Cartwright NG, Sukumar G, Dalgard CL, Schaefer BC: Controlled cortical impact and craniotomy induce strikingly similar profiles of inflammatory gene expression, but with distinct kinetics. Front Neurol 2012, 3:155.
7. Dietrich JB: The adhesion molecule ICAM-1 and its regulation in relation with the blood-brain barrier. J Neuroimmunol 2002, 128:58–68.
8. Phares TW, Fabis MJ, Brimer CM, Kean RB, Hooper DC: A peroxynitrite-dependent pathway is responsible for blood-brain barrier permeability changes during a central nervous system inflammatory response: TNF-alpha is neither necessary nor sufficient. J Immunol 2007, 178:7334–7343.
9. Walker PA, Shah SK, Jimenez F, Gerber MH, Xue H, Cutrone R, Hamilton JA, Mays RW, Deans R, Pati S, Dash PK, Cox CS Jr: Intravenous multipotent adult progenitor cell therapy for traumatic brain injury: preserving the blood brain barrier via an interaction with splenocytes. Exp Neurol 2010, 225:341–352.
10. Hailer NP: Immunosuppression after traumatic or ischemic CNS damage: it is neuroprotective and illuminates the role of microglial cells. Prog Neurobiol 2008, 84:211–233.
11. Cherry JD, Olschowka JA, O'Banion MK: Neuroinflammation and M2 microglia: the good, the bad, and the inflamed. J Neuroinflammation 2014, 11:98.
12. Turtzo LC, Lescher J, Janes L, Dean DD, Budde MD, Frank JA: Macrophagic and microglial responses after focal traumatic brain injury in the female rat. J Neuroinflammation 2014, 11:82.
13. Cabral GA, Griffin-Thomas L: Emerging role of the cannabinoid receptor CB2 in immune regulation: therapeutic prospects for neuroinflammation. Expert Rev Mol Med 2009, 11:e3.
14. Cabral GA, Raborn ES, Griffin L, Dennis J, Marciano-Cabral F: CB2 receptors in the brain: role in central immune function. Br J Pharmacol 2008, 153:240–251.
15. Buckley NE, McCoy KL, Mezey E, Bonner T, Zimmer A, Felder CC, Glass M, Zimmer A: Immunomodulation by cannabinoids is absent in mice deficient for the cannabinoid CB(2) receptor. Eur J Pharmacol 2000, 396:141–149.
16. Fraga D, Raborn ES, Ferreira GA, Cabral GA: Cannabinoids inhibit migration of microglial-like cells to the HIV protein Tat. J Neuroimmune Pharmacol 2011, 6:566–577.
17. Munro S, Thomas KL, Abu-Shaar M: Molecular characterization of a peripheral receptor for cannabinoids. Nature 1993, 365:61–65.
18. Palazuelos J, Aguado T, Pazos MR, Julien B, Carrasco C, Resel E, Sagredo O, Benito C, Romero J, Azcoitia I, Fernández-Ruiz J, Guzmán M, Galve-Roperh I: Microglial CB2 cannabinoid receptors are neuroprotective in Huntington's disease excitotoxicity. Brain 2009, 132:3152–3164.
19. Elliott MB, Tuma RF, Amenta PS, Barbe MF, Jallo JI: Acute effects of a selective cannabinoid-2 receptor agonist on neuroinflammation in a model of traumatic brain injury. J Neurotrauma 2011, 28:973–981.
20. Zhang M, Adler MW, Abood ME, Ganea D, Jallo J, Tuma RF: CB2 receptor activation attenuates microcirculatory dysfunction during cerebral ischemic/reperfusion injury. Microvasc Res 2009, 78:86–94.
21. Zhang M, Martin BR, Adler MW, Razdan RK, Jallo JI, Tuma RF: Cannabinoid CB(2) receptor activation decreases cerebral infarction in a mouse focal ischemia/reperfusion model. J Cereb Blood Flow Metab 2007, 27:1387–1396.
22. Adhikary S, Li H, Heller J, Skarica M, Zhang M, Ganea D, Tuma RF: Modulation of inflammatory responses by a cannabinoid-2-selective agonist after spinal cord injury. J Neurotrauma 2011, 28:2417–2427.
23. Amenta PS, Jallo JI, Tuma RF, Elliott MB: A cannabinoid type 2 receptor agonist attenuates blood-brain barrier damage and neurodegeneration in a murine model of traumatic brain injury. J Neurosci Res 2012, 90:2293–22305.
24. Zarruk JG, Fernandez-Lopez D, Garcia-Yebenes I, Garcia-Gutierrez MS, Vivancos J, Nombela F, Torres M, Burguete MC, Manzanares J, Lizasoain I, Moro MA: Cannabinoid type 2 receptor activation downregulates stroke-induced classic and alternative brain macrophage/microglial activation concomitant to neuroprotection. Stroke 2012, 43:211–219.
25. Price DA, Martinez AA, Seillier A, Koek W, Acosta Y, Fernandez E, Strong R, Lutz B, Marsicano G, Roberts JL, Giuffrida A: WIN55,212-2, a cannabinoid

receptor agonist, protects against nigrostriatal cell loss in the 1-methyl-4-phenyl-1,2,3,6-tetrahydropyridine mouse model of Parkinson's disease. *Eur J Neurosci* 2009, **29**:2177–2186.

26. Cabral GA, Marciano-Cabral F: Cannabinoid receptors in microglia of the central nervous system: immune functional relevance. *J Leukoc Biol* 2005, **78**:1192–1197.

27. Romero-Sandoval EA, Horvath R, Landry RP, DeLeo JA: Cannabinoid receptor type 2 activation induces a microglial anti-inflammatory phenotype and reduces migration via MKP induction and ERK dephosphorylation. *Mol Pain* 2009, **5**:25.

28. Gentleman SM, Leclercq PD, Moyes L, Graham DI, Smith C, Griffin WS, Nicoll JA: Long-term intracerebral inflammatory response after traumatic brain injury. *Forensic Sci Int* 2004, **146**:97–104.

29. Loane DJ, Byrnes KR: Role of microglia in neurotrauma. *Neurotherapeutics* 2010, **7**:366–377.

30. Norden DM, Godbout JP: Review: microglia of the aged brain: primed to be activated and resistant to regulation. *Neuropathol Appl Neurobiol* 2013, **39**:19–34.

31. Lighthall JW: Controlled cortical impact: a new experimental brain injury model. *J Neurotrauma* 1988, **5**:1–15.

32. Elliott MB, Oshinsky ML, Amenta PS, Awe OO, Jallo JI: Nociceptive neuropeptide increases and periorbital allodynia in a model of traumatic brain injury. *Headache* 2012, **52**:966–984.

33. Wiley JL, Beletskaya ID, Ng EW, Dai Z, Crocker PJ, Mahadevan A, Razdan RK, Martin BR: Resorcinol derivatives: a novel template for the development of cannabinoid CB(1)/CB(2) and CB(2)-selective agonists. *J Pharmacol Exp Ther* 2002, **301**:679–689.

34. Zhang M, Martin BR, Adler MW, Razdan RJ, Kong W, Ganea D, Tuma RF: Modulation of cannabinoid receptor activation as a neuroprotective strategy for EAE and stroke. *J Neuroimmune Pharmacol* 2009, **4**:249–259.

35. Phares TW, Kean RB, Mikheeva T, Hooper DC: Regional differences in blood-brain barrier permeability changes and inflammation in the apathogenic clearance of virus from the central nervous system. *J Immunol* 2006, **176**:7666–7675.

36. Pertwee RG: Receptors and channels targeted by synthetic cannabinoid receptor agonists and antagonists. *Curr Med Chem* 2010, **17**:1360–1381.

37. Fishbein-Kaminietsky M, Gafni M, Sarne Y: Ultralow doses of cannabinoid drugs protect the mouse brain from inflammation-induced cognitive damage. *J Neurosci Res* 2014, **92**:1669–1677.

38. Ashton JC, Glass M: The cannabinoid CB2 receptor as a target for inflammation-dependent neurodegeneration. *Curr Neuropharmacol* 2007, **5**:73–80.

39. Ramirez SH, Hasko J, Skuba A, Fan S, Dykstra H, McCormick R, Reichenbach N, Krizbai I, Mahadevan A, Zhang M, Tuma R, Son YJ, Persidsky Y: Activation of cannabinoid receptor 2 attenuates leukocyte-endothelial cell interactions and blood-brain barrier dysfunction under inflammatory conditions. *J Neurosci* 2012, **32**:4004–4016.

40. Reglero-Real N, Marcos-Ramiro B, Millan J: Endothelial membrane reorganization during leukocyte extravasation. *Cell Mol Life Sci* 2012, **69**:3079–3099.

41. Harting MT, Jimenez F, Adams SD, Mercer DW, Cox CS Jr: Acute, regional inflammatory response after traumatic brain injury: implications for cellular therapy. *Surgery* 2008, **144**:803–813.

42. Shein S, Shellington DK, Exo J, Jackson TC, Wisniewski SR, Jackson E, Vagni VA, Bayir H, Clark R, Dixon CE, Janesko-Feldman KL, Kochanek PM: Hemorrhagic shock shifts the serum cytokine profile from pro-to anti-inflammatory after experimental traumatic brain injury in mice. *J Neurotrauma* 2014, **31**:1386–1395.

43. Li GZ, Zhang Y, Zhao JB, Wu GJ, Su XF, Hang CH: Expression of myeloid differentiation primary response protein 88 (Myd88) in the cerebral cortex after experimental traumatic brain injury in rats. *Brain Res* 2011, **1396**:96–104.

44. Giambelluca MS, Rollet-Labelle E, Bertheau-Mailhot G, Laflamme C, Pouliot M: Post-transcriptional regulation of tumor necrosis factor alpha biosynthesis: relevance to pathophysiology of rheumatoid arthritis. *OA Inflammation* 2013, **1**:3.

45. Landry RP, Martinez E, Deleo JA, Romero-Sandoval EA: Spinal cannabinoid receptor type 2 agonist reduces mechanical allodynia and induces mitogen-activated protein kinase phosphatases in a rat model of neuropathic pain. *J Pain* 2012, **13**:836–848.

46. Bayir H, Kagan VE, Borisenko GG, Tyurina YY, Janesko KL, Vagni VA, Billiar TR, Williams DL, Kochanek PM: Enhanced oxidative stress in iNOS-deficient mice after traumatic brain injury: support for a neuroprotective role of iNOS. *J Cereb Blood Flow Metab* 2005, **25**:673–684.

47. Foley LM, Hitchens TK, Ho C, Janesko-Feldman KL, Melick JA, Bayir H, Kochanek PM: Magnetic resonance imaging assessment of macrophage accumulation in mouse brain after experimental traumatic brain injury. *J Neurotrauma* 2009, **26**:1509–1519.

48. Hang CH, Shi JX, Li JS, Wu W, Yin HX: Concomitant upregulation of nuclear factor-kB activity, proinflammatory cytokines and ICAM-1 in the injured brain after cortical contusion trauma in a rat model. *Neurol India* 2005, **53**:312–317.

49. Khan M, Im YB, Shunmugavel A, Gilg AG, Dhindsa RK, Singh AK, Singh I: Administration of S-nitrosoglutathione after traumatic brain injury protects the neurovascular unit and reduces secondary injury in a rat model of controlled cortical impact. *J Neuroinflammation* 2009, **6**:32.

50. Fabis MJ, Phares TW, Kean RB, Koprowski H, Hooper DC: Blood-brain barrier changes and cell invasion differ between therapeutic immune clearance of neurotrophic virus and CNS autoimmunity. *Proc Natl Acad Sci U S A* 2008, **105**:15511–15516.

51. Nag S: Pathophysiology of blood-brain barrier breakdown. *Methods Mol Med* 2003, **89**:97–119.

52. Neuwelt EA, Bauer B, Fahlke C, Fricker G, Iadecola C, Janigro D, Leybaert L, Molnar Z, O'Donnell ME, Povlishock JT, Saunders NR, Sharp F, Stanimirovic D, Watts RJ, Drewes LR: Engaging neuroscience to advance translational research in brain barrier biology. *Nat Rev Neurosci* 2011, **12**:169–182.

53. Persidsky Y, Ramirez SH, Haorah J, Kanmogne GD: Blood-brain barrier: structural components and function under physiologic and pathologic conditions. *J Neuroimmune Pharmacol* 2006, **1**:223–236.

54. Sacerdote P, Massi P, Panerai AE, Parolaro D: *In vivo* and *in vitro* treatment with the synthetic cannabinoid CP55, 940 decreases the *in vitro* migration of macrophages in the rat: involvement of both CB1 and CB2 receptors. *J Neuroimmunol* 2000, **109**:155–163.

55. Walter L, Stella N: Cannabinoids and neuroinflammation. *Br J Pharmacol* 2004, **141**:775–785.

56. Montecucco F, Burger F, Mach F, Steffens S: CB2 cannabinoid receptor agonist JWH-015 modulates human monocyte migration through defined intracellular signaling pathways. *Am J Physiol Heart Circ Physiol* 2008, **294**:H1145–H1155.

57. Correa F, Mestre L, Docagne F, Guaza C: Activation of cannabinoid CB2 receptor negatively regulates IL-12p40 production in murine macrophages: role of IL-10 and ERK1/2 kinase signaling. *Br J Pharmacol* 2005, **145**:441–448.

58. Lombard C, Nagarkatti M, Nagarkatti P: CB2 cannabinoid receptor agonist, JWH-015, triggers apoptosis in immune cells: potential role for CB2-selective ligands as immunosuppressive agents. *Clin Immunol* 2007, **122**:259–270.

59. Maresz K, Carrier EJ, Ponomarev ED, Hillard CJ, Dittel BN: Modulation of the cannabinoid CB2 receptor in microglial cells in response to inflammatory stimuli. *J Neurochem* 2005, **95**:437–445.

60. Ashton JC: Knockout controls and the specificity of cannabinoid CB2 receptor antibodies. *Br J Pharmacol* 2011, **163**:1113.

61. Ashton JC: The use of knockout mice to test the specificity of antibodies for cannabinoid receptors. *Hippocampus* 2012, **22**:643–644.

62. Atwood BK, Mackie K: CB2: a cannabinoid receptor with an identity crisis. *Br J Pharmacol* 2010, **160**:467–479.

63. Lopez-Rodriguez AB, Siopi E, Finn DP, Marchand-Leroux C, Garcia-Segura LM, Jafarian-Tehrani M, Viveros MP: CB1 and CB2 cannabinoid receptor antagonists prevent minocycline-induced neuroprotection following traumatic brain injury in mice. *Cereb Cortex* 2013. doi:10.1093/cercor/bht202

4

Low serum ficolin-3 levels are associated with severity and poor outcome in traumatic brain injury

Jian-Wei Pan[1], Xiong-Wei Gao[2], Hao Jiang[1], Ya-Feng Li[2], Feng Xiao[1] and Ren-Ya Zhan[1*]

Abstract

Background: Ficolin-mediated activation of the lectin pathway of complement contributes to the complement-independent inflammatory processes of traumatic brain injury. Lower serum ficolin-3 levels have been demonstrated to be highly associated with unfavorable outcome after ischemic stroke. This prospective observatory study was designed to investigate the relationships between serum ficolin-3 levels and injury severity and clinical outcomes after severe traumatic brain injury.

Methods: Serum ficolin-3 levels of 128 patients and 128 healthy controls were measured by sandwich immunoassays. An unfavorable outcome was defined as Glasgow Outcome Scale score of 1–3. Study endpoints included mortality at 1 week and 6 months and unfavorable outcome at 6 months after head trauma. Injury severity was assessed by Glasgow Coma Scale score. Multivariate logistic models were structured to evaluate the relationships between serum ficolin-3 levels and study endpoints and injury severity.

Results: Compared with the healthy controls, serum ficolin-3 levels on admission were statistically decreased in patients with severe traumatic brain injury. Serum ficolin-3 levels were independently correlated with Glasgow Coma Scale scores. Ficolin-3 was also identified as an independent prognostic predictor for 1-week mortality, 6-month mortality, and 6-month unfavorable outcome. Under receiver operating characteristics curves, ficolin-3 has similar prognostic predictive values for all study endpoints compared with Glasgow Coma Scale scores.

Conclusions: It was proposed that lower serum ficolin-3 levels, correlated with injury severity, had the potential to be the useful, complementary tool to predict short- or long-term clinical outcomes after severe traumatic brain injury.

Keywords: Ficolin-3, Traumatic brain injury, Clinical outcome, Mortality

Background

Severe traumatic brain injury (STBI) is a serious public health problem [1–3]. Outcome prediction is relevant for both clinical practice and research of STBI [4–6]. Low Glasgow Coma Scale (GCS) scores are associated highly with poor clinical outcomes of STBI patients [7–9]. In recent years, the application of biomarkers identified in the peripheral blood has shown potential clinical utility in neurointensive care as diagnostic, prognostic, and monitoring adjuncts [10–12]. Identifying sensitive and reliable biomarkers associated with patient outcome may improve our understanding of structural brain damage or underlying cellular pathogenesis and regenerative mechanisms after brain trauma. This information can be used to guide future basic and clinical research, therefore improving patient care and outcomes [13, 14].

The complement system is an integral part of the innate immune system and inflammation [15–17]. Three distinct pathways constitute the complement system: the classical pathway, the alternative pathway, and the lectin pathway [18]. The C1 complex initiates the classical pathway upon recognition of immune complexes and dying host cells [19]. The alternative pathway is spontaneously activated by C3 hydrolysis, but it has also been reported that properdin,

---

* Correspondence: jwpfxjsryz@163.com
[1]Department of Neurosurgery, The First Affiliated Hospital, School of Medicine, Zhejiang University, 79 Qingchun Road, Hangzhou 310003, People's Republic of China
Full list of author information is available at the end of the article

a stabilizer of the alternative pathway convertase [20], is capable of initiating the complement cascade [21]. The ficolins and mannose-binding lectin (MBL) in association with MBL/ficolin-associated serine proteases (MASPs) are the initiator molecules of the lectin pathway. Three MASPs (−1, −2, and −3) have been described so far, and the current notion is that MASP-2 is the main lectin pathway activator. Upon recognition of pathogen-associated molecular patterns or altered self by MBL and the ficolins, the associated proteases cleave C4 and C2, hereby activating the complement cascade which ultimately leads to the formation of the terminal complement complex [22]. Various studies have revealed particularly novel findings on the wide-ranging involvement of complement in neural development, synapse elimination, and maturation of neural networks, as well as the progression of pathology in a range of acute and chronic neurodegenerative disorders [23–26].

A traumatic impact to the brain induces an intracranial inflammatory response, which consequently leads to the development of brain edema and delayed neuronal death [27–29]. Evidence from experimental, clinical, and in vitro studies highlights an important role for ficolin-mediated activation of the lectin pathway of complement in contributing to inflammation within the injured brain [30–32]. To date, three different ficolins (−1, −2, and −3) derived respectively from the genes FCN1, FCN2, and FCN3 have been described in humans [33]. Ficolin-3 was firstly identified as a serum glycoprotein that reacted with autoantibodies from patients with systemic lupus erythematosus [34]. Ficolin-3 is proved to be the predominant plasma molecule and the greatest complement-activating capacity among the lectin pathway initiators [35–40]. Thus, it may possess the strongest potential to be a prognostic or diagnostic biomarker. Recently, lower serum ficolin-3 levels have been demonstrated to be highly associated with the severity and unfavorable outcome after acute ischemic stroke [41]. Moreover, low levels of plasma ficolin-3 were related to severity, vasospasm, and cerebral ischemia of aneurysmal subarachnoid hemorrhage [42]. Hence, we further investigated the ability of ficolin-3 to predict short- and long-term clinical outcomes of STBI patients.

Methods

Study populations

This is a prospective observatory study conducted during the period of 3 years from July 2011 to July 2014 at the Sanmen People's Hospital, Zhejiang Province, China. This study included the patients with isolated head trauma and postresuscitation GCS score of 8 or less. Exclusion criteria were infectious diseases; fever within recent 1 month before head trauma; an elevated white blood cell count; positive chest X-ray, less than 18 years of age;

admission time >6 h; previous head trauma; neurological disease including ischemic or hemorrhagic stroke; use of antiplatelet or anticoagulant medication; and the presence of other prior systemic diseases including diabetes mellitus, hypertension, uremia, liver cirrhosis, malignancy, and chronic heart or lung disease.

Control subjects were recruited from volunteers who attended the Sanmen People's Hospital for healthy examination between July 2011 and July 2014. They showed normal blood and biochemical laboratory tests, namely differential blood count, hemoglobin level, total serum proteins, liver function tests, erythrocytes sedimentation rate, kidney function tests, and C-reactive proteins as well as were medically tested by a specialist and found free of any other medical illness.

The study was approved by the Human Investigations Committee at the Sanmen People's Hospital, and written informed consent was obtained from the healthy controls and the legal guardians of STBI patients. This study was registered in ClinicalTrials.gov (NCT02510573) on 22 July 2015 by Xiong-Wei Gao.

Assessment

Head trauma severity was assessed using initial postresuscitation GCS score. All computerized tomography (CT) scans were performed according to the neuroradiology department protocol. Investigators who read them were blinded to clinical information. Abnormal cisterns, midline shift >5 mm, and subarachnoid hemorrhage (SAH) were recorded on initial CT scan. CT classification was performed using Traumatic Coma Data Bank criteria on initial postresuscitation CT scan according to the method of Marshall et al. Participants were followed up until death or completion of 6 months after head trauma. Clinical outcome included 1-week mortality, 6-month mortality, and 6-month functional outcome. Using structure telephone interviews, follow-up was performed by one doctor who was blinded to clinical information.

Immunoassay methods

Venous blood was drawn from patients on admission and from healthy controls at study entry. Serum was frozen at −70 °C until assayed. Serum ficolin-3 concentration was determined by enzyme-linked immunosorbent assay (Hycult Biotech, the Netherlands). The intra-assay and inter-assay variations were 3.8 and 5.9 %, respectively. All determinations were run in duplicates. The persons carrying out the assays were completely blinded to the clinical information.

Statistical analysis

The results were reported as counts (percentage) for the categorical variables, mean ± standard deviation if normally distributed, and median (interquartile range) if not normally distributed for the continuous variables. Comparisons were made by using (1) chi-square test or Fisher's exact test for categorical data, (2) Student's t test for continuous normally distributed variables, and (3) the Mann–Whitney U test for continuous non-normally distributed variables. Correlations were analyzed by Spearman's correlation coefficient or Pearson's correlation coefficient and then followed by a multivariate linear regression.

The relations of ficolin-3 levels to clinical outcomes were assessed in a logistic-regression model with calculated odds ratio (OR) and 95 % confidence interval (CI). For multivariate analysis, we included the significantly different outcome predictors as assessed in univariate analysis. Under receiver operating characteristic (ROC) curve, the area under curve (AUC) was calculated to assess the predictive performance of ficolin-3 levels for clinical outcomes. A combined logistic-regression model was configured to estimate the additive benefit of ficolin-3 levels to GCS scores.

Statistical analysis was performed with SPSS 19.0 (SPSS Inc., Chicago, IL, USA) and MedCalc 9.6.4.0. (MedCalc Software, Mariakerke, Belgium). A P value of less than 0.05 was considered statistically significant.

Results
Study populations' characteristics
During the study period, 164 patients were admitted to our emergency department with an isolated severe head trauma diagnosis. Of these, 36 patients were excluded because of the following reasons. Five cases had neurological diseases; five cases had infectious diseases; two cases, fever within recent 1 month; four cases, elevated white blood cell count; four cases, admission >6 h; four cases, the presence of other systemic diseases; two cases, previous head trauma; three cases, positive chest X-ray; two cases, less than 18 years of age; two cases, missing of follow-up; and four cases, use of antiplatelet or anticoagulant medication. Finally, 128 patients were included in the analysis.

This group of patients, consisting of 80 men and 48 women, had a mean age of 42.5 ± 15.6 years. Median initial postresuscitation GCS scores were 5 (3). Sixty-two patients (48.4 %) had unreactive pupils on admission; 58 patients (45.3 %), CT classification 5 or 6; 60 patients (46.9 %), abnormal cisterns on initial CT scan; 65 patients (50.8 %), midline shift >5 mm on initial CT scan; 70 patients (54.7 %), the presence of traumatic subarachnoid hemorrhage on initial CT scan; and 58 patients (45.3 %), intracranial surgery in the first 24 h. The mean admission time was 2.5 ± 1.3 h; the mean plasma-sampling time, 3.8 ± 1.6 h; the mean systolic arterial pressure, 129.9 ± 27.5 mmHg; the mean diastolic arterial pressure, 77.5 ± 17.9 mmHg; the mean value of mean arterial pressure

96.5 ± 18.4 mmHg; the mean plasma C-reactive protein levels, 7.9 ± 3.2 mg/L; and the mean blood glucose levels, 11.1 ± 3.9 mmol/L.

Control group, consisting of 128 healthy individuals, included 83 men and 45 women and had a mean age of 42.2 ± 16.4 years. Differences in gender and age were not shown to be statistically significant between control group and patients.

Change of serum ficolin-3 levels
Just as shown in Fig. 1, the admission serum ficolin-3 levels were significantly lower in all patients than in healthy controls, in patients dying than in patients alive within 1 week, in patients dying than in patients alive within 6 months, and in patients with unfavorable outcome than in patients with favorable outcome within 6 months.

Correlation analysis
Just as shown in Table 1, serum ficolin-3 levels were highly associated with initial postresuscitation GCS scores, pupils unreactive on admission, CT classification 5 or 6, abnormal cisterns on initial CT scan, midline shift >5 mm on initial CT scan, the presence of traumatic SAH on initial CT scan, intracranial surgery in the first 24-h blood glucose level, and plasma C-reactive protein levels. A multivariate linear regression demonstrated that serum ficolin-3 levels were still highly associated with GCS scores ($t = 4.994$, $P < 0.001$) and plasma C-reactive protein levels ($t = -3.005$, $P = 0.003$) in Fig. 2.

Prediction of 1-week mortality
In Table 2, serum ficolin-3 levels and other variables were highly associated with 1-week mortality of patients with STBI. A multivariate analysis demonstrated that GCS scores (OR 0.298, 95 % CI 0.138–0.646, $P < 0.001$) and serum ficolin-3 levels (OR 0.821, 95 % CI 0.704–0.958, $P < 0.001$) were the independent predictors for 1-week mortality of patients.

Serum ficolin-3 levels statistically significantly predicted 1-week mortality of patients under ROC curve and a cut-off value of <13.3 µg/mL predicted the prognosis with sensitivity of 85.0 % and specificity of 76.9 %. Table 3 shows that the AUC of the serum ficolin-3 levels was similar to that of GCS scores for prediction of 1-week mortality of the patients. In a combined logistic-regression model, serum ficolin-3 levels improved the AUC of GCS scores, but the difference was not statistically significant.

Prediction of 6-month mortality
In Table 2, serum ficolin-3 levels and other variables were highly associated with 6-month mortality of patients with STBI. A multivariate analysis demonstrated that GCS scores (OR 0.408, 95 % CI 0.271–0.613, $P < 0.001$) and serum ficolin-3 levels (OR 0.847, 95 % CI 0.756–0.950,

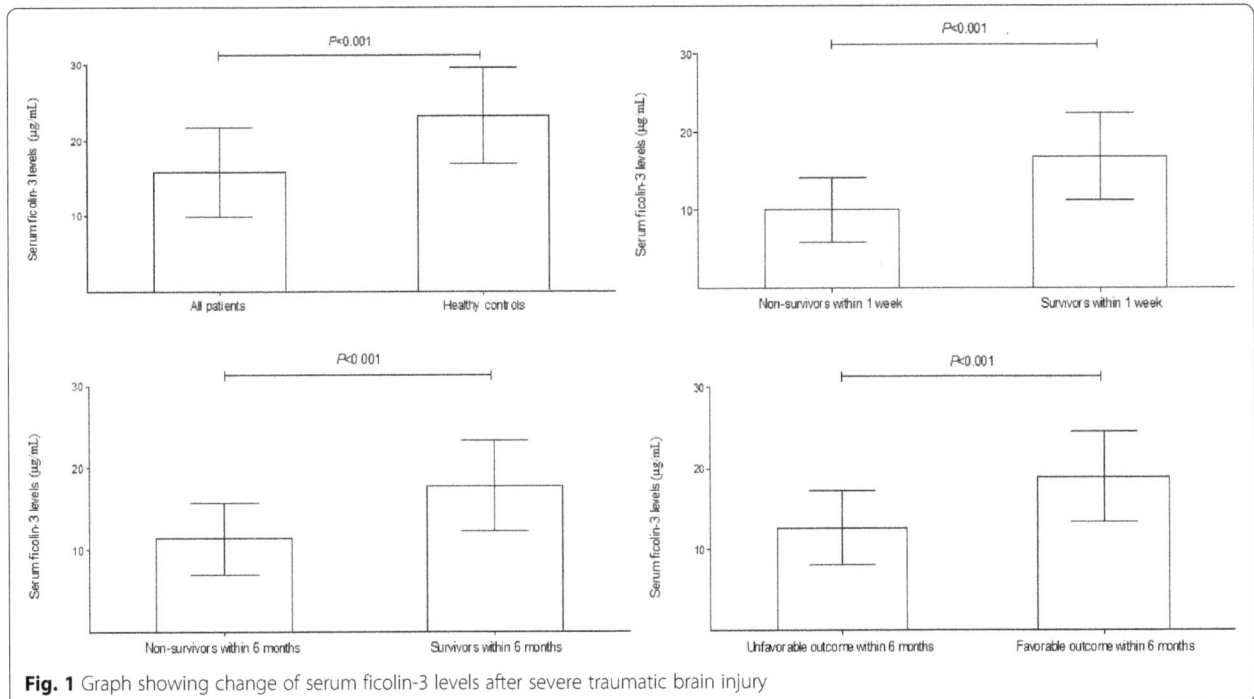

Fig. 1 Graph showing change of serum ficolin-3 levels after severe traumatic brain injury

$P < 0.001$) were the independent predictors for 6-month mortality of patients.

Serum ficolin-3 levels statistically significantly predicted 6-month mortality of patients under ROC curve, and a cutoff value of <13.4 µg/mL predicted the prognosis with

Table 1 The factors correlated with serum ficolin-3 levels in patients with severe traumatic brain injury

Characteristics	r value	P value
Sex (male/female)	0.092	0.303
Age (years)	0.046	0.606
Initial postresuscitation GCS score	0.521	<0.001
Pupils unreactive on admission	−0.414	<0.001
CT classification 5 or 6	−0.189	0.033
Abnormal cisterns on initial CT scan	−0.300	0.001
Midline shift >5 mm on initial CT scan	−0.323	<0.001
Presence of traumatic SAH on initial CT scan	−0.303	0.001
Intracranial surgery in the first 24 h	−0.245	0.005
Admission time (h)	0.090	0.310
Plasma-sampling time (h)	0.067	0.450
Systolic arterial pressure (mmHg)	0.127	0.152
Diastolic arterial pressure (mmHg)	0.120	0.179
Mean arterial pressure (mmHg)	0.132	0.137
Plasma C-reactive protein levels (mg/L)	−0.430	<0.001
Blood glucose levels (mmol/L)	−0.285	<0.001

Bivariate correlations were assessed by Spearman's or Pearson's correlation coefficient
GCS Glasgow Coma Scale, CT computerized tomography, SAH subarachnoid hemorrhage

sensitivity of 70.0 % and specificity of 83.0 %. Table 3 shows that the AUC of the serum ficolin-3 levels was similar to that of GCS scores for prediction of 6-month mortality of the patients. In a combined logistic-regression model, serum ficolin-3 levels improved the AUC of GCS scores, but the difference was not statistically significant.

Prediction of 6-month unfavorable outcome

In Table 2, serum ficolin-3 levels and other variables were highly associated with 6-month unfavorable outcome of patients with STBI. A multivariate analysis demonstrated that GCS scores (OR 0.460, 95 % CI 0.336–0.632, $P < 0.001$) and serum ficolin-3 levels (OR 0.845, 95 % CI 0.758–0.942, $P < 0.001$) were the independent predictors for 6-month unfavorable outcome of patients.

Serum ficolin-3 levels statistically significantly predicted 6-month unfavorable outcome of patients under ROC curve, and a cutoff value of <18.0 µg/mL predicted the prognosis with sensitivity of 89.1 % and specificity of 60.9 %. Table 3 shows that the AUC of the serum ficolin-3 levels was similar to that of GCS scores for prediction of 6-month unfavorable outcome of the patients. In a combined logistic-regression model, serum ficolin-3 levels improved the AUC of GCS scores, but the difference was not statistically significant.

Discussion

To our best knowledge, the current study, for the first time, investigated the serum ficolin-3 levels after STBI. Its main findings were that STBI patients had decreased

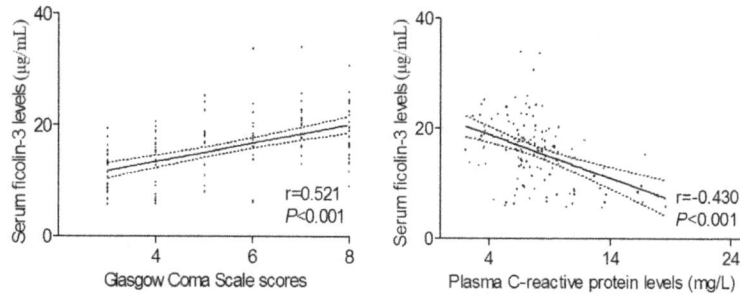

Fig. 2 Graph showing the relationships between serum ficolin-3 levels and Glasgow Coma Scale scores as well as between serum ficolin-3 levels and plasma C-reactive protein levels after severe traumatic brain injury

serum ficolin-3 levels compared with healthy controls; serum ficolin-3 levels were independently associated with GCS scores and plasma C-reactive protein levels; and ficolin-3 was identified as an independent prognostic predictor and had high predictive value.

In agreement with previous reported data regarding acute ischemic stroke and aneurysmal subarachnoid hemorrhage [41, 42], the decreased serum ficolin-3 levels were found within 6 h after STBI in the current study. In ischemic stroke, the decreased serum concentration of

Table 2 The factors associated with poor clinical outcomes in patients with severe traumatic brain injury

Characteristics	1-week mortality prediction			6-month mortality prediction			6-month functional outcome prediction		
	Non-survivors ($n = 20$)	Survivors ($n = 108$)	P value	Non-survivors ($n = 40$)	Survivors ($n = 88$)	P value	Unfavorable outcome ($n = 64$)	Favorable outcome ($n = 64$)	P value
Sex (male/female)	13/7	67/41	0.801	27/13	53/35	0.431	44/20	36/28	0.144
Age (years)	45.0 ± 14.5	42.1 ± 15.8	0.440	43.8 ± 15.5	41.9 ± 15.7	0.522	44.6 ± 16.0	40.4 ± 15.1	0.132
Initial postresuscitation GCS score	3 (1)	6 (4)	<0.001	3 (1)	6 (3)	<0.001	4 (2)	7 (3)	<0.001
Pupils unreactive on admission	18 (90.0 %)	44(40.7 %)	<0.001	32 (80.0 %)	30 (34.1 %)	<0.001	43 (80.0 %)	19 (34.1 %)	<0.001
CT classification 5 or 6	15 (75.0 %)	43 (39.8 %)	0.004	25 (62.5 %)	33 (37.5 %)	0.008	36 (56.3 %)	22 (34.4 %)	0.013
Abnormal cisterns on initial CT scan	18 (90.0 %)	42(38.9 %)	<0.001	29 (72.5 %)	31(35.2 %)	<0.001	40 (62.5 %)	20(31.3 %)	<0.001
Midline shift >5 mm on initial CT scan	17 (85.0 %)	48 (44.4 %)	0.001	30 (75.0 %)	35(39.8 %)	<0.001	42 (65.6 %)	23(35.9 %)	0.001
Presence of traumatic SAH on initial CT scan	16 (80.0 %)	54(50.0 %)	0.013	29 (72.5 %)	41(46.6 %)	0.006	41 (64.1 %)	29 (45.3 %)	0.033
Intracranial surgery in the first 24 h	12 (60.0 %)	46 (42.6 %)	0.151	21 (52.2 %)	37 (42.1 %)	0.271	31 (48.4 %)	27(42.2 %)	0.478
Admission time (h)	2.3 ± 0.9	2.5 ± 1.3	0.446	2.3 ± 0.9	2.5 ± 1.4	0.384	2.3 ± 1.1	2.6 ± 1.4	0.125
Plasma-sampling time (h)	4.2 ± 1.2	3.7 ± 1.6	0.183	3.7 ± 1.2	3.8 ± 1.7	0.627	3.6 ± 1.5	3.9 ± 1.6	0.220
Systolic arterial pressure (mmHg)	139.1 ± 22.6	128.2 ± 28.0	0.105	126.7 ± 30.7	131.4 ± 25.9	0.370	126.4 ± 31.2	133.5 ± 22.9	0.146
Diastolic arterial pressure (mmHg)	81.7 ± 12.6	76.7 ± 18.7	0.255	77.6 ± 16.5	77.4 ± 18.6	0.942	75.5 ± 20.0	79.4 ± 15.5	0.219
Mean arterial pressure (mmHg)	102.7 ± 15.1	95.4 ± 18.8	0.100	99.0 ± 16.5	95.4 ± 19.2	0.311	95.6 ± 20.4	97.4 ± 16.3	0.572
Plasma C-reactive protein level (mg/L)	11.1 ± 2.3	7.3 ± 3.1	<0.001	10.3 ± 4.1	6.8 ± 2.0	<0.001	9.3 ± 3.7	6.5 ± 1.9	<0.001
Blood glucose level (mmol/L)	12.7 ± 4.0	9.6 ± 3.1	0.002	13.6 ± 4.1	10.0 ± 3.3	<0.001	12.7 ± 4.0	9.6 ± 3.1	<0.001
Serum ficolin-3 levels (µg/mL)	10.1 ± 4.1	16.9 ± 5.6	<0.001	11.4 ± 4.4	17.8 ± 5.5	<0.001	12.7 ± 4.5	19.0 ± 5.5	<0.001

Numerical variables were presented as mean ± standard deviation or median (interquartile range) and analyzed by unpaired Student's t test or Mann–Whitney U test. Categorical variables were expressed as counts (percentage) and analyzed by chi-square test or Fisher's exact test

GCS Glasgow Coma Scale, *CT* computerized tomography, *SAH* subarachnoid hemorrhage

Table 3 Analysis and comparison of area under receiver operating characteristic curve

Variables	1-week mortality prediction		6-month mortality prediction		6-month functional outcome prediction	
	AUC (95 % CI)	P value	AUC (95 % CI)	P value	AUC (95 % CI)	P value
GCS scores	0.883 (0.814–0.933)	Ref.	0.875 (0.805–0.927)	Ref.	0.872 (0.802–0.925)	Ref.
Ficolin-3 levels	0.836 (0.760–0.896)	0.305	0.818 (0.740–0.881)	0.186	0.815 (0.736–0.878)	0.196
GCS scores + ficolin-3 levels	0.915 (0.853–0.957)	0.294	0.904 (0.839–0.949)	0.232	0.900 (0.835–0.946)	0.207

A combined logistic-regression model was configured to estimate the additive benefit of ficolin-3 to GCS score. Comparisons of AUCs were performed using z test. GCS score + ficolin-3 level indicates the combined use of GCS score and ficolin-3 level to predict prognosis
AUC area under curve, CI confidence interval, GCS Glasgow Coma Scale, Ref. reference

ficolin-3 could be observed in the very early phase and remained unchanged during the next 3–4 days [41]. Since ficolin-3 has been shown to be involved in the sequestration of dying host cells [43], it seems reasonable to surmise that this decrease of serum ficolin-3 levels should be due to consumption through the binding of the molecules to the apoptotic and necrotic cells [44], indicating that the decreased levels in sera during the acute phase of head trauma could be related to the acute traumatic event.

In ischemic stroke, serum ficolin-3 levels are inversely correlated with the severity of stroke indicated by the National Institute of Health stroke scale on admission and the concentrations of S100b, an indicator of the size of cerebral infarct [41]. In aneurysmal subarachnoid hemorrhage, low levels of plasma ficolin-3 are related to hemorrhagic severity assessed using the World Federation of Neurosurgical Societies grading scale, vasospasm defined as neuro-worsening with angiographic confirmation of vessel narrowing and cerebral ischemia defined as hypodense lesion on CT scan performed before discharge [42]. This study demonstrated that the decreased serum ficolin-3 levels were highly associated with trauma severity reflected by GCS scores. Hence, the selective ability for complement activation after the binding of ficolin-3 to dying cells might be responsible for the selective clinical correlation with the levels of this protein [45], indicating serum fiction-3 levels could reflect the severity of brain injury.

The complement activation has been confirmed as a crucial inflammatory component in a lot of diseases [36, 37]. An increasing number of clinical researches have addressed the potential role of ficolin-3 in various inflammatory status and diseases like diabetic peripheral neuropathy [46], diabetic microvascular complication [47], and pre-eclampsia [48]. The current study found that serum ficolin-3 levels were associated negatively with systemic inflammatory severity indicated by plasma C-reactive protein levels. The decrease in ficolin-3 level has been confirmed to be accompanied with increased complement activation [49]. Thus, the increased consumption of ficolin-3 might exacerbate complement activation, leading to the inflammation and tissue damage after head trauma.

Lower serum ficolin-3 levels have been demonstrated to be highly associated with the severity and unfavorable outcome after acute ischemic stroke and aneurysmal subarachnoid hemorrhage [41, 42]. In this study, ficolin-3 was identified as an independent predictor for long-term and short-term clinical outcomes including 1-week mortality, 6-month mortality, and 6-month unfavorable outcome. We further used the ROC curves to verify the prognostic predictive values of serum ficolin-3 levels. Although ficolin-3 did not improve the AUC of GCS scores under ROC curve, ficolin-3 had similar predictive performance to the GCS scores. Thus, it is more convincing that ficolin-3 may be a good prognostic predictor after STBI.

Conclusions

In this study, serum ficolin-3 levels are correlated with head trauma severity and systemic inflammatory severity, as well as independently predict short-term and long-term clinical outcomes of severe TBI. Therefore, it is suggested that serum ficolin-3 may have the potential to be a good prognostic predictive biomarker after head trauma.

Abbreviations
AUC: area under curve; CI: confidence interval; CT: computerized tomography; GCS: Glasgow Coma Scale; MASP: MBL/ficolin-associated serine proteases; MBL: mannose-binding lectin; OR: odds ratio; ROC: receiver operating characteristic; SAH: subarachnoid hemorrhage; STBI: severe traumatic brain injury.

Competing interests
The authors declare that they have no competing interests.

Authors' contributions
JWP, XWG, and RYZ were involved in the design of the study, carried out the experiments, and participated in the data analysis and manuscript preparation. HJ, YFL, and FX contributed to the data analysis and interpretation of the results. All authors read and approved the final manuscript.

Acknowledgements
The authors thank all staffs in the Department of Neurosurgery of the Sanmen People's Hospital (Sanmen, China) for their technical support. This project is supported by the National Natural Science Foundation (grant no. 81200954).

Author details
[1]Department of Neurosurgery, The First Affiliated Hospital, School of Medicine, Zhejiang University, 79 Qingchun Road, Hangzhou 310003,

People's Republic of China. [2]Department of Neurosurgery, Sanmen People's Hospital, 171 Renmin Road, Sanmen 317100, People's Republic of China.

References

1. Baguley IJ, Nott MT, Howle AA, Simpson GK, Browne S, King AC, et al. Late mortality after severe traumatic brain injury in New South Wales: a multicentre study. Med J Aust. 2012;22:40–5.
2. Frattalone AR, Ling GS. Moderate and severe traumatic brain injury: pathophysiology and management. Neurosurg Clin N Am. 2013;24:309–19.
3. Zammit C, Knight WA. Severe traumatic brain injury in adults. Emerg Med Pract. 2013;15:1–28.
4. Bosarge PL, Shoultz TH, Griffin RL, Kerby JD. Stress-induced hyperglycemia is associated with higher mortality in severe traumatic brain injury. J Trauma Acute Care Surg. 2015;79:289–94.
5. Daoud H, Alharfi I, Alhelali I, Charyk Stewart T, Qasem H, Fraser DD. Brain injury biomarkers as outcome predictors in pediatric severe traumatic brain injury. Neurocrit Care. 2014;20:427–35.
6. Zhang ZY, Zhang LX, Dong XQ, Yu WH, Du Q, Yang DB, et al. Comparison of the performances of copeptin and multiple biomarkers in long-term prognosis of severe traumatic brain injury. Peptides. 2014;60:13–7.
7. Fulkerson DH, White IK, Rees JM, Baumanis MM, Smith JL, Ackerman LL, et al. Analysis of long-term (median 10.5 years) outcomes in children presenting with traumatic brain injury and an initial Glasgow Coma Scale score of 3 or 4. J Neurosurg Pediatr. 2015;3:1–10.
8. Gorji MA, Gorji AM, Hosseini SH. Which score should be used in intubated patients' Glasgow Coma Scale or full outline of unresponsiveness? Int J Appl Basic Med Res. 2015;5:92–5.
9. Simon D, Nicol JM, Sabino Da Silva S, Graziottin C, Silveira PC, Ikuta N, et al. Serum ferritin correlates with Glasgow Coma Scale scores and fatal outcome after severe traumatic brain injury. Brain Inj. 2015;29:612–7.
10. Wang KY, Yu GF, Zhang ZY, Huang Q, Dong XQ. Plasma high-mobility group box 1 levels and prediction of outcome in patients with traumatic brain injury. Clin Chim Acta. 2012;413:1737–41.
11. Xu JF, Liu WG, Dong XQ, Yang SB, Fan J. Change in plasma gelsolin level after traumatic brain injury. J Trauma Acute Care Surg. 2012;72:491–6.
12. Dong XQ, Huang M, Yang SB, Yu WH, Zhang ZY. Copeptin is associated with mortality in patients with traumatic brain injury. J Trauma. 2011;71:1194–8.
13. Levin HS, Diaz-Arrastia RR. Diagnosis, prognosis, and clinical management of mild traumatic brain injury. Lancet Neurol. 2015;14:506–17.
14. Zetterberg H, Blennow K. Fluid markers of traumatic brain injury. Mol Cell Neurosci. 2015;66:99–102.
15. Nonaka M. Evolution of the complement system. Subcell Biochem. 2014;80:31–43.
16. Gadjeva M. The complement system. Overview. Methods Mol Biol. 2014;1100:1–9.
17. Phieler J, Garcia-Martin R, Lambris JD, Chavakis T. The role of the complement system in metabolic organs and metabolic diseases. Semin Immunol. 2013;25:47–53.
18. Walport MJ. Complement. First of two parts. N Engl J Med. 2001;344:1058–66.
19. Kishore U, Reid KB. C1q: structure, function, and receptors. Immunopharmacology. 2000;49:159–70.
20. Fearon DT, Austen KF. Properdin: binding to C3b and stabilization of the C3b-dependent C3 convertase. J Exp Med. 1975;142:856–63.
21. Spitzer D, Mitchell LM, Atkinson JP, Hourcade DE. Properdin can initiate complement activation by binding specific target surfaces and providing a platform for de novo convertase assembly. J Immunol. 2007;179:2600–8.
22. Thiel S. Complement activating soluble pattern recognition molecules with collagen-like regions, mannan-binding lectin, ficolins and associated proteins. Mol Immunol. 2007;44:3875–88.
23. Harvey H, Durant S. The role of glial cells and the complement system in retinal diseases and Alzheimer's disease: common neural degeneration mechanisms. Exp Brain Res. 2014;232:3363–77.
24. Hertle E, Stehouwer CD, van Greevenbroek MM. The complement system in human cardiometabolic disease. Mol Immunol. 2014;61:135–48.
25. Doni A, Garlanda C, Bottazzi B, Meri S, Garred P, Mantovani A. Interactions of the humoral pattern recognition molecule PTX3 with the complement system. Immunobiology. 2012;217:1122–8.
26. Brennan FH, Anderson AJ, Taylor SM, Woodruff TM, Ruitenberg MJ. Complement activation in the injured central nervous system: another dual-edged sword? J Neuroinflammation. 2012;9:137.
27. Lozano D, Gonzales-Portillo GS, Acosta S, de la Pena I, Tajiri N, Kaneko Y, et al. Neuroinflammatory responses to traumatic brain injury: etiology, clinical consequences, and therapeutic opportunities. Neuropsychiatr Dis Treat. 2015;11:97–106.
28. Corps KN, Roth TL, McGavern DB. Inflammation and neuroprotection in traumatic brain injury. JAMA Neurol. 2015;72:355–62.
29. Monaco 3rd EA, Tempel Z, Friedlander RM. Inflammation triggered by traumatic brain injury may continue to harm the brain for a lifetime. Neurosurgery. 2013;72:N19–20.
30. Balu R. Inflammation and immune system activation after traumatic brain injury. Curr Neurol Neurosci Rep. 2014;14:484.
31. Gyoneva S, Ransohoff RM. Inflammatory reaction after traumatic brain injury: therapeutic potential of targeting cell-cell communication by chemokines. Trends Pharmacol Sci. 2015;36:471–80.
32. Stahel PF, Morganti-Kossmann MC, Kossmann T. The role of the complement system in traumatic brain injury. Brain Res Brain Res Rev. 1998;27:243–56.
33. Endo Y, Matsushita M, Fujita T. Role of ficolin in innate immunity and its molecular basis. Immunobiology. 2007;212:371–9.
34. Hein E, Honore' C, Skjoedt MO, Munthe-Fog L, Hummelshøj T, Garred P. Functional analysis of ficolin-3 mediated complement activation. PLoS One. 2010;5:e15443.
35. Kjaer TR, Thiel S, Andersen GR. Toward a structure-based comprehension of the lectin pathway of complement. Mol Immunol. 2013;56:413–22.
36. Boldt AB, Goeldner I, de Messias-Reason IJ. Relevance of the lectin pathway of complement in rheumatic diseases. Adv Clin Chem. 2012;56:105–53.
37. Endo Y, Matsushita M, Fujita T. The role of ficolins in the lectin pathway of innate immunity. Int J Biochem Cell Biol. 2011;43:705–12.
38. Matsushita M, Fujita T. The lectin pathway. Res Immunol. 1996;147:115–8.
39. Gadjeva M, Thiel S, Jensenius JC. The mannan-binding-lectin pathway of the innate immune response. Curr Opin Immunol. 2001;13:74–8.
40. Nauta AJ, Raaschou-Jensen N, Roos A, Daha MR, Madsen HO, Borrias-Essers MC, et al. Mannose-binding lectin engagement with late apoptotic and necrotic cells. Eur J Immunol. 2003;33:2853–63.
41. Füst G, Munthe-Fog L, Illes Z, Széplaki G, Molnar T, Pusch G, et al. Low ficolin-3 levels in early follow-up serum samples are associated with the severity and unfavorable outcome of acute ischemic stroke. J Neuroinflammation. 2011;8:185.
42. Zanier ER, Zangari R, Munthe-Fog L, Hein E, Zoerle T, Conte V, et al. Ficolin-3-mediated lectin complement pathway activation in patients with subarachnoid hemorrhage. Neurology. 2014;82:126–34.
43. Jensen ML, Honore C, Hummelshoj T, Hansen BE, Madsen HO, Garred P. Ficolin-2 recognizes DNA and participates in the clearance of dying host cells. Mol Immunol. 2007;44:856–65.
44. Yanamadala V, Friedlander RM. Complement in neuroprotection and neurodegeneration. Trends Mol Med. 2010;16:69–76.
45. Chen H, Lu J, Chen X, Yu H, Zhang L, Bao Y, et al. Low serum levels of the innate immune component ficolin-3 is associated with insulin resistance and predicts the development of type 2 diabetes. J Mol Cell Biol. 2012;4:256–7.
46. Zhang X, Hu Y, Shen J, Zeng H, Lu J, Li L, et al. Low levels of ficolin-3 are associated with diabetic peripheral neuropathy. Acta Diabetol. 2015. doi:10.1007/s00592-015-0780-6.
47. Fujita T, Hemmi S, Kajiwara M, Yabuki M, Fuke Y, Satomura A, et al. Complement-mediated chronic inflammation is associated with diabetic microvascular complication. Diabetes Metab Res Rev. 2013;29:220–6.
48. Halmos A, Rigó Jr J, Szijártó J, Füst G, Prohászka Z, Molvarec A. Circulating ficolin-2 and ficolin-3 in normal pregnancy and pre-eclampsia. Clin Exp Immunol. 2012;169:49–56.
49. Prohászka Z, Munthe-Fog L, Ueland T, Gombos T, Yndestad A, Förhécz Z, et al. Association of ficolin-3 with severity and outcome of chronic heart failure. PLoS One. 2013;8, e60976.

5

Age exacerbates the CCR2/5-mediated neuroinflammatory response to traumatic brain injury

Josh M. Morganti[1,2], Lara-Kirstie Riparip[1], Austin Chou[1,3], Sharon Liu[4], Nalin Gupta[4,5] and Susanna Rosi[1,2,3,4*]

Abstract

Background: Traumatic brain injury (TBI) is a major risk factor for the development of multiple neurodegenerative diseases, including Alzheimer's disease (AD) and numerous recent reports document the development of dementia after TBI. Age is a significant factor in both the risk of and the incidence of acquired brain injury. TBI-induced inflammatory response is associated with activation of brain resident microglia and accumulation of infiltrating monocytes, which plays a pivotal role in chronic neurodegeneration and loss of neurological function after TBI. Despite the extensive clinical evidence implicating neuroinflammation with the TBI-related sequelae, the specific role of these different myeloid cells and the influence of age on TBI-initiated innate immune response remain unknown and poorly studied.

Methods: We used gene profiling and pathway analysis to define the effect of age on inflammatory response at the time of injury. The recruitment of peripheral CCR2+ macrophages was delineated using the $CX3CR1^{GFP/+}CCR2^{RFP/+}$ reporter mouse. These responses were examined in the context of CCR2/5 antagonism using cenicriviroc.

Results: Unsupervised gene clustering and pathway analysis revealed that age predisposes exacerbated inflammatory response related to the recruitment and activation of peripheral monocytes to the injured brain. Using a unique reporter animal model able to discriminate resident versus peripherally derived myeloid cells, we demonstrate that in the aged brain, there is an increased accumulation of peripherally derived CCR2+ macrophages after TBI compared to young animals. Exaggerated recruitment of this population of cells was associated with an augmented inflammatory response in the aged TBI animals. Targeting this cellular response with cenicriviroc, a dual CCR2/5 antagonist, significantly ameliorated injury-induced sequelae in the aged TBI animals.

Conclusions: Importantly, these findings demonstrate that peripheral monocytes play a non-redundant and contributing role to the etiology of trauma-induced inflammatory sequelae in the aged brain.

Keywords: Microglia, Macrophage, CCR2, Chemokine, Antagonist, Aging, Neurotrauma

Background

Traumatic brain injury (TBI) is an environmental risk factor for the development of many neurological disorders including degenerative diseases such as Alzheimer's and early onset dementia [1, 2]. Age significantly increases both the risk and incidence of acquired brain injury [3]. Elderly individuals are particularly vulnerable to TBI and have clinically worse outcomes after TBI

with increased morbidity and mortality, and reduced functional recovery [4, 5]. While age as a prognostic factor after TBI has long been recognized [6], limited attention has been devoted to understanding and modulating the pathologic processes that contribute to poor outcomes seen in aged individuals.

Brain injury initiates an immediate response involving multiple cellular effectors of the innate immune response, notably the brain's resident tissue macrophage and microglia, as well as the recruitment of peripherally derived monocytes/macrophages presumably through the disruption of the blood-brain barrier [7–9]. Aging in humans and rodents has been shown to alter this

* Correspondence: susanna.rosi@ucsf.edu
[1]Brain and Spinal Injury Center, University of California, 1001 Potrero Ave, Bldg. 1, Room 101, San Francisco, CA 94110, USA
[2]Department of Physical Therapy and Rehabilitation Science, University of California, San Francisco, CA, USA
Full list of author information is available at the end of the article

response [10, 11]. In the current study, we used unsupervised gene clustering and pathway analysis to define the effect of age on injury-induced inflammatory sequelae. Our data show that age predisposes the injured brain to an exaggerated inflammatory response involving the enrichment of chemotactic mediators associated with the recruitment and activation of the peripheral monocytes. Specifically, our data show that aged TBI animals have an exacerbated response in the production of ligands that bind to both CCR2 and CCR5 at a critical time point associated with migration of peripheral monocytes/macrophages to the injured brain parenchyma. This molecular response was paralleled by an increased recruitment of CCR2$^+$ macrophages to the injured brain of aged mice. Given the exacerbated CCR2/5 cellular and molecular signatures, we used a novel small molecule antagonist for CCR2/5 to abrogate this phenotype. Using a clinically relevant pharmacological approach, our data show that the age-related phenotype in response to injury is significantly mitigated in treated animals. These data implicate a new important role for the accumulation of monocyte/macrophages in the maintenance of neuroinflammatory sequelae following neurotrauma in the aged brain.

Methods

Animals

All experiments were conducted in accordance with the National Institutes of Health Guide for the Care and Use of Laboratory Animals and were approved by the Institutional Animal Care and Use Committee of the University of California (San Francisco, CA). Adult 3- (young) and 23-month-old (aged) male and female $CX3CR1^{GFP/+}CCR2^{RFP/+}$ (double heterozygous (Dbl-Het)) and $C57BL6/J$ (wild type (WT)) male mice were used for all experiments. Dbl-Het mice ($n = 16$) were generated as previously described [12] and genotyped using a commercial service (Transnetyx), while WT mice ($n = 48$) were purchased from the National Institute on Aging animal colony. Mice were group housed in environmentally controlled conditions with reverse light cycle (12:12 h light:dark cycle at 21 ± 1 °C) and provided food and water ad libitum.

Surgical procedure

All animals were randomly assigned and divided as equally possible between sexes (Dbl-Het) to their treatment group. Animals were anesthetized and maintained with 2.5 % isoflurane with a non-rebreathing nose cone and passive exhaust system connected to a stereotaxic frame (David Kopf). Once animals were secured with non-traumatic ear bars, eye ointment was applied and their heads were cleared of any hair around the scalp. Following betadine application, a midline incision was made through the scalp. TBI was reproduced using the

controlled cortical impact model in the parietal lobe as previously described [13]. A craniectomy was created using an electric microdrill with center point to the coordinates: 2.0 mm; mediolateral, 2.0 mm, with respect to the bregma. Explicit attention was paid to prevent damage to the dura during craniectomy; any animal in which the dura was disrupted, as assessed by excessive bleeding, was omitted from the study and replaced by another littermate. After craniectomy, contusion was achieved using a 3.0-mm convex tip attached to an electromagnetic impactor (Leica) mounted to the digitally calibrated manipulator arm. To impact flush with the natural curvature of the head/tissue, the manipulator arm was rotated 20° on the vertical axis. The parameters for impact were for a contusion depth of 0.95 mm (from dura), velocity was constant at 4.0 m/s, and the impact was sustained for of 300 ms. After CCI injury, the scalp was sutured and each animal received 0.5 ml of physiologic saline (i.p.) before being placed in a water-heated incubation chamber (37 °C) until they fully recovered as exhibited by resumption of movement and grooming. Sham animals were treated to the above parameters, except that the CCI injury was omitted. All animals fully recovered from surgical procedures and exhibited normal weight gain for the duration.

Tissue collection

All mice were euthanized using a mixture of ketamine (150 mg/kg)/xylazine (15 mg/kg) in accordance with standard animal protocols. For flow cytometry endpoints; once the animal was completely anesthetized, the chest cavity was opened and transcardially perfused using ice-cold Hank's balanced salt solution without calcium and magnesium (HBSS; Gibco). Immediately after perfusion, mice were decapitated and the ipsilateral brain hemisphere was placed into ice-cold RPMI-1640 medium without phenol (RPMI; Gibco). For qRT-PCR endpoints, animals were rapidly killed via cervical dislocation. Each brain was quickly removed, and the ipsilateral hippocampi were dissected and snap frozen.

Cenicriviroc administration

Cenicriviroc (CVC; Tobira Therapeutics), a small molecule dual antagonist for the human orthologs of CCR2 and CCR5 was dissolved in solution of 0.5 % hydroxypropyl methylcellulose (vehicle; HPMC + 1.0 % Tween80) to 5 mg/mL. Aged TBI animals were randomly divided between two treatment groups; vehicle and CVC. Two hours following surgery, animals were dosed at 100 mg/kg BID via oral gavage at 2 and 10 h post-surgery intervals. This treatment strategy was chosen to provide sufficient coverage of CCR2/5 through 24 h, with peak plasma concentrations of CVC reached by hour 2 (data not shown).

Flow cytometry

Brain hemispheres in RMPI were used for leukocyte isolation following standard procedures [14]. Fc receptor blocking was performed before all staining procedures using an anti-CD16/32 antibody (BD Pharmigen). The following reagents were used for labeling isolated macrophages: ZombieAqua (BD Biolegend), CD11b Alexafluor 700 (BD Pharmigen), and F4/80 APC (Invitrogen) CD45 FITC (AbD Serotec) Ly6C PE (AbD Serotec). Mandibular blood draws from naïve $CCR2^{RFP/RFP}$ and $CX3CR1^{GFP/GFP}$ mice were used as positive controls for RFP and GFP expression, respectively. Additionally, naïve WT isolated leukocytes served as negative control for RFP and GFP expression. Spectral compensation was achieved using polystyrene microparticles (BD Pharmigen) in combination with each of the above listed conjugated antibodies following manufacturer's suggested protocol. Standard staining procedures were conducted as previously described [14] before analysis on FACSAria III cell sorter (BD Biosciences). Gating parameters for both WT and Dbl-Het endpoints were used as previously described [13]. All samples were run in duplicate. Flow cytometric data were analyzed using FlowJo (Treestar; v9.9).

qRT-PCR

Dissected ipsilateral hippocampi were used for all gene expression analyses. RNA isolation and cDNA conversion were completed as previously described [13]. RNA concentration and quality were determined using a NanoDrop (Thermo Scientific). Three hundred nanograms of RNA was reverse transcribed using High-Capacity cDNA Reverse Transcription Kit (Applied Biosystems). For inflammatory profiling arrays [15], (Qiagen, #330131) equal volumes of cDNA for each sample were pooled ($n = 8$ animals/group/pool) and run on a single plate per condition (e.g., young sham, young TBI, aged sham, and aged TBI); cycling conditions were followed as suggested by manufacturer. Select analytes from the profiling arrays were validated using individual samples ($n = 8$/group) carried out in duplicate using SYBR Green Master Mix (Applied Biosystems) following manufacturer's suggested protocol. The relative expression of target genes was determined by the $2^{-\Delta\Delta Ct}$ method and normalized against beta-actin gene expression using a Statagene Mx3005P Real-Time PCR system. Specifically, the multiple genes were analyzed using the following primer sequences (5′ to 3′ sense/antisense);

CCL2 (GCTGACCCCAAGAAGGAATG/GTGCTTG AGGTGGTTGTGGA), *CCL8* (GGGTGCTGAAAAGCT ACGAGAG/GGATCTCCATGTACTCACTGACC), *CCL 7* (CAGAAGGATCACCAGTAGTCGG/ATAGCCTCCT CGACCCACTTCT), *CCL12* (CAGTCCTCAGGTATTG GCTGGA/TCCTTGGGGTCAGCACAGAT), *CCL5* (C CTGCTGCTTTGCCTACCTCTC/ACACACTTGGCG

GTTCCTTCGA), *TNFα* (TGCCTATGTCTCAGCCTC TTC/GAGGCCATTTGGGAACTTCT), *IL-1β* (TGTA ATGAAAGACGGCACACC/TCTTCTTTGGGTATTG CTTGG), *Arg1* (GAACACGGCAGTGGCTTTAAC/T GCTTAGCTCTGTCTGCTTTGC), *CD36* (GGACATT GAGATTCTTTTCCTCTG/GCAAAGGCATTGGCTG GAAGAAC), *CX3CL1* (GGCTAAGCCTCAGAGCATT G/CTGTAGTGGAGGGGGACTCA), *CXCL2* (CATCC AGAGCTTGAGTGTGACG/GGCTTCAGGGTCAAGG CAAACT), *PTX3* (CGAAATAGACAATGGACTTCATC C/CATCTGCGAGTTCTCCAGCATG), JAK2 (GCTAC CAGATGGAAACTGTGCG/GCCTCTGTAATGTTGGT GAGATC), JMJD3 (AGACCTCACCATCAGCCACTGT/ TCTTGGGTTTCACAGACTGGGC), CD86 (ACGTATT GGAAGGAGATTACAGCT/TCTGTCAGCGTTACTAT CCCGC), CD163 (GGCTAGACGAAGTCATCTGCAC/ CTTCGTTGGTCAGCCTCAGAGA), $gp91^{phox}$ (ACTC CTTGGGTCAGCACTGG/GTTCCTGTCCAGTTGTCT TCG), $p22^{phox}$ (GCTCATCTGTCTGCTGGAGTATC/C GGACGTAGTAATTCCTGGTGAG), $p40^{phox}$ (CAAAG ACCTGCTAGCGCTCATG/CCACATCCTCATCTGAC AGCAG), $p47^{phox}$ (GCTGACTACGAGAAGAGTTCGG/ CCTCGCTTTGTCTTCATCTGGC), $p67^{phox}$ (GCAG AAGAGCAGTTGGCATTGG/CTGCCTCTCATTTGGA CGGAAC). All primer pairs were independently validated using a standard curve of serially diluted mouse cDNA before use in any endpoint. In each PCR analysis, template and RT controls were included to account for contamination. Gene expression data are represented as the Log_2 fold change relative to young sham or to aged TBI-vehicle (for CVC endpoints).

Hierarchical clustering analysis

Multi Experiment Viewer (v4.8) was used for hierarchical cluster analysis. This was performed using Pearson's correlation for distance measure algorithm with average linking clustering parameters to identify multiple samples with similar expression patterns.

Ingenuity Pathway Analysis (IPA)

Data from mini arrays were analyzed using IPA. Differentially expressed genes (young TBI, aged sham, and aged TBI versus young sham) were uploaded into IPA and refined to limit only expression values of ±1.5-fold change before core analyses were commenced. Core analyses of the three groups were analyzed by comparison for the diseases and biological function analyses. These functional analyses were sorted by activation z-score of aged TBI group in a descending list, with exogenous chemicals omitted.

Statistical analyses

All analyses were performed in Prism v6.0 (GraphPad) using Student's t test and one-way ANOVA with Tukey

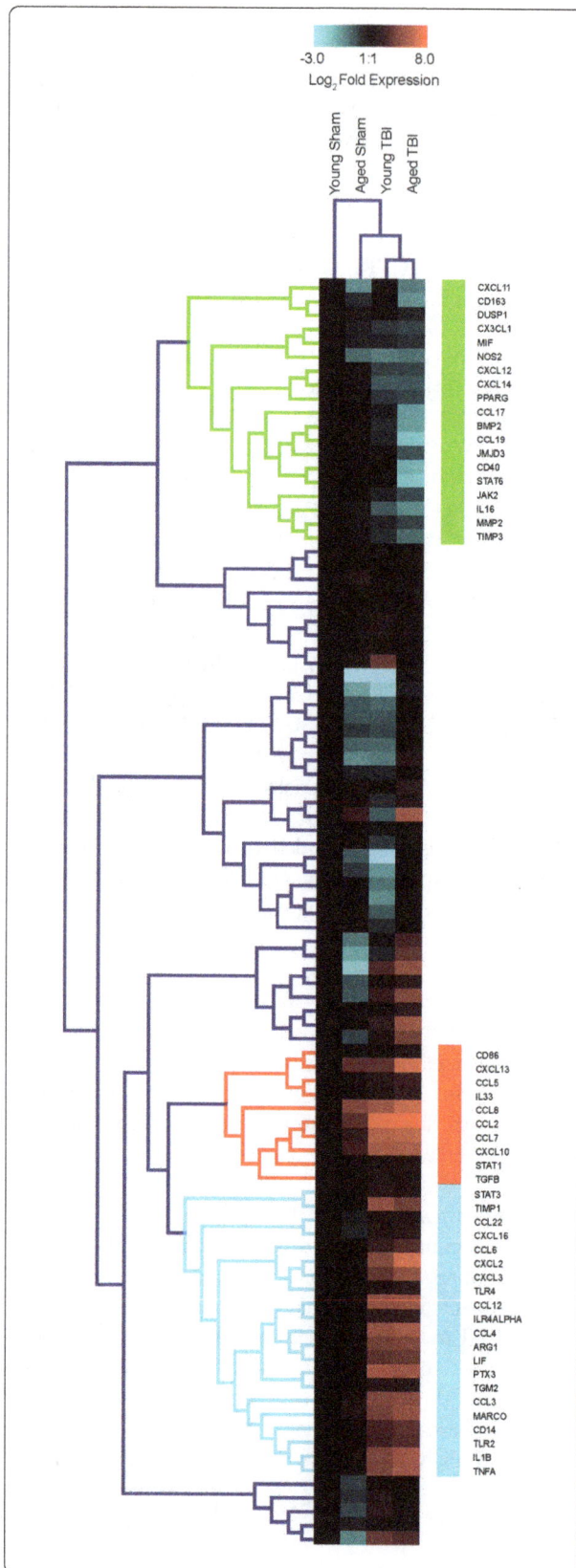

Fig. 1 Inflammatory profiling of the TBI brain. Ipsilateral hippocampi pooled from sham and injured animals (n = 8/group) of 3-month (young; Y) and 23-month (aged; A) 24 h after surgery for gene array analysis. Inflammatory profiling array revealed clusters of enrichment and downregulation of genes across three groups; young TBI, aged sham, and aged TBI, relative to young sham expression levels, all data were Log₂ transformed. Three specific clusters were examined, wherein the genes within the green cluster were downregulated in the aged TBI group, the *red gene cluster* showed marked enrichment for aged TBI, and lastly the *aquamarine cluster* showed similar enrichment of genes as a response to TBI, regardless of age. In heatmap; *teal* downregulated, *red* upregulated

HSD correction for multiple comparisons for both flow cytometry and gene expression analyses. Significance for all measures was assessed at $p < .05$.

Results

Age alters gene expression profiles as a response to injury

We first conducted gene profiling of the injured parenchyma to examine the effect of age upon neuroinflammatory response to injury. Unsupervised hierarchical clustering (Fig. 1) revealed unique arrangements of both enriched and downregulated responses as a result of injury and/or age. Of these expression clusters, we examined three that visually represented alignment of genes that were downregulated in the aged TBI group (Fig. 1; green), upregulated in the aged TBI group (Fig. 1; red), and upregulated as a result of injury (Fig. 1; aquamarine). In general, the downregulated genes of the green cluster represented a repressed inflammatory function as a combination of age and injury. By contrast, the red cluster linked a group of genes related to recruitment and activation of pro-inflammatory monocytes. Notably, within this expression cluster, our data show increased responses of several CCR2 and CCR5 cognate ligands (e.g., CCL2, CCL7, CCL8, CCL5). While the aquamarine (Fig. 1) cluster was distinct from the changes found within the red cluster, there was a similar activation profile found between both TBI groups hierarchically. There was a heterogeneous mix of chemokines, cytokines, and signal transducers, and metabolic mediators found throughout this gene cluster, which seem to be indicative of a general inflammatory response to brain injury, as there was little to no activation of these mediators in the aged sham group (Fig. 1).

Selected genes were validated within each of the green, red, and aquamarine clusters of interest. In line with the pooled observations from the array and cluster, four genes from the green cluster (Fig. 1): CD163, CX3CL1, JAK2, and JMJD3 were disproportionately downregulated in the aged TBI group, compared to young TBI (Fig. 2a). Potentially indicating that as a result of age, there is a maladaptive response to injury related to the

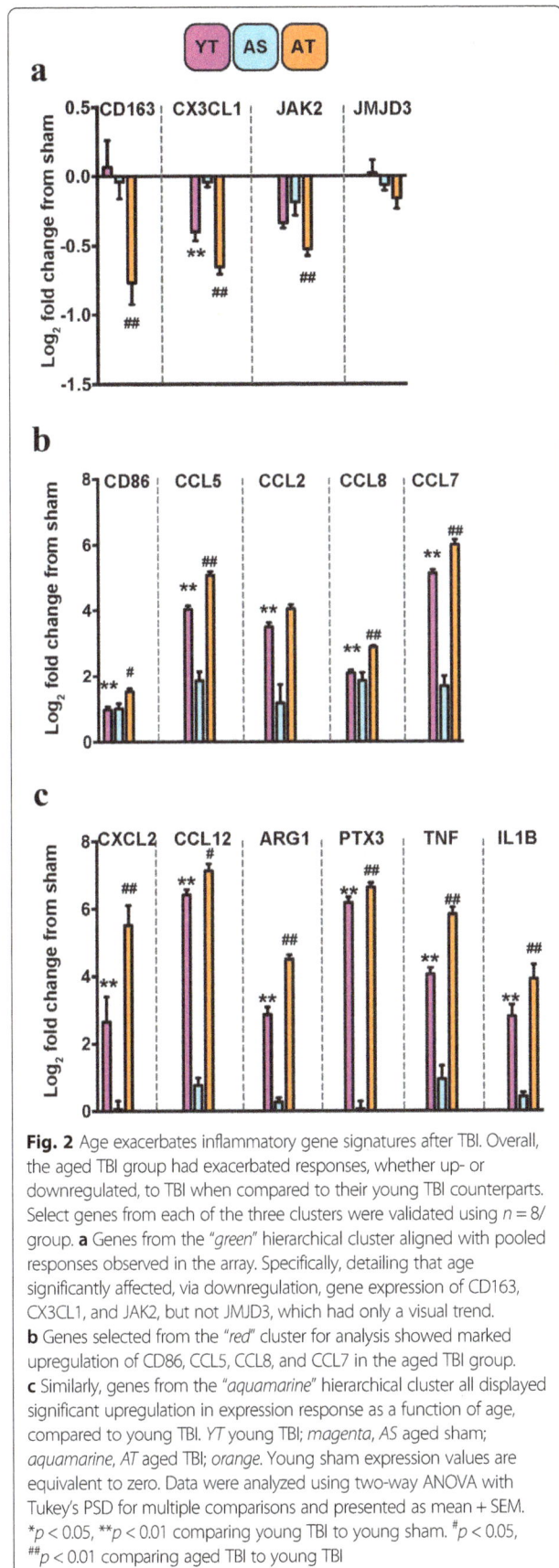

Fig. 2 Age exacerbates inflammatory gene signatures after TBI. Overall, the aged TBI group had exacerbated responses, whether up- or downregulated, to TBI when compared to their young TBI counterparts. Select genes from each of the three clusters were validated using $n = 8$/ group. **a** Genes from the "*green*" hierarchical cluster aligned with pooled responses observed in the array. Specifically, detailing that age significantly affected, via downregulation, gene expression of CD163, CX3CL1, and JAK2, but not JMJD3, which had only a visual trend. **b** Genes selected from the "*red*" cluster for analysis showed marked upregulation of CD86, CCL5, CCL8, and CCL7 in the aged TBI group. **c** Similarly, genes from the "*aquamarine*" hierarchical cluster all displayed significant upregulation in expression response as a function of age, compared to young TBI. *YT* young TBI; *magenta, AS* aged sham; *aquamarine, AT* aged TBI; *orange*. Young sham expression values are equivalent to zero. Data were analyzed using two-way ANOVA with Tukey's PSD for multiple comparisons and presented as mean + SEM. $*p < 0.05$, $**p < 0.01$ comparing young TBI to young sham. $\#p < 0.05$, $\#\#p < 0.01$ comparing aged TBI to young TBI

restraint of macrophage activation, similar to what is observed in humans [16]. Interestingly, we show that the anti-inflammatory [17] chemokine CX3CL1 is significantly downregulated in the aged TBI group compared to young animals following TBI. These findings are similar to a report on brain aging in healthy rodents that showed CX3CL1 expression is decreased with age [18], which can lead to pro-inflammatory neurotoxic responses [19, 20].

Comparatively, when we quantified selected genes from the red cluster (Fig. 1), we found that compared to young TBI, the aged TBI group had increased expression of CD86, a marker linked specifically with microglia [21], as well as CCL8, CCL7, and CCL5, which are ligands for CCR2 and/or CCR5 (Fig. 2b). However, we did not observe an increase of CCL2 gene expression in the aged TBI group, relative to young TBI as has been previously reported [22]. Although CCL2 is the strongest chemoattractant for CCR2$^+$ monocytes/macrophages, the increased presence of other constituent ligands (e.g., CCL8, CCL7, CCL5) may indicate an additive effect. As a result of age, the increased presence of multiple monocyte chemotactic mediators would allow a greater permissive environment for increased recruitment.

Similarly, validation of selected genes within the aquamarine cluster (Fig. 1) showed that there was an exacerbated response to injury due to age (Fig. 2c). Specifically, as a response to injury, aged TBI animals had significantly increased expression of the inflammatory chemokines CXCL12, and CCL12, and similarly with pro-inflammatory cytokines TNFα and IL-1β, as well as PTX3. Arg1 was also significantly induced relative to young TBI. The elevated responses we observed are analogous to gene signatures from isolated CNS monocytes/macrophages in a mouse model of EAE-induced neuroinflammation [23].

Age alters injury-induced putative upstream and downstream regulatory networks

Next, we examined the gene expression profiles for translational observations through identification of putative upstream and downstream functional analyses using IPA software. This software converts gene expression data into recognized functional matrices related to disease etiology. Using this approach, IPA software identified regulatory genes associated with predicted upstream networks (Fig. 3a). Of these putative regulators, we sorted these responses by descending activation z-score and selected the top ten regulators that were either up- or downregulated for each of the three conditions (e.g., young TBI, aged sham, aged TBI), relative to young sham animals. These analyses revealed heterogeneous regulatory responses with respect to the variety of genes identified; however, there were a few instances where these regulators were conserved between conditions.

a

Young TBI

Upregulated

Upstream Regulator	Molecule Type	z-score	p-value	Notes
TNF	cytokine	3.917	4.19E-42	
CCL2	cytokine	3.746	3.75E-27	
TGFB1	growth factor	3.718	3.76E-26	
RELA	transcription regulator	3.593	5.52E-26	
TLR7	transmembrane receptor	3.299	1.17E-20	bias
IL1A	cytokine	3.215	3.41E-26	
IRAK4	kinase	3.214	6.12E-21	
IL27	cytokine	3.116	3.95E-23	
KRT17	other	3.051	9.24E-27	
CCL5	cytokine	3.050	3.92E-17	bias

Downregulated

Upstream Regulator	Molecule Type	z-score	p-value	Notes
INSIG1	other	-2.874	6.3E-19	bias
miR-155-5p	mature microrna	-2.594	1.5E-07	bias
MEOX2	transcription regulator	-2.449	8.2E-10	
GPX1	enzyme	-2.449	1.5E-09	
VIP	other	-2.429	1.6E-22	
mir-146	microrna	-2.416	1.3E-11	bias
Alpha catenin	group	-2.414	2.7E-11	bias
CORT	other	-2.399	9.2E-17	
SIGIRR	transmembrane receptor	-2.392	2.1E-12	bias
NR1H4	nuclear receptor	-2.382	2.2E-06	

Aged Sham

Upregulated

Upstream Regulator	Molecule Type	z-score	p-value	Notes
KRT17	other	3.000	4.53E-19	
IRAK4	kinase	2.915	2.37E-17	
ERK	group	2.787	3.08E-09	
AKT1	kinase	2.578	1.04E-07	
CCL5	cytokine	2.571	2.28E-11	
CXCL3	cytokine	2.431	1.05E-13	
KLRK1	other	2.421	9.31E-17	
CXCL2	cytokine	2.414	1.05E-13	
CCL21	cytokine	2.412	2.27E-14	
AIMP1	cytokine	2.407	6.59E-14	

Downregulated

Upstream Regulator	Molecule Type	z-score	p-value	Notes
CORT	other	-2.772	2.6E-16	
ADIPOQ	other	-2.299	1.7E-14	
CRP	other	-2.236	7.8E-11	
IL37	cytokine	-2.197	1.8E-11	
CTNNB1	transcription regulator	-2.187	9.8E-05	
ZBTB16	transcription regulator	-2.177	1.6E-07	
Ins1	other	-2.177	0.00016	
NFE2L2	transcription regulator	-2.173	1.2E-08	
NCOA2	transcription regulator	-2.078	6.9E-14	
NR3C1	nuclear receptor	-2.05	3.5E-10	

Aged TBI

Upregulated

Upstream Regulator	Molecule Type	z-score	p-value	Notes
TNF	cytokine	4.139	5.91E-47	
PPIF	enzyme	3.732	6.68E-29	
TLR4	transmembrane receptor	3.541	1.93E-32	bias
AGT	growth factor	3.330	9.45E-17	
TLR7	transmembrane receptor	3.305	6.48E-24	bias
IL1B	cytokine	3.226	1.37E-46	
IL2	cytokine	3.216	2.37E-25	bias
APP	other	3.206	6.63E-25	
IL1A	cytokine	3.203	8.60E-35	bias
CCL2	cytokine	3.181	8.43E-27	

Downregulated

Upstream Regulator	Molecule Type	z-score	p-value	Notes
CD3	complex	-3.202	9.8E-23	bias
ABCG1	transporter	-2.6	1.7E-14	bias
miR-155-5p	mature microrna	-2.594	2.2E-07	bias
MEOX2	transcription regulator	-2.449	1.1E-09	bias
GPX1	enzyme	-2.449	2E-09	
FBXO32	enzyme	-2.429	1.2E-07	
ZFP36	transcription regulator	-2.415	7.1E-11	bias
IL37	cytokine	-2.403	1.1E-12	bias
CORT	other	-2.399	1.5E-16	bias
SIGIRR	transmembrane receptor	-2.392	2.8E-12	bias

b

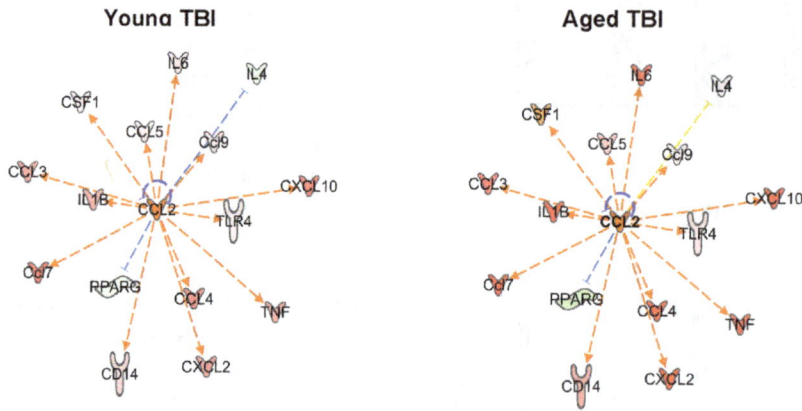

Young TBI — Aged TBI

c

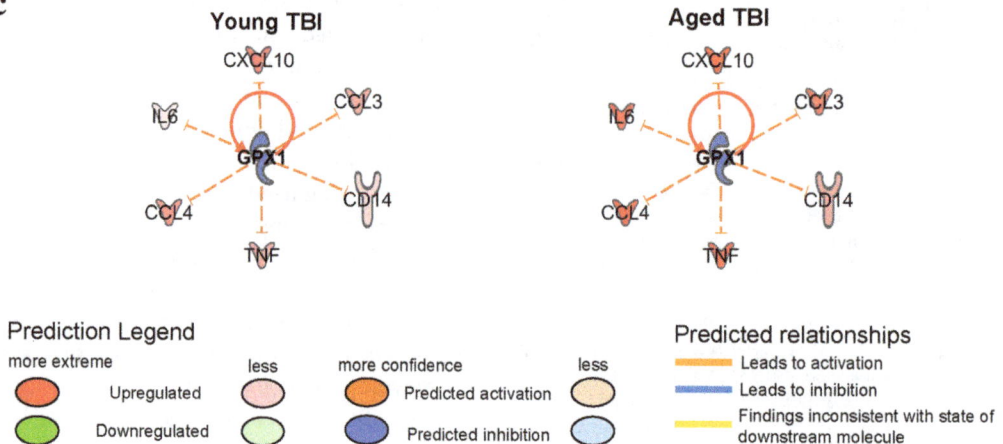

Young TBI — Aged TBI

Prediction Legend

more extreme — less
- Upregulated
- Downregulated

more confidence — less
- Predicted activation
- Predicted inhibition

Predicted relationships
- Leads to activation
- Leads to inhibition
- Findings inconsistent with state of downstream molecule

Fig. 3 (See legend on next page.)

(See figure on previous page.)
Fig. 3 IPA upstream analysis displays heterogeneous regulatory components associated with inflammatory response. Gene array data were loaded into IPA software; genes with a fold change (relative to young sham) ≥1.5 or ≤−1.5 were included for upstream regulator analysis. **a** Upregulated and downregulated molecules were sorted via their respective activation z-score and the top ten regulators (up and down) are presented for each condition. **b, c** Representative regulatory networks for putative upstream mediators associated with young TBI and aged TBI, with CCL2 representing an upregulated response and GPX1 representing a downregulated response. Both CCL2 and GPX1 show dissimilar expression responses for young TBI versus aged TBI

Interestingly, among the conserved regulators between both young and aged TBI groups were the activation of CCL2 (Fig. 3b) and downregulation of GPX1 (Fig. 3c), involved in the recruitment of $CCR2^+$ leukocytes and regulation of oxidative stress, respectively.

Comparatively, we examined if these gene expression responses were predictive of downstream disease-based functions using IPA software. Using IPA comparative analysis, we next sorted the top ten biological functions by the activation z-score in the aged TBI group. Of the top ten functions generated, there was a general theme of each related to innate immune response. In particular, there was an overrepresentation with both the differentiation and activation of monocytes in the aged TBI group, relative to young TBI (Fig. 4a; arrow). Examination of the putative response network associated with the activation of monocytes (Fig. 4a) revealed significant differential expression patterns in the mediators affecting this response system (Fig. 4b). Principal to this response was the induction of pro-inflammatory and chemotactic mediators within the CC and CXC motifs.

Age exaggerates the accumulation of $CCR2^+$ monocytes following trauma

We next sought to determine if the predictive responses generated in IPA translated to in vivo reactions. Using the Dbl-Het reporter mice, our data show that aging results in a small, but significant increase in the mean number of $CCR2^+$ infiltrated monocytes/macrophages relative to young mice (Fig. 4c). When compared to this result, following brain injury, there is a much greater recruitment and infiltration of $CD11b^+F4/80^+CCR2^+$ macrophages into the parenchyma as compared to young animals. The nature of these cells in the diseased brain remains controversial, as there are reports detailing both beneficial and detrimental actions of this population of monocytes varying among disease models [13, 24–26]. Interestingly, as a response of age, there was a visual increase in the number of resident $F4/80^+$ microglia/macrophages ($CX3CR1^+CCR2^-$; Fig. 4c), which was exaggerated in response to TBI. Recent work has shown that this subpopulation may have distinct roles in the inflammatory response to trauma [27].

Simultaneous CCR2/5 antagonism abrogates age-related response to injury

In order to abrogate this response, we treated aged TBI mice with cenicriviroc (CVC), a potent, oral, dual-antagonist of CCR2/5, which is currently being evaluated in a phase 2 clinical trial in adults with non-alcoholic fatty liver disease and liver fibrosis (NCT02217475). Separate cohorts of aged TBI animals were treated with either vehicle or CVC twice daily several hours after injury (Fig. 5a). Using this experimental approach, we observed a significant reduction in the numbers of $CD11b^+F4/80^+CD45^{hi}Ly6C^+$ macrophages (Fig. 5b,c), which are analogous to $CCR2^+$ macrophages, recruited into the diseased brain [12, 28].

CVC treatment mitigates the age-related inflammatory response to TBI

We next examined whether this treatment had any effect within the previously defined (Fig. 1) expression patterns identified by hierarchical clustering. Treatment with CVC significantly increased the expression of the genes in the green "restraint and anti-inflammatory" cluster (Fig. 6a), while significantly downregulating genes from the red "inflammatory chemotactic" cluster (Fig. 6b) and aquamarine "injury-induced inflammation" (Fig. 6c) gene clusters. The putative upstream network analysis predicted a proclivity for exaggerated oxidative stress response in the aged TBI group through downregulation of GPX1-regulated pathways (Fig. 3c). Importantly, we have recently shown that CCR2 antagonism ameliorates constituents mediating oxidative stress response following TBI through reduction of NADPH oxidase (NOX2) complex [13]. In agreement with those findings, our current data show that CVC treatment significantly downregulated multiple constituents of the neurotoxic ROS complex, NOX2 (Fig. 6d), which were previously shown to be upregulated in aged animals following TBI [22].

Discussion

The brain's response to neurotrauma initiates a wide range of molecular signaling mechanisms involving a variety of cell types [29, 30]. Of principle concern is the activation of the myeloid constituents, microglia, and monocytes, due to their involvement and propagation of

a

Diseases and Bio Functions	Young TBI	Aged Sham	Aged TBI
Immune response of cells	2.137410283	0.378200007	3.797225066
Activation of phagocytes	2.109221304	0.757928562	3.631035553
Differentiation of mononuclear leukocytes	1.336555712	-0.925694516	3.438812212
Activation of mononuclear leukocytes	1.665802187	0	3.432479095
Phagocytosis of cells	1.681625169	0.739742755	3.4196665
Accumulation of cells	1.498684733	0	3.41530725
Response of myeloid cells	2.23028562	0.994271751	3.355551739
Response of phagocytes	1.902569539	1.306244161	3.324703866
Activation of antigen presenting cells	1.876268863	0.993717667	3.286824732
Antibody response	0.618914983	-0.118573833	3.282700017

b

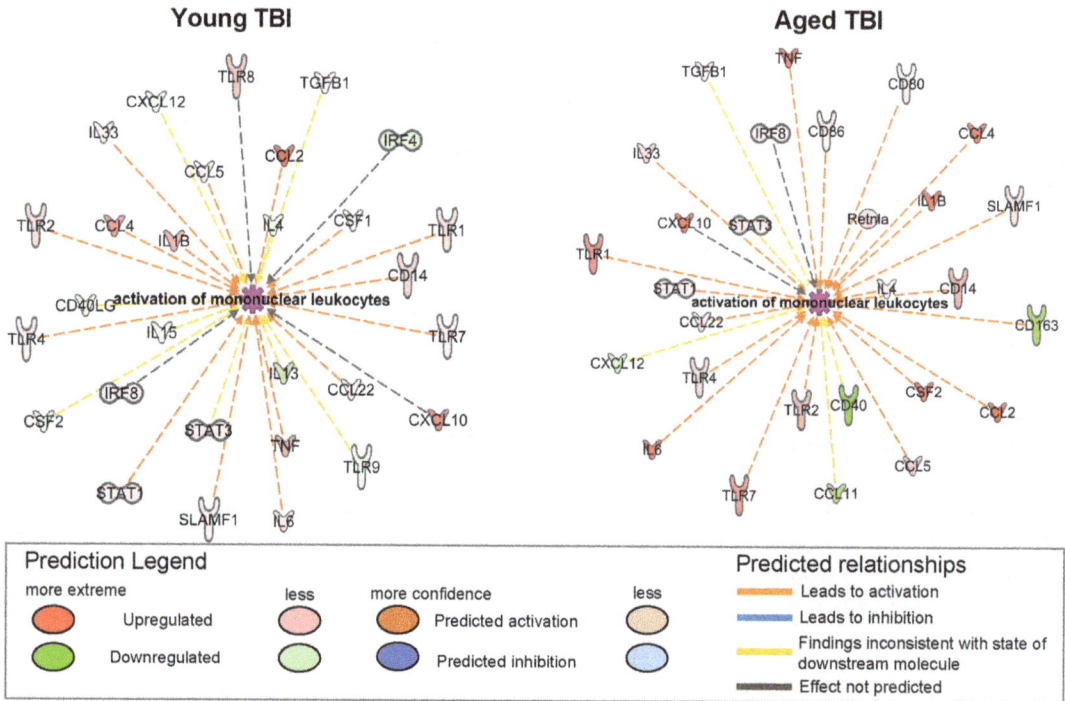

c

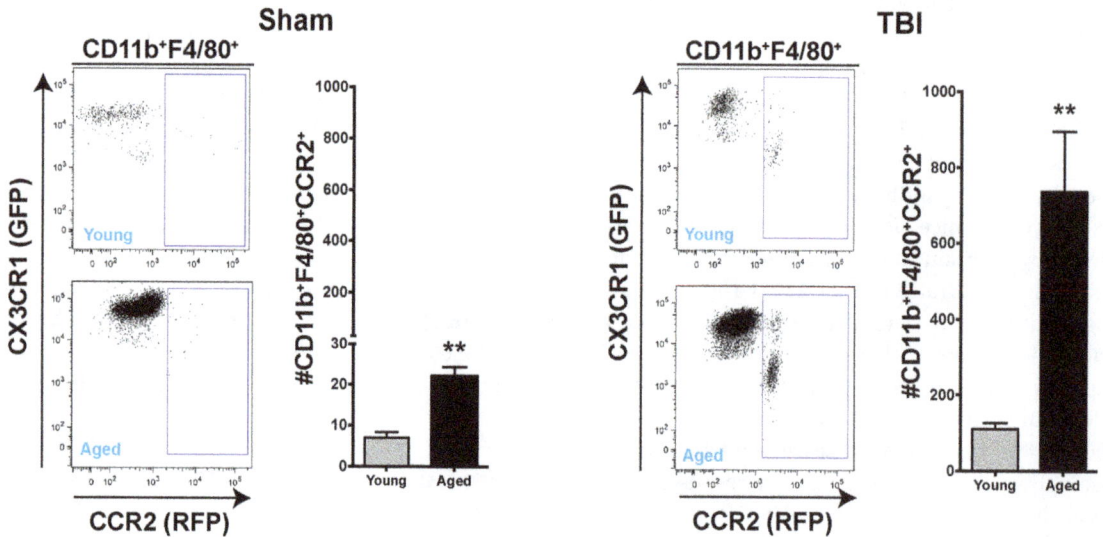

Fig. 4 (See legend on next page.)

(See figure on previous page.)
Fig. 4 Gene profiling predicts exaggerated activation and recruitment of monocytes in aged TBI. Gene array data were uploaded into IPA software, genes with a fold change (relative to young sham) ≥1.5 or ≤−1.5 were included for disease and biological function analysis. **a** Upregulated functions across all three groups were sorted by activation z-score of the aged TBI group, only the top ten functions are presented with the *black arrow* emphasizing the activation of monocytes. **b** Functional network diagram of predicted and measured regulators is presented for both young TBI and aged TBI, which highlight an overrepresented activation for this function for aged TBI group. **c** Using Dbl-Het reporter mice (*n* = 6/group), macrophages (CD11b⁺F4/80⁺) were delineated based upon their relative expression of GFP (*CX3CR1*) from RFP (*CCR2*) by flow cytometry. There were relatively very few CCR2⁺ macrophages (*blue box*) in the sham animals; however, there was a significant increase in this subpopulation due to age. However, 24 h following TBI, there was a significant increase in the mean number of CCR2⁺ macrophages (*blue box*) in the aged animals compared to young. Data were analyzed using Student's *t* test and are represented by the mean + SEM. **$p < 0.01$**

a variety of acute and chronic disorders [31]. The approaches taken in this study define the brain's inflammatory milieu in response to TBI and how these molecular patterns are altered as a function of age. The altered shift in expression patterns of chemotactic mediators in aged TBI brain created a permissive environment for the exaggerated influx of peripheral monocytes/macrophages to the brain. This, in part, may be due to redundant increases in chemokines associated with CCR2/5 signaling. While the role of these monocyte populations is diverse across various neurological diseases, we have shown that these cells augment a pro-inflammatory and potentially neurotoxic bias in the aged brain. We also used an available CCR2/5 inhibitor to reduce the accumulation of pro-inflammatory myeloid cells in the brain. Cumulatively, our findings demonstrate that the CCR2-mediated recruitment of monocytes into the injured brain is a rational therapeutic target that may abrogate TBI-induced neuroinflammatory-mediated sequelae.

We recently described the leukocyte-mediated neuroinflammatory sequelae associated with this TBI model in young animals over a detailed time course spanning acute through chronic time points [13]. Our previous findings suggest that resident microglia are responsible for the initiation of specific inflammatory mediators and infiltrated CCR2⁺ macrophages significantly augment this response. However, in the context of aging, recent work has shown that the aged brain has an altered inflammatory profile relative to basal levels of adult mice [32], potentially priming these systems for maladaptive responses to insult or injury [33]. In the context of neurotrauma, our current data suggest that age dysregulates multiple signaling networks associated with the activation, chemotaxis, and inflammatory response of innate immune effectors. We have recently shown that these responses do not fall within the dichotomous constraints of "M1/M2" polarization [15]. In agreement with or previous work, our current data indicate that as a result of age, there is dysregulation across both pro- and anti-inflammatory mediators. While we highlighted several instances of exaggerated pro-inflammatory and chemotactic gene profiles using unsupervised hierarchical clustering, we also observed pro-inflammatory mediators such as CD40, CXCL11, CCL17, CCL19, and IL16 that were downregulated in the aged TBI group, relative to young TBI. Given these opposing inflammatory responses, it is difficult to conclude that TBI in the aged predisposes a purely pro-inflammatory bias, as there are both inductions of anti-inflammatory response with

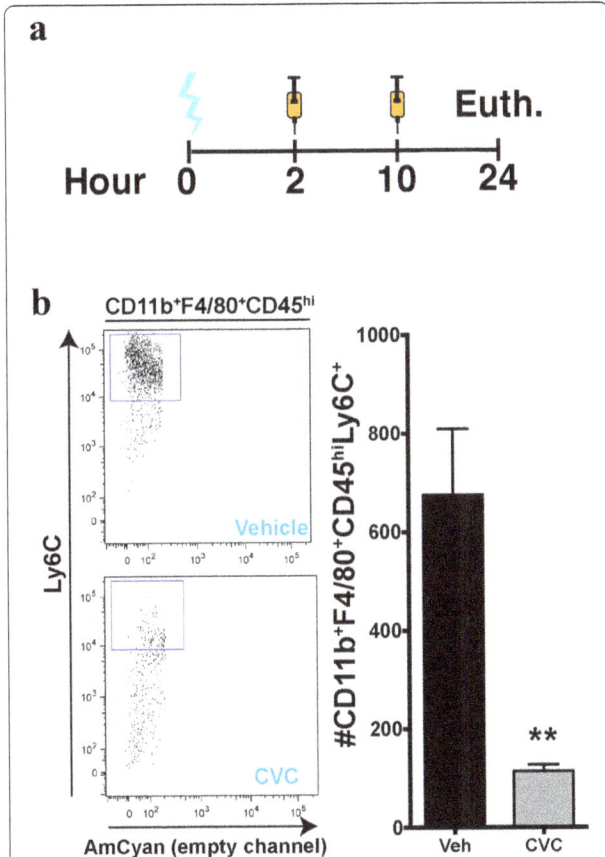

Fig. 5 Dual targeting of CCR2/5 with CVC mitigates TBI-induced macrophage recruitment. **a** In WT mice, CVC or vehicle was administered BID via oral gavage at 100 mg/kg at 2 and 10 h post surgery before animals were euthanized for various endpoints at 24 h following surgery. **b** A cohort of WT aged TBI animals (*n* = 8/group) was used for flow cytometry analysis of macrophage infiltration into the injured brain. Twenty-four hours after injury, there was a significant decrease in the number of peripheral macrophages (CD11b⁺F4/80⁺CD45^hiLy6C⁺) in the CVC-treated animals compared to their vehicle-treated counterparts

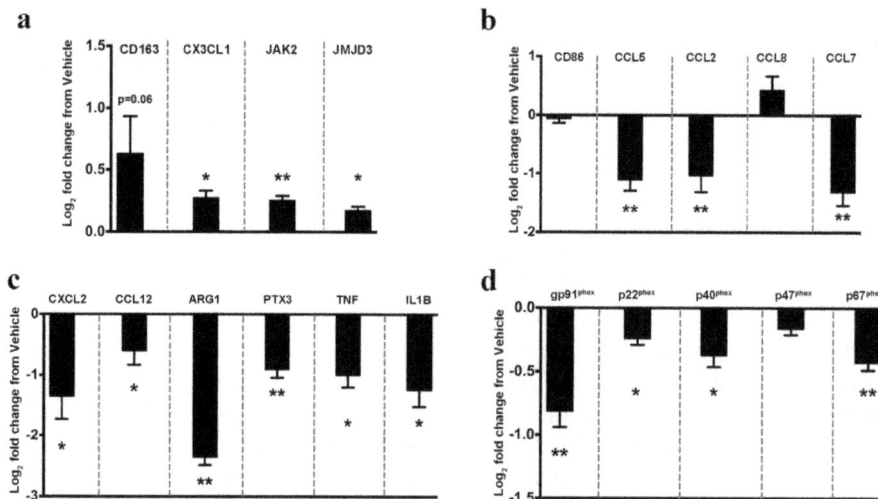

Fig. 6 Treatment with CVC attenuates age-related inflammatory and oxidative stress responses. **a–c** In a separate cohort (*n* = 8/group), inflammatory clusters were examined for their response to CVC treatment. **a–c** Correspond to the previously examined green, red, and aquamarine expression clusters, respectively. **d** Subunits of the NOX2 complex were measured as a response to CVC treatment (*n* = 8/group). Gene expression data are relative to vehicle-treated aged TBI. Vehicle expression values are equivalent to zero. Data were analyzed using Student's *t* test are represented by mean + SEM. *$p < 0.05$, **$p < 0.01$, and ***$p < 0.001$

concomitant downregulation of pro-inflammatory responses, relative to young injured animals. However, our current data attribute, in part, that cumulatively, these maladaptive responses create an overly permissive environment for the exaggerated recruitment and accumulation of CCR2$^+$ macrophages.

Although CCR2 is expressed on a variety of immune cells, circulating "inflammatory" monocytes are the main population that expresses this cytokine receptor [12]. CCR2 is currently known to have five cognate ligands; CCL2, CCL8, CCL7, CCL13 (human only), and CCL12 [34, 35]. However, there is a degree of promiscuity of the CCR2 receptor and its ligands as they are known to bind other C-C receptors; notably CCR5 [36, 37]. Expression of CCR5, like CCR2, is found on a variety of circulating immune effectors, but most relevant to our study, is co-expressed on CCR2$^+$ monocytes [38]. Overall, in the context of our current findings, the cross-talk and co-expression of CCR2/5 on monocytes, and enhanced expression of their cognate ligands may potentiate the increased recruitment we observed in aged TBI animals. Therefore, our current data are consistent with the formation of a pro-chemotactic milieu created, in part, by increased signaling through CCR2/5 expressing cells.

NOX2 activation possesses a neurotoxic nature from the production of ROS intermediates [39, 40] as well as maintaining redox pro-inflammatory signaling cascades of macrophages [41]. Recent work has detailed an increase in some subunits of the ROS-producing NOX2 complex of aged TBI animals [22]. Our treatment paradigm with CVC significantly downregulated the expression of the

multiple subunits that comprise the NOX2 complex, suggesting a decreased propensity for ROS intermediate formation relative to the vehicle-treated animals. These data align with our previous work implicating CCR2$^+$ macrophages as the predominant source for NOX2 gene expression following TBI [13]. Importantly, in rodent models of TBI, inhibiting this complex decreased neuronal damage and improved recovery [42, 43].

Conclusions

Our current study demonstrates that the aged brain's response to neurotrauma involves the exacerbated expression of multiple mediators involved in the recruitment of peripheral macrophages to the injured parenchyma. Blocking of these innate immune mediators via CCR2/5 antagonism significantly blunted their ingress, while concomitantly reducing inflammatory and potentially neurotoxic signatures. Intentionally, we limited the scope of this study to examine the period following injury where the maximum inflection of recruited CCR2$^+$ macrophages was previously known [13], in an effort to define this time point within the context of age at the time of TBI. Therefore, the conclusions garnered in this study should not be expanded beyond the presented injury paradigm. Future work is needed to define how neurotrauma in the context of age affects inflammatory response in subacute and chronic periods and whether the responses and treatment currently examined may produce tangible outcome measures in those periods.

Competing interests
The authors declare that they have no competing interests.

Authors' contributions
JMM and SR designed research studies. JMM, L-KR, AC, and SL performed the experiments. JMM, NG, and SR analyzed the data. JMM and SR wrote the manuscript. All authors read and approved the final manuscript.

Acknowledgements
Cenicriviroc was a kind gift from Tobira Therapeutics.

Funding
Research reported in this publication was supported by the National Institute Of Neurological Disorders And Stroke and National Institute on Aging of the National Institutes of Health under award numbers F32NS090805 (J.M.M.), R21NS087458 (S.R.); R21AG042016 (S.R.). The content is solely the responsibility of the authors and does not necessarily represent the official views of the National Institutes of Health.

Author details
[1]Brain and Spinal Injury Center, University of California, 1001 Potrero Ave, Bldg. 1, Room 101, San Francisco, CA 94110, USA. [2]Department of Physical Therapy and Rehabilitation Science, University of California, San Francisco, CA, USA. [3]Neuroscience Graduate Program, University of California, San Francisco, CA, USA. [4]Department of Neurological Surgery, University of California, San Francisco, CA, USA. [5]Department of Pediatrics, University of California, San Francisco, CA, USA.

References
1. Johnson VE, Stewart W, Smith DH. Traumatic brain injury and amyloid-beta pathology: a link to Alzheimer's disease? Nat Rev Neurosci. 2010;11:361–70.
2. Jellinger KA. Traumatic brain injury as a risk factor for Alzheimer's disease. J Neurol Neurosurg Psychiatry. 2004;75:511–2.
3. Stocchetti N, Paterno R, Citerio G, Beretta L, Colombo A: Traumatic brain injury in an aging population. J Neurotrauma. 2012; 29:1119-25.
4. Schonberger M, Ponsford J, Reutens D, Beare R, O'Sullivan R. The Relationship between age, injury severity, and MRI findings after traumatic brain injury. J Neurotrauma. 2009;26:2157–67.
5. Himanen L, Portin R, Isoniemi H, Helenius H, Kurki T, Tenovuo O. Longitudinal cognitive changes in traumatic brain injury: a 30-year follow-up study. Neurology. 2006;66:187–92.
6. Mushkudiani NA, Engel DC, Steyerberg EW, Butcher I, Lu J, Marmarou A, Slieker F, McHugh GS, Murray GD, Maas AI. Prognostic value of demographic characteristics in traumatic brain injury: results from the IMPACT study. J Neurotrauma. 2007;24:259–69.
7. Woodcock T, Morganti-Kossmann MC. The role of markers of inflammation in traumatic brain injury. Front Neurol. 2013;4:18.
8. Giunta B, Obregon D, Velisetty R, Sanberg PR, Borlongan CV, Tan J. The immunology of traumatic brain injury: a prime target for Alzheimer's disease prevention. J Neuroinflammation. 2012;9:185.
9. Ziebell JM, Morganti-Kossmann MC. Involvement of pro- and anti-inflammatory cytokines and chemokines in the pathophysiology of traumatic brain injury. Neurotherapeutics. 2010;7:22–30.
10. Lee DC, Ruiz CR, Lebson L, Selenica ML, Rizer J, Hunt Jr JB, Rojiani R, Reid P, Kammath S, Nash K, et al. Aging enhances classical activation but mitigates alternative activation in the central nervous system. Neurobiol Aging. 2013; 34:1610–20.
11. Inadera H, Egashira K, Takemoto M, Ouchi Y, Matsushima K. Increase in circulating levels of monocyte chemoattractant protein-1 with aging. J Interferon Cytokine Res. 1999;19:1179–82.
12. Saederup N, Cardona AE, Croft K, Mizutani M, Cotleur AC, Tsou C-L, Ransohoff RM, Charo IF. Selective chemokine receptor usage by central nervous system myeloid cells in CCR2-Red fluorescent protein knock-in mice. PLoS One. 2010;5:e13693.
13. Morganti JM, Jopson TD, Liu S, Riparip LK, Guandique CK, Gupta N, Ferguson AR, Rosi S. CCR2 antagonism alters brain macrophage polarization and ameliorates cognitive dysfunction induced by traumatic brain injury. J Neurosci. 2015;35:748–60.
14. Cardona AE, Huang D, Sasse ME, Ransohoff RM. Isolation of murine microglial cells for RNA analysis or flow cytometry. Nat Protoc. 2006;1:1947–51.
15. Morganti JM, Riparip L-K, Rosi S. Call Off the Dog(ma): M1/M2 polarization is concurrent following traumatic brain injury. PLoS One. 2016;11:e0148001.
16. Stefini R, Catenacci E, Piva S, Sozzani S, Valerio A, Bergomi R, Cenzato M, Mortini P, Latronico N. Chemokine detection in the cerebral tissue of patients with posttraumatic brain contusions. J Neurosurg. 2008;108:958–62.
17. Limatola C, Ransohoff RM: Modulating neurotoxicity through CX3CL1/CX3CR1 signaling. Front Cell Neuro 2014; 8:229.
18. Bachstetter AD, Morganti JM, Jernberg J, Schlunk A, Mitchell SH, Brewster KW, Hudson CE, Cole MJ, Harrison JK, Bickford PC, Gemma C. Fractalkine and CX 3 CR1 regulate hippocampal neurogenesis in adult and aged rats. Neurobiol Aging. 2011;32:2030–44.
19. Cardona AE, Pioro EP, Sasse ME, Kostenko V, Cardona SM, Dijkstra IM, Huang D, Kidd G, Dombrowski S, Dutta R, et al. Control of microglial neurotoxicity by the fractalkine receptor. Nat Neurosci. 2006;9:917–24.
20. Morganti JM, Nash KR, Grimmig BA, Ranjit S, Small B, Bickford PC, Gemma C. The soluble isoform of CX3CL1 is necessary for neuroprotection in a mouse model of Parkinson's disease. J Neurosci. 2012;32:14592–601.
21. Hickman SE, Kingery ND, Ohsumi T, Borowsky M, Wang L-c, Means TK, Khoury JE. The microglial sensome revealed by direct RNA sequencing. Nat Neurosci. 2013;16:1896–905.
22. Kumar A, Stoica BA, Sabirzhanov B, Burns MP, Faden AI, Loane DJ. Traumatic brain injury in aged animals increases lesion size and chronically alters microglial/macrophage classical and alternative activation states. Neurobiol Aging. 2013;34:1397–411.
23. Yamasaki R, Lu H, Butovsky O, Ohno N, Rietsch AM, Cialic R, Wu PM, Doykan CE, Lin J, Cotleur AC, et al. Differential roles of microglia and monocytes in the inflamed central nervous system. J Exp Med. 2014;211:1533–49.
24. El Khoury J, Toft M, Hickman SE, Means TK, Terada K, Geula C, Luster AD. Ccr2 deficiency impairs microglial accumulation and accelerates progression of Alzheimer-like disease. Nat Med. 2007;13:432–8.
25. Mildner A, Mack M, Schmidt H, Bruck W, Djukic M, Zabel MD, Hille A, Priller J, Prinz M. CCR2+ Ly-6Chi monocytes are crucial for the effector phase of autoimmunity in the central nervous system. Brain. 2009;132:2487–500.
26. Shechter R, Miller O, Yovel G, Rosenzweig N, London A, Ruckh J, Kim KW, Klein E, Kalchenko V, Bendel P, et al. Recruitment of beneficial M2 macrophages to injured spinal cord is orchestrated by remote brain choroid plexus. Immunity. 2013;38:555–69.
27. Donnelly DJ, Longbrake EE, Shawler TM, Kigerl KA, Lai W, Tovar CA, Ransohoff RM, Popovich PG. Deficient CX3CR1 signaling promotes recovery after mouse spinal cord injury by limiting the recruitment and activation of Ly6Clo/iNOS+ macrophages. J Neurosci. 2011;31:9910–22.
28. Auffray C, Fogg D, Garfa M, Elain G, Join-Lambert O, Kayal S, Sarnacki S, Cumano A, Lauvau G, Geissmann F. Monitoring of blood vessels and tissues by a population of monocytes with patrolling behavior. Science. 2007;317:666–70.
29. Gyoneva S, Ransohoff RM. Inflammatory reaction after traumatic brain injury: therapeutic potential of targeting cell-cell communication by chemokines. Trends Pharmacol Sci. 2015;36:471–80.
30. Hernandez-Ontiveros DG, Tajiri N, Acosta S, Giunta B, Tan J, Borlongan CV. Microglia activation as a biomarker for traumatic brain injury. Front Neurol. 2013;4:30.
31. Wynn TA, Chawla A, Pollard JW. Macrophage biology in development, homeostasis and disease. Nature. 2013;496:445–55.
32. Norden DM, Muccigrosso MM, Godbout JP. Microglial priming and enhanced reactivity to secondary insult in aging, and traumatic CNS injury, and neurodegenerative disease. Neuropharmacology. 2015;96:29–41.
33. Norden DM, Godbout JP. Review: microglia of the aged brain: primed to be activated and resistant to regulation. Neuropathol Appl Neurobiol. 2013;39:19–34.
34. Deshmane SL, Kremlev S, Amini S, Sawaya BE. Monocyte chemoattractant protein-1 (MCP-1): an overview. J Interferon Cytokine Res. 2009;29:313–26.
35. Takahashi M, Galligan C, Tessarollo L, Yoshimura T. Monocyte chemoattractant protein-1 (MCP-1), not MCP-3, is the primary chemokine required for monocyte recruitment in mouse peritonitis induced with thioglycollate or zymosan A. J Immunol. 2009;183:3463–71.
36. Mueller A, Kelly E, Strange PG. Pathways for internalization and recycling of the chemokine receptor CCR5. Blood .2002; 99:785–91.
37. Blanpain C, Migeotte I, Lee B, Vakili J, Doranz BJ, Govaerts C, Vassart G, Doms RW, Parmentier M. CCR5 binds multiple CC-chemokines: MCP-3 acts as a natural antagonist. Blood. 1999;94:1899–905.

38. Balboa L, Romero MM, Basile JI, Sabio y Garcia CA, Schierloh P, Yokobori N, Geffner L, Musella RM, Castagnino J, Abbate E, et al. Paradoxical role of CD16+ CCR2+ CCR5+ monocytes in tuberculosis: efficient APC in pleural effusion but also mark disease severity in blood. J Leukoc Biol. 2011;90:69–75.

39. Wu DC, Teismann P, Tieu K, Vila M, Jackson-Lewis V, Ischiropoulos H, Przedborski S. NADPH oxidase mediates oxidative stress in the 1-methyl-4-phenyl-1,2,3,6-tetrahydropyridine model of Parkinson's disease. Proc Natl Acad Sci U S A. 2003;100:6145–50.

40. Hernandes MS, Britto LR. NADPH oxidase and neurodegeneration. Curr Neuropharmacol. 2012;10:321–7.

41. Block ML, Zecca L, Hong JS. Microglia-mediated neurotoxicity: uncovering the molecular mechanisms. Nat Rev Neurosci. 2007;8:57–69.

42. Zhang QG, Laird MD, Han D, Nguyen K, Scott E, Dong Y, Dhandapani KM, Brann DW. Critical role of NADPH oxidase in neuronal oxidative damage and microglia activation following traumatic brain injury. PLoS One. 2012;7:e34504.

43. Loane DJ, Stoica BA, Byrnes KR, Jeong W, Faden AI. Activation of mGluR5 and inhibition of NADPH oxidase improves functional recovery after traumatic brain injury. J Neurotrauma. 2013;30:403–12.

6

Curcumin attenuates acute inflammatory injury by inhibiting the TLR4/MyD88/NF-κB signaling pathway in experimental traumatic brain injury

Hai-tao Zhu[1], Chen Bian[2], Ji-chao Yuan[1], Wei-hua Chu[1], Xin Xiang[1], Fei Chen[1], Cheng-shi Wang[1], Hua Feng[1] and Jiang-kai Lin[1*]

Abstract

Background: Traumatic brain injury (TBI) initiates a neuroinflammatory cascade that contributes to substantial neuronal damage and behavioral impairment, and Toll-like receptor 4 (TLR4) is an important mediator of thiscascade. In the current study, we tested the hypothesis that curcumin, a phytochemical compound with potent anti-inflammatory properties that is extracted from the rhizome *Curcuma longa*, alleviates acute inflammatory injury mediated by TLR4 following TBI.

Methods: Neurological function, brain water content and cytokine levels were tested in TLR4$^{-/-}$ mice subjected to weight-drop contusion injury. Wild-type (WT) mice were injected intraperitoneally with different concentrations of curcumin or vehicle 15 minutes after TBI. At 24 hours post-injury, the activation of microglia/macrophages and TLR4 was detected by immunohistochemistry; neuronal apoptosis was measured by FJB and TUNEL staining; cytokines were assayed by ELISA; and TLR4, MyD88 and NF-κB levels were measured by Western blotting. *In vitro*, a co-culture system comprised of microglia and neurons was treated with curcumin following lipopolysaccharide (LPS) stimulation. TLR4 expression and morphological activation in microglia and morphological damage to neurons were detected by immunohistochemistry 24 hours post-stimulation.

Results: The protein expression of TLR4 in pericontusional tissue reached a maximum at 24 hours post-TBI. Compared with WT mice, TLR4$^{-/-}$ mice showed attenuated functional impairment, brain edema and cytokine release post-TBI. In addition to improvement in the above aspects, 100 mg/kg curcumin treatment post-TBI significantly reduced the number of TLR4-positive microglia/macrophages as well as inflammatory mediator release and neuronal apoptosis in WT mice. Furthermore, Western blot analysis indicated that the levels of TLR4 and its known downstream effectors (MyD88, and NF-κB) were also decreased after curcumin treatment. Similar outcomes were observed in the microglia and neuron co-culture following treatment with curcumin after LPS stimulation. LPS increased TLR4 immunoreactivity and morphological activation in microglia and increased neuronal apoptosis, whereas curcumin normalized this upregulation. The increased protein levels of TLR4, MyD88 and NF-κB in microglia were attenuated by curcumin treatment.

Conclusions: Our results suggest that post-injury, curcumin administration may improve patient outcome by reducing acute activation of microglia/macrophages and neuronal apoptosis through a mechanism involving the TLR4/MyD88/NF-κB signaling pathway in microglia/macrophages in TBI.

Keywords: Toll-like receptor 4, Curcumin, Traumatic brain injury, Inflammation

* Correspondence: jklin@tmmu.edu.cn
[1]Department of Neurosurgery, Southwest Hospital, Third Military Medical University, 30 Gaotanyan Street, Chongqing 400038, China
Full list of author information is available at the end of the article

Introduction

Traumatic brain injury (TBI) is defined as damage to the brain resulting from an external mechanical force, which can lead to temporary or permanent impairment of cognitive, physical and psychosocial functions [1]. It is the leading cause of death and disability for people under the age of 45 years. Ten million deaths and/or hospitalizations annually are directly attributable to TBI, and an estimated 57 million living people worldwide have experienced such brain injury [2].

It is well known that TBI is a highly complex disorder that is caused by both primary and secondary brain injury mechanisms. Secondary brain injury, which results from delayed neurochemical, metabolic and cellular changes, can evolve over hours to days after the initial traumatic insult and cause progressive white and gray matter damage. A complex series of sterile inflammatory responses play an important role in secondary brain injury following TBI [3,4]. However, a detailed understanding of the effect of innate immunity after TBI remains limited at present. The innate immune system recognizes different pathogens via highly conserved microbial motifs, namely pathogen-associated molecular patterns (PAMPs), through pathogen-recognition receptors (PRRs) [5]. Toll-like receptors (TLRs) are a family of PRRs that recognize conserved microbial motifs in molecules such as bacterial lipopolysaccharide (LPS), peptidoglycan, flagellin, and double- and single-stranded viral RNAs. Recently, it has been shown that TLRs become activated in response to endogenous ligands released during tissue injury, such as the degradation products of macromolecules, heat shock proteins and intracellular components of ruptured cells, known as damage-associated molecular patterns (DAMPs) [6]. Microglia, the principal cells involved in the innate immune response in the CNS, express robust levels of TLR1-9 [7]. Among these TLRs, TLR4 has been shown to play an important role in initiating the inflammatory response following stroke or head trauma [8-10]. Furthermore, myeloid differentiation factor 88 (MyD88), a critical adapter protein for TLR4, leads to the activation of downstream NF-κB and the subsequent production of proinflammatory cytokines implicated in neurotoxicity [11,12].

Curcumin, a major component extracted from the rhizome *Curcuma longa*, has been consumed by humans as a curry spice for centuries. It has been extensively studied for its wide range of biological activities, including anti-inflammatory, anti-oxidant, anti-infection and anti-tumor properties [13]. *In vivo*, curcumin has been found to cross the blood-brain barrier and maintain high biological activity [14], and it has been proposed for the treatment of various neuroinflammatory and neurodegenerative conditions in the CNS. Recent studies have demonstrated that curcumin is a highly pleiotropic molecule that interacts with numerous molecular targets

[15]. Thus far, although a few studies indicate that curcumin can attenuate cerebral edema, promote membrane and energy homeostasis and influence synaptic plasticity following TBI [16-19], the modulatory effects of curcumin on the inflammatory response after TBI remain largely unknown. Recently, *in vitro*, curcumin has been shown to inhibit the homodimerization of TLR4, which is required for the activation of downstream signaling pathways [20,21]. The presumption that curcumin can attenuate inflammatory injury via the TLR4 pathway has since been tested in some models of injury [22-25], but it remains unknown whether exogenous curcumin can modulate TBI through the TLR4/MyD88/NF-κB signaling pathway. We designed this study to investigate the importance of TLR4 in initiating the acute inflammatory response following TBI, which contributes to neuronal damage and behavioral impairment, and to confirm the hypothesis that curcumin attenuates acute inflammatory damage by modulating the TLR4/MyD88/NF-κB signaling pathway in microglia/macrophages during experimental TBI.

Materials and methods

Animals

Adult male C57BL/6 mice (8 to 10 weeks, 20 to 25 g) were provided by the Animal Center of Third Military Medical University. Transgenic TLR4$^{-/-}$ mice (8 to 10 weeks, 20 to 22 g) were purchased from Jackson Laboratories (Bar Harbor, ME, USA) and were backcrossed to a C57BL/6 background more than eight times. All experiments were conducted in accordance with animal care guidelines approved by the Animal Ethics Committee of the Third Military Medical University. The animals were housed in temperature- and humidity-controlled animal quarters with a 12-hour light/dark cycle and water and food provided *ad libitum*. Mice were treated with an intraperitoneal injection of curcumin (Sigma, St. Louis, MO, USA) dissolved in 100 μL of dimethyl sulfoxide (DMSO) (50, 100, 200 mg/kg) or equal volumes of vehicle 15 minutes post-TBI. In our experiment, each test was performed independently for either three times (three mice per group) or twice (six mice per group).

Experimental traumatic brain injury model in mice

TBI was induced using a Feeney weight-drop contusion model with slight modifications [26]. Mice were anesthetized with intraperitoneal chloral hydrate (40 mg/kg) and placed in a stereotaxic frame, and a 4 mm craniotomy was performed over the right parietal cortex, centered on the coronal suture and 3 mm lateral to the sagittal suture. Considerable care was taken to avoid injury to the underlying dura. A weight-drop device was placed over the dura. An impact transducer (foot plate) was adjusted to stop at a depth of 2.5 mm below the dura. Then, one 18 g weight was dropped from 10 cm above the dura through a guide tube onto the foot plate. Body temperature was maintained with an overhead heating lamp during the experiments. Dural tears were not repaired and the bone flap was not re-inserted. If the animals demonstrated dural tears or excessive bleeding, they were excluded. After injury, the skin was closed tightly. To maintain normal body temperature during surgery and recovery, the mice were maintained with isothermic (37°C) heating. Mice in the sham-operation group were subjected to the same surgical procedure, including craniotomy, but received no cortical impact.

Neurological function evaluation

Behavioral testing was performed one day after TBI using the mNSS (modified Neurological Severity Score) assessment. The mNSS is a composite of motor, sensory, reflex and balance tests [27]. One point was scored for the inability to perform each test or for the lack of a tested reflex; thus, the higher the score was, the more severe the injury. Neurological function was graded on a scale of 0 to 18 (normal score, 0; maximal deficit score, 18).

Brain water content

Twenty-four hours post-injury, brain edema was determined using the wet/dry method:

Percent brain water = [(Wet weight−Dry weight)/Wet weight] · 100% [28]

The brains from mice in each treatment group were rapidly removed from the skull, and the brains were separated bilaterally, weighed and then placed in an oven for 72 hours at 100°C. The brains were then reweighed to obtain dry weight content.

Cortical neuronal cultures

Cortical cells were prepared from embryonic day 15 pregnant mice. Briefly, embryos were removed, the cerebral cortex was dissected, and meninges were stripped in Ca^{2+}/Mg^{2+}-free Hank's balanced saline solution (HBSS) solution. Tissues were then digested in 0.125% trypsin for 15 minutes and dispersed through the narrowed bore of a fire-polished Pasteur pipette and passed through a 40 μm cell strainer. Cells were distributed in a poly-L-lysine-coated (Sigma) culture plate containing 0.5 mL of neurobasal medium with 2% B27 supplement (Invitrogen, Carlsbad, CA, USA). The culture density was 5×10^5 cells/mL. Cultures were maintained at 37°C in a humidified incubator with 5% CO_2/95% room air. All transwell co-culture experiments were performed with neurons that had been in culture for seven days.

Microglial cultures

The cortices of the cerebral hemispheres of one-day-old post-natal mice were dissected and digested with 0.25%

trypsin. After centrifugation for five minutes at $300 \times g$, the cortical cells were seeded in DMEM-F12 with 10% FBS on a 25 cm^2 flask at a density of 3×10^5 cells/mL and cultured at 37°C in humidified 5% CO_2/95% air. The medium was replaced every four to five days, and confluency was achieved after 14 days in vitro. Microglial cells were obtained by shaking the flasks overnight. Floating cells were pelleted and subcultured at 3×10^5 cells/mL in glial-conditioned medium on poly-L-lysine pre-coated transwell inserts. Cell purity was determined by immunohistochemical staining with microglia-specific antibodies for CD11b, and purity was determined to be > 95%.

Transwell co-cultures

Transwell co-cultures were performed as previously described [29]. Microglia were plated onto the top side of the transwell inserts (0.4 μm pore size polyester membrane precoated with poly-L-lysine; Corning, NY, USA) at the cell density described above. The transwells were positioned approximately 2 mm above the neuron-enriched culture plate, and the microglia grown on the transwells were separated from the neurons by the permeable transwell membrane. Then, 1 μg/ml LPS (Sigma, St. Louis, MO, USA), curcumin, LPS plus curcumin or DMSO (Sigma, St. Louis, MO, USA) as a solvent control was added to the media below the transwells.

Cytotoxicity assay

Cell viability was evaluated by the 3-(4,5-dimethyl-thiazol-2-yl)-2,5-diphenyltetrazolium bromide (MTT) reduction assay. In brief, neurons (5×10^5 cells/mL) and microglia (3×10^5 cells/mL) were seeded in the transwell system, as described above, and treated with various concentrations of curcumin. After 24 hours of incubation, the medium was removed. The neurons and microglia were separated and then incubated with 0.5 mg/mL MTT solution. After incubation for three hours at 37°C in 5% CO_2, the supernatant was removed, and the formation of formazan crystals was measured at 490 nm with a microplate reader.

Immunofluorescence

Mice were perfused transcardially with saline, followed by 4% paraformaldehyde under deep anesthesia (100 mg/kg sodium pentobarbital) and their brains sectioned at a 20 μm thickness using a cryostat. The sections were blocked in 5% normal donkey serum diluted in PBS for one hour at room temperature and then incubated overnight at 4°C with mouse anti-TLR4 or rat anti-CD11b as the primary antibody. Donkey anti-mouse Alexa-Fluor 568 and donkey anti-rat Alexa-Fluor 488 were used as secondary fluorescent probes. The sections were viewed by confocal microscopy (LSM780, Zeiss, Jena, Germany) and analyzed as individual images for TLR4 and CD11b co-expression. Immunostained sections were quantitatively characterized by digital image analysis using Image Pro-Plus 6.0 software (Media Cybernetics, Silver Spring, MD, USA). TLR4 was quantified as the average number of positive cells per field. A negative (no antibody) control was included.

Cell cultures were fixed for 30 minutes in 4% paraformaldehyde. Cells were blocked with 1% bovine serum for one hour. Cultures were incubated overnight at 4°C with primary antibody. Microglia were incubated with mouse anti-TLR4 (1:400, ab22048;Abcam, Cambridge, MA, USA) or rat anti-CD11b (1:200, ab8878;Abcam, Cambridge, MA, USA). Neurons were incubated with mouse anti-tubulin (1:400, MAB1637; Millipore, Billerica, MA, USA). Alexa 488 and Alexa 568 secondary fluorescent antibodies (1:400, Invitrogen, Carlsbad, CA, USA) were used for one hour at 37°C, and the nuclei were stained with 4',6-diamidino-2-phenylindole(DAPI) for ten minutes. The cells were observed by confocal microscopy. The images were analyzed individually to evaluate TLR4 and CD11b co-expression, and the immunofluorescence intensity of TLR4 per field was determined using Image Pro-Plus 6.0 software(Media Cybernetics, Silver Spring, MD, USA). A negative (no antibody) control was included.

Western blot analysis

Protein was extracted from the cortex surrounding the injured area and cultured microglia or neurons using a protein extraction kit (P0027, Beyotime Biotech,Jiangsu, China). The lysate was separated by centrifugation at $12,000 \times g$ at 4°C for 15 minutes, and the supernatant was collected. The protein concentration was determined using a BCA assay kit (P0010, Beyotime Biotech, Jiangsu, China). Nuclear protein (for NF-κB p65) and other cytoplasmic proteins were diluted in the loading buffer and subjected to sodium dodecyl sulfate polyacrylamidegel electrophoresis(SDS-PAGE) followed by transfer to PVDF membranes. The membrane was blocked with 5% freshly prepared milk-TBST for two hours at room temperature and then incubated overnight at 4°C with the following primary antibodies: mouse anti-TLR4 (1:400, ab22048;Abcam, Cambridge, MA, USA), rabbit anti-MyD88 (1:400, ab2064;Abcam, Cambridge, MA, USA), mouse anti-NF-κB (1:400, sc-8008; Santa Cruz Biotechnology Inc., Santa Cruz, CA, USA), rabbit anti-cleaved caspase-3 (1:400, 9661; CST, Danvers, MA, USA), rabbit anti-IκB-α (1:400, sc-371; Santa Cruz Biotechnology Inc., Santa Cruz, CA, USA), mouse anti-phosphorylated-IκB-α (1:400, sc-8404; Santa Cruz Biotechnology Inc., Santa Cruz, CA, USA, USA) and β-actin (1:1,000, AA128; Beyotime Biotech, Jiangsu, China). After the membrane was washed in TBST, it was incubated in the appropriate AP-conjugated secondary antibody (diluted 1:2,000 in secondary antibody dilution buffer) for one hour at 37°C.

Protein bands were visualized by nickel-intensified DAB solution according to previous reports [30]. The β-actin antibody was used as an internal standard. The optical densities of the detected proteins were obtained using Image Pro-Plus software 6.0 (Media Cybernetics, Silver Spring, MD, USA).

Enzyme-linked immunosorbent assay (ELISA)

Brain tissue in the cerebral cortex around the injured area was collected and homogenized. The homogenates were centrifuged at 4°C at $12,000 \times g$ for 15 minutes, and supernatants were collected carefully and evaluated in duplicate using IL-1β, IL-6, TNF-α, MCP (monocyte chemoattractant protein)-1 and RANTES (regulated upon activation, normal T cell expressed and secreted) assay kits (R&D Systems, Minneapolis, MN, US), in accordance with the manufacturer's guidelines. Tissue cytokine concentrations are expressed as picograms per milligram of protein.

Cell culture supernatants were carefully collected at 24 hours after stimulation with LPS and centrifuged at 4°C at $12,000 \times g$ for 15 minutes. Cytokine concentrations were evaluated using protein assay kits (R&D Systems, Minneapolis, MN, US), in accordance with the manufacturer's guidelines. Cell cytokine concentrations are expressed as picograms per milliliter.

FJB histochemistry

Fluoro-Jade B (FJB) is a polyanionic fluorescein derivative that binds with high sensitivity and specificity to degenerating neurons. FJB staining of brain sections was performed as previously described with slight modifications [31]. Briefly, selected sections were first incubated in a solution of 1% NaOH in 80% ethanol for five minutes and then rehydrated in 70% ethanol and distilled water for two minutes each. The sections were then incubated in 0.06% $KMnO_4$ for ten minutes, rinsed in distilled water for two minutes and incubated in a 0.0004% solution of FJB (Chemicon, Temecula, CA, USA) for 20 minutes. Sections were observed and photographed under a confocal microscope.

TUNEL staining

The TUNEL assay was performed using a commercial kit that labels DNA strand breaks with fluorescein isothiocyanate (FITC; *In Situ* Cell Death Detection Kit, Roche Molecular Biochemicals, Mannheim, Germany). Selected sections were pretreated with 20 mg/mL proteinase-K in 10 mM Tris-HCl at 37°C for 15 minutes. These sections were then rinsed in PBS and incubated in 0.3% hydrogen peroxide dissolved in anhydrous methanol for ten minutes. The sections were then incubated in 0.1% sodium citrate and 0.1% Triton X-100 solution for two minutes at 2 to 8°C. After several washes with PBS, sections were incubated with 50 μL of TUNEL reaction mixture with terminal deoxynucleotidyltransferase (TdT) for 60 minutes at 37°C under humidified conditions, and neuronal nuclei were stained with DAPI. Each section was observed and photographed under a confocal microscope. Negative controls were obtained by omitting the TdT enzyme.

Statistical analysis

All data are presented as the mean ± SD. SPSS 11.5 was used for statistical analysis of the data. Two-way repeated-measures ANOVAs with LSD *posthoc* tests were used to determine statistical significance between behavioral measures. One-way ANOVAs with the appropriate LSD *posthoc* tests were used to compare experimental groups. For all analyses, $P < 0.05$ was considered significant.

Results

Time-dependent protein expression of TLR4

A coronal brain slice showed an obvious cavity in the injured cortex, which was surrounded by hemorrhage. The tissue examined in the experiment is indicated by a box in the figure (Figure 1A). Basal TLR4 expression was low in the sham control brains. The expression of TLR4 was significantly increased in the injured tissue at six hours post-trauma ($P < 0.05$) and reached a maximum at 24 hours ($P < 0.01$); thereafter, it decreased but remained high through 72 hours post-TBI ($P < 0.05$) (Figure 1B).

TLR4 deficiency attenuated neurological deficit, cerebral edema, cytokine release and cell death post-trauma

To confirm the role of TLR4 in TBI, TLR4$^{-/-}$ mice were used to investigate cerebral edema, neurological function impairment and the release of cytokines post-trauma in comparison with WT mice. The neurological deficit score of TLR4$^{-/-}$ mice was significantly lower than that of WT mice at 24 hours post-trauma ($P < 0.05$, Figure 1C). The brain water content of TLR4$^{-/-}$ mice was also significantly lower than that of WT mice at 24 hours post-trauma ($P < 0.05$, Figure 2A). Moreover, the IL-1β, IL-6, MCP-1 and RANTES protein concentrations in the injured brain tissue, as determined by ELISA, were also significantly decreased in TLR4$^{-/-}$ mice compared with WT mice ($P < 0.05$, Figure 2B, C, E, F), but the TNF-α concentration was not significantly different between TLR4$^{-/-}$ and WT mice ($P > 0.05$, Figure 2D). In addition, neuronal and apoptotic cell death were alleviated in TLR4$^{-/-}$ mice. Both FJB-positive cells with neuronal morphology and TUNEL-positive cells were evident 24 hours post-trauma in the pericontusional tissue (Figure 1D, E). The number of TUNEL-positive cells increased dramatically around the injured tissue in the TBI groups at 24 hours post-trauma. However, significantly fewer TUNEL-positive cells were

found in TLR4$^{-/-}$ mice than in WT mice ($P < 0.05$, Figure 1F). Furthermore, TLR4$^{-/-}$ mice also had significantly fewer FJB-positive neurons in the pericontusional tissue when compared with WT mice ($P < 0.05$, Figure 1G).

Downregulation of TLR4 expression by curcumin treatment post-trauma

Because TLR4 deficiency resulted in neuroprotection, we next examined the effects of curcumin on TLR4 protein expression. We administered different concentrations of curcumin (50, 100, or 200 mg/kg) to mice fifteen minutes post-TBI and examined TLR4 expression 24 hours post-trauma. The administration of 50 mg/kg curcumin did not significantly reduce TLR4 expression compared with TBI alone ($P > 0.05$, Figure 3A). In contrast, 100 mg/kg or 200 mg/kg curcumin significantly reduced TLR4 expression ($P < 0.01$ versus TBI alone), but TLR4 expression did not significantly differ between these two groups ($P > 0.05$). Accordingly, 100 mg/kg was selected due to the dramatic reduction of TLR4 expression and the relatively low concentration of curcumin.

Neuroprotection of curcumin post-trauma

Curcumin attenuated cerebral edema and improved neurological function following TBI. The neurological deficit scores were significantly lower in curcumin-treated mice than in vehicle-treated mice at 24 hours post-trauma ($P < 0.05$, Figure 3B). Brain water content was significantly decreased in curcumin-treated mice when compared with vehicle-treated mice at 24 hours post-trauma ($P < 0.05$, Figure 3C). In addition, curcumin reduced neuronal and apoptotic cell death. Both FJB-positive cells with neuronal morphology and TUNEL-positive cells were evident 24 hours post-trauma in the pericontusional tissue (Figure 3D, E). The number of TUNEL-positive cells was increased dramatically around the injured tissue in the TBI groups at 24 hours post-trauma. Significantly fewer TUNEL-positive cells were found in curcumin-treated mice than in vehicle-treated mice ($P < 0.05$, Figure 3F). Furthermore, curcumin-treated mice also had significantly fewer FJB-positive neurons in the pericontusional tissue than did the vehicle-treated group ($P < 0.05$, Figure 3G).

Curcumin inhibited the activation of TLR4-positive microglia/macrophages and inflammatory mediator release in injured tissue

In the pericontusional tissue of sham control mice, a few quiescent microglia with small cell bodies and fine, ramified processes were observed 24 hours post-trauma. Few or no TLR4-positive microglia were detected. However, many activated TLR4-positive microglia/macrophages (CD11b-positive cells) with large cell bodies and thickened, short processes were observed post-trauma. These

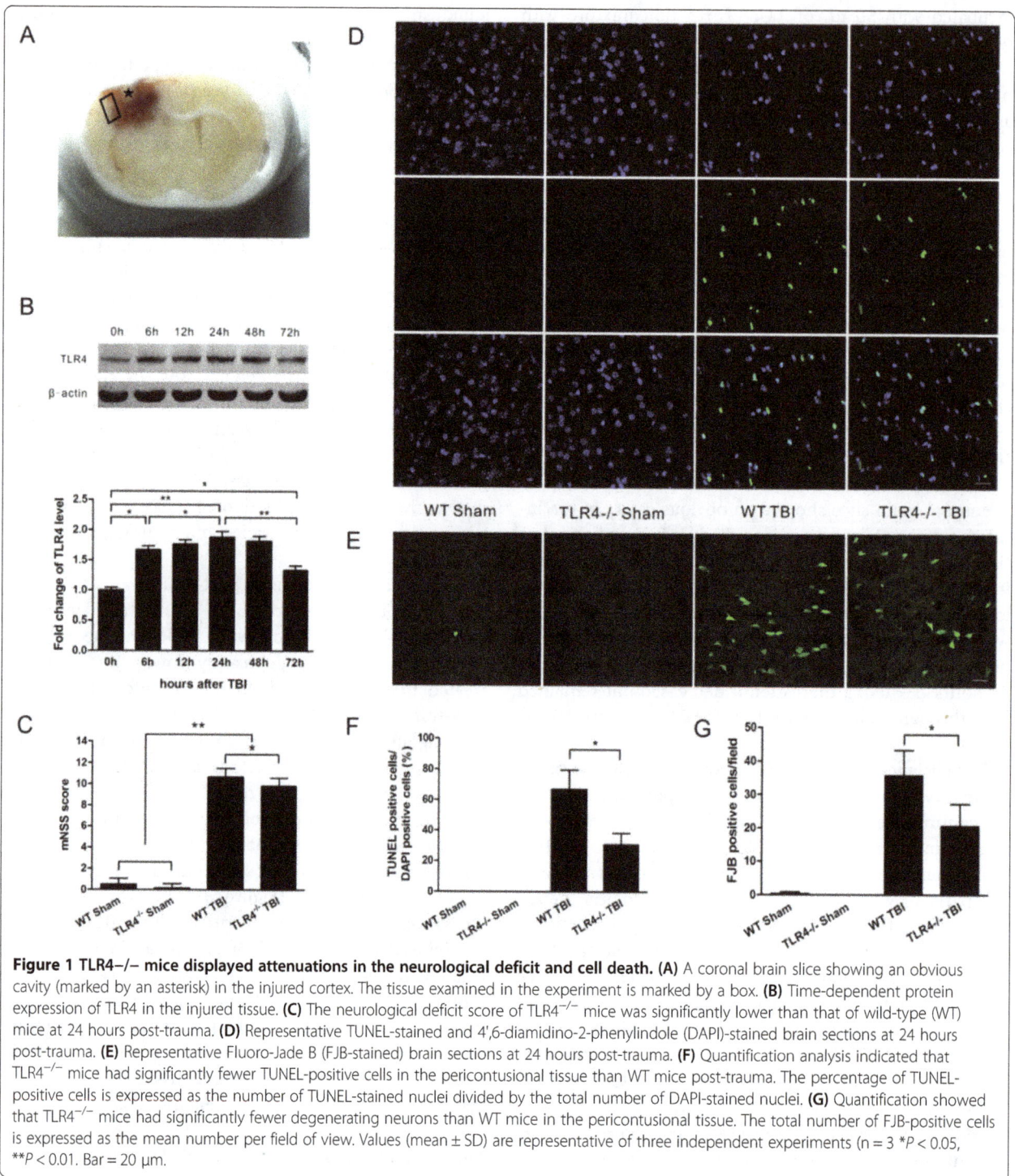

Figure 1 TLR4−/− mice displayed attenuations in the neurological deficit and cell death. (A) A coronal brain slice showing an obvious cavity (marked by an asterisk) in the injured cortex. The tissue examined in the experiment is marked by a box. **(B)** Time-dependent protein expression of TLR4 in the injured tissue. **(C)** The neurological deficit score of TLR4$^{-/-}$ mice was significantly lower than that of wild-type (WT) mice at 24 hours post-trauma. **(D)** Representative TUNEL-stained and 4′,6-diamidino-2-phenylindole (DAPI)-stained brain sections at 24 hours post-trauma. **(E)** Representative Fluoro-Jade B (FJB-stained) brain sections at 24 hours post-trauma. **(F)** Quantification analysis indicated that TLR4$^{-/-}$ mice had significantly fewer TUNEL-positive cells in the pericontusional tissue than WT mice post-trauma. The percentage of TUNEL-positive cells is expressed as the number of TUNEL-stained nuclei divided by the total number of DAPI-stained nuclei. **(G)** Quantification showed that TLR4$^{-/-}$ mice had significantly fewer degenerating neurons than WT mice in the pericontusional tissue. The total number of FJB-positive cells is expressed as the mean number per field of view. Values (mean ± SD) are representative of three independent experiments (n = 3 *$P < 0.05$, **$P < 0.01$. Bar = 20 μm.

microglia/macrophages exhibited robust TLR4 immuno-reactivity (Figure 4A). The administration of 100 mg/kg curcumin inhibited the increase in TLR4-positive microglia/macrophages post-trauma ($P < 0.05$, Figure 4B), although microglia/macrophages still exhibited reactive morphology. Moreover, the concentrations of inflammatory mediators (IL-1β, IL-6, TNF-α, MCP-1 and RANTES) in the injured brain tissue, determined using ELISA, were significantly increased in the two TBI groups when compared with the two sham groups ($P < 0.01$), and these mediators were all dramatically decreased in curcumin-treated mice when compared with vehicle-treated mice, with the exception of IL-6 ($P < 0.05$, Figure 4C-G).

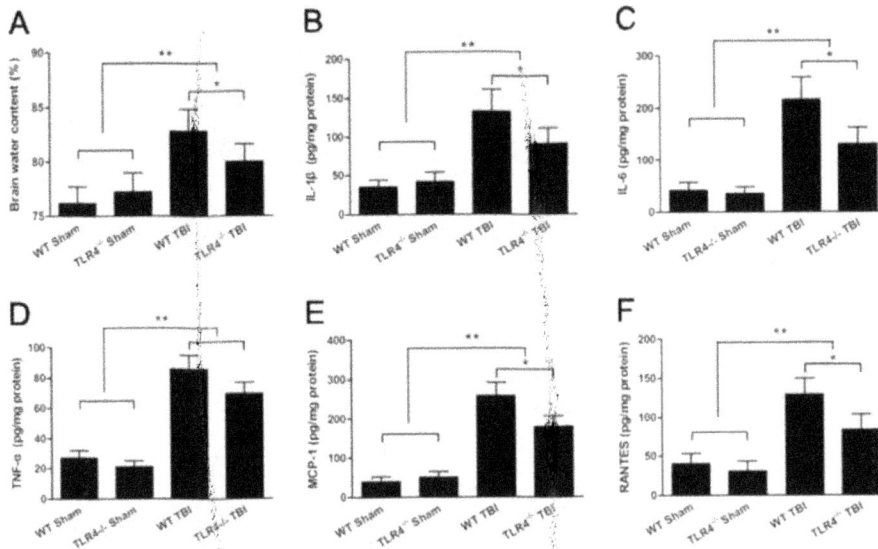

Figure 2 TLR4⁻/⁻mice displayed attenuated brain edema and neuroinflammation post-trauma. (A) TLR4⁻/⁻ mice displayed decreased brain water content compared with WT mice. ELISA showed a change in the release of IL-1β, IL-6, TNF-α, MCP-1 and RANTES **(B, C, D, E, F)** in TLR4⁻/⁻ mice brain tissue 24 hours post-trauma. Values (mean ± SD) are representative of three independent experiments (n = 3 mice/group). *$P < 0.05$, **$P < 0.01$.

Curcumin suppressed protein expression in the TLR4/MyD88/NF-κB signaling pathway *in vivo*

Western blotting showed that TLR4 and MyD88 protein expression in the injured tissue was increased dramatically in the TBI groups when compared with the sham control groups ($P < 0.01$) and that it was significantly lower in curcumin-treated mice than in vehicle-treated mice at 24 hours post-trauma ($P < 0.05$, Figure 5A). NF-κB p65 and p-IκB-α protein expression in the injured tissue was also increased dramatically in the TBI groups but was significantly decreased in curcumin-treated mice compared to the vehicle-treated mice at 24 hours post-trauma ($P < 0.05$, Figure 5B). In contrast, IκB-α protein expression was decreased in the TBI groups but was significantly increased in curcumin-treated mice when compared with vehicle-treated mice at 24 hours post-trauma ($P < 0.05$, Figure 5B).

Curcumin reduced neuronal damage induced by LPS *in vitro*

To directly observe the interaction of microglia and neurons, we used a transwell co-culture system including primary neurons and microglia and stimulated the cells with LPS. Microglia were plated onto the transparent polyester membrane of the transwell inserts, and neurons were placed on the wells below the polyester membrane; as a result, the microglia grown on the transwells were separated from the neuron-enriched cultures by the permeable transwell membrane (Figure 6A). To determine the optimal concentration of curcumin for cell co-culture, 0.5, 1, 2, 5 and 10 μM were applied

separately. The administration of 10 μM curcumin significantly reduced microglial viability compared with the no-curcumin control ($P < 0.05$), whereas the cell viability in the 0.5, 1, 2 and 5 μM curcumin treatment groups did not significantly differ from that in the control group ($p > 0.05$, Figure 6B). However, 5 and 10 μM curcumin both significantly reduced neuronal viability when compared with the no-curcumin control ($P < 0.05$, Figure 6B). Accordingly, 2 μM was chosen as the optimal concentration for the transwell co-culture system.

We then examined neuronal damage under various conditions. The protein levels of cleaved caspase-3 in neurons were significantly increased 24 hours after LPS stimulation ($P < 0.01$), and the protein level in co-cultured neurons was significantly higher than that in the single-culture group ($P < 0.05$). In the co-culture groups, curcumin treatment after LPS administration significantly decreased the upregulation of cleaved caspase-3 ($P < 0.05$). In contrast, in the single-culture groups, curcumin treatment after LPS stimulation did not significantly decrease the upregulation of cleaved caspase-3 ($P > 0.05$, Figure 6C). Similar results were observed using immunofluorescence. At 24 hours after LPS administration, many neuronal bodies and processes were destroyed or no longer evident, and more serious neuronal damage was observed in the co-culture group than in the single-culture group. However, when the cells were treated with curcumin after LPS stimulation, less serious neuronal damage was observed in the co-culture groups, whereas no marked change in neuronal damage was observed in the single-culture groups (Figure 6D).

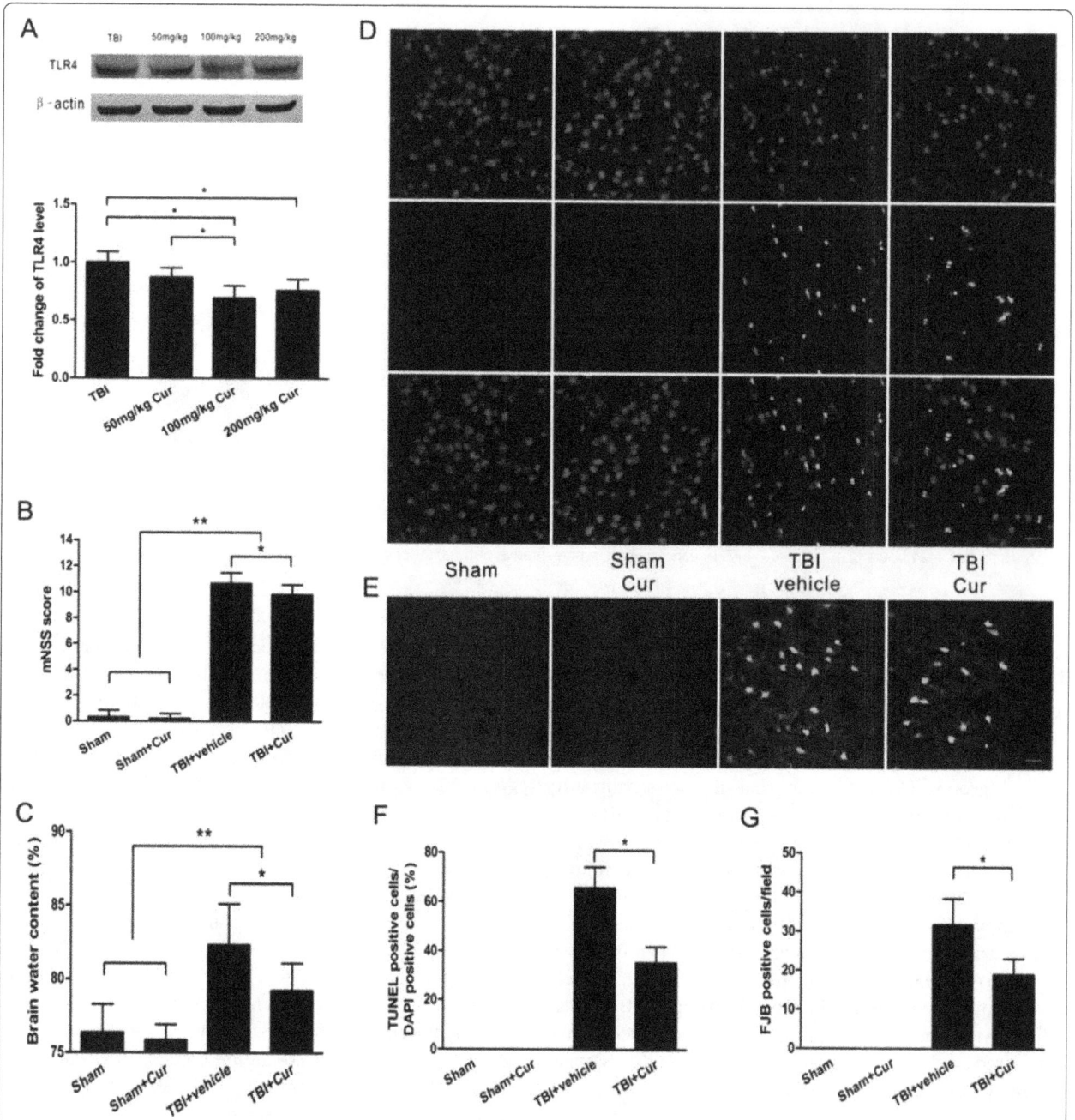

Figure 3 Curcumin attenuated brain injury post-trauma. (A) The effect of different concentrations of curcumin on TLR4 expression in injured tissue at 24 hours post-trauma. Curcumin treatment decreased the neurological deficit scores **(B)** and brain water content **(C)**. **(D)** Representative TUNEL-stained and 4',6-diamidino-2-phenylindole (DAPI)-stained brain sections at 24 hours post-trauma. **(E)** Representative Fluoro-Jade B (FJB)-stained brain sections at 24 hours post-trauma. **(F)** Quantification analysis indicated that curcumin-treated mice had significantly fewer TUNEL-positive cells in the pericontusional tissue than vehicle-treated mice. The percentage of TUNEL-positive cells is expressed as the number of TUNEL-stained nuclei divided by the total number of DAPI-stained nuclei. **(G)** Quantification showed that curcumin-treated mice had significantly fewer degenerating neurons than vehicle-treated mice in the pericontusional tissue. The total number of FJB-positive cells is expressed as the mean number per field of view. Values (mean ± SD) are representative of two independent experiments (n = 6 mice/group). *$P < 0.05$, **$P < 0.01$. Bar = 20 μm.

Curcumin attenuated the microglial activation and inflammatory mediator release induced by LPS *in vitro*

In the transwell co-culture experiments, LPS stimulation induced a reactive state in the microglia, which was demonstrated by a larger cell body and thickened, shorter processes, and these microglia also showed robust TLR4 immunofluorescence intensity. In contrast, in cells treated with curcumin after LPS stimulation, a less reactive state of the microglia and lower TLR4 immunofluorescence intensity were observed (Figure 7A, B). We next characterized

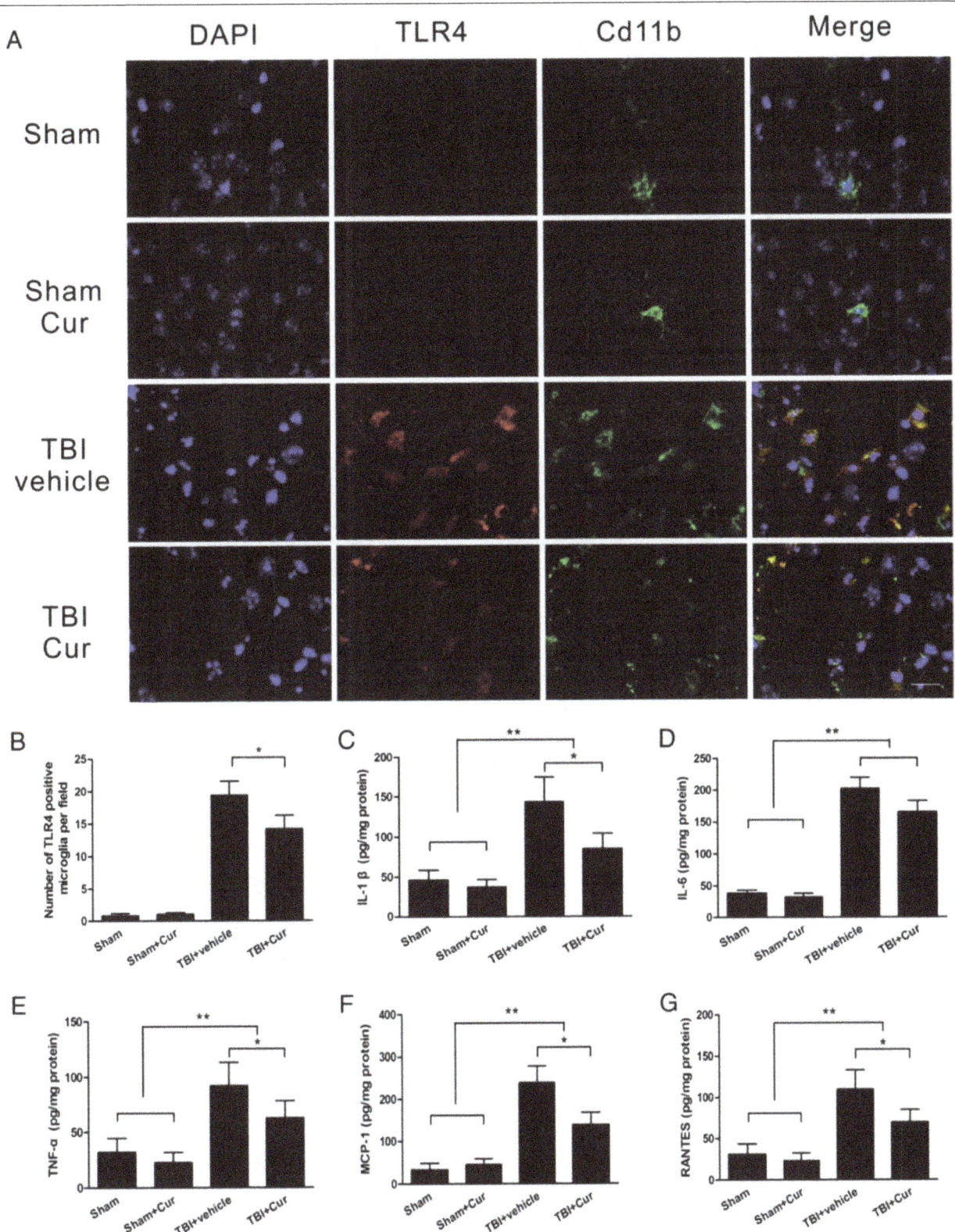

Figure 4 (See legend on next page.)

(See figure on previous page.)
Figure 4 Curcumin decreased neuroinflammation and the activation of CD11b-positive cells co-labeled with TLR4 post-trauma. (A)
Representative CD11b-positive cells co-labeled with TLR4 in the pericontusional tissue at 24 hours post-trauma. **(B)** Quantification showed that
curcumin-treated mice had significantly fewer CD11b-positive cells co-labeled with TLR4 in the pericontusional tissue than vehicle-treated mice.
The total number of CD11b-positive cells co-labeled with TLR4 is expressed as the mean number per field of view. ELISA showed that curcumin
treatment resulted in a change in the release of IL-1β, IL-6, TNF-α, MCP-1 and RANTES **(C, D, E, F, G)** at 24 hours post-trauma. Values (mean ± SD)
are representative of two independent experiments (n = 6 mice/group). *$P < 0.05$, **$P < 0.01$. Bar = 20 μm.

the release of inflammatory mediators in the co-culture supernatants by ELISA. These mediators were all increased
dramatically 24 hours after LPS stimulation ($P < 0.01$), but
only IL-1β, IL-6 and RANTES were significantly decreased
in the curcumin-treated group compared with the vehicle-
treated group ($P < 0.05$, Figure 7C, D, G); the differences in
TNF-α and MCP-1 between the curcumin-treated group

and the vehicle-treated group were not significant following
LPS stimulation ($P > 0.05$, Figure 7E, F).

Curcumin suppressed microglial TLR4/MyD88/NF-κB signaling pathway protein expression *in vitro*

To further understand the effect of curcumin treatment
on TLR4 downstream signaling pathways in microglia,

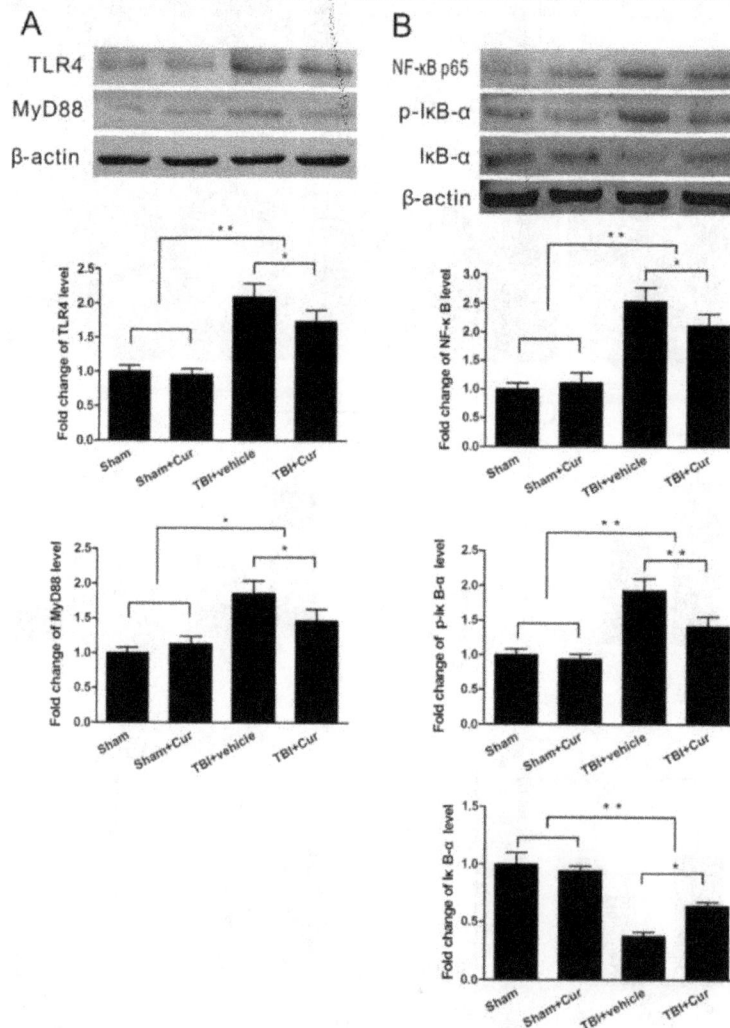

Figure 5 Curcumin suppressed TLR4/MyD88/NF-κB signaling pathway protein expression *in vivo*. (A) TLR4 and MyD88 protein expression
in the injured tissue was significantly lower in curcumin-treated mice than in vehicle-treated mice at 24 hours post-trauma. **(B)** NF-κB p65 and
p-IκB-α protein expression in the injured tissue was also significantly lower in curcumin-treated mice than in vehicle-treated mice at 24 hours
post-trauma. In contrast, IκB-α protein expression was significantly higher in curcumin-treated mice than in vehicle-treated mice post-trauma.
Values (mean ± SD) are representative of three independent experiments (n = 3 mice/group). *$P < 0.05$, **$P < 0.01$.

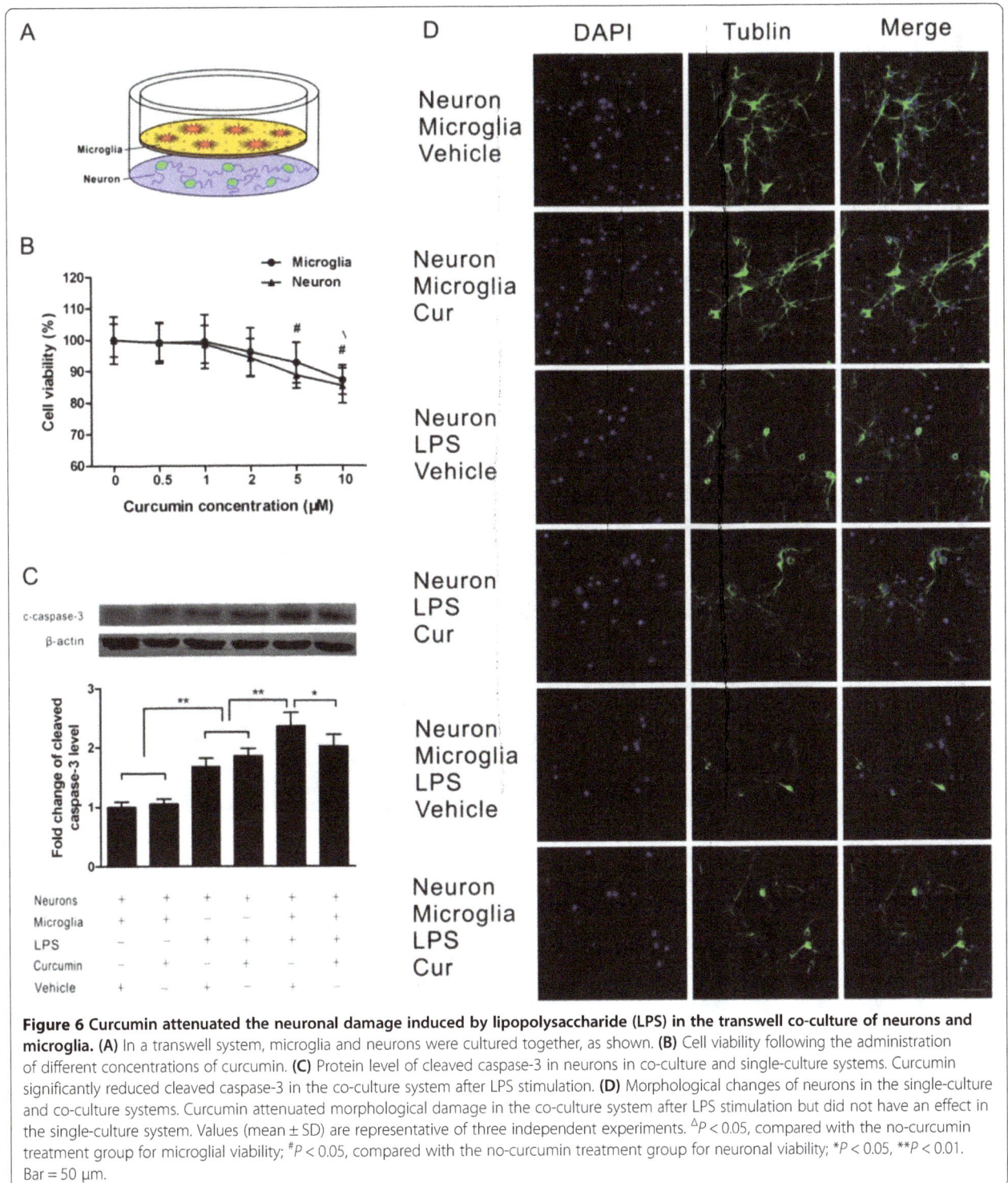

Figure 6 Curcumin attenuated the neuronal damage induced by lipopolysaccharide (LPS) in the transwell co-culture of neurons and microglia. (A) In a transwell system, microglia and neurons were cultured together, as shown. **(B)** Cell viability following the administration of different concentrations of curcumin. **(C)** Protein level of cleaved caspase-3 in neurons in co-culture and single-culture systems. Curcumin significantly reduced cleaved caspase-3 in the co-culture system after LPS stimulation. **(D)** Morphological changes of neurons in the single-culture and co-culture systems. Curcumin attenuated morphological damage in the co-culture system after LPS stimulation but did not have an effect in the single-culture system. Values (mean ± SD) are representative of three independent experiments. $^{\Delta}P < 0.05$, compared with the no-curcumin treatment group for microglial viability; $^{\#}P < 0.05$, compared with the no-curcumin treatment group for neuronal viability; $^{*}P < 0.05$, $^{**}P < 0.01$. Bar = 50 μm.

Western blotting was performed to detect the expression of TLR4 and its adapter proteins at 24 hours post-trauma. In the transwell co-cultures of primary neurons and microglia stimulated by LPS, the levels of TLR4 and MyD88 protein expression in microglia were significantly increased compared with those in the two control groups ($P < 0.01$); further, they were significantly decreased in the curcumin-treated group compared with the vehicle-treated group following LPS stimulation ($P < 0.05$, Figure 8A). Similar changes in p-IκB-a and NF-κB p65 were observed. In contrast, IκB-a protein expression was significantly decreased in the two LPS-

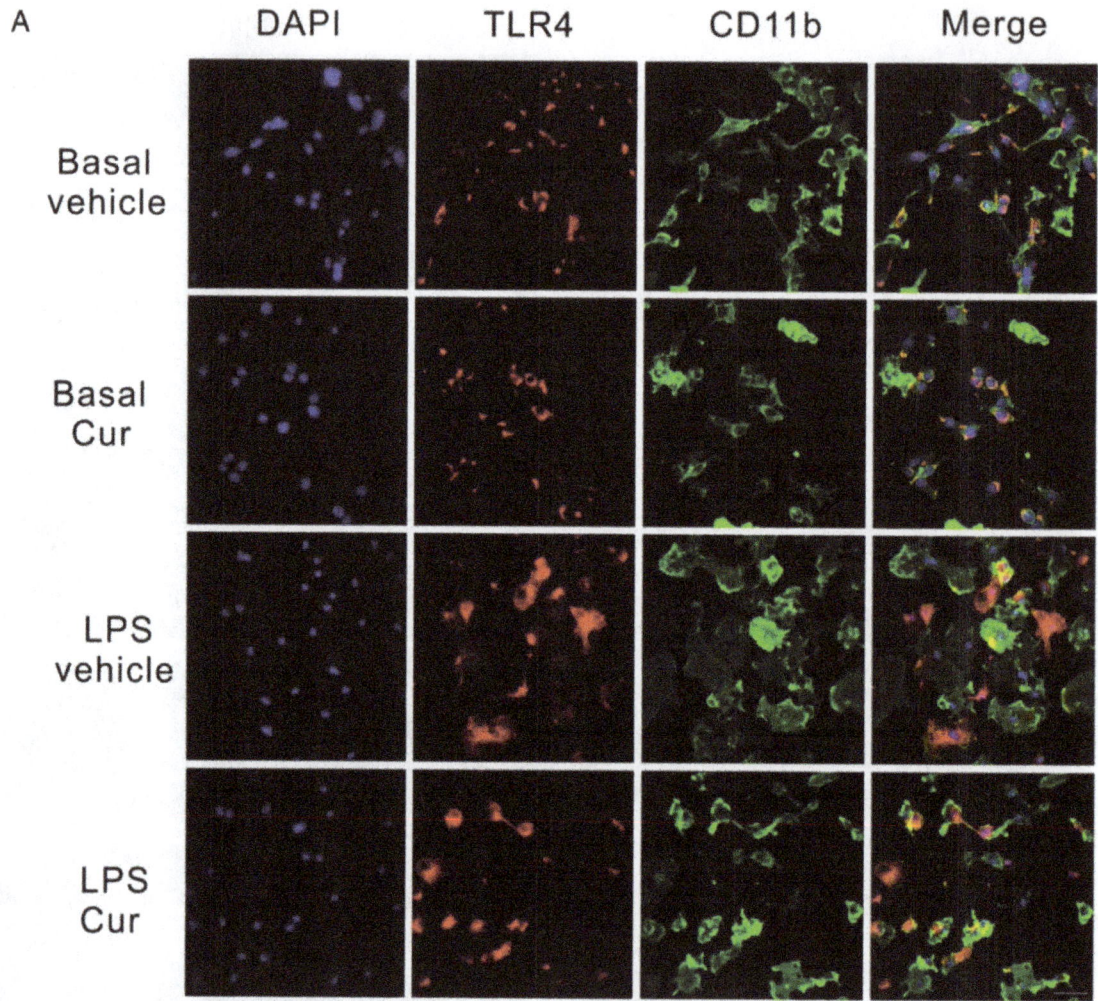

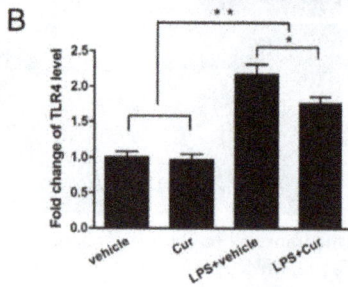

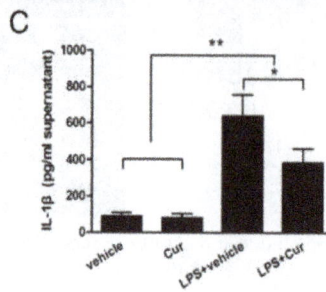

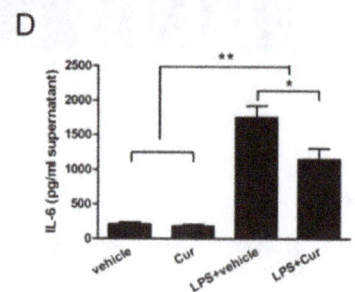

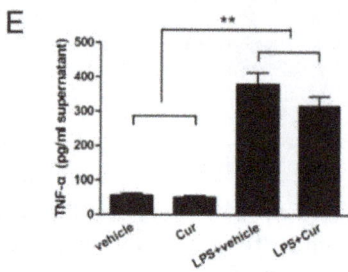

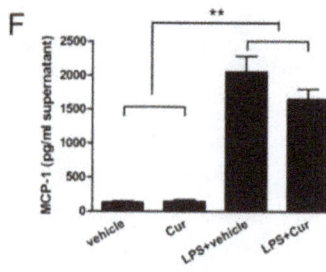

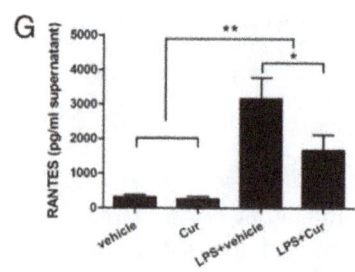

Figure 7 (See legend on next page.)

(See figure on previous page.)
Figure 7 Curcumin reduced microglial activation and inflammatory mediator release induced by lipopolysaccharide (LPS) in the transwell co-culture of neurons and microglia. (A) Colocalization of CD11b and TLR4 was evident. Treatment with curcumin after LPS stimulation resulted in a less reactive state of the microglia, as shown. **(B)** TLR4 immunofluorescence intensity in microglia was also reduced after curcumin treatment. ELISA showed that curcumin-treated cells had a change in the release of IL-1β, IL-6, TNF-α, MCP-1 and RANTES **(C, D, E, F, G)** at 24 hours after LPS administration. Values (mean ± SD) are representative of three independent experiments. *$P < 0.05$, **$P < 0.01$. Bar = 50 μm.

stimulated groups when compared with the two control groups ($P < 0.05$) and was significantly increased in the curcumin-treated group when compared with the vehicle-treated group following LPS stimulation ($P < 0.05$, 8B).

Discussion

In this study, we used TLR4$^{-/-}$ mice to investigate the role of TLR4 during the acute stage of TBI and observed reductions in cerebral edema, neurological deficit and neuronal apoptosis at 24 hours post-injury in TLR4$^{-/-}$ mice compared with WT mice. We administered curcumin (100 mg/kg) to WT mice after TBI and observed decreases in microglia/macrophages, inflammatory factor release, neurological deficit and neuronal apoptosis at 24 hours post-injury by inhibiting the TLR4/MyD88/NF-κB signaling cascade. *In vitro*, in a co-culture system of microglial and neuronal cells, LPS administration induced microglial activation and neuronal damage, while 2 μM curcumin could inhibit microglial activation and neuronal apoptosis by suppressing the microglial TLR4 signaling pathway. To our knowledge, we report for the first time that one possible molecular mechanism whereby curcumin attenuates brain injury is the modulation of acute neuroinflammation mediated by the TLR4/MyD88/NF-κB signaling pathway in microglia/macrophages during experimental TBI.

One key factor in secondary brain injury is a complex series of inflammatory responses that is initiated largely through TLRs that possibly interact with endogenous ligands released from damaged cells [32,33]. Furthermore, TLR4, which is widely expressed on the plasma membranes of neural cells, has been demonstrated to play an important role in initiating the cerebral inflammation related to cerebral ischemia-reperfusion injury and intracerebral hemorrhage in TLR4$^{-/-}$ mice [34,35]. Along these lines, neuroinflammatory responses initiated by TLR4 may also be an important factor underlying secondary brain injury after TBI. Indeed, TLR4 protein expression was significantly increased at six hours after brain trauma and remained high at 72 hours compared with the levels observed in the control group in our study, which is consistent with the report of Chen and colleagues [36]. Furthermore, a critical role of TLR4 was demonstrated by our observations that brain water content, neurological deficit score and neuronal death were significantly decreased in TLR4$^{-/-}$ mice in comparison

to WT mice suffering a similar severity of head trauma. The neuroprotective effect of TLR4 deficiency in TBI can be partially attributed to the suppression of acute neuroinflammation induced by the inhibition of microglial or peripheral leukocyte activation and the subsequent cytokine release. In Helmy's clinical study, the release of many cytokines, such as IL-1β, TNF-α and RANTES, peaked at 24 hours post-trauma, and notably, the concentrations of some cytokines (for example, IL-1β, IL-6, MCP-1) were significantly higher in brain tissue than in plasma [37]. In the present study, the upregulation of IL-1β, IL-6, MCP-1 and RANTES in injured brain tissue was dramatically attenuated in injured TLR4$^{-/-}$ mice, although TNF-α was not significantly decreased. Some anti-inflammatory therapies aimed at inhibiting TLR4 activation have displayed neuroprotective effects at 24 hours in animal TBI models [38,39]. Recently, another study of TBI, which showed lower infarct volumes and better outcomes on neurological and behavioral tests in TLR4$^{-/-}$ mice at 24 hours post-injury, has also validated the important role of TLR4 in TBI [10].

We focused on curcumin, which is used as a spice or a pigment, because of its numerous pharmacological activities, very low toxicity and widespread availability. Unfortunately, curcumin exhibits relatively poor oral bioavailability and a short serum half-life (< 45 minutes), which could contribute to its limited therapeutic window (less than one hour post-injury) in head trauma [17,40]. One study reported that in mice, peak plasma concentrations (approximately 1.6 μM) were achieved 15 minutes after the intraperitoneal administration of 100 mg/kg curcumin, followed by brain accumulation within one hour [41]. A much better curcumin bioavailability has been reported in many articles following intraperitoneal injection [41-43]. Thus, we chose an intraperitoneal injection at 15 minutes post-trauma in our study because of the better bioavailability and the limited effective window of curcumin. A 100 mg/kg dose was selected due to its dramatic reduction of TLR4 expression at 24 hours and the relatively low concentration in the three different concentrations administered to mice. In addition, the use of liposomes or nanoparticles may improve drug delivery, overcome bioavailability issues and extend the therapeutic window [40].

In TBI experiments, cognitive disability tested by the Morris water maze has been ameliorated by treatment

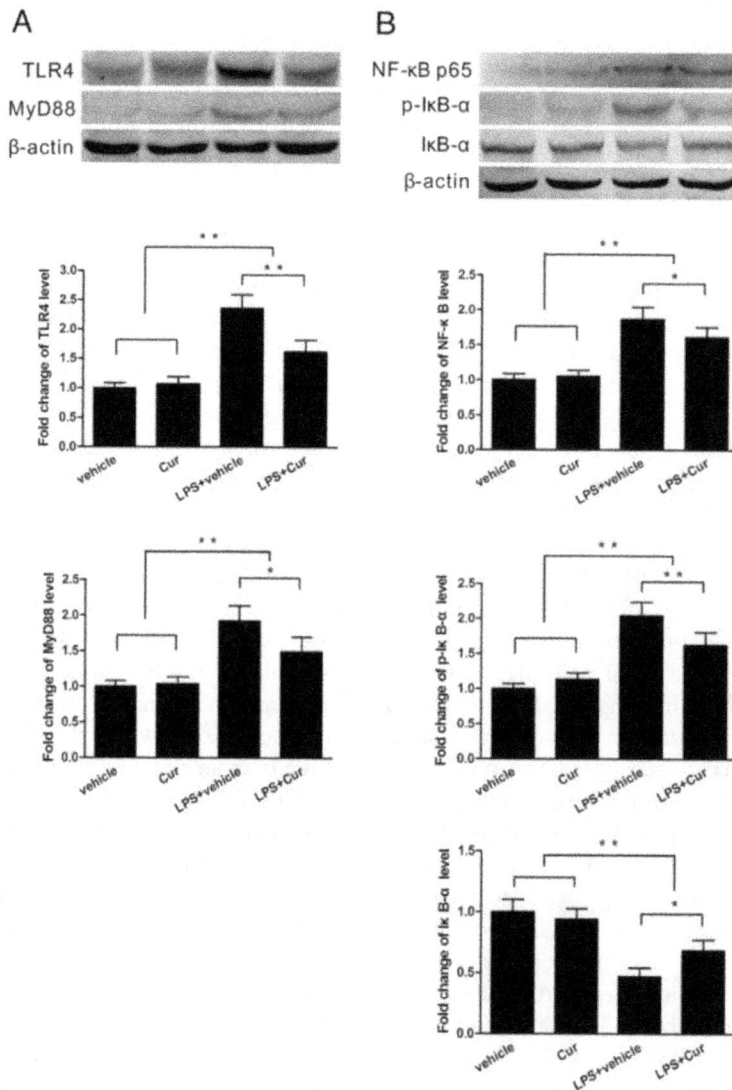

Figure 8 Curcumin suppressed the expression of proteins in the microglial TLR4/MyD88/NF-κB signaling pathway in co-culture system.
(A) TLR4 and MyD88 protein expression in microglia was significantly lower in the curcumin-treated group than in the vehicle-treated group at 24 hours after lipopolysaccharide (LPS) stimulation. **(B)** NF-κB p65 and p-IκB-α protein expression in microglia was also significantly lower in the curcumin-treated group than in the vehicle-treated group at 24 hours following LPS stimulation. In contrast, IκB-α protein expression was significantly higher in the curcumin-treated group than in the vehicle-treated group after LPS stimulation. Values (mean ± SD) are representative of three independent experiments. *$P < 0.05$, **$P < 0.01$.

with curcumin or curcumin derivatives [16,44]; the cognitive protection conferred by curcumin is partially related to the restoration of membrane homeostasis or to normalized levels of brain-derived neurotrophic factor (BDNF) and its downstream effectors of synaptic plasticity (cAMP-response element binding protein, synapsin1). In addition to the cognitive functions described above, locomotor function and brain edema have also been improved with curcumin treatment due to the decrease in the induction of NF-κB and its downstream production of IL-1β in the brain [17]. In mice with intracerebral hemorrhage, the attenuation of hematoma size and neurological injury was also associated with the

decreased induction of cytokine expression after curcumin treatment [45]. These findings suggest that immune modulation by curcumin is a promising approach to the treatment of brain injury. Furthermore, TLR4, a critical membrane receptor mediating innate immunity, can induce NF-κB upregulation when it is activated by stimuli [46]. Therefore, for immunomodulation following TBI, TLR4 may be an important target of curcumin. Notably, Youn *et al.* have demonstrated that the TLR4 receptor complex is a molecular target of curcumin and that curcumin can inhibit TLR4 homodimerization [20]. In the present study, the upregulation of TLR4 expression and inflammatory mediator release (IL-1β, TNF-α, MCP-1 and RANTES) was attenuated by curcumin treatment following TBI. Among these mediators, RANTES has been suggested as a significant early marker of severe TBI in critically injured trauma patients [47]. Furthermore, the curcumin-treated group, which exhibited suppressed acute inflammatory responses after TBI, showed ameliorated brain damage, including reduced neurological impairment, brain edema and neuronal and apoptotic cell death. Thus, curcumin could reduce TLR4-mediated post-traumatic acute neuroinflammation, thereby attenuating secondary brain injury. A few studies have also reported that curcumin can attenuate inflammation and subsequent inflammatory injury by inhibiting TLR4 expression in colitis [48], hepatic fibrosis [49] and lung injury [50]. Within the TLR4 signaling pathway, the MyD88-dependent signaling pathway is an important activator of NF-κB and the subsequent regulatory effects of NF-κB signaling [51,52]. In accordance with these reports, the levels of MyD88 and NF-κB were observed to decrease following curcumin administration. These data suggest that the protective effects of curcumin on the brain against excessive inflammatory responses may be mediated by the TLR4/MyD88/NF-κB signaling cascade following TBI.

Microglia, which when activated by exogenous or endogenous ligands produce a number of proinflammatory cytokines implicated in neurotoxicity, are the principal cells involved in the innate immune response in the CNS [53]. In the present study, CD11b-positive cells were reduced in injured brain tissue following curcumin treatment. However, CD11b positivity does not imply that these cells are exclusively microglia; CD11b-positive cells can also include monocytes/macrophages and lymphocytes, which permeated the injured tissue. Peripheral immune infiltration and alterations can also have a significant impact in TBI [54]. However, microglia were our primary interest, and we therefore used a transwell co-culture system with microglia and neurons to further investigate the role of microglia in immunomodulation.

In our experiments *in vitro*, LPS resulted in obvious neuronal damage in both the single-culture and co-culture systems. However, the observation that the damage was more serious in neurons co-cultured with microglia indicates that microglia play an important role in neuronal injury. This was consistent with another report [55], in which low concentrations of LPS induced significant neuronal death in a co-culture system that allowed direct microglial-neuronal contact; however, high concentrations of LPS were necessary to induce neurotoxicity in a transwell system permitting only cell contact-independent communication. Nevertheless, the critical role of microglia in neuronal damage was evident.

Curcumin treatment dramatically alleviated neuronal damage in the co-culture system but had no obvious effect in neuron-only cell culture after LPS stimulation.

These results suggest that the protective effect of curcumin on neurons was mediated through microglia. Similarly, a previous study showed that curcumin protected dopaminergic neurons from MPP+-induced neurotoxicity in rat mid-brain neuron-glia co-cultures and that the protective effect of curcumin disappeared in microglia-depleted cultures [56]. Furthermore, curcumin had an inhibitory effect on microglial migration in a BV-2 cell scratch model and transwell migration model [57]. The TLR-induced activation of microglia and the release of proinflammatory molecules are responsible for neurotoxic processes in the course of some CNS diseases [58,59]. In the present transwell co-culture system, curcumin treatment inhibited TLR4 expression in microglia, the morphological activation of microglia and inflammatory mediator release following LPS stimulation, and these findings are consistent with the observed attenuated neuronal damage. These *in vitro* observations suggest that the inhibition of microglial TLR4 may be one reason underlying the suppression of neuroinflammation and the protection of neurons following curcumin treatment. In regard to the TLR4 pathway, one study reported that a functional TLR4/MyD88 cascade in microglia was essential for neuronal injury induced by HSP60 via the co-culture of WT neurons with MyD88[−/−] or Lps[d] microglia (hyporesponsiveness to LPS as a consequence of a point mutation rendering the cytosolic domain of TLR4 incapable of signal transduction) [60]. In another study of rat vascular smooth muscle cells (VSMCs), curcumin suppressed the LPS-induced overexpression of inflammatory mediators in VSMCs by inhibiting the TLR4/NF-κB pathway [24]. In our co-culture system including primary WT neurons and microglial cells, the protein levels of TLR4 and downstream molecules (MyD88, p-IκB-α and NF-κB) in microglia were increased by LPS, and curcumin attenuated the upregulation of these molecules in the TLR4 pathway. These data further indicate that curcumin regulates a complex series of inflammatory responses contributing to neuronal damage, in part through the microglial TLR4/MyD88/NF-κB signaling pathway.

Interestingly, in contrast to LPS administration after brain injury, LPS preconditioning protected the brain from ischemic injury through the redirection of TLR4 signaling, including the suppression of NF-κB activity, enhancement of interferon regulatory factor 3 (IRF3) activity and an increase in anti-inflammatory/type I interferon gene expression [61,62]. In TBI, LPS preconditioning has also been shown to confer a long-lasting neuroprotective effect associated with the modulation of microglia/macrophage activity and cytokine production [63]. In a study of cold-induced cortical injury, microglial activation in response to peripheral LPS preconditioning largely depended on nonhematogenous TLR4 receptors, and these activated microglia resulted in reduced inhibitory axosomatic synapses for neuroprotection [64]. The role of the microglial TLR4 signaling pathway in this type of neuroprotection warrants further investigation. Notably, immune modulation by curcumin is robust, and the TLR4 signaling pathway may not be an exclusive mechanism through which curcumin modulates neuroinflammation and contributes to secondary brain injury. However, modulation of the TLR4 pathway was undeniably critical for the neuroprotection mediated by curcumin post-TBI.

In conclusion, our findings demonstrated a critical role for TLR4 of microglia/macrophages in acute neuroinflammation following TBI. Post-injury treatment with curcumin attenuated TLR4-mediated acute activation of microglia/macrophages, proinflammatory mediator release and neuronal apoptosis in the injured brain tissue via inhibition of the MyD88/NF-κB signaling cascade, and this may be an important mechanism through which curcumin improves outcome following TBI. All the data support modulation of the TLR4/MyD88/NF-κB signaling pathway in microglia/macrophages as a potential therapeutic target in TBI and suggest that curcumin should be considered a candidate for clinical trials in TBI.

Abbreviations
BDNF: brain-derived neurotrophic factor; DAMP: damage-associated molecular pattern; DAPI: 4',6-diamidino-2-phenylindole; DMSO: dimethyl sulfoxide; DMEM: Dulbecco's modified Eagle's medium; ELISA: Enzyme-Linked Immunosorbent Assay; FJB: Fluoro-Jade B; IRF3: interferon regulatory factor 3; HBSS: Hank's balanced saline solution; LPS: lipopolysaccharide; MCP: monocyte chemoattractant protein; MTT: 3-(4,5-dimethylthiazol-2-yl)-2,5- diphenyltetrazolium bromide; MyD88: myeloid differentiation factor 88; NF-κB: nuclear factor-kappa B; PAMP: pathogen-associated molecular pattern; PBS: phosphate-buffered saline; PRR: pathogen-recognition receptors; RANTES: regulated upon activation, normal T cell expressed and secreted; SDS-PAGE: sodium dodecyl sulfate polyacrylamidegel electrophoresis; TBI: traumatic brain injury; TdT: terminal deoxynucleotidyltransferase; TLR: Toll-like receptor; TNF-α: tumor necrosis factor alpha; VSMC: vascular smooth muscle cell; WT: wild-type.

Competing interests
The authors declare that they have no competing interests.

Authors' contributions
This study was based on the original idea of JKL and HF. HTZ and CB carried out the molecular biology and morphological studies and drafted the manuscript. XX and FC carried out the behavioral studies. JCY and CSW performed data analyses. JKL and HTZ were responsible for supervising all experiments, data analyses and the drafting of the manuscript. WHC read and revised the manuscript. All authors read and approved the final manuscript.

Acknowledgments
We gratefully thank MD Peng-fei Wang and MD Huang Fang for their generous assistance. This work was supported by the National Science Foundation of China (NSFC, number 81070979, 81000531) and National '973' Project of China (2014CB541605).

Author details
[1]Department of Neurosurgery, Southwest Hospital, Third Military Medical University, 30 Gaotanyan Street, Chongqing 400038, China. [2]Department of Neurobiology, Third Military Medical University, 30 Gaotanyan Street, Chongqing 400038, China.

References
1. Maas AI, Stocchetti N, Bullock R: Moderate and severe traumatic brain injury in adults. Lancet Neurol 2008, 7:728–741.
2. Xiong Y, Mahmood A, Chopp M: Animal models of traumatic brain injury. Nat Rev Neurosci 2013, 14:128–142.
3. Helmy A, De Simoni MG, Guilfoyle MR, Carpenter KL, Hutchinson PJ: Cytokines and innate inflammation in the pathogenesis of human traumatic brain injury. ProgNeurobiol 2011, 95:352–372.
4. Ziebell JM, Morganti-Kossmann MC: Involvement of pro- and anti-inflammatory cytokines and chemokines in the pathophysiology of traumatic brain injury. Neurotherapeutics 2010, 7:22–30.
5. Takeuchi O, Akira S: Pattern recognition receptors and inflammation. Cell 2010, 140:805–820.
6. Lin Q, Li M, Fang D, Fang J, Su SB: The essential roles of Toll-like receptor signaling pathways in sterile inflammatory diseases. Int Immunopharmacol 2011, 11:1422–1432.
7. Carpentier PA, Duncan DS, Miller SD: Glial toll-like receptor signaling in central nervous system infection and autoimmunity. Brain Behav Immun 2008, 22:140–147.
8. Fang H, Wang PF, Zhou Y, Wang YC, Yang QW: Toll-like receptor 4 signaling in intracerebral hemorrhage-induced inflammation and injury. J Neuroinflammation 2013, 10:27.
9. Hyakkoku K, Hamanaka J, Tsuruma K, Shimazawa M, Tanaka H, Uematsu S, Akira S, Inagaki N, Nagai H, Hara H: Toll-like receptor 4 (Tlr4), but not Tlr3 or Tlr9, knock-out mice have neuroprotectiveeffects against focal cerebral ischemia. Neuroscience 2010, 171:258–267.
10. Ahmad A, Crupi R, Campolo M, Genovese T, Esposito E, Cuzzocrea S: Absence of TLR4 reduces neurovascular unit and secondary inflammatory process after traumatic brain injury in mice. PLoS One 2013, 8:e57208.
11. Li GZ, Zhang Y, Zhao JB, Wu GJ, Su XF, Hang CH: Expression of myeloid differentiation primary response protein 88 (Myd88) in the cerebral cortex after experimental traumatic brain injury in rats. Brain Res 2011, 1396:96–104.
12. Wang X, Stridh L, Li W, Dean J, Elmgren A, Gan L, Eriksson K, Hagberg H, Mallard C: Lipopolysaccharide sensitizes neonatal hypoxic-ischemic brain injury in a MyD88-dependent manner. J Immunol 2009, 183:7471–7477.
13. Agarwal NB, Jain S, Agarwal NK, Mediratta PK, Sharma KK: Modulation of pentylenetetrazole-induced kindling and oxidative stress by curcumin in mice. Phytomedicine 2011, 18:756–759.
14. Yang F, Lim GP, Begum AN, Ubeda OJ, Simmons MR, Ambegaokar SS, Chen PP, Kayed R, Glabe CG, Frautschy SA, Cole GM: Curcumin inhibits formation of amyloid beta oligomers and fibrils, binds plaques, and reduces amyloid in vivo. J BiolChem 2005, 280:5892–5901.
15. Heger M, Van Golen RF, Broekgaarden M, Michel MC: The molecular basis for the pharmacokinetics and pharmacodynamics of curcumin and its metabolites in relation to cancer. Pharmacol Rev 2014, 66:222–307.
16. Sharma S, Ying Z, Gomez-Pinilla F: A pyrazolecurcumin derivative restores membrane homeostasis disrupted after brain trauma. Exp Neurol 2010, 226:191–199.
17. Laird MD, Sukumari-Ramesh S, Swift AE, Meiler SE, Vender JR, Dhandapani KM: Curcumin attenuates cerebral edema following traumatic brain injury in mice: a possible role for aquaporin-4? J Neurochem 2010, 113:637–648.
18. Wu A, Ying Z, Schubert D, Gomez-Pinilla F: Brain and spinal cord interaction: a dietary curcumin derivative counteracts locomotor and cognitive deficits after brain trauma. Neurorehabil Neural Repair 2011, 25:332–342.
19. Sharma S, Zhuang Y, Ying Z, Wu A, Gomez-Pinilla F: Dietary curcumin supplementation counteracts reduction in levels of molecules involved in energy homeostasis after brain trauma. Neuroscience 2009, 161:1037–1044.
20. Youn HS, Saitoh SI, Miyake K, Hwang DH: Inhibition of homodimerization of Toll-like receptor 4 by curcumin. Biochem Pharmacol 2006, 72:62–69.
21. Zhao L, Lee JY, Hwang DH: Inhibition of pattern recognition receptor-mediated inflammation by bioactive phytochemicals. Nutr Rev 2011, 69:310–320.
22. Zeng Z, Zhan L, Liao H, Chen L, Lv X: Curcumin improves TNBS-induced colitis in rats by inhibiting IL-27 expression via the TLR4/NF-kappaB signaling pathway. Planta Med 2013, 79:102–109.
23. Tu CT, Han B, Yao QY, Zhang YA, Liu HC, Zhang SC: Curcumin attenuates Concanavalin A-induced liver injury in mice by inhibition of Toll-like

receptor (TLR) 2, TLR4 and TLR9 expression. *Int Immunopharmacol* 2012, **12**:151–157.

24. Meng Z, Yan C, Deng Q, Gao DF, Niu XL: Curcumin inhibits LPS-induced inflammation in rat vascular smooth muscle cells *in vitro* via ROS-relative TLR4-MAPK/NF-kappaB pathways. *Acta Pharmacol Sin* 2013, **34**:901–911.

25. Chearwae W, Bright JJ: 15-deoxy-Delta(12,14)-prostaglandin J(2) and curcumin modulate the expression of toll-like receptors 4 and 9 in autoimmune T lymphocyte. *J Clin Immunol* 2008, **28**:558–570.

26. Feeney DM, Boyeson MG, Linn RT, Murray HM, Dail WG: Responses to cortical injury: I. Methodology and local effects of contusions in the rat. *Brain Res* 1981, **211**:67–77.

27. Chen SF, Hsu CW, Huang WH, Wang JY: Post-injury baicalein improves histological and functional outcomes and reduces inflammatory cytokines after experimental traumatic brain injury. *Br J Pharmacol* 2008, **155**:1279–1296.

28. Roof RL, Duvdevani R, Heyburn JW, Stein DG: Progesterone rapidly decreases brain edema: treatment delayed up to 24 hours is still effective. *Exp Neurol* 1996, **138**:246–251.

29. Carlson NG, Rojas MA, Black JD, Redd JW, Hille J, Hill KE, Rose JW: Microglial inhibition of neuroprotection by antagonists of the EP1 prostaglandin E2 receptor. *J Neuroinflammation* 2009, **6**:5.

30. Bian C, Zhu K, Yang L, Lin S, Li S, Su B, Zhang J: Gonadectomy differentially regulates steroid receptor coactivator-1 and synaptic proteins in the hippocampus of adult female and male C57BL/6 mice. *Synapse* 2012, **66**:849–857.

31. Schmued LC, Hopkins KJ: Fluoro-Jade B: a high affinity fluorescent marker for the localization of neuronal degeneration. *Brain Res* 2000, **874**:123–130.

32. Lee H, Lee S, Cho IH, Lee SJ: Toll-like receptors: sensor molecules for detecting damage to the nervous system. *Curr Protein Pept Sci* 2013, **14**:33–42.

33. Hanke ML, Kielian T: Toll-like receptors in health and disease in the brain: mechanisms and therapeutic potential. *Clin Sci (Lond)* 2011, **121**:367–387.

34. Lin S, Yin Q, Zhong Q, Lv FL, Zhou Y, Li JQ, Wang JZ, Su BY, Yang QW: Heme activates TLR4-mediated inflammatory injury via MyD88/TRIF signaling pathway in intracerebral hemorrhage. *J Neuroinflammation* 2012, **9**:46.

35. Yang QW, Lu FL, Zhou Y, Wang L, Zhong Q, Lin S, Xiang J, Li JC, Fang CQ, Wang JZ: HMBG1 mediates ischemia-reperfusion injury by TRIF-adaptor independent Toll-like receptor 4 signaling. *J Cereb Blood Flow Metab* 2011, **31**:593–605.

36. Chen CC, Hung TH, Wang YH, Lin CW, Wang PY, Lee CY, Chen SF: Wogonin improves histological and functional outcomes, and reduces activation of TLR4/NF-kappaB signaling after experimental traumatic brain injury. *PLoS One* 2012, **7**:e30294.

37. Helmy A, Carpenter KL, Menon DK, Pickard JD, Hutchinson PJ: The cytokine response to human traumatic brain injury: temporal profiles and evidence for cerebral parenchymal production. *J Cereb Blood Flow Metab* 2011, **31**:658–670.

38. Mao SS, Hua R, Zhao XP, Qin X, Sun ZQ, Zhang Y, Wu YQ, Jia MX, Cao JL, Zhang YM: Exogenous administration of PACAP alleviates traumatic brain injury in rats through a mechanism involving the TLR4/MyD88/NF-kappaB pathway. *J Neurotrauma* 1941–1959, **2012**:29.

39. Chen G, Zhang S, Shi J, Ai J, Qi M, Hang C: Simvastatin reduces secondary brain injury caused by cortical contusion in rats: possible involvement of TLR4/NF-kappaB pathway. *Exp Neurol* 2009, **216**:398–406.

40. Anand P, Kunnumakkara AB, Newman RA, Aggarwal BB: Bioavailability of curcumin: problems and promises. *Mol Pharm* 2007, **4**:807–818.

41. Pan MH, Huang TM, Lin JK: Biotransformation of curcumin through reduction and glucuronidation in mice. *Drug Metab Dispos* 1999, **27**:486–494.

42. Ravindranath V, Chandrasekhara N: Absorption and tissue distribution of curcumin in rats. *Toxicology* 1980, **16**:259–265.

43. Shoba G, Joy D, Joseph T, Majeed M, Rajendran R, Srinivas PS: Influence of piperine on the pharmacokinetics of curcumin in animals and human volunteers. *Planta Med* 1998, **64**:353–356.

44. Wu A, Ying Z, Gomez-Pinilla F: Dietary curcumin counteracts the outcome of traumatic brain injury on oxidative stress, synaptic plasticity, and cognition. *Exp Neurol* 2006, **197**:309–317.

45. King MD, McCracken DJ, Wade FM, Meiler SE, Alleyne CH Jr, Dhandapani KM: Attenuation of hematoma size and neurological injury with curcumin following intracerebral hemorrhage in mice. *J Neurosurg* 2011, **115**:116–123.

46. Covert MW, Leung TH, Gaston JE, Baltimore D: Achieving stability of lipopolysaccharide-induced NF-kappaB activation. *Science* 1854–1857, **2005**:309.

47. Lumpkins K, Bochicchio GV, Zagol B, Ulloa K, Simard JM, Schaub S, Meyer W, Scalea T: Plasma levels of the beta chemokine regulated upon activation, normal T cell expressed, and secreted (RANTES) correlate with severe brain injury. *J Trauma* 2008, **64**:358–361.

48. Lubbad A, Oriowo MA, Khan I: Curcumin attenuates inflammation through inhibition of TLR-4 receptor in experimental colitis. *Mol Cell Biochem* 2009, **322**:127–135.

49. Tu CT, Yao QY, Xu BL, Wang JY, Zhou CH, Zhang SC: Protective effects of curcumin against hepatic fibrosis induced by carbon tetrachloride: modulation of high-mobility group box 1, Toll-like receptor 4 and 2 expression. *Food ChemToxicol* 2012, **50**:3343–3351.

50. Liu K, Shen L, Wang J, Dong G, Wu H, Shao H, Jing H: The preventative role of curcumin on the lung inflammatory response induced by cardiopulmonary bypass in rats. *J Surg Res* 2012, **174**:73–82.

51. Buchanan MM, Hutchinson M, Watkins LR, Yin H: Toll-like receptor 4 in CNS pathologies. *J Neurochem* 2010, **114**:13–27.

52. Barton GM, Medzhitov R: Toll-like receptor signaling pathways. *Science* 2003, **300**:1524–1525.

53. Rivest S: Regulation of innate immune responses in the brain. *Nat Rev Immunol* 2009, **9**:429–439.

54. Walker PA, Shah SK, Jimenez F, Aroom KR, Harting MT, Cox CS Jr: Bone marrow-derived stromal cell therapy for traumatic brain injury is neuroprotective via stimulation of non-neurologic organ systems. *Surgery* 2012, **152**:790–793.

55. Zujovic V, Taupin V: Use of cocultured cell systems to elucidate chemokine-dependent neuronal/microglial interactions: control of microglial activation. *Methods* 2003, **29**:345–350.

56. Yang S, Zhang D, Yang Z, Hu X, Qian S, Liu J, Wilson B, Block M, Hong JS: Curcumin protects dopaminergic neuron against LPS induced neurotoxicity in primary rat neuron/glia culture. *Neurochem Res* 2044–2053, **2008**:33.

57. Karlstetter M, Lippe E, Walczak Y, Moehle C, Aslanidis A, Mirza M, Langmann T: Curcumin is a potent modulator of microglial gene expression and migration. *J Neuroinflammation* 2011, **8**:125.

58. Lehnardt S: Innate immunity and neuroinflammation in the CNS: the role of microglia in Toll-like receptor-mediated neuronal injury. *Glia* 2010, **58**:253–263.

59. Yao L, Kan EM, Lu J, Hao A, Dheen ST, Kaur C, Ling EA: Toll-like receptor 4 mediates microglial activation and production of inflammatory mediators in neonatal rat brain following hypoxia: role of TLR4 in hypoxic microglia. *J Neuroinflammation* 2013, **10**:23.

60. Lehnardt S, Schott E, Trimbuch T, Laubisch D, Krueger C, Wulczyn G, Nitsch R, Weber JR: A vicious cycle involving release of heat shock protein 60 from injured cells and activation of toll-like receptor 4 mediates neurodegeneration in the CNS. *J Neurosci* 2008, **28**:2320–2331.

61. Vartanian KB, Stevens SL, Marsh BJ, Williams-Karnesky R, Lessov NS, Stenzel-Poore MP: LPS preconditioning redirects TLR signaling following stroke: TRIF-IRF3 plays a seminal role in mediating tolerance to ischemic injury. *J Neuroinflammation* 2011, **8**:140.

62. Marsh B, Stevens SL, Packard AE, Gopalan B, Hunter B, Leung PY, Harrington CA, Stenzel-Poore MP: Systemic lipopolysaccharide protects the brain from ischemic injury by reprogramming the response of the brain to stroke: a critical role for IRF3. *J Neurosci* 2009, **29**:9839–9849.

63. Longhi L, Gesuete R, Perego C, Ortolano F, Sacchi N, Villa P, Stocchetti N, De Simoni MG: Long-lasting protection in brain trauma by endotoxin preconditioning. *J Cereb Blood Flow Metab* 1919–1929, **2011**:31.

64. Chen Z, Jalabi W, Shpargel KB, Farabaugh KT, Dutta R, Yin X, Kidd GJ, Bergmann CC, Stohlman SA, Trapp BD: Lipopolysaccharide-induced microglial activation and neuroprotection against experimental brain injury is independent of hematogenous TLR4. *J Neurosci* 2012, **32**:11706–11715.

7

Trovafloxacin attenuates neuroinflammation and improves outcome after traumatic brain injury in mice

Charu Garg[1], Joon Ho Seo[1], Jayalakshmi Ramachandran[1], Ji Meng Loh[2], Frances Calderon[1*] and Jorge E. Contreras[1*]

Abstract

Background: Trovafloxacin is a broad-spectrum antibiotic, recently identified as an inhibitor of pannexin-1 (Panx1) channels. Panx1 channels are important conduits for the adenosine triphosphate (ATP) release from live and dying cells that enhances the inflammatory response of immune cells. Elevated extracellular levels ATP released upon injury activate purinergic pathways in inflammatory cells that promote migration, proliferation, phagocytosis, and apoptotic signals. Here, we tested whether trovafloxacin administration attenuates the neuroinflammatory response and improves outcomes after brain trauma.

Methods: The murine controlled cortical impact (CCI) model was used to determine whether in vivo delivery of trovafloxacin has anti-inflammatory and neuroprotective actions after brain trauma. Locomotor deficit was assessed using the rotarod test. Levels of tissue damage markers and inflammation were measured using western blot, qPCR, and immunofluorescence. In vitro assays were used to evaluate whether trovafloxacin blocks ATP release and cell migration in a chemotactic-stimulated microglia cell line.

Results: Trovafloxacin treatment of CCI-injured mice significantly reduced tissue damage markers and improved locomotor deficits. In addition, trovafloxacin treatment significantly reduced mRNA levels of several pro-inflammatory cytokines (IL-1β, IL-6, and TNF-α), which correlates with an overall reduction in the accumulation of inflammatory cell types (neutrophils, microglia/macrophages, and astroglia) at the injury zone. To determine whether trovafloxacin exerted these effects by direct action on immune cells, we evaluated its effect on ATP release and cell migration using a chemotactic-stimulated microglial cell line. We found that trovafloxacin significantly inhibited both ATP release and migration of these cells.

Conclusion: Our results show that trovafloxacin administration has pronounced anti-inflammatory and neuroprotective effects following brain injury. These findings lay the foundation for future studies to directly test a role for Panx1 channels in pathological inflammation following brain trauma.

Keywords: Brain injury, Neuroinflammation, Microglia, Pannexin, Hemichannel

* Correspondence: calderfr@njms.rutgers.edu; contrejo@njms.rutgers.edu
[1]Department of Pharmacology, Physiology and Neurosciences, New Jersey Medical School, Rutgers University, 185 South Orange Ave, Newark, NJ 07103, USA
Full list of author information is available at the end of the article

Background

Trovafloxacin is a fluoroquinolone antibiotic that exerts bactericidal activity by inhibiting prokaryotic topoisomerase enzymes, which are important for cellular division [1]. Recently, trovafloxacin was demonstrated to target human pannexin 1 (Panx1) channels at therapeutic concentrations reached in blood plasma [2]. Studies in mice have shown that Panx1 inhibition by trovafloxacin leads to dysregulated fragmentation of dying cells and blockade of ATP release [2]. Panx1 channels are large transmembrane pores that, besides ions, are permeable to small molecules such as ATP; they are expressed in various cell types [3, 4]. Recently, Panx1 channels have emerged as important players in response to injury and inflammation [5–7]. ATP release via Panx1 channels enhances inflammatory responses in peripheral immune cells and is implicated in the activation of the inflammasome [4, 6, 8]. Additionally, Panx1 channels expressed in endothelial cells can regulate the acute vascular inflammation by potentiating leukocyte emigration via ATP release [9]. In the brain, neuronal Panx1 channel activation during ischemia or cortical spreading depression is thought to be an important mechanism for mediating neuronal dysfunction and death [10–13]. Although it is likely that Panx1 channels also contribute to neuroinflammatory responses upon brain injury, their potential as therapeutic targets in traumatic brain injury (TBI) remains elusive.

The primary damage induced by mechanical brain trauma results in necrotic death of neurons, glial cells, and blood vessels [14–16]. The dying tissue produces damage-associated molecular pattern molecules (DAMPs, including ATP), which initiate and maintain an inflammatory response. The neuroinflammatory response is characterized by activation and migration of microglia and glial cells, leukocyte infiltration, and upregulation of inflammatory mediators [17, 18]. Elevated extracellular levels of ATP released upon injury have been shown to enhance the inflammatory response [19, 20]. ATP activates the purinergic pathway in inflammatory cells, thus playing an important role in migration, proliferation, phagocytosis, and apoptotic signals [21–24]. There is compelling evidence demonstrating that Panx1 channels, in part, represent a cellular mechanism for ATP release to the external milieu during inflammation [7, 25].

By taking advantage of previous work assessing the pharmacological properties of trovafloxacin in mice [2, 26, 27], we aimed to evaluate the potential role of trovafloxacin administration on curtailing inflammation in the controlled cortical impact (CCI) model of TBI. We found that in vivo administration of trovafloxacin significantly attenuated the inflammatory response in CCI injured mice. In addition, it decreased

tissue damage and improved locomotor deficits. Our results also indicate that trovafloxacin diminish the accumulation of microglia and macrophages at the injury zone. In vitro studies showed that trovafloxacin as well as other Panx1 channel blockers inhibited ATP release and cell migration of a stimulated microglia cell line. We propose that a reduced number of pro-inflammatory cells at the injury site in trovafloxacin treated mice might be related to lesser migration and could contribute to improve outcomes after TBI.

Methods

Animal handling and CCI

All procedures were performed in accordance with the institutional guidelines and approved by the Institutional Animal Care and Use Committee of Rutgers-New Jersey Medical School. C57BL/6 mice (Charles River, USA) were housed two per cage during pre- and postoperative procedures with a 12-h light-dark cycle with ad libitum access to water and chow.

Ten-week-old-male mice were subjected to CCI injury using the stereotaxic impactor Impact One™ (Leica Biosystems, USA). Animals were secured in a stereotaxic frame and anesthetized with isoflurane (induction at 3% and maintenance at 2%) administered through a nose mask. A midline incision was made over the skull. A unilateral craniectomy was performed between Bregma and Lambda using a hand drill with a 5-mm-diameter trephine. Special care was taken to prevent any damage to the dura mater, therefore assuring it was intact after each craniotomy. Animals were impacted using a 4.0-mm stainless steel flat impactor tip, at stereotaxic coordinates AP − 2.26, ML + 2.0 and 0.65 mm deep at a rate of 4.0 m/s and a dwell time of 200 ms, at an angle of 0.4°. After injury, any bleeding was cleaned up, the incision was sutured with clips, and the animals were immediately removed from anesthesia. Post-surgery, the mouse was placed on its back in a cage, which was set over a heating pad. The recovery of each mouse was observed until they were standing on their four paws. Sham animals went through the same procedures as CCI-injured animals, including anesthesia and skin incision over the skull, but not craniotomy, as it has been shown that the craniotomy procedure alone stimulates production of pro-inflammatory cytokines at 24 h after surgery [28], which would confound our analyses. The stock of trovafloxacin (100 mM) was prepared in DMSO and was then diluted to 1:10 in saline. Trovafloxacin-treated group was given intraperitoneal injections of 60 mg/kg at 1, 24, and 48 h post-CCI injury. Non-treated CCI-injured animals received vehicle only.

Total RNA extraction, reverse transcription, and real-time PCR (RT-qPCR)

Injured cortex was carefully dissected from the ipsilateral hemisphere using an adult mouse brain slicer. Total RNA was isolated using Trizol (Thermo Fisher scientific, USA) according to the manufacturer's protocol. Two micrograms of RNA was reverse transcribed using High Capacity RNA-to-cDNA kit (Thermo Fisher scientific, USA). TaqMan® Universal PCR Master Mix and TaqMan® FAM™ conjugated primers (Thermo Fisher Scientific, USA) were used to evaluate mRNA using the ABI 7500 Sequence Detection System (Applied Biosystems, USA). mRNA expression was normalized to GAPDH as endogenous control, and the relative fold difference in expression was calculated using the comparative $2^{-\Delta\Delta CT}$, a widely used method to present relative expression respect to controls (shams) [29, 30]. The following primer genes were assessed: IL-1β (Accession#Mm00434228_m1), TNF-α (Accession#Mm00443258_m1), IL-6 (Accession #Mm00446190_m1), MPO (Accession #Mm01298424_m1), GAFP (Accession #Mm01253033_m1), CD68 (Accession #Mm03047343_m1), and Iba1 (Accession #Mm00520165_m1). GAPDH (Accession #Mm99999915_g1) was used as an endogenous control. The ΔΔCT method was used to calculate the relative gene expression levels respect to shams.

Total protein extraction and western blot analysis

Brain tissues enclosing the injury were carefully dissected from the ipsilateral cortex under a dissecting microscope and then homogenized in buffer containing M-PER Mammalian protein extraction reagent 5 mM Na_3VO_4, 1 mM NaF, 1 mM $Na_2P_2O_7$, 1 mM Bezamidine, 5 mM EDTA, and Halt Protease Inhibitor Cocktail (Thermo Fisher scientific, USA). Protein concentrations were estimated using a BCA kit (Pierce, USA). Equal amounts of protein (20 μg) per sample was separated on 4–20% gradient gels (Bio-Rad, USA) and run under the same experimental conditions, transferred to PVDF membranes, and probed with the following antibodies: GFAP (Cell Signaling, USA), CD68 (Abcam, USA), α–II spectrin (Santa Cruz Biotechnology, USA), MMP-9 (NeuroMab, USA), and GAPDH (Cell Signaling, USA). Blots were developed using enhanced chemiluminescence, and densitometric analysis was performed using Fuji Images or Bio-Rad Image Lab software.

Cell culture

BV-2 cell line was previously generated by others through infection of murine primary microglial cells with a v-raf/v-myc oncogene carrying retrovirus [31]. This cell line has been found to retain some of the morphological, phenotypical, and functional properties of freshly isolated microglial cells and is considered immortalized microglial cells [32]. BV-2 cells were seeded at a density of 7.5×10^5 cells/ml and maintained in DMEM/F-12 supplemented with 5% FBS, penicillin 100 IU/ml, and streptomycin 100 μg/mL. Cell cultures were kept in a cell incubator at 37 °C with 95% air and 5% CO_2 and saturated humidity.

ATP release measurements

Extracellular ATP release was measured using the ATP bioluminescence assay kit (Molecular Probe, USA) following the manufacturer's instructions. BV-2 cells were seeded in 24-well culture plates at a cell density of 1.5×10^5 cells/well in serum-free DMEM media supplemented with 4 mM L-glutamine. After 24 h, cells were treated with C5a (10 nM) in the presence or absence of Panx1 channel blockers trovafloxacin (1 μM), Brilliant Blue FCF (5μM) or ^{10}Panx1 (200 μM) in serum-free DMEM medium. Extracellular ATP was measured before C5a stimulation and every 10 min thereafter. At the indicated time points, 10 μl aliquots from a total volume of 300 μl were collected from the culture supernatants for ATP determinations.

Transmigration assay

Migration assay was performed using 24-well plates and 8.0-μm pore size transwell inserts (Corning Costar, NY, USA). BV-2 cells suspended in serum-free medium were seeded at a density of 1.5×10^5 cells/ml/well in the upper chamber of the transwell insert. Cells were allowed to attach overnight. Then, the cells were stimulated with C5a (10 nM) or ATP (200 μM) in the presence or absence of pannexin channel blockers trovafloxacin (1 μM), Brilliant Blue FCF (5μM) or ^{10}Panx1 (200 μM). At 4 or 24 h post treatment, cells were fixed with 4% paraformaldehyde (PFA) and stained with 0.05% crystal violet. BV-2 cells that did not migrate were removed from upper chamber by wiping with cotton swabs. Cells that migrated to the bottom of the filters were quantified from at least 5 images taken from different fields taken at 20× using an Olympus AX70 microscope.

Brain sample preparation for histology and immunofluorescence

For morphological analysis, CCI-injured mice were anesthetized with ketamine/xylazine at 6 days post-injury and transcardially perfused with RPMI media containing heparin (1000 USP units/ml) at a rate of 4 ml/min followed by 4% PFA in PBS, pH 7.4 at a rate of 5 ml/min. Once the animals were fixed, mice were decapitated and the whole brains were removed, taking care to keep the contusion region intact. After fixation, brains were immersed in 30% sucrose for 24 h and frozen – 80 °C until sectioning. Twenty micrometer coronal sections were made from whole brains using a cryostat.

Immunostaining

Brain sections were taken at room temperature for 20 min. Then, they were washed twice with tris buffer 1× (TBS), pH 7.4 and permeabilized with 0.3% triton X-100 in TBS in a humid chamber at room temperature for 30 min. Sections were washed again with TBS and incubated in TBS buffer containing 10% BSA, 10% Normal Donkey Serum, pH 7.4 (TDB) in humid chamber at room temperature for 1 h. Primary antibody against CD68 (Bio-Rad, USA) diluted 1:300 in TDB diluent containing 20% TDB solution, 0.2% triton X-100, and 80% TBS pH 7.4 were applied to the slides and kept in a humid chamber at 4 °C for 12 h. The sections were washed for 5 min in TBS and then incubated with secondary antibodies (Cy3™ or Alexa Fluor 488 Donkey Anti-Rabbit IgG) from Jackson Immunoresearch (West Grove, USA) diluted 1:300 in TDB diluent were applied on the sections at room temperature for 2 h. Tissue slides were washed with 1× TBS buffer for 5 min. Samples were counterstained with 4′,6-diamidino-2-phenylindole (DAPI) for nuclear staining at 1:10,000 dilution for 10 min at room temperature in a humid chamber. Slides were rinsed twice with 1× TBS for 5 min each. Glass cover slips were mounted on the samples on glass slides with fluorescent mounting medium containing anti-fade (Gelvatol containing DABCO). Slides were left to dry at room temperature for 24 h and then stored at 4 °C. Images were captured using 10× objective in up-right fluorescence BX51 Olympus microscope and injury areas were evaluated using ImageJ software.

Quantification of areas for high-density immunofluorescence of CD68 positive microglial/macrophage cells

The core of the injury was morphologically identified as the region with the deepest damage in serial sections. At 6 days post injury, we identified a lesion zone with a bottom of approximately 600-μm diameter centered around the stereotactic coordinates of the epicenter (AP − 2.26, ML 2.0). This lesion zone was filled with a high density of CD68+ cells. The areas of high-density CD68+ cells were measured using the ImageJ 1× software [33]. Using a slide scale under 4× objective in the fluorescence microscope, the pixels equivalent to 1 mm (388 pixels) were identified and set to scale in the ImageJ software. Using the polygon selection tool, high-density immunofluorescence of CD68+ cells were selected to enclose an area of injury. This area was measured in square millimeter and plotted against the distance from Bregma. To keep the fluorescence intensity levels uniform across all slides, they were stained all at the same time and images were acquired using the same settings and time exposure to minimize threshold bias.

Rotarod performance test

Mice were placed on a rotarod machine (IITC Life Sciences, USA) that has an accelerating rotating cylinder suspended over a platform. When the animal falls the platform is displaced and the machine records the latency in seconds for the animal to fall. This acquisition phase was performed at days 1, 3, and 5 after injury, (3 trials per day). Mice were trained in the rotarod for 3 days before CCI injury; last training day was considered the baseline testing. Sham, CCI vehicle, and CCI + trovafloxacin mice were evenly grouped on the basis of their average latency to fall.

Statistical analysis

One-way or two-way ANOVA followed by Tukey's HSD (honest significant difference) test was used to determine statistical significance in migration assay and western blot analysis, respectively. Linear regression analysis was performed for time series of measurements using treatment and the interaction between treatment and time as factors. These analyses include ATP assays, RT-qPCR, and behavior. For immunofluorescence of CD68 analysis, linear regression was performed using treatment and the interaction of treatment and distance from Bregma as factors. Analyses were performed using SPSS 15.0 (IBM) or R statistical software. All experiments were performed at least three times. The values were expressed as the means ± SEM. The differences with $p < 0.05$ were considered statistically significant. Values are represented as means ± SEM. Differences with p values < 0.05 were considered statistically significant.

Results

Trovafloxacin improves locomotor recovery and reduces tissue damage in CCI-injured mice

We conducted locomotor behavioral analysis using the rotarod coordination test at 1, 3, and 5 days post-injury in sham and CCI-injured mice treated with vehicle or trovafloxacin. Vehicle-treated CCI-injured mice showed a significant decrease in the latency to fall at 1 day post-injury (Fig. 1a), and their performance remained greatly impaired at 3 and 5 days post injury. Conversely, trovafloxacin-treated mice showed longer latencies to fall as compared to the vehicle-treated CCI-injured group. At 3 and 5 days post injury, trovafloxacin-treated animals display a recovery in locomotor performance (Fig. 1a). Importantly, sham animals treated with vehicle or trovafloxacin do not display differences in locomotor activity.

To determinate whether the improvements observed in the behavioral outcome of trovafloxacin-treated mice correlate with neuroprotective actions after CCI, we analyzed protein levels of matrix metallopeptidase 9 (MMP9) and neuronal α–II spectrin breakdown products (SBDPs) in

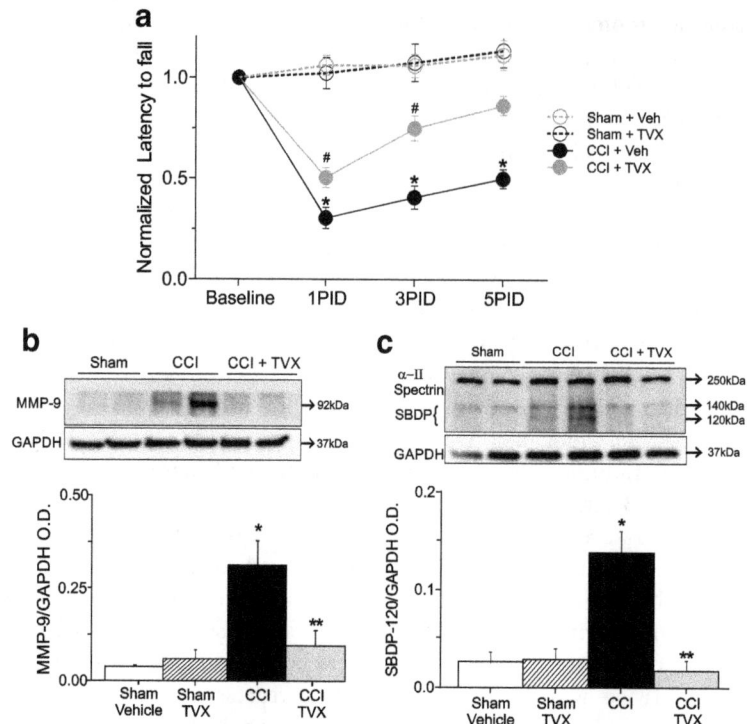

Fig. 1 Trovafloxacin treatment improves locomotor behavior and attenuates brain damage. **a** The rotarod test was used to evaluate latency (time) to fall in sham treated with vehicle (gray open circles), sham treated with trovafloxacin (TVX, black open circles), CCI-injured mice treated with vehicle (gray closed circles), or trovafloxacin (TVX, black closed circles) for up to 5 days post-CCI. Latency to fall was normalized to the baseline behavior for each group. Values are represented as mean ± SEM (n = 8 per group). Linear regression analysis was used to determine statistical difference between different groups at each time point (p values calculated for treatment and treatment*time). *p < 0.05, sham vehicle vs. CCI + vehicle; #p < 0.05 sham vehicle vs. CCI + TVX. Identical p values at their respective PDI were found for sham + TVX vs. CCI vehicle or CCI + TVX (not symbols display). **b** Representative western blots images showing MMP-9 protein levels at 6 days post-injury in sham treated with vehicle and CCI-injured mice treated with vehicle or trovafloxacin. Bottom western blot corresponds to the GAPDH, which was used as housekeeping gene. Note that sham mice treated with TVX are not display in the western blots. Graph shows to densitometric quantification of MMP-9 normalized to GAPDH values. Values are represented as mean ± SEM (n = 5 per group). **c** α–II spectrin and SPDBs (140 and 120 kDa) expression levels at 6 days post-injury in sham and CCI-injured mice treated with vehicle or trovafloxacin. Bottom western blot shows GAPDH. Note that sham mice treated with TVX are not displayed in the western blots. Graph shows densitometric quantification of SPDB 120 kDa normalized to GAPDH expression. Values are represented as mean ± SEM. (n = 5 per group). Two-way ANOVA followed by Tukey's HSD test was used to determine statistical significance. *p < 0.01, sham vehicle vs. CCI group; **p < 0.01, CCI vehicle vs. CCI + TVX. No differences were found between sham vehicle and sham TVX (see also Additional file 1: Figure S1)

CCI-injured mice treated with vehicle or trovafloxacin. MMP9 and SBDPs are general biomarkers for brain injury, such as TBI, in rodents and humans [34, 35]. Figure 1b shows that MMP-9 levels were sixfold higher in the CCI-injured group as compared to the sham group. Conversely, mice treated with a daily *i.p.* injection of trovafloxacin for up to 3 days post CCI showed a significant reduction in MMP-9 levels when compared to vehicle-treated CCI animals. The protein levels of full-length α–II spectrin (250 kDa) and SBDP (140 and 120 kDa) were also examined at the cortex at 6 days post CCI (Fig. 1c). Full α–II spectrin and SBDP 140 kDa remain unchanged in all three groups; conversely, the levels SBDP 120 kDa levels were noticeable higher in vehicle-treated CCI mice when compared to sham and trovafloxacin-treated mice. This suggests that brain injury-induced neuronal proteolysis in CCI-injured mice is reduced

by trovafloxacin treatment. We also did not find differences in biomarker levels in sham mice treated with vehicle or trovafloxacin (Additional file 1: Figure S1).

In addition to biochemical analysis of TBI biomarker protein levels, visual observation of fixed CCI-injured brains from mice treated with vehicle or trovafloxacin clearly indicated that trovafloxacin treatment reduces damage. Qualitative analysis shows that the size of a CCI-induced hematoma is smaller in trovafloxacin-treated mice as compared to those treated with vehicle (Fig. 2a). To confirm that trovafloxacin treatment protects the integrity of the blood brain barrier after trauma, we performed western blot analysis against immunoglobulin G (IgG) chains to assess its infiltration into the parenchyma in ipsilateral brains from sham, vehicle, and trovafloxacin-treated mice 6 days post injury.

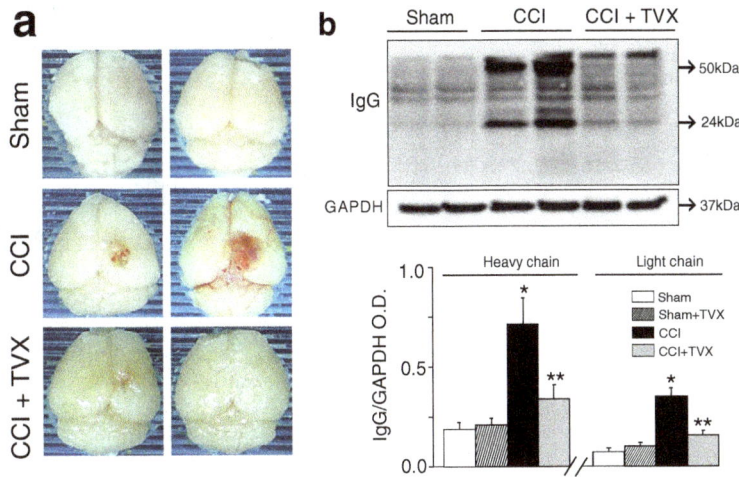

Fig. 2 Trovafloxacin treatment attenuates blood brain barrier leakage in CCI-injured mice. **a** Representative images of perfused and fixed mice brains from sham and CCI-injured mice treated with vehicle or trovafloxacin (TVX) after 6 days post-CCI. **b** Representative western blot showing IgG protein levels from injury of sham and CCI-injured mice treated with vehicle or TVX 6 days post-injury. Bottom western blot corresponds to GAPDH. **b** Densitometric quantification of IgG levels for each group ($n \geq 5$ per group) relative to their corresponding GAPDH expression levels. Note that sham mice treated with TVX are not displayed in the western blots. Values are represented as mean $\pm$ SEM. Two-way ANOVA followed by Tukey's HSD test was used to determine statistical significance. *$p < 0.01$, sham vs. CCI group; **$p < 0.01$, CCI vehicle vs. CCI + TVX. No differences were found between sham vehicle and sham TVX (see also Additional file 1: Figure S1)

Figure 2b shows that while the levels of heavy and light chain of IgG are not noticeable in sham cortex, both proteins are significantly elevated in vehicle treated CCI-injured mice. Conversely, those CCI-injured mice treated with trovafloxacin show a twofold decrease in the protein levels of heavy and light IgG chains as compared to vehicle-treated CCI mice (Fig. 2b). Taken together, our results indicate that treatment with trovafloxacin improves tissue integrative and behavioral outcomes after CCI injury.

Trovafloxacin decreases mRNA levels of pro-inflammatory cytokines and activated innate immune and glia cells after CCI

Neuroinflammation is a major component of secondary traumatic brain injury, which contributes to the ongoing neurodegeneration associated with brain damage. The levels of pro-inflammatory cytokines are significantly upregulated in response to TBI and play central roles in the initiation and propagation of the inflammatory response [36]. We performed RT-qPCR to evaluate whether treatment with trovafloxacin reduces mRNA levels of the pro-inflammatory cytokines IL-1β, TNF-α, and IL-6 after CCI injury. Figure 3 shows that mRNA levels of IL-1β, TNF-α, and IL-6 are increased several fold in the vehicle-treated CCI group at 1 day post-CCI when values were normalized with respect to sham values. Subsequently, we observed a reduction in mRNA levels of all three

cytokines at 6 days post-CCI when compared to 1 day post-CCI. Conversely, trovafloxacin treatment (i.p. injection, 60 mg/kg) markedly reduced IL-1β, TNF-α, and IL-6 mRNA by at least 2.5 fold at 1 day post-injury when compared to vehicle-treated CCI animals (Fig. 3a–c). IL-6 mRNA levels remained significantly reduced in trovafloxacin treated mice 6 days post-injury as compared to vehicle-treated CCI mice. Similar results were found for all three cytokines tested 1 day post-injury in mice treated with another Panx1 channel blocker, the food dye Brilliant Blue FCF [37] (Additional file 2: Figure S2).

Leukocyte infiltration, microglia accumulation, and glial cell proliferation at the injury zone are key components of the neuroinflammatory response after brain trauma. Accordingly, we examined the extent of neutrophil infiltration (myeloperoxidase; MPO), levels of activated astrocytes (glial fibrillary acidic protein, GFAP), and accumulation of microglia/macrophage cells (ionized calcium-binding adapter molecule 1, Iba1; and cluster of differentiation 68, CD68) in the injury site. mRNA levels of these markers are known to increase after TBI [14, 38–41]. Figure 4a shows that mRNA levels of MPO in CCI-injured animals significantly increased with respect to sham animals; however, a single trovafloxacin i.p. injection at 1 h post-CCI significantly reduced MPO expression levels. mRNA levels of MPO were decreased in both vehicle and trovafloxacin-treated CCI mice 6 days post-injury.

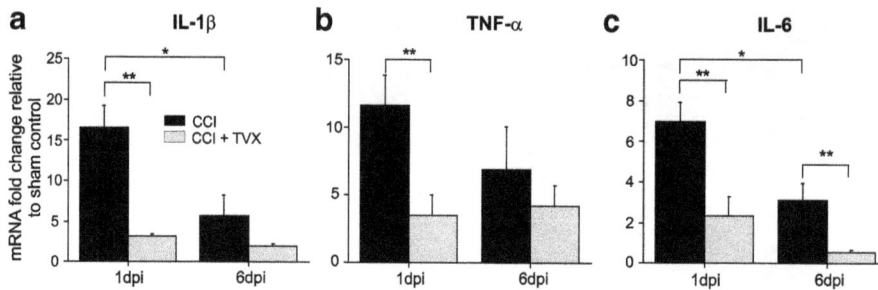

Fig. 3 Pro-inflammatory cytokines mRNA levels are decreased in trovafloxacin-treated CCI mice. RNA was isolated from ipsilateral cortex from sham and CCI-injured mice treated with vehicle or trovafloxacin (TVX). Gene expression levels for **a** IL-1β, **b** TNF-α, and **c** IL-6 were measured at 1 and 6 days post-injury by qPCR. Values are expressed as mean fold change (± SEM) relative to sham ($n = 5$), and GAPDH was used as endogenous control. Linear regression analyses were used to determine statistical significance. (p values calculated for dpi and treatment, for IL-1β, TNF-α, and IL-6 separately). *$p < 0.01$, CCI 1 dpi vs. CCI 6 dpi, **$p < 0.05$, CCI vehicle vs. CCI + TVX

This is consistent with previous observations showing that the presence of neutrophils at the injury zone diminished 6 days post-CCI [42]. In contrast, microglia and macrophage accumulation, as well as astrogliosis, have been shown to steadily increase up to 6 days post-injury [43]. In line with this, Fig. 4b–d shows that expression levels of GFAP, Iba1, and CD68 in CCI-injured animals increased in a time-dependent manner when compared to sham animals. Strikingly, trovafloxacin administration significantly attenuated the levels of these markers in CCI-injured animals by at least twofold (Fig. 4b–d). Together, our results indicate that trovafloxacin treatment reduced the neuroinflammatory response triggered by CCI.

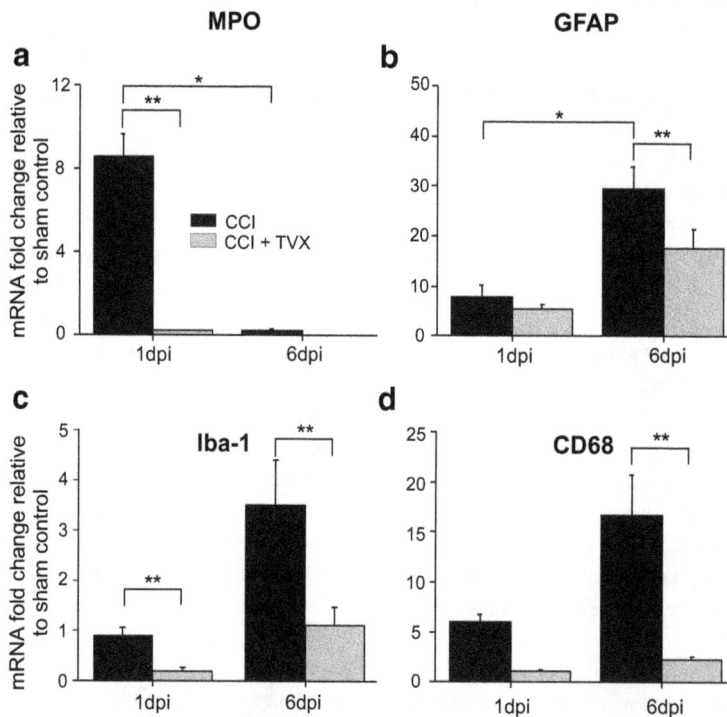

Fig. 4 Trovafloxacin treatment attenuates the expression levels of markers for leukocytes and glia cells in the injured brain. RNA was isolated from ipsilateral cortex from each group, and gene expression levels were determined by qPCR at 1 and 6 days post-injury: **a** myeloperoxidase (MPO), marker of neutrophils; **b** glial fibrillary protein (GFAP), marker of astrocytes; **c** ionized calcium-binding adapter molecule 1 (Iba-1), marker of microglia; and **d** cluster of differentiation 68 (CD68), marker of activated microglia. Values are expressed as mean fold change (± SEM) relative to sham, and GAPDH was used as endogenous control. Linear regression analyses were used to determine statistical significance. (p values calculated for dpi and treatment, for MPO, GFAP, Iba-1, and CD68 separately). *$p < 0.01$, CCI 1 dpi vs. CCI 6 dpi, **$p < 0.05$, CCI vehicle vs. CCI + TVX

Microglia and macrophage accumulation is reduced in CCl-injured mice treated with trovafloxacin

Sustained activation of pro-inflammatory microglia is one of the detrimental processes leading to neuronal damage during brain injury [44]. CD68 is a transmembrane glycoprotein that expresses in activated microglia and macrophages serving as a marker of inflammation. To further demonstrate that trovafloxacin administration diminishes accumulation of microglia and macrophage cells at the injury site, we analyzed protein levels and expression of CD68 in the ipsilateral hemisphere using western blot and immunofluorescence, respectively. Previous work has shown that CD68 expression levels reach maximum at 6 days post-injury [41]; consistent with this, Fig. 5 shows a significant increase in CD68 protein levels in CCI-injured animals when compared to the sham group at this time point. Trovafloxacin-treated CCI mice, however, display a fourfold decrease in CD68 protein levels at the ipsilateral cortex compared to vehicle-treated animals (Fig. 5). This result is in agreement with RT-qPCR data, supporting the notion that trovafloxacin reduces accumulation of microglia and macrophage cells.

To further confirm whether accumulation of microglia/macrophages from CCI-injured animals is attenuated by trovafloxacin, we quantified the high-density areas of CD68 immunoreactive cells in the ipsilateral

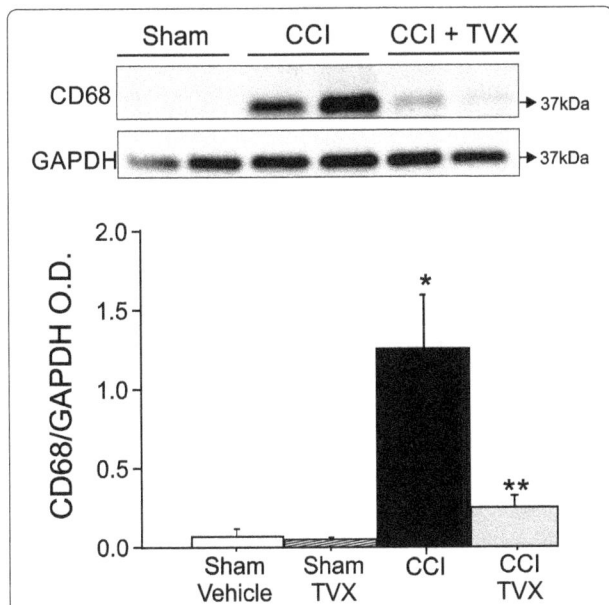

Fig. 5 Trovafloxacin treatment reduces CD68 protein expression levels at 6 days post-injury. Representative western blots showing CD68 protein levels expressions at 6 days post-injury in sham or CCI-injured mice treated with vehicle or trovafloxacin (TVX). Graph shows densitometric quantification of CD68 is represented in each group (n = 5 per group). Values are represented as mean ± SEM. Two-way ANOVA followed by Tukey's HSD test was used to determine statistical significance. *p < 0.01, sham vs. CCI group; **p < 0.01, CCI vehicle vs. CCI + TVX

cortex from vehicle-treated and trovafloxacin-treated CCI-injured mice at 6 days post-injury (Fig. 6). We analyzed the core of the injury, which was identified in serial sections stained with DAPI as a cavity with a flat bottom of approximately 600-μm diameter centered on the epicenter at AP − 2.26 and ML 2.0 in CCI-injured mice. The lesion or cavity was filled with CD68+ cells and was visibly less pronounced in trovafloxacin-treated animals (Fig. 6a, compared ipsilateral hemispheres). Quantification of the high-density CD68+ cells area show that administration of trovafloxacin in CCI-injured mice significantly attenuated the accumulation of microglia/macrophage cells at the core of the injury in the ipsilateral cortex (Fig. 6b) reducing the number of CD68 + cells by up to 50 % (AP − 2.06 and AP − 2.46).

Trovafloxacin inhibits ATP release and microglial migration in vitro by inhibition of Panx1 channels

Accumulation of activated microglia and macrophages in the ipsilateral cortex depends, at least in part, of microglia migration to the injury site and infiltration of monocytes. These processes are related to purinergic signaling and have also been linked to Panx1 channel activation, which acts as a conduit for ATP release in various cell types [9, 45]. Therefore, we next tested whether trovafloxacin attenuates acute ATP release and migration in a stimulated murine microglial cell line (BV-2 cells). Cells were stimulated with the complement component 5a (C5a), an extracellular soluble protein that forms part of a complement component activated upon tissue injury. C5a is a potent mediator of the innate immune response [46], and blockade of the C5a receptors have been shown to improve outcomes in rodent models of TBI [47]. Figure 7a shows that incubation of BV-2 cells (open circles) with C5a (10 nM) promotes extracellular ATP release as compared to non-stimulated cells (closed circles). Extracellular ATP release was significantly inhibited when C5a-stimulated BV-2 cells were co-incubated with 1 μM trovafloxacin (upright triangles), 5 μM BBFCF (upside down triangles), or 200 μM [10]Panx1, a specific Panx1 mimetic blocker peptide (open diamonds). To reliably measure extracellular ATP levels in each experiment, these measurements were performed in the presence of 10 μM POM 1, a generic ecto-ATPase inhibitor that prevents breakdown of ATP. Importantly, the action of these different known Panx1 channel blockers on ATP release in this culture system strongly suggests that the ATP is release via Panx1 channels.

Because extracellular ATP release promotes migration of microglial cells both in vitro and in vivo [9, 48], we assessed whether trovafloxacin treatment reduces C5a-induced BV-2 cell migration in a transwell migration assay. POM 1 was not used in these experiments because ATP byproducts

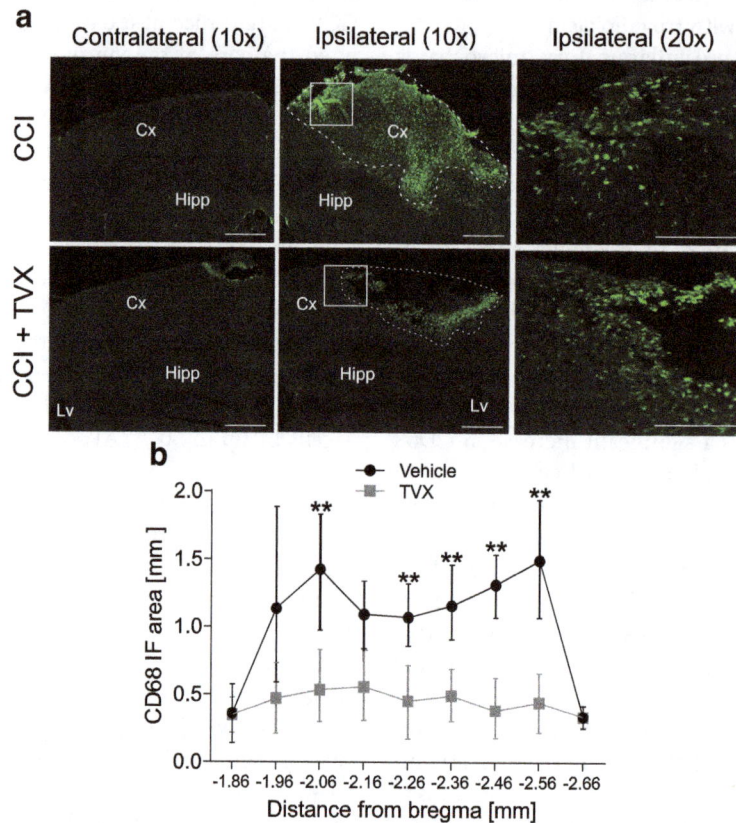

Fig. 6 Microglia/macrophage accumulation is reduced in trovafloxacin-treated CCI mice. Mice that received CCI injury where treated with trovafloxacin (TVX) or vehicle and were sacrificed at 6 dpi for histology analysis. **a** Representative images of CD68 immunoreactivity of brain sections from non-treated or TVX-treated CCI-injured mice at the core of the injury (AP − 1.96 to AP − 2.56). These areas were examined in the same anatomical location for each animal. Scale bar = 0.5 mm. Dotted lines demarcated high-density areas of CD68+ staining. **b** Correspond to the quantification of high-density areas of CD68+ cells ($n = 5$ per group). Error bars indicate SE of the mean. Linear regression analysis was performed to analyze statistical differences. (p values calculated for distance from Bregma and treatment). **$p < 0.05$ CCI vehicle vs. CCI + TVX

also activate different purinergic receptors involved in chemotaxis [49]. Figure 7b shows lack of BV-2 cell migration in the absence of stimulation with C5a. Conversely, after a 4-h incubation with 10 nM C5a, a significant number of cells migrate through the pores, as detected by crystal violet staining (Fig. 7b). Co-incubation with 1-μM trovafloxacin or 5-μM Brilliant Blue FCF drastically reduced migration of BV-2 cells when compared with cells exposed to C5a alone (Fig. 7b). Quantitative analysis indicated that C5a treatment shows 131 ± 9 migrating cells per field versus 8 ± 2 or 3 ± 2 cells per field when BV-2 cells were co-incubated with trovafloxacin or Brilliant Blue FCF, respectively (Fig. 7b). A potential mechanism that could mediate this reduction in C5a-induced migration by trovafloxacin is blockade of Panx1 channels and thereby reduced ATP release. To confirm whether the reduction in the number of migrating BV-2 cells is due to the blockade of ATP release and not through downstream effects (i.e., trovafloxacin block of purinergic receptor signaling), we evaluated BV-2 cell migration by directly applying 200 μM ATP to the cell culture medium in the absence or presence

of 1 μM trovafloxacin. No significant changes in the number of ATP-stimulated migrating BV-2 cells were observed in the presence or absence of trovafloxacin or Brilliant Blue FCF (Fig. 8). These data support the notion these blockers reduce extracellular ATP release potentially via the blockade of Panx1 channels, without affecting ATP signaling downstream of purinergic receptor activation.

Discussion

In the present study, we found that administration of trovafloxacin to CCI-injured mice produced anti-inflammatory and neuroprotective effects and, importantly, ameliorated CCI-induced locomotor impairment. The beneficial effects of trovafloxacin treatment in this animal model of TBI are supported by (1) decreased tissue damage that correlated with improved locomotor behavioral outcomes; (2) significantly reduced mRNA levels of pro-inflammatory cytokines (IL-1β, IL-6, and TNF-α) at their corresponding expression peaks; (3) reduced mRNA levels of infiltrating neutrophils (MPO), reactive astrocytes (GFAP), microglia and macrophage

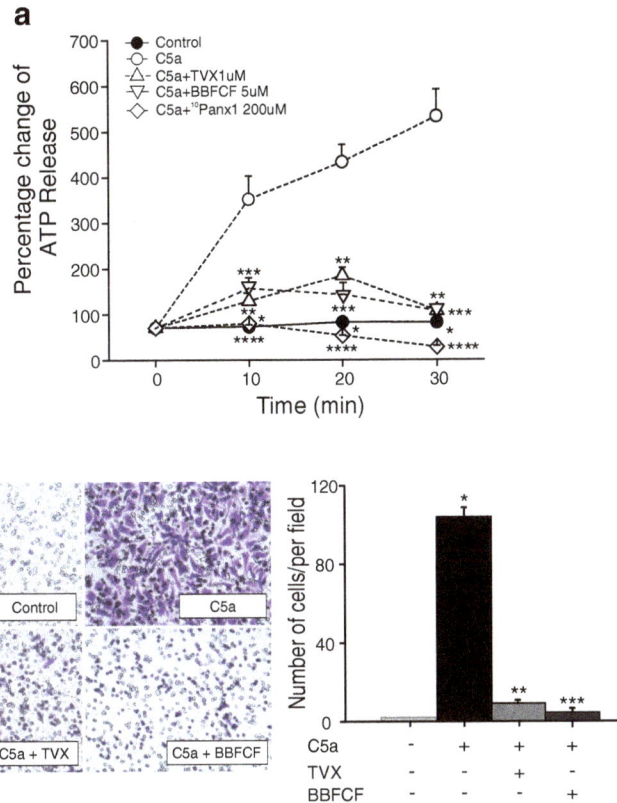

Fig. 7 Trovafloxacin inhibits ATP release and migration in C5a-stimulated BV-2 cells. **a** BV-2 cells were stimulated with 10 nM of C5a in the presence or absence of Panx1 channel blockers, trovafloxacin (TVX, 1 µM), Brilliant Blue FCF (BBFCF, 5 µM), or [10]Pnx1 (200 µM) for 30 min. Aliquots were collected from the medium every 10 min for ATP measurement. ATP was measured using the luciferin–luciferase assay. Values are represented as mean ± SEM. Percentage values were estimated with respect to basal ATP release before simulation at each condition. Each experiment was repeated at least three times in triplicates. Statistical difference was determined using linear regression with log(ATP) as the response. (p values calculated for treatment and treatment*time). *$p < 0.05$, C5a vs. control; **$p < 0.05$, C5a vs. TVX; ***$p < 0.05$, C5a vs. BBFCF, ****$p < 0.05$, C5a vs. [10]Panx1. **b** Left panel shows representative images of BV-2 cells that were seeded in the upper compartment of the transwells for transmigration assay and treated with C5a in the absence or presence of TVX (1 µM) or BBFCF (5 µM). After 4 h, cells that had migrated to the bottom of the transwell were fixed, stained with crystal violet, and counted. The images are representative of the control treated with vehicle solutions, C5a, C5a + TVX, and C5a + BBFCF-treated cells. Graph corresponds to the quantification of transmigrated BV-2 cells after 4 h stimulation from images taken in five different fields at 20× per condition. Each experiment was repeated at least three times. One-way ANOVA with Tukey's HSD test was used to measure statistical differences among groups. Values are expressed as mean ± SEM, *$p < 0.05$, control vs. C5a; **$p < 0.05$ C5a vs. C5a + TVX, or ***$p < 0.05$, C5a vs. C5a + BBFCF

cells (CD68, Iba-1), which was corroborated by immunofluorescence, and western blot analyses; and (4) in vitro assays demonstrating a trovafloxacin-dependent reduction in migration of stimulated microglial cell lines via blockade of extracellular ATP release.

Although trovafloxacin was originally described as a broad-spectrum antibiotic, it has been recently shown that it is a blocker for Panx1 channels. Thus, it is possible to hypothesize that Panx1 channel activation after brain trauma enhances the neuroinflammatory responses via ATP release. Other potential routes of ATP release that are involved in stroke-induced neurodegeneration [11, 50] implicated Cx43 hemichannels or Panx2 channels; however, these channels are not blocked by trovafloxacin [2]. Moreover, data from our laboratory indicate that trovafloxacin does not block other large ATP permeable pores

including Cx26, Cx46, and CALHM-1 channels (unpublished results). It is important to note, however, that trovafloxacin was withdrawn from the market relatively soon after its release as a generic antibiotic due to the risk of hepatotoxicity [51]. Trovafloxacin-induced hepatotoxicity appears to occur in conjunction with episodes of inflammatory stress associated with high levels of TNF-α in blood plasma. For example, a single trovafloxacin dose of 80 mg/kg or greater caused hepatotoxicity in LPS-treated mice, but 1000 mg/kg trovafloxacin in mice non-treated with LPS did not exert toxic effects [26]. In the present study, we used daily doses of 60 mg/kg via *i.p* that was not extended for more than 3 days post-injury. Interestingly, this dosage was enough to attenuate TBI-induced neuroinflammatory events that peak at 6 days post-injury suggesting that early action of trovafloxacin is critical in

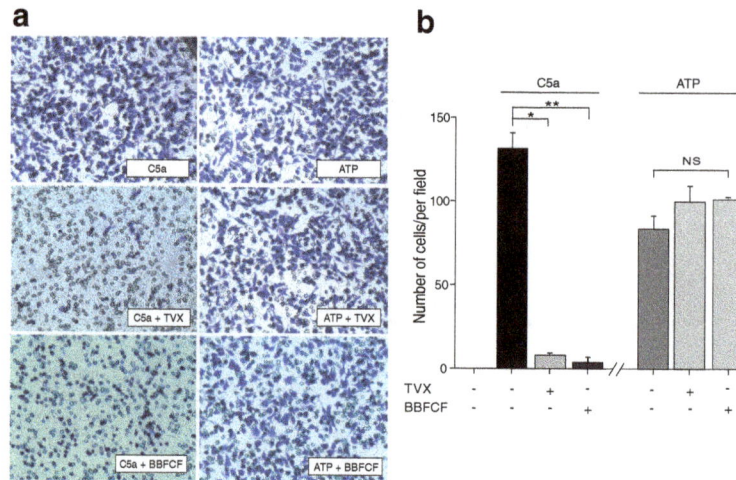

Fig. 8 Trovafloxacin does not affect downstream of ATP signaling. **a** Representative images of BV-2 cells that were seeded for transmigration assay and stimulated with C5a (10 nM) or ATP (200 μM) for 24 h in the presence or absence of trovafloxacin (TVX, 1 μM) or Brilliant Blue FCF (BBFCF, 5 μM). Cells were fixed and stained with crystal violet. **b** Quantification of transmigrated BV-2 cells at 24 h from five different fields at 20× per condition. Each experiment was repeated at least three times. One-way ANOVA with Tukey's HSD test was used to measure statistical differences among groups. Values are expressed as mean ± SEM. *$p < 0.05$, C5a vs. C5a + trovafloxacin. **$p < 0.05$, C5a vs. C5a + BBFCF. No significant changes in the number of migrated cells were observed between ATP, ATP + TVX, and ATP + BBFCF ($p > 0.05$)

affecting the later progression of the neuroinflammatory response.

Fluoroquinoline antibiotics including alatrofloxacin and trovafloxacin have previously been shown to have immunosuppression effects in infected monocytes and macrophages [52–54]; however, no mechanisms of actions have been described. More recent work has shown that trovafloxacin might inhibit α-adrenoreceptors and suppress the activation of the peroxisome proliferator-activated receptor alpha (PPARα) in the liver [55, 56]. While the blockade of α-adrenoreceptors by trovafloxacin seems to be mediated by direct interactions, the mechanism by which trovafloxacin suppresses PPARα activation is still unclear. The role of these two receptors in brain trauma has also been well documented; crucially, it has been shown that activation, but not inhibition, of these receptors is neuroprotective after brain injury [57–60]. For example, there is compelling evidence that activation of PPARα promotes anti-inflammatory and neuroprotective effects in several models of brain trauma [61–64]. Moreover, blockade of α-adrenoreceptors increases behavioral deficits in traumatic brain injury [57]. Therefore, it is unlikely that inhibition of α-adrenoreceptors and PPARα by trovafloxacin contributes to neuroprotection in our model of brain injury since, then, we would expect opposite results. Moreover, the fact that another Panx1 channel blocker like Brilliant Blue FCF has similar effects to trovafloxacin, at least at 1 day post-CCI supports the idea that trovafloxacin may have neuroprotective actions by inhibiting Panx1 channels. However, this hypothesis needs to be tested directly in future studies.

Several studies indicate that blockade or global deletion of Panx1 after stroke is neuroprotective [11–13, 65]. Panx1 is ubiquitously expressed in the brain, identified in both neurons and astrocytes. Also, leukocytes, microglia, and endothelial cells express Panx1 protein. Thus, it is possible that the beneficial effects exerted by trovafloxacin involve multiple neuronal and non-neuronal cell types. For instance, neuronal Panx1 activation via src-kinase has been recently shown to be deleterious in ischemia-induced excitotoxicity in vitro and in vivo [66, 67]. Moreover, endothelial Panx1 is also essential for leukocyte emigration in the acute inflammatory response by acting as a conduit for ATP release [9], whereas neuronal and astrocytic activation of Panx1 induces inflammasome activation in vitro [6].

Among the multiple cell types that could be targeted by trovafloxacin in our model of TBI, we focused on the accumulation of pro-inflammatory microglia and macrophages at the core of the injury site. In addition to cell proliferation, the accumulation of inflammatory cells requires infiltration of leukocytes (neutrophils and monocytes) and microglial migration. These events are mediated by activation of purinergic signaling via extracellular ATP and its byproducts [22]. Several sources for ATP release upon injury have been described; an important contributor is the Panx1 pathway activated by dying cells. These cells function as a signal beacon to direct or point innate immune cells towards apoptotic cell death activity [24, 45]. Autocrine release of ATP from infiltrating innate immune cells is also associated with Panx1 channel activation and might contribute to cellular migration [68]. Consistent with this idea, we found that trovafloxacin significantly reduced extracellular ATP release from C5a-stimulated BV-2 cells. It also prevented cell migration without affecting purinergic receptor activation and downstream signaling. Thus, our in vitro data may partially explain the decreased accumulation of leukocytes and microglial cells observed at the injury site of CCI animals treated with trovafloxacin. A reduction in the number of pro-inflammatory cells at the ipsilateral side in CCI mice treated with trovafloxacin also correlates with the lower mRNA levels detected for pro-inflammatory cytokines (IL-1β, IL-6, and TNF-α) when compared to vehicle-treated CCI mice. Accumulation of activated pro-inflammatory microglia and macrophage cells can promote the release of various pro-inflammatory factors, which in turn are detrimental to neuronal health and eventually causes cell death [69, 70]. Microglial cells in the activated state, in the cortical area, persist for at least 1 year in animal models of TBI, indicating a chronic inflammatory process induced by brain trauma [71]. Indeed, the inflammatory-based progression of TBI in human postmortem studies shows that microglial activation remains for up to 17 years after TBI in subcortical brain areas [72, 73]. Thus, further studies are necessary to evaluate the role of Panx1 in the acute and chronic activation states of microglia and macrophage cells.

SBPD 120 kDa and MMP9, two well-known biomarkers associated with the worsening of brain injury after trauma, were found at high levels in vehicle-treated CCI mice, but were significantly reduced in trovafloxacin-treated CCI mice. SBPD 120 kDa is a byproduct of the neuronally expressed α–II spectrin and is generated from sequential cleavage by caspase-3 proteases, which are activated upon neuronal injury and indicative of apoptotic cell death [74, 75]. Furthermore, pathological activation of MMPs, in particular MMP-9, has been shown to promote detrimental outcomes after brain injury, including blood brain barrier disruption, hemorrhage, and neuronal apoptosis [76, 77]. Hence, a reduction of the levels of MMP-9 in CCI mice treated with trovafloxacin might also contribute to the smaller hematomas observed in fixed brain from this group when compared to those that were treated only with vehicle.

To further link the actions of trovafloxacin with the blockade of Panx1 channel, we used Brilliant blue FCF another well-known Panx1 channel blocker [37]. As expected, Brilliant Blue FCF markedly reduced C5a-induced ATP release and migration in BV-2 cells in vitro further supporting a role for Panx1 channels. Importantly, Brilliant Blue FCF is a derivative of Brilliant Blue G; the latter has been shown to have anti-inflammatory and neuroprotective actions in mice and rats after traumatic brain injury [78, 79]. While

Brilliant Blue G blocks both P2X7 channels and Panx1 channels, Brilliant Blue FCF only inhibits Panx1 channels [37]. Here, we found that mice treated with Brilliant blue FCF 1 h post-injury showed significant reduction of mRNA levels of pro-inflammatory cytokines IL-1β, IL-6, and TNF-α (Additional file 2: Figure S2). Lastly, our preliminary data show that mice treated daily with Brilliant Blue FCF (i.p. injection, 60 mg/kg) display a trend towards improved locomotor outcomes after 5 days post-injury (unpublished results). Unlike trovafloxacin, previous studies have shown that Brilliant Blue FCF is poorly absorbed from the gastrointestinal tract, and following absorption, it goes through extensive and rapid biliary and urinary excretion [80, 81]. Hence, further studies are necessary to find optimal doses and frequency of administration of Brilliant Blue FCF to establish a neuroprotective role in our model of brain trauma.

Conclusions

Trovafloxacin treatment reduces inflammation and brain damage in a model of moderate TBI. We propose that the anti-inflammatory and neuroprotective actions of trovafloxacin are linked to the blockade of Panx1 channels due to the known roles of Panx1 channels in neuronal death during ischemia and infiltration of leukocytes during acute inflammation [9, 67, 11]. It is therefore possible that opening of Panx1 channels might potentiate the secondary damage response triggered by brain trauma. Future studies addressing the cell-type specific role of Panx1 in TBI will enhance our understanding and contribute to the development of Panx1 channels as a therapeutic target to improve outcome after brain injury.

Additional files

Additional file 1: Figure S1. No detectable protein levels of MMP9, SPDBs, IgG, and CD68 in sham mice treated with trovafloxacin. Western blot analysis was performed to detect expression of SPDBs (140 and 120 kDa), MMP9, IgG, and CD68 in sham + trovafloxacin (TVX), sham + vehicle, and CCI-injured mice treated with vehicle. Only CCI-injured mice display protein expression of MMP9, SPDB120, IgG, and CD68 at the injury site. Bottom western blots below each protein marker correspond to GAPDH levels. Each lane corresponds to samples from different animals.

Additional file 2: Figure S2. Blue Brilliant FCF treatment reduced CCI-induced pro-inflammatory cytokines. Administration of Blue Brilliant FCF via intraperitoneal injection (60 mg/kg) was performed 1 h post-CCI. Gene expression levels determined by qPCR for IL-1b, TNF-α, and IL-6 were measured 1 day post-injury. Values are expressed as mean fold change (± SEM) relative to sham (n = 8). GAPDH was used as an endogenous control. Statistical significance was evaluated using one-way ANOVA followed by Tukey's HSD.

Abbreviations

ATP: Adenosine triphosphate; BBFCF: Brilliant Blue FCF; CCI: Controlled cortical impact; CD68: Cluster of differentiation; Cx: Connexin;

DMEM: Dulbecco 's Modified Eagle Medium; GAFP: Glial fibrillary acidic protein; GAPDH: Glyceraldehyde 3-phosphate dehydrogenase; Iba1: Ionized calcium-binding adapter molecule 1; IL-1β: Interleukin-1β; IL-6: Interleukin-6; MMP9: Matrix metalloproteinase 9; MPO: Myeloperoxidase; Panx1: Pannexin 1; PBS: Phosphate-buffered saline; PFA: Paraformaldehyde; TBI: Traumatic brain injury; TNF-α: Tumor necrosis factor alpha; TVX: Trovafloxacin

Acknowledgements
We thank Ms. Yu Liu for her technical support.

Funding
This research was supported by the New Jersey Commission for Brain Injury Research (Pre-doctoral CBIR14FEL006 to C. Garg, CBIR13IRG015 to F. Calderon, CBIR15IRG018 to J.E. Contreras) and Health Resources and Services Administration through grant D34HP26020 to New Jersey Medical School Hispanic Center of Excellence (to support F. Calderon and J.E. Contreras).

Authors' contributions
Study concept and design were contributed by FC and JEC. Experiments were performed by CG, JHS, JR, and FC. Analysis and interpretation of data were contributed by CG, JHS, FC, and JEC. Statistical analyses were performed by JMH. The manuscript was written by FC and JEC. Study supervision was contributed by FC and JEC. All authors read and approved the final manuscript.

Consent for publication
Not applicable.

Competing interests
The authors declare that they have no competing interests.

Author details
[1]Department of Pharmacology, Physiology and Neurosciences, New Jersey Medical School, Rutgers University, 185 South Orange Ave, Newark, NJ 07103, USA. [2]Department of Mathematical Sciences, New Jersey Institute of Technology, University Heights, Newark, NJ 07102, USA.

References
1. Gootz TD, Zaniewski R, Haskell S, Schmieder B, Tankovic J, Girard D, Courvalin P, Polzer RJ. Activity of the new fluoroquinolone trovafloxacin (CP-99,219) against DNA gyrase and topoisomerase IV mutants of Streptococcus pneumoniae selected in vitro. Antimicrob Agents Chemother. 1996;40:2691–7.
2. Poon IK, Chiu YH, Armstrong AJ, Kinchen JM, Juncadella IJ, Bayliss DA, Ravichandran KS. Unexpected link between an antibiotic, pannexin channels and apoptosis. Nature. 2014;507:329–34.
3. Chiu YH, Ravichandran KS, Bayliss DA. Intrinsic properties and regulation of pannexin 1 channel. Channels (Austin). 2014;8:103–9.
4. Dahl G. ATP release through pannexon channels. Philos Trans R Soc Lond Ser B Biol Sci. 2015;370
5. Brough D, Pelegrin P, Rothwell NJ. Pannexin-1-dependent caspase-1 activation and secretion of IL-1beta is regulated by zinc. Eur J Immunol. 2009;39:352–8.
6. Silverman WR, de Rivero Vaccari JP, Locovei S, Qiu F, Carlsson SK, Scemes E, Keane RW, Dahl G. The pannexin 1 channel activates the inflammasome in neurons and astrocytes. J Biol Chem. 2009;284:18143–51.
7. Garre JM, Yang G, Bukauskas FF, Bennett MV. FGF-1 triggers pannexin-1 hemichannel opening in spinal astrocytes of rodents and promotes inflammatory responses in acute spinal cord slices. J Neurosci. 2016; 36:4785–801.
8. Woehrle T, Yip L, Elkhal A, Sumi Y, Chen Y, Yao Y, Insel PA, Junger WG. Pannexin-1 hemichannel-mediated ATP release together with P2X1 and P2X4 receptors regulate T-cell activation at the immune synapse. Blood. 2010;116:3475–84.
9. Lohman AW, Leskov IL, Butcher JT, Johnstone SR, Stokes TA, Begandt D, DeLalio LJ, Best AK, Penuela S, Leitinger N, et al. Pannexin 1 channels regulate leukocyte emigration through the venous endothelium during acute inflammation. Nat Commun. 2015;6:7965.
10. Karatas H, Erdener SE, Gursoy-Ozdemir Y, Lule S, Eren-Kocak E, Sen ZD, Dalkara T. Spreading depression triggers headache by activating neuronal Panx1 channels. Science. 2013;339:1092–5.
11. Bargiotas P, Krenz A, Hormuzdi SG, Ridder DA, Herb A, Barakat W, Penuela S, von Engelhardt J, Monyer H, Schwaninger M. Pannexins in ischemia-induced neurodegeneration. Proc Natl Acad Sci U S A. 2011;108:20772–7.
12. Thompson RJ. Pannexin channels and ischaemia. J Physiol. 2015;593:3463–70.
13. Cisneros-Mejorado A, Gottlieb M, Cavaliere F, Magnus T, Koch-Nolte F, Scemes E, Perez-Samartin A, Matute C. Blockade of P2X7 receptors or pannexin-1 channels similarly attenuates postischemic damage. J Cereb Blood Flow Metab. 2015;35:843–50.
14. Lumpkins KM, Bochicchio GV, Keledjian K, Simard JM, McCunn M, Scalea T. Glial fibrillary acidic protein is highly correlated with brain injury. J Trauma. 2008;65:778–82. discussion 782–774
15. Raghupathi R. Cell death mechanisms following traumatic brain injury. Brain Pathol. 2004;14:215–22.
16. Meaney DF, Smith DH. Cellular biomechanics of central nervous system injury. Handb Clin Neurol. 2015;127:105–14.
17. Morganti-Kossmann MC, Satgunaseelan L, Bye N, Kossmann T. Modulation of immune response by head injury. Injury. 2007;38:1392–400.
18. Nortje J, Menon DK. Traumatic brain injury: physiology, mechanisms, and outcome. Curr Opin Neurol. 2004;17:711–8.
19. Fredholm BB. Adenosine, an endogenous distress signal, modulates tissue damage and repair. Cell Death Differ. 2007;14:1315–23.
20. Bours MJ, Swennen EL, Di Virgilio F, Cronstein BN, Dagnelie PC. Adenosine 5'-triphosphate and adenosine as endogenous signaling molecules in immunity and inflammation. Pharmacol Ther. 2006;112:358–404.
21. Avanzato D, Genova T, Fiorio Pla A, Bernardini M, Bianco S, Bussolati B, Mancardi D, Giraudo E, Maione F, Cassoni P, et al. Activation of P2X7 and P2Y11 purinergic receptors inhibits migration and normalizes tumor-derived endothelial cells via cAMP signaling. Sci Rep. 2016;6:32602.
22. Sáez PJ, Vargas P, Shoji KF, Harcha PA, Lennon-Duménil AM, Sáez JC. ATP promotes the fast migration of dendritic cells through the activity of pannexin 1 channels and P2X(7) receptors. Sci Signal. 2017;10(506).
23. Marques-da-Silva C, Burnstock G, Ojcius DM, Coutinho-Silva R. Purinergic receptor agonists modulate phagocytosis and clearance of apoptotic cells in macrophages. Immunobiology. 2011;216:1–11.
24. Chen J, Zhao Y, Liu Y. The role of nucleotides and purinergic signaling in apoptotic cell clearance—implications for chronic inflammatory diseases. Front Immunol. 2014;5:656.
25. Iglesias R, Dahl G, Qiu F, Spray DC, Scemes E. Pannexin 1: the molecular substrate of astrocyte "hemichannels". J Neurosci. 2009;29:7092–7.
26. Shaw PJ, Hopfensperger MJ, Ganey PE, Roth RA. Lipopolysaccharide and trovafloxacin coexposure in mice causes idiosyncrasy-like liver injury dependent on tumor necrosis factor-alpha. Toxicol Sci. 2007;100:259–66.
27. Ng W, Lutsar I, Wubbel L, Ghaffar F, Jafri H, McCracken GH, Friedland IR. Pharmacodynamics of trovafloxacin in a mouse model of cephalosporin-resistant Streptococcus pneumoniae pneumonia. J Antimicrob Chemother. 1999;43:811–6.
28. Cole JT, Yarnell A, Kean WS, Gold E, Lewis B, Ren M, McMullen DC, Jacobowitz DM, Pollard HB, O'Neill JT, et al. Craniotomy: true sham for traumatic brain injury, or a sham of a sham? J Neurotrauma. 2011;28:359–69.
29. Schmittgen TD, Livak KJ. Analyzing real-time PCR data by the comparative C(T) method. Nat Protoc. 2008;3:1101–8.
30. Livak KJ, Schmittgen TD. Analysis of relative gene expression data using real-time quantitative PCR and the 2(−Delta Delta C(T)) method. Methods. 2001;25:402–8.
31. Blasi E, Barluzzi R, Bocchini V, Mazzolla R, Bistoni F. Immortalization of murine microglial cells by a v-raf/v-myc carrying retrovirus. J Neuroimmunol. 1990;27:229–37.

32. Henn A, Lund S, Hedtjarn M, Schrattenholz A, Porzgen P, Leist M. The suitability of BV2 cells as alternative model system for primary microglia cultures or for animal experiments examining brain inflammation. ALTEX. 2009;26:83–94.

33. Schneider CA, Rasband WS, Eliceiri KW. NIH image to ImageJ: 25 years of image analysis. Nat Methods. 2012;9:671–5.

34. Aikman J, O'Steen B, Silver X, Torres R, Boslaugh S, Blackband S, Padgett K, Wang KK, Hayes R, Pineda J. Alpha-II-spectrin after controlled cortical impact in the immature rat brain. Dev Neurosci. 2006;28:457–65.

35. Vafadari B, Salamian A, Kaczmarek L. MMP-9 in translation: from molecule to brain physiology, pathology, and therapy. J Neurochem. 2016;139(Suppl 2):91–114.

36. Woodcock T, Morganti-Kossmann MC. The role of markers of inflammation in traumatic brain injury. Front Neurol. 2013;4:18.

37. Wang J, Jackson DG, Dahl G. The food dye FD&C Blue no. 1 is a selective inhibitor of the ATP release channel Panx1. J Gen Physiol. 2013;141:649–56.

38. Clark RS, Schiding JK, Kaczorowski SL, Marion DW, Kochanek PM. Neutrophil accumulation after traumatic brain injury in rats: comparison of weight drop and controlled cortical impact models. J Neurotrauma. 1994;11:499–506.

39. Scholz M, Cinatl J, Schadel-Hopfner M, Windolf J. Neutrophils and the blood-brain barrier dysfunction after trauma. Med Res Rev. 2007;27:401–16.

40. Gatson JW, Liu MM, Abdelfattah K, Wigginton JG, Smith S, Wolf S, Minei JP. Resveratrol decreases inflammation in the brain of mice with mild traumatic brain injury. J Trauma Acute Care Surg. 2013;74:470–4. discussion 474–475

41. Turtzo LC, Lescher J, Janes L, Dean DD, Budde MD, Frank JA. Macrophagic and microglial responses after focal traumatic brain injury in the female rat. J Neuroinflammation. 2014;11:82.

42. Jin X, Ishii H, Bai Z, Itokazu T, Yamashita T. Temporal changes in cell marker expression and cellular infiltration in a controlled cortical impact model in adult male C57BL/6 mice. PLoS One. 2012;7:e41892.

43. Susarla BT, Villapol S, Yi JH, Geller HM, Symes AJ. Temporal patterns of cortical proliferation of glial cell populations after traumatic brain injury in mice. ASN Neuro. 2014;6:159–70.

44. Streit WJ, Mrak RE, Griffin WS. Microglia and neuroinflammation: a pathological perspective. J Neuroinflammation. 2004;1:14.

45. Chekeni FB, Elliott MR, Sandilos JK, Walk SF, Kinchen JM, Lazarowski ER, Armstrong AJ, Penuela S, Laird DW, Salvesen GS, et al. Pannexin 1 channels mediate 'find-me' signal release and membrane permeability during apoptosis. Nature. 2010;467:863–7.

46. Monk PN, Scola AM, Madala P, Fairlie DP. Function, structure and therapeutic potential of complement C5a receptors. Br J Pharmacol. 2007;152:429–48.

47. Fluiter K, Opperhuizen AL, Morgan BP, Baas F, Ramaglia V. Inhibition of the membrane attack complex of the complement system reduces secondary neuroaxonal loss and promotes neurologic recovery after traumatic brain injury in mice. J Immunol. 2014;192:2339–48.

48. Qiu F, Wang J, Spray DC, Scemes E, Dahl G. Two non-vesicular ATP release pathways in the mouse erythrocyte membrane. FEBS Lett. 2011;585:3430–5.

49. Domercq M, Vazquez-Villoldo N, Matute C. Neurotransmitter signaling in the pathophysiology of microglia. Front Cell Neurosci. 2013;7:49.

50. Freitas-Andrade M, Naus CC. Astrocytes in neuroprotection and neurodegeneration: the role of connexin43 and pannexin1. Neuroscience. 2016;323:207–21.

51. Sun Q, Zhu R, Foss FW Jr, Macdonald TL. Mechanisms of trovafloxacin hepatotoxicity: studies of a model cyclopropylamine-containing system. Bioorg Med Chem Lett. 2007;17:6682–6.

52. Hall IH, Schwab UE, Ward ES, Ives TJ. Effects of alatrofloxacin, the parental prodrug of trovafloxacin, on phagocytic, anti-inflammatory and immunomodulation events of human THP-1 monocytes. Biomed Pharmacother. 2003;57:359–65.

53. Khan AA, Slifer TR, Remington JS. Effect of trovafloxacin on production of cytokines by human monocytes. Antimicrob Agents Chemother. 1998;42:1713–7.

54. Rubin BK, Tamaoki J. Antibiotics as anti-inflammatory and immunomodulatory agents. Basel ; Boston: Birkhäuser; 2005.

55. Oshida K, Vasani N, Thomas RS, Applegate D, Rosen M, Abbott B, Lau C, Guo G, Aleksunes LM, Klaassen C, Corton JC. Identification of modulators of the nuclear receptor peroxisome proliferator-activated receptor alpha (PPARalpha) in a mouse liver gene expression compendium. PLoS One. 2015;10:e0112655.

56. Angus JA, Wright CE. Novel alpha1-adrenoceptor antagonism by the fluroquinolone antibiotic trovafloxacin. Eur J Pharmacol. 2016;791:179–84.

57. Dunn-Meynell AA, Yarlagadda Y, Levin BE. Alpha 1-adrenoceptor blockade increases behavioral deficits in traumatic brain injury. J Neurotrauma. 1997; 14:43–52.

58. Stibick DL, Feeney DM. Enduring vulnerability to transient reinstatement of hemiplegia by prazosin after traumatic brain injury. J Neurotrauma. 2001;18: 303–12.

59. Prasad MR, Tzigaret CM, Smith D, Soares H, McIntosh TK. Decreased alpha 1-adrenergic receptors after experimental brain injury. J Neurotrauma. 1992;9:269–79.

60. Kapadia R, Yi JH, Vemuganti R. Mechanisms of anti-inflammatory and neuroprotective actions of PPAR-gamma agonists. Front Biosci. 2008; 13:1813–26.

61. Chen XR, Besson VC, Beziaud T, Plotkine M, Marchand-Leroux C. Combination therapy with fenofibrate, a peroxisome proliferator-activated receptor alpha agonist, and simvastatin, a 3-hydroxy-3-methylglutaryl-coenzyme A reductase inhibitor, on experimental traumatic brain injury. J Pharmacol Exp Ther. 2008;326:966–74.

62. Chen XR, Besson VC, Palmier B, Garcia Y, Plotkine M, Marchand-Leroux C. Neurological recovery-promoting, anti-inflammatory, and anti-oxidative effects afforded by fenofibrate, a PPAR alpha agonist, in traumatic brain injury. J Neurotrauma. 2007;24:1119–31.

63. Liu H, Rose ME, Culver S, Ma X, Dixon CE, Graham SH. Rosiglitazone attenuates inflammation and CA3 neuronal loss following traumatic brain injury in rats. Biochem Biophys Res Commun. 2016;472:648–55.

64. Yao J, Zheng K, Zhang X. Rosiglitazone exerts neuroprotective effects via the suppression of neuronal autophagy and apoptosis in the cortex following traumatic brain injury. Mol Med Rep. 2015;12:6591–7.

65. Bargiotas P, Krenz A, Monyer H, Schwaninger M. Functional outcome of pannexin-deficient mice after cerebral ischemia. Channels (Austin). 2012;6:453–6.

66. Weilinger NL, Lohman AW, Rakai BD, Ma EM, Bialecki J, Maslieieva V, Rilea T, Bandet MV, Ikuta NT, Scott L, et al. Metabotropic NMDA receptor signaling couples Src family kinases to pannexin-1 during excitotoxicity. Nat Neurosci. 2016;19:432–42.

67. Weilinger NL, Tang PL, Thompson RJ. Anoxia-induced NMDA receptor activation opens pannexin channels via Src family kinases. J Neurosci. 2012; 32:12579–88.

68. Bao Y, Chen Y, Ledderose C, Li L, Junger WG. Pannexin 1 channels link chemoattractant receptor signaling to local excitation and global inhibition responses at the front and back of polarized neutrophils. J Biol Chem. 2013; 288:22650–7.

69. Hanisch UK. Microglia as a source and target of cytokines. Glia. 2002; 40:140–55.

70. Hanisch UK, Kettenmann H. Microglia: active sensor and versatile effector cells in the normal and pathologic brain. Nat Neurosci. 2007;10:1387–94.

71. Loane DJ, Kumar A, Stoica BA, Cabatbat R, Faden AI. Progressive neurodegeneration after experimental brain trauma: association with chronic microglial activation. J Neuropathol Exp Neurol. 2014;73:14–29.

72. Ramlackhansingh AF, Brooks DJ, Greenwood RJ, Bose SK, Turkheimer FE, Kinnunen KM, Gentleman S, Heckemann RA, Gunanayagam K, Gelosa G, Sharp DJ. Inflammation after trauma: microglial activation and traumatic brain injury. Ann Neurol. 2011;70:374–83.

73. Giunta B, Obregon D, Velisetty R, Sanberg PR, Borlongan CV, Tan J. The immunology of traumatic brain injury: a prime target for Alzheimer's disease prevention. J Neuroinflammation. 2012;9:185.

74. Nicholson DW, Ali A, Thornberry NA, Vaillancourt JP, Ding CK, Gallant M, Gareau Y, Griffin PR, Labelle M, Lazebnik YA, et al. Identification and inhibition of the ICE/CED-3 protease necessary for mammalian apoptosis. Nature. 1995;376:37–43.

75. Jacobsen MD, Weil M, Raff MC. Role of Ced-3/ICE-family proteases in staurosporine-induced programmed cell death. J Cell Biol. 1996;133: 1041–51.

76. Hadass O, Tomlinson BN, Gooyit M, Chen S, Purdy JJ, Walker JM, Zhang C, Giritharan AB, Purnell W, Robinson CR 2nd, et al. Selective inhibition of matrix metalloproteinase-9 attenuates secondary damage resulting from severe traumatic brain injury. PLoS One. 2013;8:e76904.

77. Chen ZL, Strickland S. Neuronal death in the hippocampus is promoted by plasmin-catalyzed degradation of laminin. Cell. 1997;91:917–25.

78. Wang YC, Cui Y, Cui JZ, Sun LQ, Cui CM, Zhang HA, Zhu HX, Li R, Tian YX, Gao JL. Neuroprotective effects of brilliant blue G on the brain following traumatic brain injury in rats. Mol Med Rep. 2015;12:2149–54.

79. Kimbler DE, Shields J, Yanasak N, Vender JR, Dhandapani KM. Activation of P2X7 promotes cerebral edema and neurological injury after traumatic brain injury in mice. PLoS One. 2012;7:e41229.
80. Brown JP, Dorsky A, Enderlin FE, Hale RL, Wright VA, Parkinson TM. Synthesis of 14C-labelled FD & C Blue no. 1 (Brilliant Blue FCF) and its intestinal absorption and metabolic fate in rats. Food Cosmet Toxicol. 1980;18:1–5.
81. Phillips JC, Mendis D, Eason CT, Gangolli SD. The metabolic disposition of 14C-labelled green S and Brilliant Blue FCF in the rat, mouse and guinea-pig. Food Cosmet Toxicol. 1980;18:7–13.

8

Progesterone treatment reduces neuroinflammation, oxidative stress and brain damage and improves long-term outcomes in a rat model of repeated mild traumatic brain injury

Kyria M. Webster[1], David K. Wright[2,3], Mujun Sun[1], Bridgette D. Semple[1], Ezgi Ozturk[1], Donald G. Stein[4], Terence J. O'Brien[1] and Sandy R. Shultz[1*]

Abstract

Background: Repeated mild traumatic brain injuries, such as concussions, may result in cumulative brain damage, neurodegeneration and other chronic neurological impairments. There are currently no clinically available treatment options known to prevent these consequences. However, growing evidence implicates neuroinflammation and oxidative stress in the pathogenesis of repetitive mild brain injuries; thus, these may represent potential therapeutic targets. Progesterone has been demonstrated to have potent anti-inflammatory and anti-oxidant properties after brain insult; therefore, here, we examined progesterone treatment in rats given repetitive mild brain injuries via the repeated mild fluid percussion injury model.

Methods: Male Long-Evans rats were assigned into four groups: sham injury + vehicle treatment, sham injury + progesterone treatment (8 mg/kg/day), repeated mild fluid percussion injuries + vehicle treatment, and repeated mild fluid percussion injuries + progesterone treatment. Rats were administered a total of three injuries, with each injury separated by 5 days. Treatment was initiated 1 h after the first injury, then administered daily for a total of 15 days. Rats underwent behavioural testing at 12-weeks post-treatment to assess cognition, motor function, anxiety and depression. Brains were then dissected for analysis of markers for neuroinflammation and oxidative stress. Ex vivo MRI was conducted in order to examine structural brain damage and white matter integrity.

Results: Repeated mild fluid percussion injuries + progesterone treatment rats showed significantly reduced cognitive and sensorimotor deficits compared to their vehicle-treated counterparts at 12-weeks post-treatment. Progesterone treatment significantly attenuated markers of neuroinflammation and oxidative stress in rats given repeated mild fluid percussion injuries, with concomitant reductions in grey and white matter damage as indicated by MRI.

Conclusions: These findings implicate neuroinflammation and oxidative stress in the pathophysiological aftermath of mild brain injuries and suggest that progesterone may be a viable treatment option to mitigate these effects and their detrimental consequences.

Keywords: Concussion, Chronic traumatic encephalopathy, Animal model, DTI, MRI, Treatment, Microglia, Macrophages, Astrogliosis, Lipid peroxidation

* Correspondence: sshultz@unimelb.edu.au
[1]Department of Medicine, The Royal Melbourne Hospital, The University of Melbourne, Parkville, VIC 3050, Australia
Full list of author information is available at the end of the article

Background

Mild traumatic brain injuries (mTBI), including concussions, are a common medical problem worldwide [1]. mTBI is defined as a complex pathophysiological process induced by traumatic biomechanical forces to the brain and often occurs in motor vehicle accidents, assaults, slips, and falls and in combative sports and military settings [1]. Although a patient will typically recover within hours to weeks after a single mTBI [1, 2], there is growing evidence that repeated mTBI (rmTBI) can have cumulative and persisting neurological consequences. For example, rmTBI has been associated with chronic cognitive impairments and an increased risk of depression [3–5]. Furthermore, rmTBI has been linked with a number of neurodegenerative conditions, such as chronic traumatic encephalopathy (CTE), and is implicated in connection with severe cognitive, emotional and motor abnormalities [6].

Although a number of pathophysiological mechanisms have been postulated to contribute to the cumulative and chronic effects of rmTBI, there is growing evidence suggesting important roles for neuroinflammation and oxidative stress [7, 8]. Neuroinflammation is common in TBI patients, as well as in other neurodegenerative conditions associated with mTBI, including Alzheimer's disease and motor neuron disease [8, 9]. Furthermore, both our laboratory and others have observed elevated and persisting neuroinflammation and oxidative stress in experimental models of mTBI, which coincides with progressive brain damage and chronic behavioural abnormalities [7, 10–17].

To date, there is no clinically available intervention known to prevent the cumulative and chronic consequences of rmTBI. However, considering the possible role of neuroinflammation and oxidative stress in the pathogenesis of rmTBI, an intervention that targets these secondary injury pathways may have therapeutic effects. Progesterone (PROG), a neurosteroid originally named due to its progestational role during pregnancy, exerts neuroprotective effects in experimental brain insults, including TBI [18–22]. Of particular relevance here, PROG is safe for clinical use and has been demonstrated to have potent anti-inflammatory and anti-oxidant properties [18, 21, 22].

Considering the high incidence of mTBI, the cumulative and chronic consequences of rmTBI, the lack of an effective treatment strategy, as well as the likely pathological involvement of neuroinflammation and oxidative stress in the aftermath of rmTBI, we here investigated the use of PROG treatment in a rat model of rmTBI. With the hypothesis that PROG treatment would ameliorate long-term behavioural impairments via the attenuation of post-traumatic inflammation and oxidative stress, rmTBI and sham-operated rats were treated with

PROG or vehicle control and assessed after a 12-week post-treatment recovery period. We herein report that PROG treatment in rmTBI significantly reduced neuroinflammation, oxidative stress, brain damage and cognitive and motor impairments.

Methods

Animals

Fifty young adult male Long-Evans hooded rats were obtained from the animal breeding service of the Melbourne Brain Centre and were used as subjects. All rats were 8–12 weeks of age, weighed 250–300 g, and were experimentally naïve prior to surgical procedures. After surgery, all rats were housed individually under a 12 h:12 h light/dark cycle with ad libitum access to food and water. All procedures were performed in accordance with the guidelines of the Australian Code of Practice for the Care and Use of Animals for Scientific Purposes written by the Australian National Health and Medical Research Council and were approved by the University of Melbourne Animal Ethics Committee (#1112173).

Experimental groups and treatment

Rats were assigned into two injury groups: repeated mild fluid percussion injury (rFPI) or sham injury (SHAM). Rats were then further assigned to two treatment groups: cyclodextrin 22.5 % vehicle treatment (VEH; Sigma, Sydney, Australia) or PROG treatment (8 mg/kg in 22.5 % cyclodextrin; Sigma, Sydney, Australia). Thus, there were a total of four experimental groups: SHAM + VEH, SHAM + PROG, rFPI + VEH, and rFPI + PROG.

After each injury, the rat received an intraperitoneal injection of their assigned treatment at 1 h post-injury. This was followed by a daily subcutaneous injection of their assigned treatment for 5 days. This occurred after each of their three injuries. The dose and treatment regimen was based on previous studies reporting neuroprotective effects with PROG treatment after brain injury [18–22].

Injury model

Previous studies report that a single mild fluid percussion injury (FPI) in the rat induces transient behavioural and pathophysiological changes that occur in the absence of significant neuronal loss or structural brain damage [23–25], which is consistent with what may occur after a single mTBI in humans [1]. Furthermore, our laboratory [10, 11] and others [12, 24] have found that rFPI results in cumulative and long-term neurological changes in rats that bear resemblance to those reported in humans who have suffered rmTBI and CTE.

All of the surgical and rFPI procedures used in this study were based on standard protocols as previously described and used by our group [10, 11]. Briefly, rats were placed in a sealed Plexiglas box into which 4 % isoflurane and 2 L/min oxygen flow was introduced for anaesthesia. Rats were then placed in a stereotaxic frame via ear bars, with anaesthesia maintained at 2 % isoflurane and 1 L/min oxygen, and given a subcutaneous injection of analgesic (carprofen 5 mg/kg). A craniotomy (5 mm diameter) was performed on all rats, centred over the following coordinates with reference to the bregma: anterior/posterior −3.0 mm, medial/lateral 4.0 mm. A hollow plastic injury cap was sealed over the craniotomy, and a removable plug was inserted into the injury cap to seal the craniotomy at all times except during mild FPI or sham injury. Immediately after the surgery, rats were attached to the FPI device. At the first response of a hind limb withdrawal to a toe pinch, rats assigned to the rFPI groups were administered a mild FPI that was induced by a 1–1.5 atm fluid pulse to the brain. Rats from the SHAM groups were administered a sham injury, which involved identical procedures as those for a FPI except that the fluid pulse was not administered. Two subsequent injuries were performed in the same manner at 5-day intervals. Apnea, return of toe pinch reflex, and self-righting reflexes were monitored after each of the injuries as indicators of injury severity [10, 11, 23] (Table 1).

Behavioural testing

Behavioural testing began 12 weeks after the final day of treatment. Testing was carried out over five consecutive days and was completed by a researcher blinded to experimental conditions on all 50 rats. Rats first underwent testing in the elevated plus maze to assess anxiety-like behaviours as previously described [10, 11, 26, 27]. Briefly, rats were placed into the maze facing an open arm and allowed 5 min to freely explore the maze. An overhead camera recorded behaviours, and the number of entries into and the amount of time spent in open or closed arms were quantified by *EthoVision* Tracking Software (Noldus™, Netherlands). A percentage score was calculated for the time spent in the open arm, as this is decreased in rats experiencing heightened anxiety [26, 27]. Entries into the closed arm were calculated as a

measure of locomotion and were defined by all four paws having entered the arm [11].

Rats were next tested in the open field to assess locomotor and anxiety-like behaviours as previously described [10, 11, 23]. Briefly, the rats were individually placed in a circular open arena (100 cm diameter, 20 cm high wall) and allowed to freely explore for 10 min. An overhead video camera recorded behaviour, and *EthoVision* software was used to calculate the total distance travelled (cm), as well as the time spent and number of entries into the inner area (50 cm diameter) of the open field.

To assess cognition, water maze testing was conducted as previously described [27]. A circular pool (163 cm diameter) was filled with tap water (29 °C), and a hidden acrylic escape platform (10 cm diameter) was submerged 2 cm below the water surface in one of the quadrants of the pool. Water maze testing involved an acquisition session (day 1) and a reversal session (day 2), with each day consisting of ten trials with a maximum time of 60 s given for each trial. Each trial began at one of the four locations in the pool (north, south, east or west) that were pseudo-randomized to prevent sequential starts from the same location. A trial began when a rat was placed in the pool next to and facing the pool wall and ended when either the rat reached and stood on the hidden platform or 60 s elapsed, at which point the experimenter would guide the rat onto the platform. An overhead video camera recorded behaviour and *EthoVision* software used to calculate the search time to locate the platform and the number of direct and circle swims as measures of spatial place memory [27]. Swim speed (cm/s) was also calculated as a measure of motor ability. All the settings for the acquisition session and reversal session were the same, with the exception of the escape platform, which was moved to the opposite quadrant [11, 28].

The beam task was used to assess sensorimotor function as previously described [27, 28]. During beam training, rats were given five trials to traverse a 100-cm-long beam with a width of 4 cm and an additional five trials to traverse a 100-cm-long beam with a width of 2 cm. Beam testing occurred 24 h after beam training and consisted of ten trials on the 2-cm-wide, 100-cm-long beam.

Table 1 Acute post-injury outcomes

	Injury 1		Injury 2		Injury 3	
	Hind limb	Self-righting	Hind limb	Self-righting	Hind limb	Self-righting
SHAM + VEH	0 ± 0	98.9 ± 5.2	0 ± 0	98.1 ± 6.5	0 ± 0	93.3 ± 5.0
SHAM + PROG	0 ± 0	101.8 ± 5.8	0 ± 0	99.2 ± 6.4	0 ± 0	96.1 ± 7.4
rFPI + VEH	0.83 ± .56*	149.2 ± 13.4*	2.08 ± .96*	159.9 ± 13.7*	1.25 ± .90*	160.2 ± 9.6*
rFPI + PROG	1.15 ± .61*	158.7 ± 13.0*	1.54 ± .67*	150.2 ± 10.5*	1.54 ± .87*	154.5 ± 8.0*

Regardless of the assigned treatment, rFPI resulted in worse acute injury severity outcomes as indicated by increased hind limb withdrawal and self-righting reflex times compared to the SHAM groups. There was no apnea observed after any of the injuries

*rFPI significantly greater than sham-injured groups, $p < 0.001$

A maximum of 60 s was permitted for each trial. Traverse times and the number of slips and falls were scored [10]. Rats that fell off the beam were scored with the maximum time.

Depression-like behaviour was assessed using the forced swim task [12, 29]. Rats underwent forced swim training on day 4 of behavioural testing. For training, the rat was placed in the forced swim apparatus, which consisted of a clear cylinder (diameter = 30 cm, height = 40 cm) filled to a depth of 30 cm with water at 25 °C for 15 min. Forced swim testing occurred 24 h after forced swim training. Each rat was placed in the apparatus for 5 min. Behaviour was recorded by a video camera from a horizontal angle and later scored to calculate the time each rat spent immobile, the time spent escaping and the time spent swimming. Only behaviours that persisted longer than 2 s were scored.

Brain tissue preparation

One day after completion of behavioural testing, rats were killed to obtain either fresh brain tissue for measurement of lipid peroxidation ($n = 5$/group) or fixed brain tissue for MRI and immunofluorescence analyses ($n = 7$–8/group). For fresh tissue collection, rats were deeply anaesthetised and decapitated, and the ipsilateral cortex was rapidly dissected. Fresh tissue was then immediately frozen in liquid nitrogen and later stored at $-80°C$. For fixed brain tissue collection, rats were deeply anaesthetised and transcardially perfused with ice-cold phosphate-buffered saline followed by 4 % paraformaldehyde in phosphate-buffered saline. Whole brains were removed and stored in 4 % paraformaldehyde at 4 °C until MRI scanning. After MRI, fixed brains were embedded in paraffin for immunofluorescence procedures [23, 30, 31]. All analyses were conducted by investigators blinded to injury or treatment group allocation.

MRI data acquisition

A 4.7 T Bruker Avance III scanner (Bruker™ Biospec®, USA) with a 30-cm horizontal bore was used for MRI scanning. The magnet was fitted with a BGA12S2 gradient set and actively decoupled volume transmit and four-channel surface receive coils for imaging. Ex vivo brains were placed in 15-ml falcon tubes filled with paraformaldehyde and taped to the surface coil to be scanned.

The protocol for scanning consisted of a three-plane localizer sequence followed by multi-slice axial, coronal and sagittal images to accurately determine the orientation of the rat brain. A rapid acquisition with relaxation enhancement (RARE) sequence was used to acquire T_2-weighted images with the following imaging parameters: RARE factor = 8, effective echo time = 36 ms, repetition time = 12 s, matrix size = 144×72, field of view = 28.8×14.4 mm^2, number of axial slices = 60, isotropic spatial resolution = $200 \times 200 \times 200$ μm^3, and number of excitations = 32.

A 3D echo planar sequence was used to perform diffusion-weighted imaging with the following parameters: repetition time = 2500 ms, field of view = $32 \times 16 \times 12$ mm^3, echo time = 62 ms, matrix size = $128 \times 64 \times 48$, and isotropic resolution = $250 \times 250 \times 250$ μm^3. Diffusion weighting was performed with the diffusion duration (δ) = 7 ms, the diffusion gradient separation (Δ) = 20 ms, and b value = 8000 s/mm^2 in 81 non-collinear directions with 9 non-diffusion images (b_0).

MRI analysis

MRI analysis was completed by two researchers, both of whom were blinded to the experimental conditions. As previously described [27, 31, 32], one researcher used FSL View (Analysis group, Oxford, UK) to manually trace eight a priori regions of interest (ROIs) on T_2-weighted images. ROIs included the ipsilateral and contralateral hippocampus, cortex, corpus callosum and lateral ventricles. ROIs were traced on consecutive coronal MRI slices, and only slices containing hippocampus were analysed. The second researcher confirmed the accuracy of the ROI traces and processed the MRI data. The total volume for each ROI was calculated using MATLAB® (The MathWorks®, Natick, MA, USA).

Diffusion tensor imaging (DTI) analysis was conducted in order to assess the integrity of the corpus callosum, a major white matter tract commonly affected by TBI [27, 32]. ROI masks of the corpus callosum were transformed into the diffusion image space using Advanced Normalization Tools (ANTs, http://stnava.github.io/ANTs/), and mean DTI measures including fractional anisotropy (FA), mean diffusivity, radial diffusivity and axial diffusivity were calculated using the FSL diffusion toolbox (FDT, http://fsl.fmrib.ox.ac.uk/fsl/fslwiki/FDT) and MATLAB® software.

Immunofluorescence analysis

As previously described [31–33], immunofluorescence staining and analysis was performed to assess neuroinflammation. Three 4-μm coronal sections from each rat were selected and obtained at the level of injury (–3.0 mm bregma). The sections were deparaffinized and rehydrated [31, 33, 34], then immersed in 0.21 % citric acid buffer (pH 6.0) at boiling temperature in a 1250-W microwave oven for 15 min for antigen retrieval. The sections were then permeabilized with 0.1 % Triton X-100 in phosphate-buffered saline for 10 min and covered in 5 % bovine serum albumin for 60 min at room temperature, followed by incubation with primary antibodies overnight at 4 °C [31, 33]. Anti-GFAP antibody (1:500, rabbit Dako®, Carpentaria, CA, USA) was used as a marker for reactive astrocytes, which have increased expression of GFAP, enlarged cytoplasm and bear elongated and hypertrophic processes [35]. Anti-CD68 (1:500, mouse Abcam®, Cambridge, UK) antibody was used as a marker for activated microglia/macrophages with an amoeboid morphology/phagocytic function [36–38]. The sections were washed in PBS then incubated for 60 min with goat anti-rabbit secondary antibody (1:800, Alexafluor® 488, USA), for GFAP staining, or goat anti-mouse secondary antibody (1:500, Alexafluor® 488, USA), for CD68 staining. The sections were washed again and incubated at room temperature with Sudan Black for 10 min. Slides were then dehydrated and coverslipped [31, 33].

For analysis, photomicrographs of GFAP and CD68 staining were captured using a Carl Zeiss® fluorescence Axioplan-2 microscope at ×20 magnification, under fixed exposure times and light illumination settings to ensure objectivity in image quality and position. One photomicrograph of the most immunoreactive position in the ipsilateral cortex for a total of three photomicrographs for each rat was captured, for a total of three photomicrographs per rat.

GFAP was quantified using the threshold function on ImageJ software (NIH, USA) to create a semi-quantitative index of immunoreactivity by summing the immunopositive area within the digital image, expressed in square micrometers [31, 33]. CD68-positive cells were manually counted on each photomicrograph, and the numbers from the three sections were summed for each rat [31, 33].

Measurement of lipid peroxidation
The relative levels of malondialdehyde (MDA), an indicator of lipid peroxidation, were measured using a thiobarbituric acid reactive substances (TBARS) assay as previously described [11, 28]. Tissue samples were prepared as directed from the MDA assay kit (MAK085; Sigma-Aldrich®, St Louis, MO, USA).

Statistical analysis
SPSS 21.0 was used for all statistical analyses. Water maze search time was analysed using a repeated measures analysis of variance (ANOVA) with injury and treatment as between-subjects factors and trial as the within-subjects factors. Two-way ANOVAs, with injury and treatment as between-subjects factors, were used for all other analyses. Bonferonni post hoc comparisons were used when appropriate. Statistical significance was set at $p \leq 0.05$.

Results
PROG treatment reduces cognitive and sensorimotor deficits in rFPI
ANOVA indicated a significant injury × treatment interaction on the measure of direct and circle swims during water maze testing ($F_{1, 46} = 4.133$, $p < 0.05$, Fig. 1a). Post hoc analysis found that rFPI + VEH rats performed fewer direct and circle swims than all other groups ($p < 0.05$), whereas the rFPI + PROG group did not significantly differ from either of the SHAM groups. There was also a significant treatment effect found for the measure of search time ($F_{1, 46} = 4.387$, $p < 0.05$, Fig. 1b), indicating that rats treated with PROG located the platform faster than those treated with VEH. Significant effects for injury were also found for both direct and circle swims ($F_{1, 46} = 8.474$, $p < 0.01$) and search time ($F_{1, 46} = 5.607$, $p < 0.05$). There were no statistically significant differences on the measure of swim speed (Fig. 1c), suggesting that motor impairments did not confound the cognitive measures.

ANOVA revealed a significant injury × treatment interaction on the measure of slips and falls on the beam task ($F_{1, 46} = 51.533$, $p < 0.05$, Fig. 2a). Post hoc analysis indicated that the rFPI + VEH group had significantly more slips and falls than all other groups ($p < 0.01$), whilst the rFPI + PROG group did not significantly differ from either of the SHAM groups. There were no statistically significant findings on the measurement of average traverse times (Fig. 2b).

There were no statistically significant findings for the elevated plus maze, open field or forced swim task (all $p > 0.05$).

PROG treatment reduces brain damage in rFPI
MRI volumetrics
As shown in the representative MRI images (Fig. 3a–d), there was a loss of ipsilateral cortex and ipsilateral hippocampus volumes in rFPI + VEH rats as compared to all other groups. ANOVA revealed a significant injury × treatment interaction in the ipsilateral cortex ($F_{1, 26} = 4.237$, $p < 0.05$, Fig. 3e) and ipsilateral hippocampus ($F_{1, 26} = 4.697$, $p < 0.05$, Fig. 3f). Post hoc analysis indicated a significant reduction of ipsilateral cortex and ipsilateral hippocampus volumes in rFPI + VEH group compared to all other groups ($p < 0.01$), whereas the rFPI + PROG group did not differ significantly from either SHAM group.

Significant treatment effects were found in the ipsilateral corpus callosum ($F_{1, 26} = 16.801$, $p < 0.001$, Fig. 3g), contralateral cortex ($F_{1, 26} = 5.357$, $p < 0.05$, Fig. 3e), and contralateral corpus callosum ($F_{1, 26} = 5.659$, $p < 0.05$, Fig. 3g), indicating that PROG-treated rats had significantly more volume of these brain structures compared to VEH-treated rats. There were also significant treatment effects in the ipsilateral ($F_{1, 26} = 9.626$, $p < 0.005$, Fig. 3h) and contralateral lateral ventricles ($F_{1, 26} = 10.687$, $p < 0.01$, Fig. 3h), indicating that PROG-treated rats had smaller lateral ventricle volumes than rats treated with VEH.

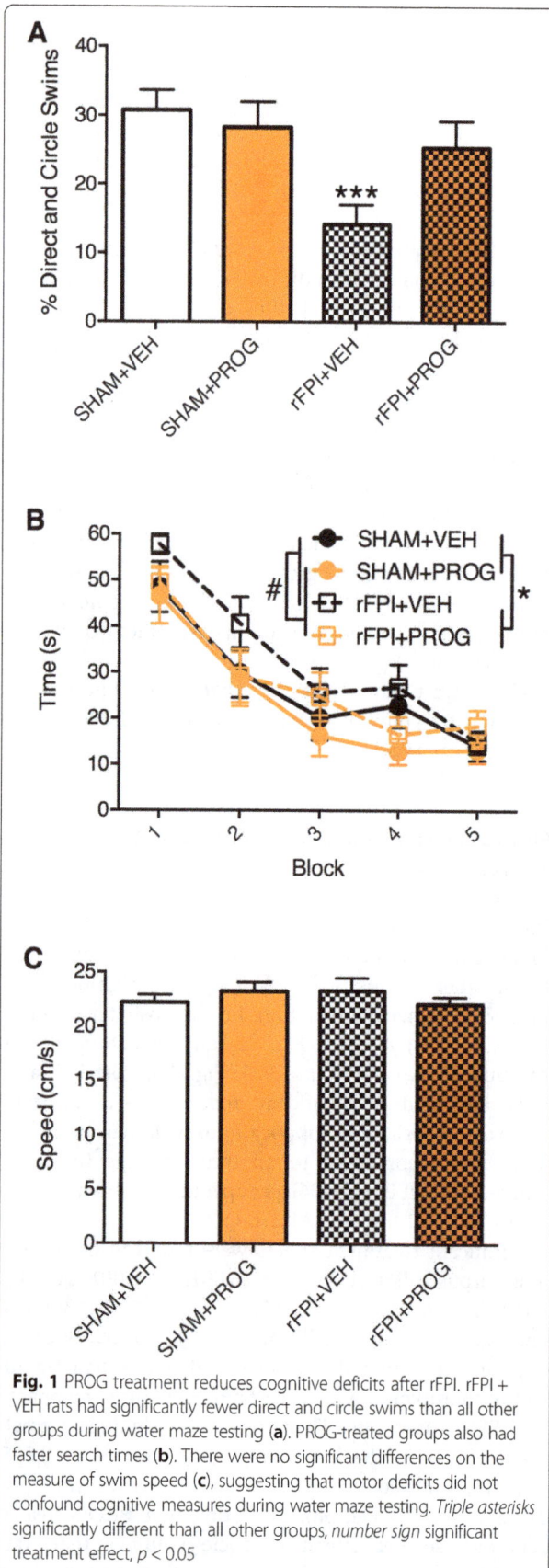

Fig. 1 PROG treatment reduces cognitive deficits after rFPI. rFPI + VEH rats had significantly fewer direct and circle swims than all other groups during water maze testing (**a**). PROG-treated groups also had faster search times (**b**). There were no significant differences on the measure of swim speed (**c**), suggesting that motor deficits did not confound cognitive measures during water maze testing. *Triple asterisks* significantly different than all other groups, *number sign* significant treatment effect, $p < 0.05$

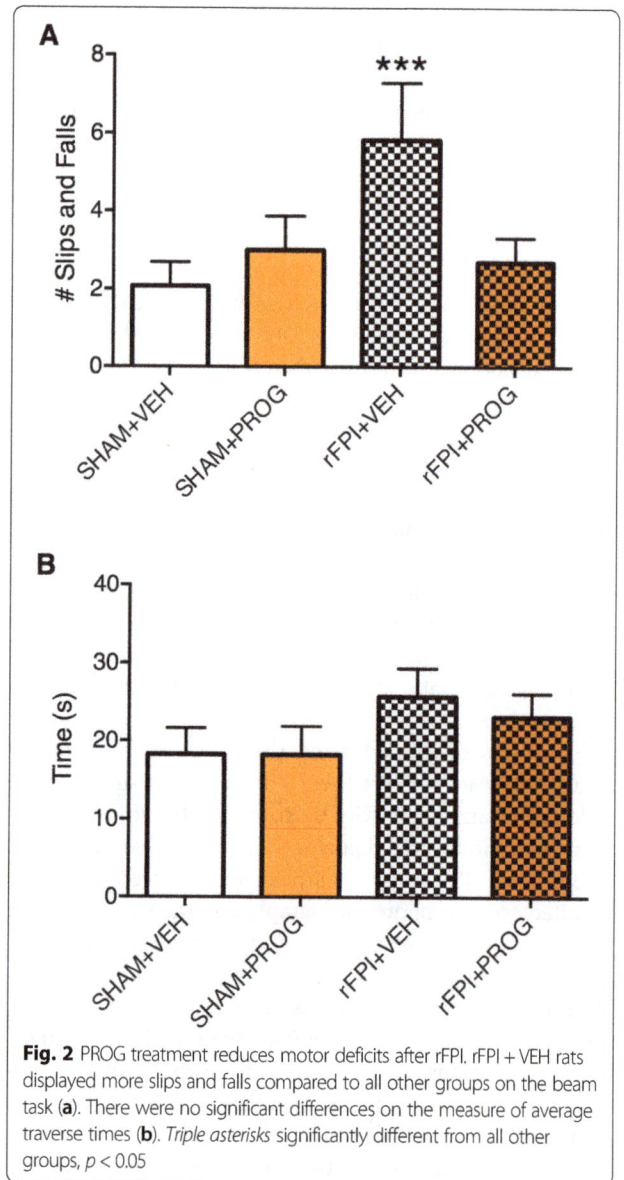

Fig. 2 PROG treatment reduces motor deficits after rFPI. rFPI + VEH rats displayed more slips and falls compared to all other groups on the beam task (**a**). There were no significant differences on the measure of average traverse times (**b**). *Triple asterisks* significantly different from all other groups, $p < 0.05$

Significant injury effects were found in the ipsilateral corpus callosum ($F_{1, 26} = 4.887$, $p < 0.05$), contralateral hippocampus ($F_{1,26} = 5.190$, $p < 0.05$), and contralateral corpus callosum ($F_{1, 26} = 9.220$, $p < 0.005$), indicating that rFPI rats had significantly less volume of these structures than SHAM rats. There were also significant injury effects in the ipsilateral ($F_{1, 26} = 11.812$, $p < 0.005$) and contralateral ($F_{1, 26} = 6.727$, $p < 0.05$) lateral ventricles indicating that rFPI rats had significantly larger lateral ventricles than SHAM rats.

DTI

The integrity of the corpus callosum, a major white matter tract commonly affected by mTBI, was assessed using DTI. ANOVA found a significant injury × treatment interaction ($F_{1, 26} = 4.340$, $p < 0.05$, Fig. 4e) on the

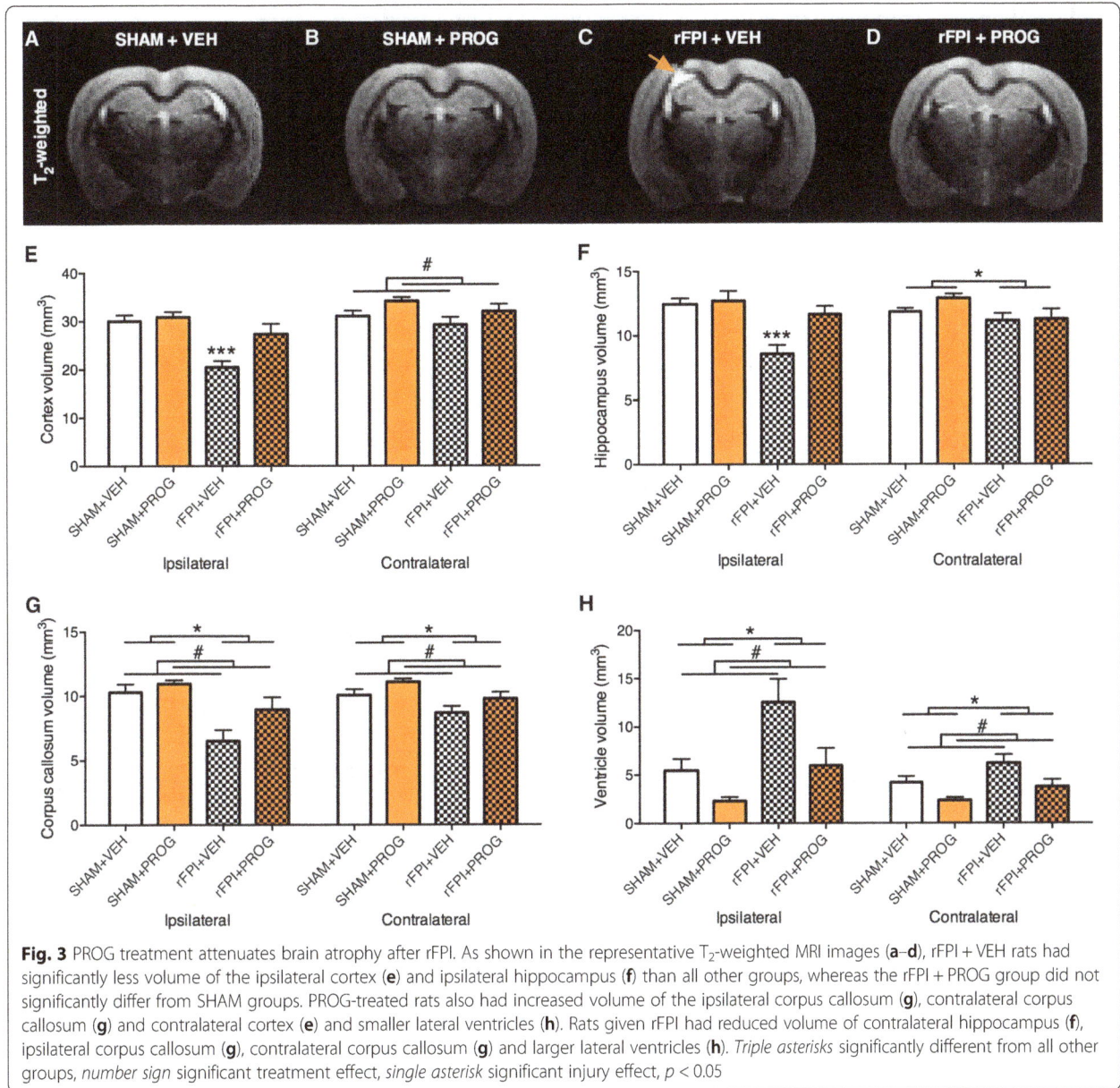

Fig. 3 PROG treatment attenuates brain atrophy after rFPI. As shown in the representative T_2-weighted MRI images (**a–d**), rFPI + VEH rats had significantly less volume of the ipsilateral cortex (**e**) and ipsilateral hippocampus (**f**) than all other groups, whereas the rFPI + PROG group did not significantly differ from SHAM groups. PROG-treated rats also had increased volume of the ipsilateral corpus callosum (**g**), contralateral corpus callosum (**g**) and contralateral cortex (**e**) and smaller lateral ventricles (**h**). Rats given rFPI had reduced volume of contralateral hippocampus (**f**), ipsilateral corpus callosum (**g**), contralateral corpus callosum (**g**) and larger lateral ventricles (**h**). *Triple asterisks* significantly different from all other groups, *number sign* significant treatment effect, *single asterisk* significant injury effect, $p < 0.05$

measure of FA in the ipsilateral corpus callosum. Post hoc analysis found that rFPI + VEH rats had a significant reduction in FA compared to all other groups ($p < 0.01$), suggesting axonal injury. Notably, rFPI + PROG rats were not significantly different than shams. There were no differences in FA findings in the contralateral corpus callosum.

In addition, significant treatment effects indicated that VEH-treated rats had increased mean diffusivity (ipsilateral corpus callosum, $F_{1, 26} = 7.876$, $p < 0.005$; contralateral corpus callosum, $F_{1, 26} = 4.313$, $p < 0.05$; Fig. 4f), radial diffusivity (ipsilateral corpus callosum, $F_{1, 26} = 8.127$, $p < 0.01$; contralateral corpus callosum, $F_{1, 26} = 4.443$, $p < 0.05$; Fig. 4g), and axial diffusivity (ipsilateral corpus callosum, $F_{1, 26} =$

6.897, $p < 0.05$, Fig. 4h). Significant injury effects further revealed that rats given rFPI also had increased mean diffusivity (ipsilateral corpus callosum, $F_{1, 26} = 10.570$, $p < 0.005$; contralateral corpus callosum, $F_{1, 26} = 10.047$, $p < 0.005$; Fig. 4f), radial diffusivity (ipsilateral corpus callosum, $F_{1, 26} = 13.924$, $p < 0.001$; contralateral corpus callosum, $F_{1, 26} = 14.225$, $p < 0.001$; Fig. 4g), and axial diffusivity (ipsilateral corpus callosum, $F_{1, 26} = 6.001$, $p < 0.05$; contralateral corpus callosum, $F_{1, 26} = 5.124$, $p < 0.05$; Fig. 4h).

PROG treatment reduces neuroinflammation and oxidative stress in rFPI

There was a significant injury × treatment interaction for GFAP immunoreactive area in the injured cortex

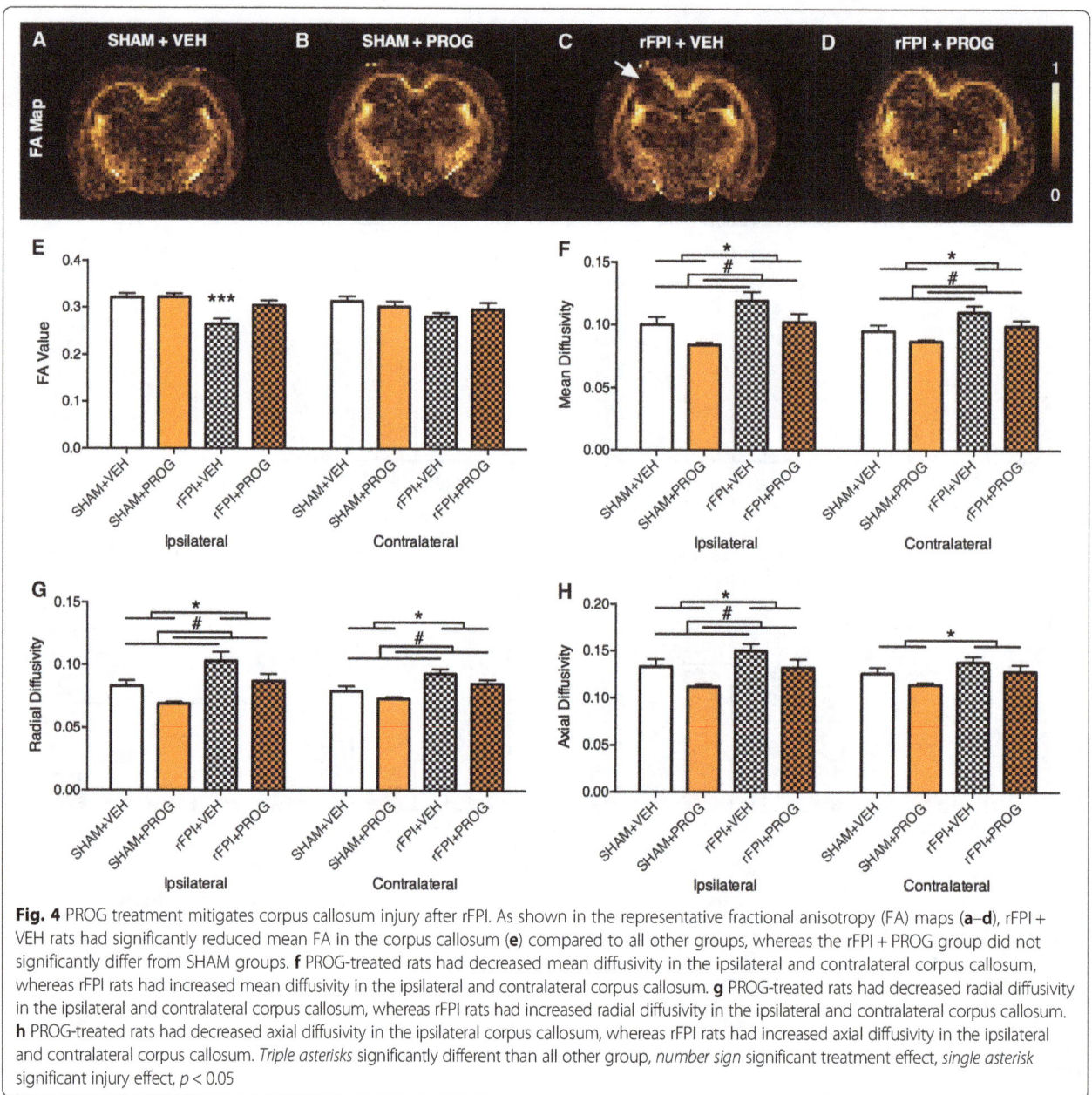

Fig. 4 PROG treatment mitigates corpus callosum injury after rFPI. As shown in the representative fractional anisotropy (FA) maps (**a–d**), rFPI + VEH rats had significantly reduced mean FA in the corpus callosum (**e**) compared to all other groups, whereas the rFPI + PROG group did not significantly differ from SHAM groups. **f** PROG-treated rats had decreased mean diffusivity in the ipsilateral and contralateral corpus callosum, whereas rFPI rats had increased mean diffusivity in the ipsilateral and contralateral corpus callosum. **g** PROG-treated rats had decreased radial diffusivity in the ipsilateral and contralateral corpus callosum, whereas rFPI rats had increased radial diffusivity in the ipsilateral and contralateral corpus callosum. **h** PROG-treated rats had decreased axial diffusivity in the ipsilateral corpus callosum, whereas rFPI rats had increased axial diffusivity in the ipsilateral and contralateral corpus callosum. *Triple asterisks* significantly different than all other group, *number sign* significant treatment effect, *single asterisk* significant injury effect, $p < 0.05$

$(F_{1, 17} = 7.642$, $p < 0.05$, Fig. 5i). Post hoc analysis found that rFPI + VEH rats had a significant increase of GFAP compared to all other groups ($p < 0.01$), whereas there was no difference between rFPI + PROG and SHAM groups. As shown in Fig. 5c, rFPI + VEH rats had densely stained and hypertrophic astrocytes with long and overlapping processes. These findings suggest that treatment with PROG attenuated rFPI-induced reactive astrogliosis.

There was a significant injury × treatment interaction for the number of CD68-positive cells in the injured cortex ($F_{1, 17} = 5.206$, $p < 0.05$, Fig. 5j). Post hoc analysis found that rFPI + VEH rats had significantly more

CD68-positive cells than all other groups ($p < 0.05$), whereas there was no difference between rFPI + PROG and SHAM groups. As shown in Fig. 5g, these CD68-postive cells had an amoeboid morphology typical of phagocytic macrophages. These findings suggest that treatment with PROG attenuated the rFPI-induced activation of macrophages/microglia.

ANOVA found a significant injury × treatment interaction ($F_{1, 13} = 7.177$, $p < 0.05$, Fig. 5k) in MDA, an indicator of lipid peroxidation. Post hoc analysis found that rFPI + VEH rats had significantly higher levels of MDA than all other groups, including the rFPI + PROG group ($p < 0.05$). However, it was also found that rFPI + PROG

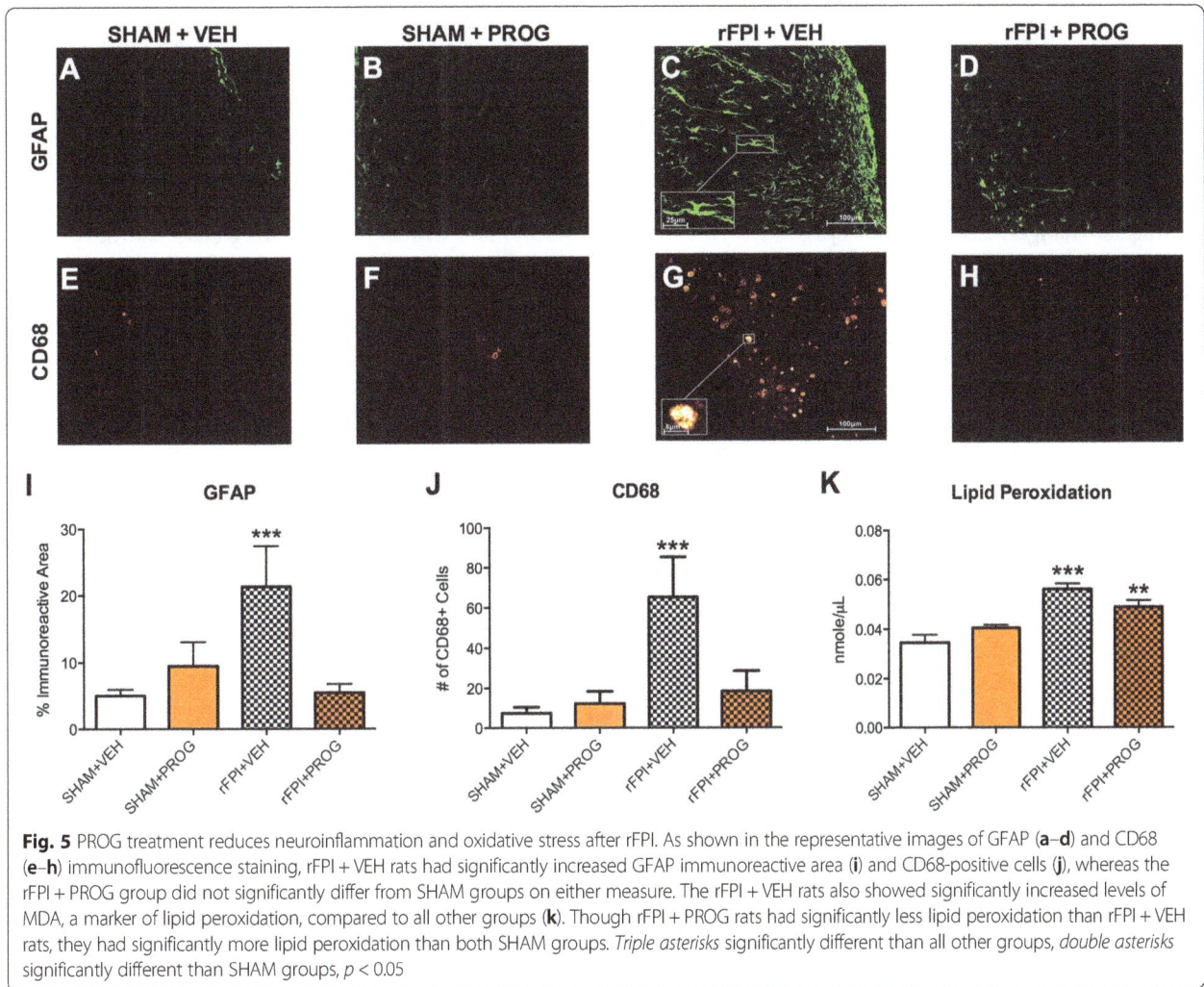

Fig. 5 PROG treatment reduces neuroinflammation and oxidative stress after rFPI. As shown in the representative images of GFAP (**a–d**) and CD68 (**e–h**) immunofluorescence staining, rFPI + VEH rats had significantly increased GFAP immunoreactive area (**i**) and CD68-positive cells (**j**), whereas the rFPI + PROG group did not significantly differ from SHAM groups on either measure. The rFPI + VEH rats also showed significantly increased levels of MDA, a marker of lipid peroxidation, compared to all other groups (**k**). Though rFPI + PROG rats had significantly less lipid peroxidation than rFPI + VEH rats, they had significantly more lipid peroxidation than both SHAM groups. *Triple asterisks* significantly different than all other groups, *double asterisks* significantly different than SHAM groups, $p < 0.05$

rats had significantly higher levels of MDA than both SHAM groups ($p < 0.05$), suggesting that treatment with PROG reduced rFPI-induced lipid peroxidation but did not prevent it.

Discussion

Repetitive mild brain injuries can result in cumulative brain damage and neurodegeneration that has been linked to neuroinflammation and oxidative stress, and there are currently no clinically available treatment options known to mitigate these effects in rmTBI patients. Therefore, here, we conducted the first study to evaluate the potential of PROG to reduce neuroinflammation and oxidative stress, and the associated neurodegeneration and neurological impairments, in experimental rmTBI. Rats given rFPI and treated with VEH had increased neuroinflammation and oxidative stress, with concomitant damage to grey and white matter brain structures, and cognitive and motor deficits at 12 weeks post-injury. Importantly, rats given rFPI and treated with PROG had significantly less neuroinflammation, oxidative stress and

brain damage, in addition to improved cognitive and sensorimotor function compared to their VEH-treated counterparts. These novel data demonstrate that PROG treatment has anti-inflammatory, anti-oxidant and neuroprotective effects in experimental rmTBI and thus presents potential as a therapeutic intervention for the clinical presentation of this syndrome.

The role of neuroinflammation and oxidative stress in rmTBI

The pathogenesis of rmTBI likely involves a number of secondary injury processes. Growing evidence, supported by our findings here, implicates neuroinflammation and oxidative stress as key contributing factors [7, 8]. Sustained neuroinflammation, characterized by activation of microglia and astrocytes, is known to be a key mediator of progressive secondary injury after brain insult and other neurodegenerative conditions [8]. With regard to mTBI, we and others have reported transient neuroinflammation after a single mild FPI in rats that becomes exacerbated and sustained upon repeated insults [10–12, 23, 25, 30].

Consistent with these findings, we observed astrogliosis, as indicated by increased GFAP immunoreactivity, and increased activated microglia and macrophages, as evidenced by increased CD68-positive cells with amoeboid morphologies, in the injured cortex of rFPI + VEH rats at 12 weeks post-injury.

Once activated, astrocytes and microglia undergo morphological changes. Reactive astrocytosis involves cellular hypertrophy, lengthened processes and increased expression of GFAP [35]. Activated microglia undergo a morphological change, taking on an amoeboid shape resembling peripheral macrophages, and scavenge the damaged CNS, performing phagocytic functions [39, 40]. Activated astrocytes and microglia produce and release a number of pro-inflammatory mediators, including the cytokine tumour necrosis factor-alpha (TNF-α) and interleukin-1 beta (IL-1β) that may contribute to secondary brain damage through mechanisms such as apoptosis [39, 40]. Activated microglia/macrophages, reactive astrocytes and other immune cells can also produce and release reactive oxygen species, such as nitric oxide, that contribute to oxidative stress—an imbalance of reactive oxygen species and endogenous anti-oxidants agents [11, 28, 39–43]. Neuroinflammatory factors such as NF-κB, signaling downstream of TNF-α and nitric oxide, are robustly elevated after TBI and likely contribute to oxidative stress and neuronal loss, which in turn further exacerbate the inflammatory response [44, 45]. One consequence of oxidative stress is lipid peroxidation, which involves the oxidative degradation of lipids in cell membranes [11, 21, 28, 46]. We also detected an increase in lipid peroxidation in rats given rFPI + VEH.

Our findings of persisting neuroinflammation and oxidative stress occurred in the presence of structural brain damage and functional impairments, which suggests a role for these secondary injury pathways in the pathogenesis of rmTBI. Further supporting this notion, we found that PROG attenuated the persisting neuroinflammation and oxidative stress and that these changes were associated with decreased brain damage and improved long-term cognitive and motor outcomes in rats given rmTBI. These results of anti-inflammatory and anti-oxidant effects of PROG treatment in rmTBI are consistent with previous experiments in moderate to severe TBI studies [19–22]. Whilst the exact mechanisms remain unclear, PROG is thought to act on inflammation and oxidative stress both directly [47, 48] and indirectly by the modulation of toll-like receptors and NF-κB signaling with a concurrent reduction in cytokines [49, 50]. Nitric oxide has also been shown to be reduced by post-injury treatment with PROG, possibly through the prevention of inducible nitric oxide synthase, an isoform that abundantly produces nitric oxide during secondary injury [51, 52]. It should be noted that although rFPI +

PROG rats had significantly reduced levels of lipid peroxidation than the rFPI + VEH group, MDA levels were still elevated compared to both SHAM groups. This remaining oxidative stress may have contributed to the relatively mild MRI-detected brain damage that was still evident in the rFPI + PROG rats. That PROG treatment was not able to fully negate oxidative stress may be due to a number of reasons, including dose and duration of the PROG treatment or the potential contribution of other mechanisms not targeted by PROG, and requires further exploration. For example, future experimentation could look at a combinatorial therapy, with the addition of agents targeting other secondary pathways.

The nature of cognitive and motor deficits after rmTBI
Spatial cognition, as assessed in the water maze [53, 54], was shown to be impaired in rFPI + VEH rats through the measure of direct and circle swims, consistent with previous data [10, 11]. Direct and circle swims represent the most efficient route to a known escape position in the water maze, indicating that rFPI + VEH rats were less efficient at the task than the other groups [10, 11, 53, 54]. As there were no group differences on the measure of swim speed during water maze testing, or any anxiety-related outcomes in other tasks, the deficits observed in the rFPI + VEH rats were likely cognitive in nature. Notably, the rFPI + PROG group did not significantly differ from the two SHAM groups on the measure of direct and circle swims, suggesting that PROG was able to preserve cognitive function after rFPI. There was also a significant treatment effect indicating that PROG-treated rats located the hidden platform faster than VEH-treated rats, which further supports the notion that PROG preserved cognitive function in the water maze.

Consistent with previous studies [10, 11], the rFPI + VEH rats displayed significant sensorimotor deficits, as indicated by more slips and falls on the beam task compared to all other groups [55]. In contrast, the rFPI + PROG rats did not show any significant sensorimotor deficits relative to the SHAM groups. As there were no differences found in average beam traverse times, nor in other gross motor measures from the other behavioural tasks between groups, these sensorimotor deficits occurring in the rFPI + VEH rats was likely mild in nature. Nonetheless, these findings indicate that PROG treatment is able to attenuate both sensorimotor and cognitive dysfunction after rFPI.

The cognitive and sensorimotor deficits in the rFPI + VEH rats, and the preservation of these functions in the rFPI + PROG rats, may be related to the degree of brain damage in these animals. MRI-based volumetric analysis of the ipsilateral cortex and ipsilateral hippocampus revealed significant atrophy of these structures in the rFPI + VEH rats that did not occur in the rFPI + PROG rats. Of particular note, the sensorimotor cortex is situated near the FPI impact area [27, 56, 57], and damage to the cortex and hippocampus has been linked to cognitive and sensorimotor deficits in TBI [27, 58–61]. DTI analyses of the corpus callosum, a major white matter tract commonly affected by TBI [62], showed significant diffusion abnormalities suggestive of axonal injury in the rFPI + VEH group but not in the rFPI + PROG group. Finally, a previous study found that rats given a TBI had increased cell proliferation and survival of immature neurons in the dentate gyrus of the hippocampus and that PROG treatment normalized these effects [63]. Because the hippocampus is an important structure involved in cognitive function, it is interesting to speculate whether abnormalities in neurogenesis may be involved in the cognitive outcomes we found here. Taken together, it is likely that changes to each of the abovementioned brain structures may have contributed to the behavioural findings in this study. However, further research is required to determine the precise mechanisms underlying the functional deficits occurring in rmTBI.

PROG as a treatment for mTBI patients?

To our knowledge, this is the first study to demonstrate that PROG reduces neuroinflammation, oxidative stress, brain damage and functional deficits in experimental rmTBI, particularly in the more chronic stage of injury. Considering that there is currently no effective treatment known to reduce the detrimental long-term effects caused by rmTBI, these findings hold important implications for the future treatment of mTBI patients. In this study, we began PROG treatment after the first mTBI and continued treatment until 5 days after the third injury. As such, PROG treatment was given prophylactically for the second and third injuries, and this may have contributed to the protective effects. In the clinical setting, this could be comparable to a high-risk individual (e.g., athlete or soldier) who has already suffered one mTBI and continues treatment for the remaining duration of their high-risk activity (e.g., season or tour of duty). As the recommended time window for PROG treatment after a brain insult is within 2 h [64, 65], this preventative treatment paradigm may be advantageous within these high-risk environments. However, there are other possible scenarios where PROG treatment may be beneficial as a therapy for mTBI. For example, it is possible that PROG treatment acutely after a single mTBI may improve recovery, prevent post-concussion syndrome or reduce vulnerability to a second brain insult. PROG treatment in the chronic stages post-mTBI may also be beneficial for the minority of mTBI patients who do suffer a persisting post-concussion syndrome or for individuals who have suffered past mTBIs and have persisting neuroinflammation. Of particular interest, a recent study utilizing PET imaging found that retired NFL players with a history of mTBI had increased binding of [^{11}C]DPA-713 to translocator protein, an indicator of neuroinflammation, as well as concomitant brain atrophy [66]. Therefore, treatment with PROG at chronic stages post-injury should also be explored, and the use of neuroinflammatory biomarkers (e.g., PET) could allow for a more precise medical approach. Taken together, there are a number of clinical mTBI settings where PROG treatment may be applicable; however, future studies are clearly required to investigate whether PROG treatment is beneficial in these various scenarios and to determine the optimal therapeutic windows and dose.

Importantly, PROG has a long history of clinical use and safe administration in both male and female patients [67, 68]. This includes recent phase III clinical trials with PROG treatment in severe TBI patients [69, 70]. Unfortunately, these trials did not show improvement on the Glasgow Outcome Scale and Extended Glasgow Outcome Scale at 3 and 6 months post-injury in moderate and severe TBI patients treated acutely with PROG [69, 70]. Though these trials failed to demonstrate efficacy for PROG treatment in more severe TBI, the authors of these studies raised a number of limitations that are important to consider including limited/insensitive outcome measures, unidimensional TBI characterization approaches (e.g., Glasgow coma scale) and the heterogeneity of severe TBI [69–73]. It has also been suggested that sub-optimal doses were used in the PROG trials [71–73], which highlight the need to measure PROG levels in future clinical and pre-clinical studies. It is also worth speculating whether PROG, which targets secondary injury processes, may be better suited to attenuate responses in the more subtle pathological environment occurring in mTBI and rmTBI, where there is little to no irreversible primary injury. This is in contrast to moderate and severe TBI, where the primary injury incurred at the moment of impact contributes to a large part of the deficits seen in patients, and initiates a robust secondary injury response resulting in considerable swelling, cell death and tissue loss [74].

Conclusions

Here, we examined whether PROG treatment in rats given rmTBI improved long-term outcomes. Progesterone treatment significantly attenuated markers of neuroinflammation and oxidative stress in rats given rmTBI, with concomitant reductions in behavioural impairments and brain damage. These findings further implicate neuroinflammation and oxidative stress in the pathophysiological aftermath of mild brain injuries. Furthermore, the proven safety and limited negative side effects of PROG, along with our findings here, suggest that PROG may be a viable treatment option within the context of mTBIs and their more chronic consequences.

Abbreviations

ANOVA: analysis of variance; CTE: chronic traumatic encephalopathy; DTI: diffusion tensor imaging; FA: fractional anisotropy; MDA: malondialdehyde; mTBI: mild traumatic brain injury; PROG: progesterone; rFPI: repeated mild fluid percussion injury; rmTBI: repeated mild traumatic brain injuries; ROI: regions of interest; SHAM: sham injury; TBARS: thiobarbituric acid reactive substances; VEH: cyclodextrin vehicle.

Competing interests

DGS along with Emory University retains patents related to the use of progesterone in TBI and certain forms of CNS tumours but has no financial gains, royalties or licensing agreements from research on progesterone. None of the other authors have competing interests.

Authors' contributions

SRS, TOB, DGS and BDS conceptualized and designed the study. SRS completed all surgeries and injuries. KMW completed all injections and behavioural testing. KMW, MS and EO completed immunofluorescence and lipid peroxidation assays. KMW and DW completed MRI analysis. All authors were involved in data interpretation and writing the manuscript. All authors read and approved the final manuscript.

Acknowledgements

We would like to thank Dr. Iqbal Sayeed (Emory University) for his contributions towards this project. This study was funded by a grant to SRS from the National Health and Medical Research Council (NHMRC #1062653) and fellowships to SRS from the Canadian Institute of Health Research and NHMRC.

Author details

[1]Department of Medicine, The Royal Melbourne Hospital, The University of Melbourne, Parkville, VIC 3050, Australia. [2]Anatomy and Neuroscience, The University of Melbourne, Parkville, VIC 3010, Australia. [3]The Florey Institute of Neuroscience and Mental Health, Parkville, VIC 3052, Australia. [4]Department of Emergency Medicine, Emory University, Atlanta, GA 30322, USA.

References

1. McCrory P, Meeuwisse W, Aubry M, Cantu B, Dvorak J, Echemendia RJ, et al. Consensus statement on concussion in sport: the 4th International Conference on Concussion in Sport held in Zurich, November 2012. Br J Sports Med. 2013; 47:250–8.
2. Signoretti S, Lazzarino G, Tavazzi B, Vagnozzi R. The pathophysiology of concussion. PM R. 2011;3:S359–68.
3. Guskiewicz KM, Marshall SW, Bailes J, McCrea M, Cantu RC, Randolph C, et al. Association between recurrent concussion and late-life cognitive impairment in retired professional football players. Neurosurgery. 2005;57: 719–26.
4. Guskiewicz KM, Marshall SW, Bailes J, McCrea M, Harding Jr HP, Matthews A, et al. Recurrent concussion and risk of depression in retired professional football players. Med Sci Sports Exerc. 2007;39:903–9.
5. Guskiewicz KM, McCrea M, Marshall SW, Cantu RC, Randolph C, Barr W, et al. Cumulative effects associated with recurrent concussion in collegiate football players: the NCAA concussion study. JAMA. 2003;290:2549–55.
6. DeKosky ST, Blennow K, Ikonomovic MD, Gandy S. Acute and chronic traumatic encephalopathies: pathogenesis and biomarkers. Nat Rev Neurol. 2013;9:192–200.
7. Roth TL, Nayak D, Atanasijevic T, Koretsky AP, Latour LL, McGavern DB. Transcranial amelioration of inflammation and cell death after brain injury. Nature. 2014;505:223–8.

8. Faden AI, Loane DJ. Chronic neurodegeneration after traumatic brain injury: Alzheimer disease, chronic traumatic encephalopathy, or persistent neuroinflammation? Neurotherapeutics. 2015;12:143–50.
9. Ramlackhansingh AF, Brooks DJ, Greenwood RJ, Bose SK, Turkheimer FE, Kinnunen KM, et al. Inflammation after trauma: microglial activation and traumatic brain injury. Ann Neurol. 2011;70:374–83.
10. Shultz SR, Bao F, Omana V, Chiu C, Brown A, Cain DP. Repeated mild lateral fluid percussion brain injury in the rat causes cumulative long-term behavioral impairments, neuroinflammation, and cortical loss in an animal model of repeated concussion. J Neurotrauma. 2012;29:281–94.
11. Shultz SR, Bao F, Weaver LC, Cain DP, Brown A. Treatment with an anti-CD11d integrin antibody reduces neuroinflammation and improves outcome in a rat model of repeated concussion. J Neuroinflammation. 2013;15:26.
12. Aungst SL, Kabadi SV, Thompson SM, Stoica BA, Faden AI. Repeated mild traumatic brain injury causes chronic neuroinflammation, changes in hippocampal synaptic plasticity, and associated cognitive deficits. J Cereb Blood Flow Metab. 2014;34:1223–32.
13. Mouzon BC, Bachmeier C, Ferro A, Ojo JO, Crynen G, Acker CM, et al. Chronic neuropathological and neurobehavioral changes in a repetitive mild traumatic brain injury model. Ann Neurol. 2014;75:241–54.
14. Mouzon B, Chaytow H, Crynen G, Bachmeier C, Stewart J, Mullan M, et al. Repetitive mild traumatic brain injury in a mouse model produces learning and memory deficits accompanied by histological changes. J Neurotrauma. 2012;29:2761–73.
15. Laurer HL, Bareyre FM, Lee VM, Trojanowski JQ, Longhi L, Hoover R, et al. Mild head injury increasing the brain's vulnerability to a second concussive impact. J Neurosurg. 2001;95:859–70.
16. Uryu K, Laurer H, McIntosh T, Pratico D, Martinez D, Leight S, et al. Repetitive mild brain trauma accelerates Abeta deposition, lipid peroxidation, and cognitive impairment in a transgenic mouse model of Alzheimer amyloidosis. J Neurosci. 2002;22:446–54.
17. Creeley CE, Wozniak DF, Bayly PV, Olney JW, Lewis LM. Multiple episodes of mild traumatic brain injury result in impaired cognitive performance in mice. Academic emergency medicine: Acad Emerg Med. 2004;11:809–19.
18. Stein DG, Wright DW. Progesterone in the clinical treatment of acute traumatic brain injury. Expert Opin Investig Drugs. 2010;19(7):847–57.
19. Roof RL, Duvdevani R, Braswell L, Stein DG. Progesterone facilitates cognitive recovery and reduces secondary neuronal loss caused by cortical contusion injury in male rats. Exp Neurol. 1994;129:64–9.
20. Shear DA, Galani R, Hoffman SW, Stein DG. Progesterone protects against necrotic damage and behavioral abnormalities caused by traumatic brain injury. Exp Neurol. 2002;178:59–67.
21. Roof RL, Hoffman SW, Stein DG. Progesterone protects against lipid peroxidation following traumatic brain injury in rats. Mol Chem Neuropathol. 1997;31:1–11.
22. He J, Evans CO, Hoffman SW, Oyesiku NM, Stein DG. Progesterone and allopregnanolone reduce inflammatory cytokines after traumatic brain injury. Exp Neurol. 2004;189:404–12.
23. Shultz SR, MacFabe DF, Foley KA, Taylor R, Cain DP. A single mild fluid percussion injury induces short-term behavioral and neuropathological changes in the Long-Evans rat: support for an animal model of concussion. Behav Brain Res. 2011;224:326–35.
24. DeRoss AL, Adams JE, Vane DW, Russell SJ, Terella AM, Wald SL. Multiple head injuries in rats: effects on behavior. J Trauma. 2002;52:708–14.
25. Hylin MJ, Orsi SA, Zhao J, Bockhorst K, Perez A, Moore AN, et al. Behavioral and histopathological alterations resulting from mild fluid percussion injury. J Neurotrauma. 2013;30:702–15.
26. Walf AA, Frye CA. The use of the elevated plus maze as an assay of anxiety-related behavior in rodents. Nat Protoc. 2007;2:322–8.
27. Johnstone VPA, Wright DK, Wong K, O'Brien TJ, Rajan R, Shultz SR. Experimental traumatic brain injury results in long-term recovery of functional responsiveness in sensory cortex but persisting structural changes and sensorimotor, cognitive, and emotional deficits. J Neurotrauma. 2015;32:1333–46.
28. Bao F, Shultz SR, Hepburn JD, Omana V, Weaver LC, Cain DP, et al. A CD11d monoclonal antibody treatment reduces tissue injury and improves neurological outcome after fluid percussion brain injury in rats. J Neurotrauma. 2012;29:2375–92.
29. Porsolt RD, Le Pichon M, Jalfre M. Depression: a new animal model sensitive to antidepressant treatments. Nature. 1977;266:730–2.

30. Shultz SR, MacFabe DF, Foley KA, Taylor R, Cain DP. Sub-concussive brain injury in the Long-Evans rat induces acute neuroinflammation in the absence of behavioral impairments. Behav Brain Res. 2012;229:145–52.

31. Shultz SR, Tan XL, Wright DK, Liu SJ, Semple BD, Johnston L, et al. Granulocyte-macrophage colony-stimulating factor (GM-CSF) is neuroprotective in experimental traumatic brain injury. J Neurotrauma. 2014;31:976–83.

32. Shultz SR, Wright DK, Zheng P, Stuchbery R, Liu SJ, Sashindranath M, et al. Sodium selenate reduces hyperphosphorylated tau and improves outcomes after traumatic brain injury. Brain. 2015;138:1297–313.

33. Shultz SR, Aziz NA, Yang L, Sun M, MacFabe DF, O'Brien TJ. Intracerebroventricular injection of propionic acid, an enteric metabolite implicated in autism, induces social abnormalities that do not differ between seizure-prone (FAST) and seizure-resistant (SLOW) rats. Behav Brain Res. 2015;278:542–8.

34. Shi SR, Cote RJ, Taylor CR. Antigen retrieval techniques: current perspectives. J Histochem Cytochem. 2001;49:931–7.

35. Laird MD, Vender JR, Dhandapani KM. Opposing roles for reactive astrocytes following traumatic brain injury. Neurosignals. 2008;16:154–64.

36. Rabinowitz SS, Gordon S. Macrosialin, a macrophage-restricted membrane sialoprotein differentially glycosylated in response to inflammatory stimuli. J Exp Med. 1991;174:827–36.

37. Zotova E, Bharambe V, Cheaveau M, Morgan W, Holmes C, Harris S, et al. Inflammatory components in human Alzheimer's disease and after active amyloid-β_{42} immunization. Brain. 2013;136:2677–96.

38. Ferrer-Martin RM, Martin-Oliva D, Sierra A, Carrasco M-C, Martin-Estebane M, Calvente R, et al. Microglial cells in organotypic cultures of developing and adult mouse retina and their relationship with cell death. Exp Eye Res. 2014; 121:42–57.

39. Morganti-Kossman MC, Satgunaseelan NB, Kossman T. Modulation of immune response by head injury. Injury Int J. 2007;38:1392–400.

40. Kadhim HJ, Duchateau J, Sebire G. Cytokines and brain injury. J Intensive Care Med. 2009;23:236–49.

41. Lewen A, Matz P, Chan PH. Free radical pathways in CNS injury. J Neurotrauma. 2000;17:871–90.

42. Block ML, Zecca L, Hong J-S. Microglia-mediated neurotoxicity: uncovering the molecular mechanisms. Nat Rev Neurosci. 2007;8:57–69.

43. Sheng WS, Hu S, Feng A, Rock RB. Reactive oxygen species from human astrocytes induced functional impairment and oxidative damage. Neurochem Res. 2013;38:2148–59.

44. Cornelius C, Crupi R, Calabrese V, Graziano A, Milone P, Pennisi G, et al. Traumatic brain injury: oxidative stress and neuroprotection. Antioxid Redox Signal. 2013;19:836–53.

45. Abdul-Muneer PM, Chandra N, Haorah J. Interactions of oxidative stress and neurovascular inflammation in the pathogenesis of traumatic brain injury. Mol Neurobiol. 2015;51:966–79.

46. Tavazzi B, Vagnozzi R, Signoretti S, Amorini AM, Belli A, Cimatti M, et al. Temporal window of metabolic brain vulnerability to concussions: oxidative and nitrosative stresses—part II. Neurosurgery. 2007;61:390–5.

47. Ishihara Y, Takemoto T, Ishida A, Yamazaki T. Protective actions of 17β-estradiol and progesterone on oxidative neuronal injury induced by organometallic compounds. Oxid Med Cell Longev. 2015;2015: 343706.

48. Cai J, Cao S, Chen J, Yan F, Chen G, Dai Y. Progesterone alleviates acute brain injury via reducing apoptosis and oxidative stress in a rat experimental subarachnoid hemorrhage model. Neurosci Lett. 2015;600:238–43.

49. Roberston CL, Fidan E, Stanley RM, Noje C, Bayir H. Progesterone for neuroprotection in pediatric traumatic brain injury. Pediatr Crit Care Med. 2015;16:236–44.

50. Wang J, Zhao Y, Liu C, Jiang C, Zhao C, Zhu Z. Progesterone inhibits inflammatory respeonse pathways after permanent middle cerebral artery occlusion in rats. Mol Med Rep. 2011;4:319–24.

51. Gibson CL, Constantin D, Prior MJ, Bath PM, Murphy SP. Progesterone suppresses the inflammatory response and nitric oxide synthase-2 expression following cerebral ischemia. Exp Neurol. 2005;193:522–30.

52. Coughlan T, Gibson C, Murphy S. Modulatory effects of progesterone on inducible nitric oxide synthase expression in vivo and in vitro. J Neurochem. 2005;93:932–42.

53. Morris RGM. Synaptic plasticity and learning—selective impairment of learning in rats and blockade of long-term potentiation in vivo by the n-methyl-d-aspartate receptor anatagonist AP5. J Neurosci. 1989;9:3040–57.

54. Whishaw IQ, Jarrard LE. Similarities vs differences in place learning and circadian activity in rats after fimbria-fornix section or ibotenate removal of hippocampal cells. Hippocampus. 1995;5:595–604.

55. Kolb B, Whishaw IQ. Earlier is not always better: behavioral dysfunction and abnormal cerebral morphogenesis following neonatal cortical lesions in the rat. Behav Brain Res. 1985;17:25–43.

56. Paxinos G, Watson C. The rat brain in stereotaxic coordinates. 6th ed. Amsterdam: Elsevier; 2007.

57. Johnstone VPA, Shultz SR, Yan EB, O'Brien TJ, Rajan R. The acute phase of mild traumatic brain injury is characterized by a distance-dependent neuronal hypoactivity. J Neurotrauma. 2014;31:1881–95.

58. Pierce JES, Smith DH, Trojanowski JQ, McIntosh TK. Enduring cognitive, neurobehavioral and histopathological changes persist for up to one year following severe experimental brain injury in rats. Neuroscience. 1998;87: 359–69.

59. Scheff SW, Baldwin SA, Brown RW, Kraemer PJ. Morris water maze deficits in rats following traumatic brain injury: lateral controlled cortical impact. J Neurotrauma. 1997;14:615–27.

60. Gould KR, Ponsford JL, Johnston L, Schonberger M. The nature, frequency and course of psychiatric disorders in the first year after traumatic brain injury: a prospective study. Psychol Med. 2011;41:2099–109.

61. Arciniegas DB, Held K, Wagner P. Cognitive impairment following traumatic brain injury. Curr Treat Options Neurol. 2002;4:43–57.

62. Aoki Y, Inokuchi R, Gunshin M, et al. Diffusion tensor imaging studies of mild traumatic brain injury: a meta-analysis. J Neurol Neurosurg Psychiatry. 2012;83:870–6.

63. Barha CK, Ishrat T, Epp JR, Galea LA, Stein DG. Progesterone treatment normalizes the levels of cell proliferation and cell death in the dentate gyrus of the hippocampus after traumatic brain injury. Exp Neurol. 2011;231:72–81.

64. Roof RL, Duvdevani R, Heyburn JW, Stein DG. Progesterone rapidly decreases brain edema: treatment delayed up to 24 hours is still effective. Exp Neurol. 1996;138:246–51.

65. Wright DW, Kellermann AL, Hertzberg VS, Clark PL, Frankel M, Goldstein FC, et al. ProTECT: a randomized clinical trial of progesterone for acute traumatic brain injury. Ann Emerg Med. 2007;49:391–402.

66. Coughlin JM, Wang Y, Munro CA, Ma S, Yue C, Chen S, et al. Neuroinflammation and brain atrophy in former NFL players: an in vivo multimodal imaging pilot study. Neurobiol Dis. 2015;74:58–65.

67. Aebi S, Schnider TW, Los G, Heath DD, Darrah D, Kirmani S, et al. A phase II/ pharmacokinetic trial of high-dose progesterone in combination with paclitaxel. Cancer Chemother Pharmacol. 1999;44:259–65.

68. Allolio B, Oremus M, Reincke M, Schaeffer HJ, Winkelmann W, Heck G, et al. High-dose progesterone infusion in healthy males: evidence against antiglucocorticoid activity of progesterone. Eur J Endocrinol. 1995;133: 696–700.

69. Wright DW, Yeatts SD, Silbergleit R, Paleshc YY, Hertzberg VS, Frankel M, et al. Very early administration of progesterone for acute traumatic brain injury. N Engl J Med. 2014;371:2457–66.

70. Skolnick BE, Maas AI, Narayan RK, van der Hoop RG, MacAllister T, Ward JD, et al. A clinical trial of progesterone for severe traumatic brain injury. N Engl J Med. 2014;371:2467–76.

71. Stein DG. Embracing failure: what the phase III progesterone studies can teach about TBI clinical trials. Brain Inj. 2015;29:1259–72.

72. Howard RB, Sayeed I, Stein DG. Suboptimal dosing parameters as possible factors in the negative phase III clinical trials of progesterone for TBI. J Neurotrauma 2015; epub ahead of print.

73. Stein DG. Lost in translation: understanding the failure of the progesterone/ TBI phase III trials. Future Neurol 2015; epub ahead of print.

74. Blennow K, Hardy J, Zetterberg H. The neuropathology and neurobiology of traumatic brain injury. Neuron. 2012;76:886–99.

9

Novel TNF receptor-1 inhibitors identified as potential therapeutic candidates for traumatic brain injury

Rachel K. Rowe[1,2,3*], Jordan L. Harrison[4], Hongtao Zhang[5], Adam D. Bachstetter[6], David P. Hesson[5], Bruce F. O'Hara[7], Mark I. Greene[5] and Jonathan Lifshitz[1,2,3,4]

Abstract

Background: Traumatic brain injury (TBI) begins with the application of mechanical force to the head or brain, which initiates systemic and cellular processes that are hallmarks of the disease. The pathological cascade of secondary injury processes, including inflammation, can exacerbate brain injury-induced morbidities and thus represents a plausible target for pharmaceutical therapies. We have pioneered research on post-traumatic sleep, identifying that injury-induced sleep lasting for 6 h in brain-injured mice coincides with increased cortical levels of inflammatory cytokines, including tumor necrosis factor (TNF). Here, we apply post-traumatic sleep as a physiological bio-indicator of inflammation. We hypothesized the efficacy of novel TNF receptor (TNF-R) inhibitors could be screened using post-traumatic sleep and that these novel compounds would improve functional recovery following diffuse TBI in the mouse.

Methods: Three inhibitors of TNF-R activation were synthesized based on the structure of previously reported TNF CIAM inhibitor F002, which lodges into a defined TNFR1 cavity at the TNF-binding interface, and screened for in vitro efficacy of TNF pathway inhibition (IκB phosphorylation). Compounds were screened for in vivo efficacy in modulating post-traumatic sleep. Compounds were then tested for efficacy in improving functional recovery and verification of cellular mechanism.

Results: Brain-injured mice treated with Compound 7 (C7) or SGT11 slept significantly less than those treated with vehicle, suggesting a therapeutic potential to target neuroinflammation. SGT11 restored cognitive, sensorimotor, and neurological function. C7 and SGT11 significantly decreased cortical inflammatory cytokines 3 h post-TBI.

Conclusions: Using sleep as a bio-indicator of TNF-R-dependent neuroinflammation, we identified C7 and SGT11 as potential therapeutic candidates for TBI.

Keywords: Diffuse brain injury, Midline fluid percussion, Mouse, Concussion, Cytokines, Tumor necrosis factor

Background

There are approximately 1.7 million TBIs in the USA annually, with approximately 1.36 million that seek medical treatments [1]. The primary injury caused by a TBI occurs at the time of the mechanical impact, with limited possibilities to mitigate this damage; however, secondary injury processes, such as inflammation, oxidative stress, and excitotoxicity, amplify the primary damage

and represent plausible targets for pharmaceutical intervention [2]. The development of an effective pharmacological therapy for acute TBI could prevent, restrict, or reverse the emergence of chronic post-traumatic morbidities. Such therapy may also require a systematic pre-clinical paradigm to translate pharmacological neuroprotection into improving neurological performance, as proposed by Janowitz and Menon [3].

Following TBI, the pathophysiological inflammation as part of secondary injury processes can contribute to worsening outcome [4, 5], particularly with unregulated inflammatory cytokine signaling [4–6]. Tumor necrosis factor (TNF)-α has central nervous system function by

* Correspondence: rkro222@email.arizona.edu
[1]BARROW Neurological Institute at Phoenix Children's Hospital, Phoenix, AZ, USA
[2]Department of Child Health, University of Arizona College of Medicine—Phoenix, Phoenix, AZ, USA
Full list of author information is available at the end of the article

contributing to the activation of microglia and astrocytes and release of inflammation mediating cytokines and can influence blood-brain barrier permeability and synaptic plasticity [7]. TNF functions through interaction with two members of the TNF-receptor (TNFR) family, TNFR1 and TNFR2. TNFR1 has been associated with inflammation and degeneration, whereas TNFR2 has been identified as neuroprotective [8, 9], for review see [10]. For this reason, we chose to spare the effects of TNF through TNFR2 signaling and selectively inhibit TNF function through TNFR1.

In vitro studies have revealed complex and divergent TNFR signaling pathways that account for TNF's ability to induce cell death, co-stimulation, and cell activation [11]. TNFR signaling results in the phosphorylation and degradation of the inhibitor of NF-κB (IκB), which allows for the translocation of NF-κB to the nucleus where it binds DNA and functions as a transcription factor [11]. Thus, TNF-induced NF-κB is a master regulator of inflammation since NFκB is a global activator of pro-inflammatory cytokines, chemokines, and their receptors [11].

TNF-α is pleiotropic in its actions regarding the regulation of inflammation. Relevant to the current study, substantial evidence also supports the involvement of TNF-α in the physiological process of sleep [12–16]. An increase in sleep is temporally associated with the acute increase in inflammation following TBI [17]. Therefore, sleep can be used as a sensitive bio-indicator of the ability of novel TNFR1 inhibitor compounds to modulate TBI-induced neuroinflammation and behavioral phenotypes. Herein, we report that the novel allosteric modulators of TNFR1 inhibitors improved functional recovery following diffuse TBI in the mouse. In addition, we validated sleep as a bio-indicator of TNFR1-dependent neuroinflammation, which could be applied as a minimally invasive approach to show therapeutic efficacy in future clinical studies.

Methods
Study design
In a controlled laboratory experiment, this study tested a refined pre-clinical strategy to identify and confirm the utility of experimental compounds with therapeutic potential for treating acute TBI pathophysiology. All animal studies were conducted in accordance with the guidelines established by the internal IACUC (Institutional Animal Care and Use Committee) and the NIH guidelines for the care and use of laboratory animals. Studies are reported following the ARRIVE (Animal Research: Reporting In Vivo experiments) guidelines [18]. Randomization of animals was achieved by assigning animals to treatment groups before the initiation of the study to ensure equal distribution across groups. A

power analysis was performed to calculate group sizes that enable statistically robust detection of injury-induced deficits while minimizing the number of animals needed. This calculation was based on preliminary data and previously published work from our group. Data collection stopped at pre-determined final endpoints based on days post-injury for each animal. Animals were excluded from the study if post-operative weight decreased by 15% of pre-surgical weight ($n = 3$), or pre-injury baseline rotarod score was not met ($n = 5$). All animal behavior was scored by investigators blinded to the treatment groups and blinded to drug groups. Data sets were screened using the extreme studentized deviate method for significant outliers. One significant outlier treated with C7 was found and excluded from the cytokine analyses.

Compound design and synthesis
F002 was the first highly active lead in a series of rigid propeller-like compounds identified from commercial databases by docking to a cavity-induced allosteric modifier (CIAM) algorithm identified pocket on TNFR1. Further modeling efforts combined the propeller-like arrangement of the aryl groups with the goal of improved solubility, using a propane diol backbone. These changes led to two novel compounds, C7 and SGT11. C7 had a slightly better SYBYL-X docking score (2.68), but possessed a higher molecular weight (567.99) and more lipophilicity, with a CLogP score of 5.45. Removal of the benzyl alcohol acetates from C7 yielded the corresponding bis-benzyl alcohol SGT11 with significantly improved SYBYL-X score (6.15), reduced molecular weight, and a 2-log drop in CLogP. The total calculated surface area for all of the molecules were similar and ranged from 75.53 to 87.67, with SGT11 being smallest. The compounds were synthesized by Shanghai Medicilion (Shanghai, China).

In vitro screening
NFκB activity reporter gene assay
To study TNFα-mediated NFκB activity, a luciferase reporter system was established. The stable cell line A549-LUC-14 was derived from human A549 cells with chromosomal integration of a luciferase reporter construct regulated by six copies of the NFκB response element. This clonal cell line was obtained by co-transfection of pNFκB-TA-luc and pFLAG-TNFR1-neo followed by G418 selection at 800 μg/ml. A549-LUC-14 cells were seeded, at 3000 cells per well, in a 96-well flat-bottom cell culture plate. After incubation at 37 °C for 24 h, cells were changed into fresh medium with indicated compounds for 1 h pre-incubation. Then, 50 μl of medium containing TNF-α or control was added to each well for a 4-h incubation at 37 °C. The final TNF-α was 5 ng/ml. After 4 h, media

were removed and cells were gently washed twice with 200 μl DPBS. Twenty-five microliters of 1× reporter lysis buffer was added to each well at room temperature and incubated for 5 min, followed with incubation at – 80 °C for 1 h. The plate was thawed at room temperature, and 20 μl of each sample was transferred into an opaque 96-well plate to measure luminescence using a Luminoskan Ascent luminometer (Thermo Labsystems, Franklin, MA).

Western blot

L929 cells were grown on tissue culture plastic in complete DMEM supplemented with 5% FBS, non-essential amino acids, and glutamine. To obtain cell lysates for western blot, cells treated with TNF-α and inhibitors were lysed in a RIPA-based buffer consisting of 20 mM Tris-HCl (pH 7.4), 150 mM NaCl, 1 mM EDTA, 1 mM EGTA, 1% Nonidet P-40, 1% sodium deoxycholate, 10 mM NaF, 1 mM sodium orthovanadate, and Complete Mini Protease Inhibitors (Roche Diagnostics) on ice for 15 min and lysates were clarified by centrifugation ($16,000 \times g$) for 10 min. Supernatant was used for western blot analysis after separation by SDS-PAGE and was subsequently transferred to a nitrocellulose membrane. Membranes were subsequently blocked with 5% non-fat dry milk in PBS buffer for 1 h at room temperature. Membranes were then washed and incubated with primary antibodies (Cell Signaling Technology, 1:10,000 dilution), followed by the appropriate HRP-conjugated secondary antibody. The membrane was then treated with chemiluminescent HRP substrate (Millipore) and exposed to Hyblot CL autoradiography film (Denville Scientific Inc.).

Animals

Male C57BL/6 mice (20–24 g) (Harlan Laboratories, Inc., Indianapolis, IN) were used for all experiments ($n = 103$). Mice were housed in a 14-h light/10-h dark cycle at a constant temperature (23 °C ± 2 °C) with food and water available ad libitum according to the Association for Assessment and Accreditation of Laboratory Animal Care International. All mice used in this study were singly housed. Mice were acclimated to their environment following shipment for at least 3 days prior to any experiments. After surgery, mice were evaluated daily during post-operative care via a physical examination and documentation of each animal's condition. Animal care was approved by the Institutional Animal Care and Use Committees at the University of Arizona (Tucson, AZ).

Midline fluid percussion injury (mFPI)

Since human TBI is a markedly heterogeneous disease, no single animal model of TBI can reproduce the entire spectrum of clinical TBI features and symptoms. For this study, we used the midline fluid percussion injury (mFPI) model for its clinical relevance (for review see Lifshitz et al.) [19]. mFPI can model diffuse TBI resulting in acute behavioral deficits and late-onset behavioral morbidities in the absence of a focal component, gross histopathology, and cavitation, as seen with controlled cortical impact (CCI) [19, 20]. In the current study, adult male mice (2 months of age) were subjected to midline fluid percussion injury consistent with methods previously described [17, 21–25]. Group sizes are indicated in the "Results" section and figure legends for individual studies. Mice were anesthetized using 5% isoflurane in 100% oxygen for 5 min, and the head of the mouse was placed in a stereotaxic frame with continuously delivered isoflurane at 2.5% via nosecone. While anesthetized, body temperature was maintained using a Deltaphase® isothermal heating pad (Braintree Scientific Inc., Braintree, MA). A midline incision was made exposing bregma and lambda, and fascia was removed from the surface of the skull. A trephine (3 mm outer diameter) was used for the craniotomy, centered on the sagittal suture between bregma and lambda without disruption of the dura. An injury cap prepared from the female portion of a Luer-Loc needle hub was fixed over the craniotomy using cyanoacrylate gel and methyl-methacrylate (Hygenic Corp., Akron, OH). The incision was sutured at the anterior and posterior edges, and topical Lidocaine ointment was applied. The injury hub was closed using a Luer-Loc cap, and mice were placed in a heated recovery cage and monitored until ambulatory before being returned to their piezoelectric sleep cage.

For injury induction 24 h post-surgery (approximately 11:00), mice were re-anesthetized with 5% isoflurane delivered for 5 min. The cap was removed from the injury hub assembly, and the dura was visually inspected through the hub to make sure it was intact with no debris. The hub was then filled with normal saline and attached to an extension tube connected to the male end of the fluid percussion device (Custom Design and Fabrication, Virginia Commonwealth University, Richmond, VA). An injury of moderate severity for our injury model (1.1–1.2 atm) was administered by releasing the pendulum onto the fluid-filled cylinder. Sham-injured mice underwent the same procedure except the pendulum was not released. Mice were monitored for the presence of a forearm fencing response, and righting reflex times were recorded for the injured mice as indicators of injury severity [26]. The righting reflex time is the total time from the initial impact until the mouse spontaneously rights itself from a supine position. The fencing response is a tonic posturing characterized by extension and flexion of opposite arms that has been validated as an overt indicator of injury severity

[26]. The injury hub was removed, and the brain was inspected for uniform herniation and integrity of the dura. The dura was intact in all mice, so none were excluded as technical failures. The incision was cleaned using saline and closed using sutures. Diffuse brain-injured mice had righting reflex recovery times greater than 5 min, less than 11 min, and a positive fencing response. Sham-injured mice recovered a righting reflex within 20 s. After spontaneously righting, mice were placed in a heated recovery cage and monitored until ambulatory (approximately 5 to 15 additional min) before being returned to their individual sleep cage (vide infra). Adequate measures were taken to minimize pain or discomfort [27].

Pharmacological treatment

Mice were treated with vehicle (10% DMSO), C7, SGT-11, or F002. Compounds were administered intraperitoneally at (20 mg/kg) or (2 mg/kg) immediately following injury. In the subsequent functional and histological studies, compounds (2 mg/kg) were administered intraperitoneally twice: immediately following the injury and 24 h post-injury. Dosing was selected with regard to published studies using F002 in mice [28] and the solubility of the novel compounds. High doses (20 mg/kg) were maximum solubility, whereas low doses were one tenth of that dose (2 mg/kg).

Sleep recordings

The non-invasive sleep cage system (Signal Solutions, Lexington, KY) used in this study consisted of 16 separate units that simultaneously monitored sleep and wake states, as previously published [22, 29, 30]. Each cage unit housed a single mouse inside 18×18-cm walled compartments with attached food and water structures [29]. The cages had open bottoms resting on polyvinylidine difluoride (PVDF) sensors serving as the cage floor [29]. The non-invasive high-throughput PVDF sensors were coupled to an input differential amplifier, and pressure signals were generated and classified by the classifier as motions consistent with either activity related to wake or inactivity and regular breathing movements associated with sleep [22, 29]. Briefly, sleep was characterized primarily by periodic (3 Hz) and regular amplitude signals recorded from the PVDF sensors, which is typical of respiration from a sleeping mouse. In contrast, signals characteristic of wake were both the absence of characteristic sleep signals and higher amplitude, irregular signals associated with volitional movements, even during quiet wake. The piezoelectric signals in 2-s epochs were classified by a linear discriminant classifier algorithm based on multiple signal variables to assign a binary label of "sleep" or "wake" [29]. Mice sleep in a polycyclic manner (often more than 40 sleep episodes per hour if

short arousals are recorded) [31], and therefore, mouse sleep was quantified as the minutes spent sleeping per hour, presented as a percentage for each hour. Data collected from the cage system were binned over specified time periods (e.g., 1 h) using the average of percent sleep, as well as binned by length of individual bouts of sleep. Where applicable, sleep metrics were compared between 6 h of light and 6 h of dark.

Rotarod

Sensorimotor function was assessed using the Economex Rotarod system from Columbus Instruments (Columbus, OH). Mice were acclimated 3 days prior to surgery/injury. The mice were placed on the stationary rod and allowed to explore for 30 s. Following exploration, the mice were placed on the rod at a constant speed of 5 revolutions per minute (rpm). If the mouse fell off the rod, it was placed back on the rod and the timer was restarted (until the mice could walk 15 s at 5 rpm). Next, mice were placed on the rod with a rotation of 5 rpm and an acceleration of 0.2 rpm/s. The trial ended when the mouse fell off the rod; after two trials, the acclimation period ended. The testing phase occurred over 3 consecutive days prior to surgery/injury (last test before surgery was recorded as baseline) and 1, 3, 5, and 7 days post-injury (DPI). For the post-injury testing phase, mice were placed on the stationary rod and the instrument was started at 5 rpm with an acceleration of 0.2 rpm/s. Two trials were run back to back, after which mice were returned to holding cages. After 10 min, mice performed a third trial. The times from the best two trials were averaged to generate a latency to fall from the rotating rod for each mouse.

Neurological severity score (NSS)

Post-traumatic neurological impairments were assessed at 24 h post-injury using an eight-point NSS paradigm implemented from those previously used in experimental models of TBI [32–35]. One point was given for failure on an individual task, and no points were given if a mouse completed a task successfully. Mice were observed for hindlimb flexion, startle reflex, and seeking behavior (presence of these behaviors was considered successful task completion). Mice traversed in sequence, 3-, 2-, and 1-cm beams. The beams were elevated, and mice were given 1 min to travel 30 cm on the beams. The task was scored as a success if the mouse traveled 30 cm with normal forelimb and hindlimb position (forelimb/hindlimb did not hang from the beam). Mice were also required to balance on a 0.5-cm beam and a 0.5-cm round rod for 3 s in a stationary position with front paws between hind paws. Non-parametric data are presented as a composite score ranging from zero to eight representing performance on all tasks combined.

High final NSS scores were indicative of task failures and interpreted as neurological impairment.

Novel object recognition (NOR)

Cognitive function was tested using the NOR test as previously published [22, 36, 37]. The test consisted of three phases: habituation, training, and testing. On day 6 post-injury, mice were placed in an open field ($21 \times 21 \times 42$ cm) for 1 h of habituation. Mice were removed and two identical objects were placed in opposing quadrants of the field for the training phase. Mice were placed in the center of the open field and given 5 min to explore the objects. Following training, mice were returned to their individual sleep cages. Testing began 4 h after training. One familiar object was placed in an original location, and one novel object was placed in the opposing quadrant of the open field. Mice were placed into the center and given 5 min to explore. For testing, the times spent actively investigating the novel and familiar object were quantified. Investigation of an object included sniffing, touching, or climbing onto an object while the mouse was facing the object. If an animal climbed onto an object and sniffed into the air, this time was not calculated into the exploration of the novel object. Testing data are reported as the percentage of total investigation time spent with each object and as a discrimination index (DI) in which $DI = (T_{novel} - T_{familiar})/(T_{novel} + T_{familiar})$. A discrimination index of zero indicates no object preference, and positive values show preference for the novel object.

Tissue preparation for cytokine measurement and immunofluorescence

At selected time points (3 h or 7 days) post-injury or sham operation, mice were given an overdose of sodium pentobarbital (i.p.) and transcardially perfused with 4% paraformaldehyde after a phosphate-buffered saline (PBS) flush. For cytokine measurement, brains were dissected on ice and snap frozen in liquid nitrogen and then stored at -80 °C until used. For immunofluorescence, brains were removed and placed in 4% paraformaldehyde overnight. Brains were immersed in serial dilutions (15 and 30%) of sucrose for 24 h each. The brains were removed from the 30% sucrose and frozen at -20 °C. After freezing, brains were cryosectioned in the coronal plane at 20 μm, mounted onto glass slides, and stored at -80 °C.

Cytokine measurement

The protein levels of a panel of inflammatory cytokines were measured in the neocortex by Meso Scale Discovery (MSD) multiplex immunoassay (sector imager 2400, Meso Scale Discovery; Gaithersburg, MD) as previously described [38]. Brain cortex was homogenized using high shear homogenizer (Omni TH115), in a 1:10 (w/v) of ice-cold lysis buffer consisting of PBS containing 1 μg/ml Leupeptin, 1 mM PMSF, and 1 mM EDTA. The cortical homogenate was centrifuged at $14,000 \times g$ for 20 min at 4 °C in a microcentrifuge. Fifty microliters of the resulting supernatant was loaded per well of the custom MSD plate, and cortical cytokine levels were determined by MSD assay (Mouse Proinflammatory 7-Plex Ultra-Sensitive (K15012C)). Cytokine levels in the cortex were normalized to the total amount of protein in the sample loaded as determined by BCA Protein Assay (Pierce).

Iba-1 immunofluorescence

Slides were removed from -80 °C, placed in an oven at 60 °C for approximately 4 h, and then rinsed three times for 5 min each in PBS. Next, the slides were incubated in 4% goat serum blocking solution for 1 h. Slides were incubated with the primary antibody (rabbit anti-ionized calcium-binding adaptor molecule 1, IBA-1; 1:1000, Item # 0199-19741, Wako Chemicals, Richmond, VA) and stored at 4 °C overnight. Slides were rinsed three times in PBS and the secondary antibody (biotinylated horse anti-rabbit; 1:250, Vector Laboratories, Burlingame, CA) was added and slides were incubated on a rocker at room temperature for 1 h. Slides were washed in PBS three times for 5 min each, tertiary stain was applied (streptavidin Alexa© Fluor 594; 1:1000, Jackson Immunoresearch, Westgrove, PA), and slides were incubated for 1 h at room temperature. Lastly, slides were rinsed three times in PBS and coverslipped with anti-fade medium (Fluoromount G; Southern Biotech, Birmingham, AL).

Microglial identification and quantification

Stained sections (four sections per animal; $n = 8$ per group) were analyzed following Iba-1 staining to determine the proportion of microglial morphologies post-injury. The area of interest, the primary somatosensory barrel fields (S1BF), was chosen based on previous work demonstrating a focus of neuropathology and microglial activation in the S1BF following midline fluid percussion brain injury in the rodent [39–42]. Sections were screened using a Zeiss (AXIO imager A2) microscope with an attached digital camera (AxioCam MRc5). Images were captured with proprietary Zen software (Carl Zeiss, Germany) at $\times 20$ magnification. The area of interest was examined in both hemispheres and in two different coronal sections: an anterior section (~Bregma -1.555 mm) and a posterior section (~Bregma -2.255 mm). A total of four photos per brain ($n = 8$ animals per group) per area of interest were analyzed. Photomicrographs were analyzed using Image J software (National Institutes of Health, Bethesda, MD). On each photomicrograph, $250,000$ pixel^2 grid lines were placed and quantification was limited to four pre-defined boxes. Microglia within these boxes were classified by a blinded investigator as either having ramified (small soma, high defined processes) or activated (hypertrophied soma, fewer processes) morphologies. A minimum of 50 microglia were counted per section per region. Sham treatment groups were combined.

Statistical analysis

Results are shown as mean ± SEM and analyzed using GraphPad Prism 6, with statistical significance assigned at the 95% confidence level ($\alpha < 0.05$), unless otherwise indicated. For each test, sham animals receiving each treatment were compared. No differences were detected between sham groups (treated and vehicle), so shams were combined from each treatment. Percent sleep and differences in rotarod performance were analyzed using a repeated measure two-way analysis of variance (ANOVA) followed by Tukey's multiple comparisons test. Improvement on the rotarod was analyzed using a one-way ANOVA with a Sidak's multiple comparisons test. Cumulative sleep measured in minutes and cytokine levels were analyzed with a one-way ANOVA followed by Tukey's multiple comparisons test. Non-parametric Kruskal-Wallis tests implemented in the statistical program R [43] were used to investigate if median NSS scores differed among groups (including shams) across and within injury-specific time points. If Kruskal-Wallis tests were significant ($p < 0.05$), a post hoc Dunn test implemented in the R package DescTools [44] was performed with p values adjusted using a Bonferroni correction for multiple comparisons to determine which groups differed. Identical analytical methods were also used to investigate if median NSS scores differed among injury-specific time points without considering a group effect. Proportional differences in microglia were compared using a one-way ANOVA. For all parametric analyses, the assumption that data were normally distributed was verified using density and q-q plots and Shapiro-Wilk's tests to ensure the validity of the analytical approaches used. Resulting test values are included in the figure legends.

Results

Novel TNF-R1 inhibitors demonstrate target engagement by blocking TNF-R1 signaling pathways

We have previously reported a novel TNFR1 inhibitor, F002, which is a cavity-induced allosteric modifier (CIAM) of TNFR1 that inhibits TNF-α binding to TNFR1 and subsequent pathway activation [45]. To extend properties of F002, two new analogues were rationally designed and synthesized by Shanghai Medicilon (Shanghai, China). The two new compounds, called C7 and SGT11, differed in the R1 position (SGT11, R1 = OH; C7, R1 = OAc;

Fig. 1a) and efficiently inhibited TNF pathway activation (Fig. 1b, c). CIAM compounds concentration-dependently inhibited NF-κB activation as demonstrated by the western blots of IκBα phosphorylation.

Upon binding to TNFRs, TNFα induces inflammation through the activation of NFκB and p38 MAPK signaling pathways. The novel CIAM compounds were tested for

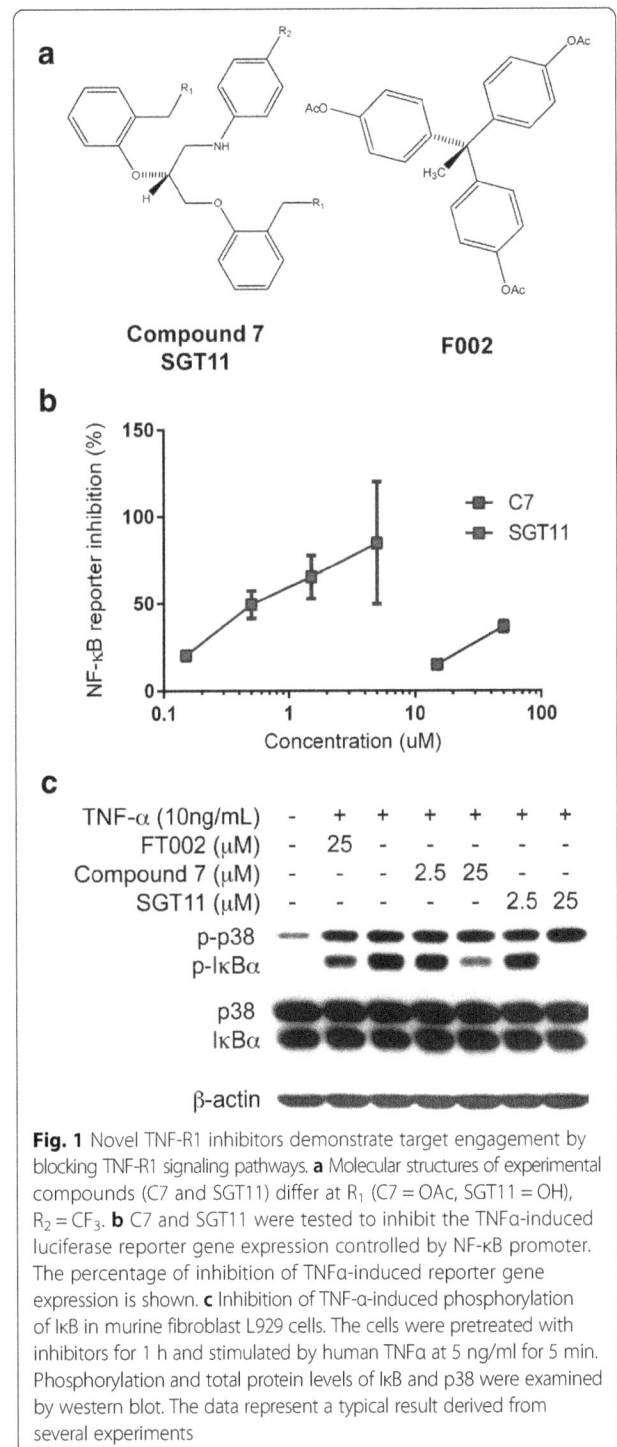

Fig. 1 Novel TNF-R1 inhibitors demonstrate target engagement by blocking TNF-R1 signaling pathways. **a** Molecular structures of experimental compounds (C7 and SGT11) differ at R₁ (C7 = OAc, SGT11 = OH), R₂ = CF₃. **b** C7 and SGT11 were tested to inhibit the TNFα-induced luciferase reporter gene expression controlled by NF-κB promoter. The percentage of inhibition of TNFα-induced reporter gene expression is shown. **c** Inhibition of TNF-α-induced phosphorylation of IκB in murine fibroblast L929 cells. The cells were pretreated with inhibitors for 1 h and stimulated by human TNFα at 5 ng/ml for 5 min. Phosphorylation and total protein levels of IκB and p38 were examined by western blot. The data represent a typical result derived from several experiments

activity to inhibit TNFα-induced NF-κB signaling and p38 MAPK signaling. An NF-κB reporter gene system was generated in the human A549 cell line by chromosomal integration of a luciferase reporter construct under the transcriptional control of the NF-κB response element. In this system, TNFα treatment activates NF-κB and results in luciferase expression. As shown in Fig. 1b, both C7 and SGT11 inhibited the luciferase activity concentration-dependently. However, SGT11, which had an IC50 of 5.5 μM, showed greater inhibition than C7, which did not reach 50% inhibition at 50 μM. These compounds, which were confirmed to inhibit NF-κB phosphorylation (Fig. 1c), were selected to move to in vivo testing. At 25 μM, F002 minimally inhibited the TNF-α-induced phosphorylation of IκBα (p-IκBα). In contrast, at 25 μM, both C7 and SGT11 limited p-IκBα phosphorylation (Fig. 1c). None of these inhibitors displayed significant activity on TNF-α-induced p38 phosphorylation.

Novel TNF-R1 inhibitors modulated post-traumatic sleep

In a preliminary cohort of mice, two doses of the three compounds were tested for their efficacy of modulating post-traumatic sleep, which is proposed to be a physiological bio-indicator of inflammation. As expected, diffuse TBI resulted in a significant increase in the percent of post-traumatic sleep over the first 6 h post-injury in vehicle-treated mice compared to uninjured shams [23] (Fig. 2a, b). While both doses of compound C7 modulated post-traumatic sleep compared to vehicle sleep profile, there were no significant differences compared to vehicle-treated brain-injured mice in the percent sleep during the first 6 h post-injury or the cumulative minutes slept (Fig. 2c, d). Both doses of compound SGT modulated the percent of post-traumatic sleep compared to vehicle-treated brain-injured mice (Fig. 2e). There was a significant decrease in the cumulative minutes slept by the SGT-treated brain-injured mice given a high dose, compared to the mice given a low dose (Fig. 2f). Compound F002 did not significantly modulate the percent of post-traumatic sleep, or cumulative minutes slept, regardless of the dose given (Fig. 2g, h). Uninjured sham mice showed no significant drug-induced change in sleep compared to baseline or the vehicle-treated group (Additional file 1: Figure S1). Using the modulation of post-traumatic sleep as an indicator of efficacy, compound C7 and SGT, but not F002, were selected for further study.

Novel TNF-R1 inhibitors improved functional outcome measures following TBI

To assess sensorimotor function, the rotarod task was used as previously published [22, 42, 46]. Motor function was tested as the latency to fall from the rotating rod

out to 7 days post-injury, with significant effects for time post-injury and between treatment groups (Fig. 3a, b). By 3 days post-injury (DPI), SGT attenuated motor deficits compared to vehicle treatment (Fig. 3a) and increased latency to fall from the rod (Fig. 3b). Compound C7 showed no difference from the vehicle treatment group. Diffuse TBI led to immediate neurological deficits measured by a modified Neurological Severity Score (NSS) at 1, 3, and 5 DPI (Fig. 3c, d). At 3 and 5 DPI, SGT attenuated neurological deficits observed in vehicle-treated animals, and by 7 DPI, all injured groups recovered to uninjured sham performance, as expected. Cognitive function was measured using the novel object recognition task (Fig. 3e) [42]. SGT improved cognitive performance to uninjured sham levels, with SGT-treated brain-injured mice having a discrimination index higher than uninjured shams, indicating recall of the familiar object (Fig. 3f). To extend findings from the preliminary screening cohort, we measured sleep immediately following injury in the behavior cohort. TBI led to increased sleep during the first light cycle with C7-treated brain-injured mice sleeping significantly more at 15:00, and SGT-treated brain-injured mice sleeping significantly more at 15:00 and 17:00 (Fig. 3g). TBI did not significantly alter sleep during the transition from light to dark cycle (Fig. 3g, h). Following the light/dark change (19:00) sham mice, C7-treated, and SGT11-treated mice had an increase in sleep. Inversely, vehicle-treated mice had a decrease in sleep (Fig. 3h); however, this was not statistically significant. There were no alterations in sleep during the first dark cycle (Fig. 3h) and no changes during the transition from dark to light (Fig. 3h). Overall, SGT-treated brain-injured mice slept more cumulative minutes than uninjured shams during the light (sleep) cycle (Fig. 3i), but mice slept similarly during the dark (wake) cycle (Fig. 3i).

Novel TNF-R1 inhibitors reduce neuroinflammation following TBI

Diffuse TBI increased inflammatory cytokines in the cortex at 3 h post-injury, and these increases were attenuated by treatment with C7 and SGT to levels that were not different from uninjured sham (Fig. 4a–d). Overall, diffuse TBI increased cortical levels of IL-10 and IL-1β in vehicle-treated brain-injured mice compared to uninjured shams (Fig. 4a, b), but not for cortical TNF-α and CCL2 levels (Fig. 4c, d). With the administration of either compound, cytokine levels were reduced to levels neither significantly elevated from uninjured sham nor lower than vehicle-treated brain-injured animals. Treatment with TNF-α receptor inhibitors did not prevent TBI-induced activation of microglia in the somatosensory cortex among brain-injured animals (Fig. 4e–h). All brain-injured groups demonstrated a reduced proportion

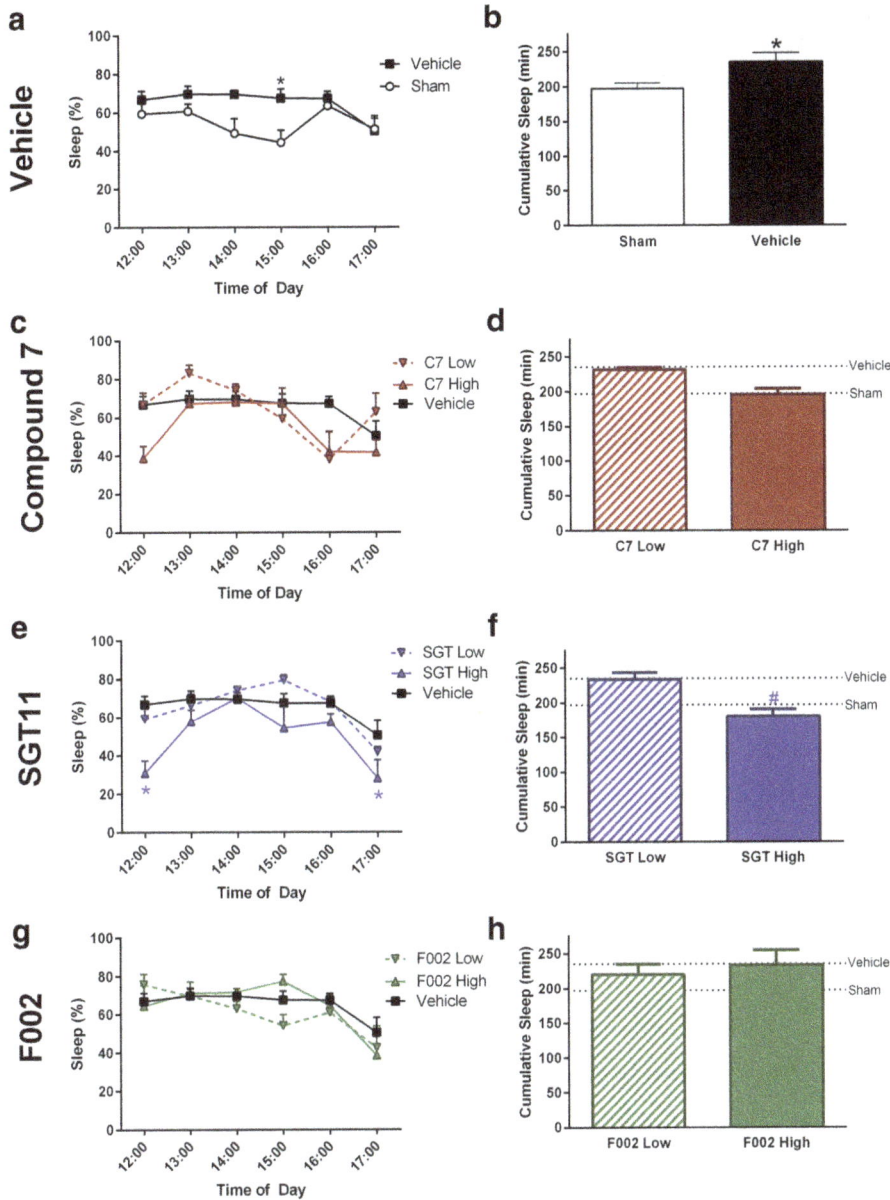

Fig. 2 Screening of novel TNF-R1 inhibitors showed modulated post-traumatic sleep. Compounds were screened at two doses (high dose 20 mg/kg; low dose 2 mg/kg) for efficacy in modulating post-traumatic sleep compared to vehicle-treated and uninjured sham mice. Compounds were administered immediately following injury or sham procedure. A repeated measure two-way ANOVA was used to analyze main effect of treatment on percent sleep followed by Sidak's multiple comparisons test when appropriate. Cumulative minutes slept was analyzed between sham and vehicle-treated using an un-paired t test, and across treatment groups using a one-way ANOVA followed by Tukey's multiple comparisons test where appropriate. **a, b** Vehicle-treated brain-injured mice had a significant main effect of treatment on percent sleep ($F_{1,11} = 6.835$, $p = 0.0241$) and cumulative minutes spent sleeping ($t_{11} = 2.614$, $p = 0.0241$) compared to uninjured shams. **c, d** While both high- and low-dose compound C7 modulated post-traumatic sleep, there was no significant treatment effect between brain-injured mice treated with C7 compared to vehicle on percent sleep ($F_{2,9} = 3.135$, $p = 0.0926$) but there was an overall effect on cumulative minutes spent sleeping ($F_{3,15} = 3.917$, $p = 0.0300$). **e, f** There was an overall significant treatment effect between brain-injured mice treated with SGT compared to vehicle on percent sleep ($F_{2,10} = 5.274$, $p = 0.0273$) and cumulative minutes spent sleeping ($F_{3,16} = 5.641$, $p = 0.0078$). **g, h** Compound F002 did not significantly modulate percent sleep ($F_{2,10} = 0.2786$, $p = 0.7625$) or cumulative minutes spent sleeping ($F_{3,16} = 2.252$, $p = 0.1217$). Sleep groups; sham $n = 7$, vehicle-treated $n = 6$, C7-low $n = 2$, C7-high $n = 4$, SGT-low $n = 4$, SGT-high $n = 3$, F002-low $n = 4$, F002-low $n = 3$

of ramified microglia compared to uninjured sham mice at 7 DPI (Fig. 4e, f). All brain-injured groups demonstrated a greater proportion of activated microglia than uninjured sham mice (Fig. 4g, h).

Discussion

Accumulated and published data indicate that inflammation contributes to secondary damage following TBI and therefore represents a plausible therapeutic target for

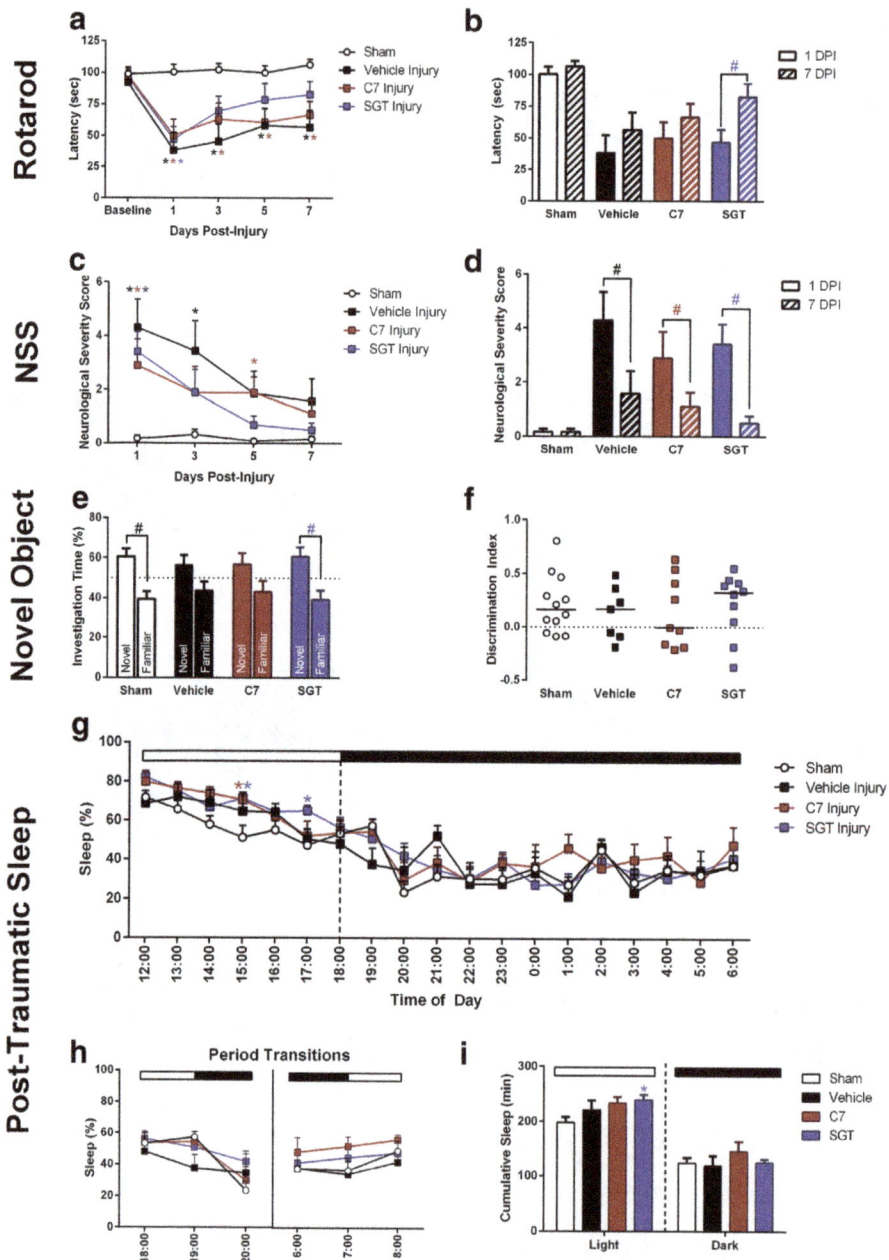

Fig. 3 Novel TNF-R1 inhibitors modulated post-traumatic sleep and improved functional outcome measures following TBI. Following preliminary sleep screening, a second cohort of mice was tested for functional outcome following administration of low-dose (2 mg/kg) compounds given immediately following injury or sham procedure. **a** The rotarod was used to test motor function. There was a significant effect of time after injury ($F_{3,102} = 9.612$, $p < 0.0001$) and group effect on the latency to fall from the rotarod ($F_{3,34} = 6.646$, $p = 0.0012$). SGT attenuated motor deficits by 3 days post-injury (DPI). **b** There was a significant time effect ($F_{1,34} = 17.14$, $p = 0.0002$) and treatment effect ($F_{3,34} = 8.450$, $p = 0.0002$). Sidak's post hoc analysis indicated SGT led to a significant improvement at 7 DPI compared to 1 DPI. **c** Neurological deficits were measured by a modified Neurological Severity Score (NSS). Median NSS scores differed among groups with a treatment effect ($\chi_3^2 = 32.669$; $p < 0.001$) and time effect ($\chi_3^2 = 10.178$; $p = 0.021$). At 3 and 5 DPI, SGT attenuated neurological deficits. **d** All injured groups showed improvement on the NSS task by 7 DPI. **e** Cognitive impairment was measured by novel object recognition (NOR). Differences in time spent exploring the novel versus familiar object revealed a significant difference between investigation times among sham ($t_{11} = 2.686$, $p = 0.0212$) and SGT-treated brain-injured mice ($t_9 = 2.277$, $p = 0.0488$), indicating recall of the familiar object. Vehicle-treated brain-injured mice ($t_6 = 1.371$, $p = 0.2195$) and C7 treated brain-injured mice ($t_8 = 1.259$, $p = 0.2435$) spent similar times investigating both objects. **f** There were no significant differences in discrimination indices between groups ($F_{3,34} = 0.2276$, $p = 0.8766$). **g** TBI led to increased sleep during the first light cycle ($F_{3,25} = 3.933$, $p = 0.0199$). **h** TBI did not alter sleep during the transition from light to dark cycle ($F_{3,25} = 0.5272$, $p = 0.6677$). **i** There was an overall effect on cumulative sleep during the light cycle ($F_{3,25} = 3.233$, $p = 0.0393$) mice slept similarly during the dark cycle ($F_{3,25} = 0.8089$, $p = 0.5009$). Behavior groups: sham $n = 12$, vehicle-treated $n = 7$, C7-treated $n = 9$, SGT-treated $n = 10$. Sleep groups: sham $n = 9$, vehicle-treated $n = 5$, C7-treated $n = 6$, SGT-treated $n = 9$

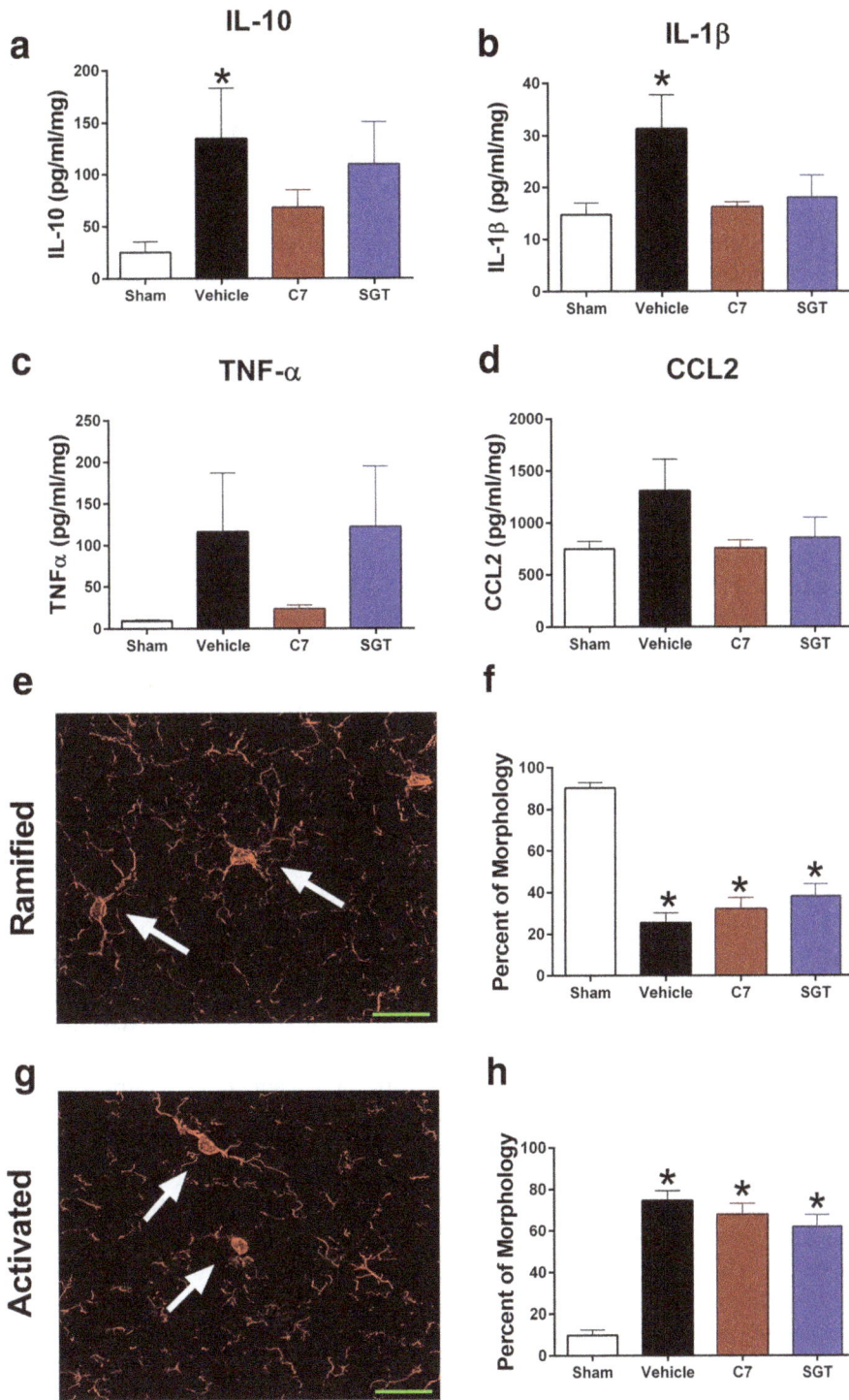

Fig. 4 Novel TNF-R1 inhibitors reduce neuroinflammation following TBI. **a** Vehicle-treated mice, but not C7-treated or SGT-treated brain-injured mice, had significantly increased IL-10 ($F_{3,19}$ = 3.217, p = 0.0460) and **b** IL-1β ($F_{3,19}$ = 3.831, p = 0.0266) compared to uninjured shams at 3 h post-injury. **c** There was an injury-induced increase in TNF-α ($F_{3,19}$ = 1.977, p = 0.1516) and **d** CCL2 ($F_{3,19}$ = 2.340, p = 0.1057) but these increases failed to reach statistical significance. **e, f** Iba-1 immunohistochemistry revealed diffuse TBI significantly reduced ramified microglia in the cortex regardless of drug treatment ($F_{3,26}$ = 33.57, p < 0.0001). Representative ramified microglia indicated by arrows. **g, h** All brain-injured groups had a significant increase in activated microglia compared to uninjured shams ($F_{3,26}$ = 33.57, p < 0.0001). Representative activated microglia indicated by arrows. Cytokine groups: sham n = 9, vehicle-treated n = 5, C7-treated n = 4, SGT-treated n = 5. Immunohistochemistry groups: sham n = 7, vehicle-treated n = 7, C7-treated n = 8, SGT-treated n = 8; scale bar is 20 μm

intervention. Universally across rodent models, TNF-α levels (systemic and central) increase within hours of injury and return to basal levels as early as 24 h post-injury [24, 46]. TNF-α is an inflammatory cytokine that stimulates monocyte and glial activation and infiltration, neuronal and myelin loss, and blood-brain barrier permeability [47, 48]. TNFR-induced NF-κB activation can transcriptionally induce TNF and thus, amplify TNF and TNFR signaling pathways, including the expression of over 20 different cytokines and chemokines and receptors involved in immune regulation [49]. TNF-α binding to the TNF receptor can be blocked pharmacologically and thereby inhibit subsequent activation of downstream inflammatory signaling pathways. In the current study, three compounds (C7, SGT11, and F002) were synthesized to act as cavity-induced allosteric modifiers, binding to the TNF receptor and preventing downstream signaling. Since neuroinflammation and TNF signaling are pathophysiological hallmarks of clinical TBI [50], these studies set the stage for a pharmacological pipeline based on therapeutic biomarkers.

The use of sleep as a bio-indicator of inflammation is a novel approach to screen potential therapeutics. In the current study, we employ sleep as a valid indicator of inflammation. We have previously reported that acute sleep increases following experimental diffuse TBI and this increase is temporally associated with increased cytokine levels [17]. The current findings show diffuse TBI increased cumulative sleep, which was attenuated by C7 and SGT11. Furthermore, we were able to investigate two doses of each compound on their efficacy to modulate a physiological bio-indicator, sleep. We also showed diffuse TBI increased cortical cytokine levels, which was attenuated by C7 and SGT11. These data support the use of sleep as a bio-indicator of acute inflammation for screening potential therapeutic compounds, particularly anti-inflammatory compounds.

The novel TNFR1 inhibitors modulated inflammation via the TNFR1 signaling pathway, as predicted from molecular modeling. In vivo, compounds with efficacy to modulate post-traumatic sleep showed efficacy towards improved motor function following diffuse TBI. Our data are in line with pre-clinical studies using etanercept (Enbrel®), a biopharmaceutical marketed to treat autoimmune diseases by acting as a TNF inhibitor. Rats systemically injected with etanercept and subjected to fluid percussion brain injury demonstrated reduced motor and neurological deficits by 3 days post-injury, which was attributed to the attenuation of microglia activation and TNF production in the cortex, white matter, hippocampus, and hypothalamus [51]. A similar study using a weight-drop injury model indicated a single systemic injection of TNF-α synthesis inhibitor 3,6′-dithiothalidomide (DT) prevented injury-induced increases in TNF-α

and ameliorated neuronal loss and cognitive impairments in the mouse [52]. DT injected in rats for 14 consecutive days has also been shown to reverse cognitive deficits induced by chronic inflammation [53]. A comprehensive review of studies using selective TNF inhibitors to treat brain injury and stroke has been previously published, for review see Tuttolomondo et al. [7].

TNF-α has pleiotropic actions in the brain. TNF-α can regulate host response to disease, control chemotaxis through the production of chemokines, regulate monocyte adhesion molecules, and contribute to microglia activation [7, 47]. As a potent pro-inflammatory cytokine, TNF promotes inflammatory signaling and injury-mediated microglial activation in the central nervous system [6]. In the current study, TNFR1 inhibiting compounds were used to prevent TNFR-induced NF-κB activation and the subsequent inflammatory surge [49], as demonstrated in vitro. We show a decrease in inflammatory cytokines in the cortex measured at 3 h post-injury, without a change in microglia activation between vehicle-treated brain-injured mice and brain-injured mice treated with C7 or SGT. We found C7 and SGT did not reduce microglia activation at 3 h post-injury in the cortex, possibly indicating that TNF inhibition was too transient to affect morphological inhibition of microglial activation, despite an impact on functional outcomes. Extended dosing strategies can test whether these novel compounds can modulate microglial activation. Although all measured cytokines and chemokines in the current study were reduced 3 h post-injury in brain-injured mice treated with C7 or SGT11 compared to vehicle, the decrease in TNF-α levels in the cortex did not reach significance. TNF-α stimulates the NF-κB signaling pathway directly, which can amplify inflammation and TNF production [49]. It is possible that TNF produced in response to TBI then induced NF-κB activation, leading to TNF transcription, thereby amplifying TNF and TNFR signaling pathways; these compounds would not necessarily inhibit TNF-induced TNF amplification, even though downstream inflammatory signals were dampened [11]. This positive auto-regulatory loop may overall affect TNF levels in the brain while other pro-inflammatory cytokines attenuate by the inhibition of TNFR-induced NF-κB activation.

Limitations of this study identified by the data require further support for (i) the role of sleep as predictive biomarker of underlying inflammation in the brain and (ii) the therapeutic efficacy of the candidate compounds. First, cumulative sleep was increased in SGT-treated brain-injured mice compared to uninjured shams across the 6-h light cycle immediately following injury, but at 3 h post-injury, we observed an attenuation of IL-1β, a sleep regulatory substance, in SGT-treated brain-injured mice. Also, the uninjured shams had a higher percent sleep than previously published from our lab [17], which may have

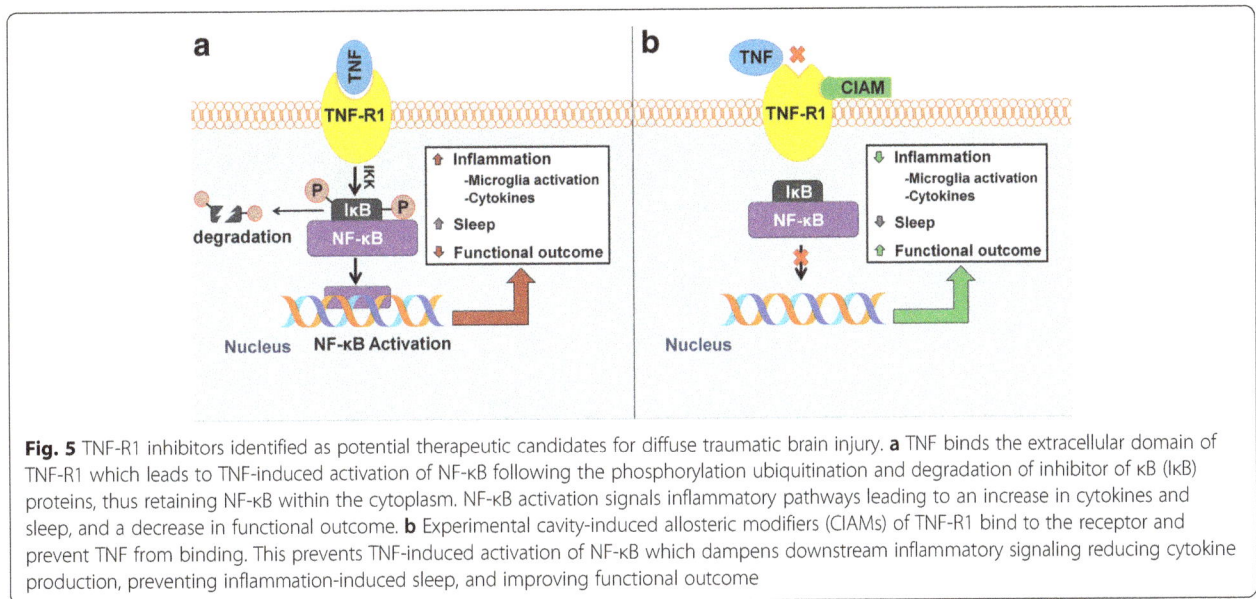

Fig. 5 TNF-R1 inhibitors identified as potential therapeutic candidates for diffuse traumatic brain injury. **a** TNF binds the extracellular domain of TNF-R1 which leads to TNF-induced activation of NF-κB following the phosphorylation ubiquitination and degradation of inhibitor of κB (IκB) proteins, thus retaining NF-κB within the cytoplasm. NF-κB activation signals inflammatory pathways leading to an increase in cytokines and sleep, and a decrease in functional outcome. **b** Experimental cavity-induced allosteric modifiers (CIAMs) of TNF-R1 bind to the receptor and prevent TNF from binding. This prevents TNF-induced activation of NF-κB which dampens downstream inflammatory signaling reducing cytokine production, preventing inflammation-induced sleep, and improving functional outcome

reduced power to detect differences among groups. In the current study, the DMSO vehicle itself could have contributed to changes in sleep architecture [54]. Cavas et al. reported an increase in sleep following 15 and 20% DMSO (in saline) administration to rats [54]. Although the current study used 10% DMSO in saline as a solvent, this concentration may produce physiological alterations in sleep architecture in mice, and further investigation into the effects of DMSO on sleep in the mouse is necessary. We also note that TNF itself is a modulator of sleep. The combined sham group for this study included those treated with vehicle, C7, or SGT11, since sleep was not significantly different among groups. The experimental compounds could affect sleep architecture independent of injury-induced inflammation. To control for this, we analyzed the change in sleep after compound administration compared to baseline and the change from vehicle-treated sham cumulative minutes of sleep (Additional file 1: Figure S1). All three sham groups slept less in the post-surgery period compared to the baseline period, but this change was not dependent on the compound. Handling of the animals and surgical anesthesia likely contributed to the mice spending more time awake during the initial hours upon being returned to their cage. Although targeting TNF in the absence of TBI might influence sleep, uninjured sham mouse sleep was unaffected by the experimental compounds.

Further, the route and timing of administration requires further exploration to investigate clinical efficacy. We also acknowledge that the high dose contributed to the greatest modulation of post-traumatic sleep; however, availability and cost of the high dose warranted this exploratory study with low dose. Lastly, the increase in sleep could possibly be a result of decreased

wakefulness. Orexin, a pleiotropic neuropeptide, is produced by neurons in the lateral hypothalamus and governs survival behaviors, including sleep/wake cycles, through the promotion of wakefulness [55]. A reduction in orexin-producing neurons could contribute to a reduction in wakefulness observed as an increase in sleep. Although we do not anticipate a loss in orexin neurons acutely at 6 h post-injury, further experiments are likely necessary to investigate brain injury-induced death of orexin neurons. To increase the efficiency of the proposed systematic pre-clinical approach, flow cytometry could report on microglial phenotypes in response to drug treatment as an alternate outcome measure. Using flow cytometry to quantify cells may prove advantageous over immunohistochemistry and cell count analyses.

Conclusions

These findings are consistent with improved functional outcome from brain injury by inhibiting TNFR-induced NF-κB signaling [7, 51–53, 56–59]. In concordance with previous reports, our results show an accelerated improvement in sensorimotor, neurological, and cognitive function when brain-injured mice are treated with compounds that inhibit TNFR1 (Fig. 5). On the basis of these observations, we add evidence that pharmacological inhibition of TNF-α is a plausible treatment for acute diffuse brain injury [56]. Furthermore, our results raise the consideration that post-traumatic sleep can be used as a bio-indicator of neuroinflammation and operate as a therapeutic biomarker; therefore, sleep could serve as a predictive biomarker of therapeutic efficacy. We posit that sleep should be considered as a valuable screening tool for the development and testing of drugs that target brain injury-induced inflammation in the laboratory and possibly the clinic.

Acknowledgements
The authors wish to thank Dr. Linda Van Eldik and Dr. Sean Murphy at the University of Kentucky for their contribution to the analyses and editing of this manuscript.

Funding
Research reported in this manuscript was supported, in part, by the National Institute of Neurological Disorders and Stroke of the National Institutes of Health under award numbers R21 NS072611 and PCH Mission Support Funds. The generosity of the Diane and Bruce Halle Foundation and NIH fellowship F31-NS090921 supported JLH during the conduct of these studies. RKR was supported by a Science Foundation Arizona Bisgrove Scholarship during the conduct of these studies.

Authors' contributions
RKR prepared the manuscript. RKR and JLH performed the surgeries and injuries, sleep and behavior, tissue preparation, immunofluorescence staining, and microglia semi-quantification. ADB and LVE measured cytokines. HZ, DPH, and MIG synthesized the compounds and performed in vitro experiments. BFO helped with the analysis and interpretation of the sleep data. JL helped with the study design, interpretation of all data, figure preparation, and manuscript preparation. All authors read and approved the final manuscript.

Competing interests
MIG is an inventor of the molecules presented in this manuscript on a patent owned by the University of Pennsylvania, but has no financial interest. BFO is an owner of Signal Solutions LLC.

Author details
[1]BARROW Neurological Institute at Phoenix Children's Hospital, Phoenix, AZ, USA. [2]Department of Child Health, University of Arizona College of Medicine—Phoenix, Phoenix, AZ, USA. [3]Phoenix Veteran Affairs Healthcare System, Phoenix, AZ, USA. [4]Basic Medical Sciences, University of Arizona College of Medicine—Phoenix, Phoenix, AZ, USA. [5]University of Pennsylvania Perelman School of Medicine, Philadelphia, PA, USA. [6]Sanders-Brown Center on Aging, Spinal Cord and Brain Injury Research Center, and Department of Neuroscience, University of Kentucky, Lexington, KY, USA. [7]Department of Biology, University of Kentucky, Lexington, KY, USA.

References
1. Coronado VG, McGuire LC, Sarmiento K, Bell J, Lionbarger MR, Jones CD, Geller AI, Khoury N, Xu L. Trends in traumatic brain injury in the U.S. and the public health response: 1995-2009. J Saf Res. 2012;43:299–307.
2. Werner C, Engelhard K. Pathophysiology of traumatic brain injury. Br J Anaesth. 2007;99:4–9.
3. Janowitz T, Menon DK. Exploring new routes for neuroprotective drug development in traumatic brain injury. Sci Transl Med. 2010;2:27rv21.
4. Ziebell JM, Morganti-Kossmann MC. Involvement of pro- and anti-inflammatory cytokines and chemokines in the pathophysiology of traumatic brain injury. Neurotherapeutics. 2010;7:22–30.
5. Morganti-Kossmann MC, Rancan M, Stahel PF, Kossmann T. Inflammatory response in acute traumatic brain injury: a double-edged sword. Curr Opin Crit Care. 2002;8:101–5.
6. McCoy MK, Tansey MG. TNF signaling inhibition in the CNS: implications for normal brain function and neurodegenerative disease. J Neuroinflammation. 2008;5:45.
7. Tuttolomondo A, Pecoraro R, Pinto A. Studies of selective TNF inhibitors in the treatment of brain injury from stroke and trauma: a review of the evidence to date. Drug Des Devel Ther. 2014;8:2221–38.
8. Dong Y, Fischer R, Naude PJ, Maier O, Nyakas C, Duffey M, Van der Zee EA, Dekens D, Douwenga W, Herrmann A, et al. Essential protective role of tumor necrosis factor receptor 2 in neurodegeneration. Proc Natl Acad Sci U S A. 2016;113:12304–9.
9. Wang Y, Han G, Chen Y, Wang K, Liu G, Wang R, Xiao H, Li X, Hou C, Shen B, et al. Protective role of tumor necrosis factor (TNF) receptors in chronic intestinal inflammation: TNFR1 ablation boosts systemic inflammatory response. Lab Investig. 2013;93:1024–35.
10. Aggarwal BB. Signalling pathways of the TNF superfamily: a double-edged sword. Nat Rev Immunol. 2003;3:745–56.
11. Sedger LM, McDermott MF. TNF and TNF-receptors: from mediators of cell death and inflammation to therapeutic giants—past, present and future. Cytokine Growth Factor Rev. 2014;25:453–72.
12. Krueger JM. Central cytokines and sleep. J Immunol. 1993;150:A82.
13. Krueger JM, Takahashi S, Kapas L, Bredow S, Roky R, Fang JD, Floyd R, Renegar KB, Guhathakurta N, Novitsky S, Obal F. Cytokines in sleep regulation. Adv Neuroimmunol. 1995;5:171–88.
14. Krueger JM, Obal F, Fang JD, Kubota T, Taishi P. The role of cytokines in physiological sleep regulation. Ann N Y Acad Sci. 2001;933:211–21.
15. Krueger JM. The role of cytokines in sleep regulation. Curr Pharm Design. 2008;14:3408–16.
16. Krueger JM, Rector DM, Churchill L. Sleep and cytokines. Sleep Med Clin. 2007;2:161–9.
17. Rowe RK, Striz M, Bachstetter AD, Van Eldik LJ, Donohue KD, O'Hara BF, Lifshitz J. Diffuse brain injury induces acute post-traumatic sleep. PLoS One. 2014;9:e82507.
18. Kilkenny C, Browne WJ, Cuthill IC, Emerson M, Altman DG. Improving bioscience research reporting: the ARRIVE guidelines for reporting animal research. PLoS Biol. 2010;8:e1000412.
19. Lifshitz J, Rowe RK, Griffiths DR, Evilsizor MN, Thomas TC, Adelson PD, McIntosh TK. Clinical relevance of midline fluid percussion brain injury: acute deficits, chronic morbidities and the utility of biomarkers. Brain Inj. 2016;30(11):1293–301.
20. Rowe RK, Griffiths DR, Lifshitz J. Midline (central) fluid percussion model of traumatic brain injury. In: Kobeissy HF, Dixon EC, Hayes LR, Mondello S, editors. Injury models of the central nervous system: methods and protocols. New York: Springer New York; 2016. p. 211–30.
21. Lifshitz J. Fluid percussion injury. In: Chen ZX J, Xu X-M, Zhang J, editors. Animal models of acute neurological injuries. Totowa: The Humana Press Inc; 2008.
22. Rowe RK, Harrison JL, O'Hara BF, Lifshitz J. Recovery of neurological function despite immediate sleep disruption following diffuse brain injury in the mouse: clinical relevance to medically untreated concussion. Sleep. 2014;37:743–52.
23. Rowe RK, Harrison JL, O'Hara BF, Lifshitz J. Diffuse brain injury does not affect chronic sleep patterns in the mouse. Brain Inj. 2014;28:504–10.
24. Harrison JL, Rowe RK, O'Hara BF, Adelson PD, Lifshitz J. Acute over-the-counter pharmacological intervention does not adversely affect behavioral outcome following diffuse traumatic brain injury in the mouse. Exp Brain Res. 2014;232(9):2709–19.
25. Rowe RK, Griffiths DR, Lifshitz J. Midline (central) fluid percussion model of traumatic brain injury. Methods Mol Biol. 2016;1462:211–30.
26. Hosseini AH, Lifshitz J. Brain injury forces of moderate magnitude elicit the fencing response. Med Sci Sports Exerc. 2009;41:1687–97.
27. Rowe RK, Harrison JL, Thomas TC, Pauly JR, Adelson PD, Lifshitz J. Using anesthetics and analgesics in experimental traumatic brain injury. Lab Anim (NY). 2013;42:286–91.
28. Nakachi H, Aoki K, Tomomatsu N, Alles N, Nagano K, Yamashiro M, Zhang H, Murali R, Greene MI, Ohya K, Amagasa T. A structural modulator of tumor necrosis factor type 1 receptor promotes bone formation under lipopolysaccharide-induced inflammation in a murine tooth extraction model. Eur J Pharmacol. 2012;679:132–8.
29. Donohue KD, Medonza DC, Crane ER, O'Hara BF. Assessment of a non-invasive high-throughput classifier for behaviours associated with sleep and wake in mice. Biomed Eng Online. 2008;7:14.
30. Mang GM, Nicod J, Emmenegger Y, Donohue KD, O'Hara BF, Franken P. Evaluation of a piezoelectric system as an alternative to electroencephalogram/ electromyogram recordings in mouse sleep studies. Sleep. 2014;37:1383–92.
31. McShane BB, Galante RJ, Jensen ST, Naidoo N, Pack AI, Wyner A. Characterization of the bout durations of sleep and wakefulness. J Neurosci Methods. 2010;193:321–33.
32. Ziebell JM, Bye N, Semple BD, Kossmann T, Morganti-Kossmann MC. Attenuated neurological deficit, cell death and lesion volume in Fas-mutant mice is associated with altered neuroinflammation following traumatic brain injury. Brain Res. 2011;1414:94–105.
33. Semple BD, Bye N, Rancan M, Ziebell JM, Morganti-Kossmann MC. Role of CCL2 (MCP-1) in traumatic brain injury (TBI): evidence from severe TBI

patients and CCL2–/– mice. J Cereb Blood Flow Metab. 2010;30:769–82.

34. Chen Y, Constantini S, Trembovler V, Weinstock M, Shohami E. An experimental model of closed head injury in mice: pathophysiology, histopathology, and cognitive deficits. J Neurotrauma. 1996;13:557–68.

35. Pleasant JM, Carlson SW, Mao H, Scheff SW, Yang KH, Saatman KE. Rate of neurodegeneration in the mouse controlled cortical impact model is influenced by impactor tip shape: implications for mechanistic and therapeutic studies. J Neurotrauma. 2011;28:2245–62.

36. Han X, Tong J, Zhang J, Farahvar A, Wang E, Yang J, Samadani U, Smith DH, Huang JH. Imipramine treatment improves cognitive outcome associated with enhanced hippocampal neurogenesis after traumatic brain injury in mice. J Neurotrauma. 2011;28:995–1007.

37. Ennaceur A, Aggleton JP. The effects of neurotoxic lesions of the perirhinal cortex combined to fornix transection on object recognition memory in the rat. Behav Brain Res. 1997;88:181–93.

38. Bachstetter AD, Xing B, de Almeida L, Dimayuga ER, Watterson DM, Van Eldik LJ. Microglial p38alpha MAPK is a key regulator of proinflammatory cytokine up-regulation induced by toll-like receptor (TLR) ligands or beta-amyloid (Abeta). J Neuroinflammation. 2011;8:79.

39. Cao T, Thomas TC, Ziebell JM, Pauly JR, Lifshitz J. Morphological and genetic activation of microglia after diffuse traumatic brain injury in the rat. Neuroscience. 2012;225:65–75.

40. Ziebell JM, Taylor SE, Cao T, Harrison JL, Lifshitz J. Rod microglia: elongation, alignment, and coupling to form trains across the somatosensory cortex after experimental diffuse brain injury. J Neuroinflammation. 2012;9:247.

41. Lifshitz J, Lisembee AM. Neurodegeneration in the somatosensory cortex after experimental diffuse brain injury. Brain Struct Funct. 2012;217:49–61.

42. Harrison JL, Rowe RK, Ellis TW, Yee NS, O'Hara BF, Adelson PD, Lifshitz J. Resolvins AT-D1 and E1 differentially impact functional outcome, post-traumatic sleep, and microglial activation following diffuse brain injury in the mouse. Brain Behav Immun. 2015;47:131–40.

43. R: a language and environment for stastical computing [http://www.cran.r-project.org//]. Accesed 19 Sept 2016.

44. Signorell A: DescTools: tools for descriptive statistics. 0.99.18 edition; 2016.

45. Murali R, Cheng X, Berezov A, Du X, Schon A, Freire E, Xu X, Chen YH, Greene MI. Disabling TNF receptor signaling by induced conformational perturbation of tryptophan-107. Proc Natl Acad Sci U S A. 2005;102:10970–5.

46. Bachstetter AD, Rowe RK, Kaneko M, Goulding D, Lifshitz J, Van Eldik LJ. The p38alpha MAPK regulates microglial responsiveness to diffuse traumatic brain injury. J Neurosci. 2013;33:6143–53.

47. Chio CC, Lin MT, Chang CP. Microglial activation as a compelling target for treating acute traumatic brain injury. Curr Med Chem. 2015;22:759–70.

48. Rochfort KD, Cummins PM. The blood-brain barrier endothelium: a target for pro-inflammatory cytokines. Biochem Soc Trans. 2015;43:702–6.

49. Yamamoto Y, Gaynor RB. Therapeutic potential of inhibition of the NF-kappaB pathway in the treatment of inflammation and cancer. J Clin Invest. 2001;107:135–42.

50. Di Battista AP, Rhind SG, Hutchison MG, Hassan S, Shiu MY, Inaba K, Topolovec-Vranic J, Neto AC, Rizoli SB, Baker AJ. Inflammatory cytokine and chemokine profiles are associated with patient outcome and the hyperadrenergic state following acute brain injury. J Neuroinflammation. 2016;13:40.

51. Chio CC, Chang CH, Wang CC, Cheong CU, Chao CM, Cheng BC, Yang CZ, Chang CP. Etanercept attenuates traumatic brain injury in rats by reducing early microglial expression of tumor necrosis factor-alpha. BMC Neurosci. 2013;14:33.

52. Baratz R, Tweedie D, Wang JY, Rubovitch V, Luo W, Hoffer BJ, Greig NH, Pick CG. Transiently lowering tumor necrosis factor-alpha synthesis ameliorates neuronal cell loss and cognitive impairments induced by minimal traumatic brain injury in mice. J Neuroinflammation. 2015;12:45.

53. Belarbi K, Jopson T, Tweedie D, Arellano C, Luo W, Greig NH, Rosi S. TNF-alpha protein synthesis inhibitor restores neuronal function and reverses cognitive deficits induced by chronic neuroinflammation. J Neuroinflammation. 2012;9:23.

54. Cavas M, Beltran D, Navarro JF. Behavioural effects of dimethyl sulfoxide (DMSO): changes in sleep architecture in rats. Toxicol Lett. 2005;157:221–32.

55. Clark IA, Vissel B. Inflammation-sleep interface in brain disease: TNF, insulin, orexin. J Neuroinflammation. 2014;11:51.

56. Tobinick E, Kim NM, Reyzin G, Rodriguez-Romanacce H, DePuy V. Selective TNF inhibition for chronic stroke and traumatic brain injury: an observational study involving 629 consecutive patients treated with perispinal etanercept. CNS Drugs. 2012;26:1051–70.

57. Baratz R, Tweedie D, Rubovitch V, Luo W, Yoon JS, Hoffer BJ, Greig NH, Pick CG. Tumor necrosis factor-alpha synthesis inhibitor, 3,6′-dithiothalidomide, reverses behavioral impairments induced by minimal traumatic brain injury in mice. J Neurochem. 2011;118:1032–42.

58. Sun YX, Dai DK, Liu R, Wang T, Luo CL, Bao HJ, Yang R, Feng XY, Qin ZH, Chen XP, Tao LY. Therapeutic effect of SN50, an inhibitor of nuclear factor-kappaB, in treatment of TBI in mice. Neurol Sci. 2013;34:345–55.

59. Wang YX, You Q, Su WL, Li Q, Hu ZQ, Wang ZG, Sun YP, Zhu WX, Ruan CP. A study on inhibition of inflammation via p75TNFR signaling pathway activation in mice with traumatic brain injury. J Surg Res. 2013;182:127–33.

10

Hydrogen sulfide-releasing cyclooxygenase inhibitor ATB-346 enhances motor function and reduces cortical lesion volume following traumatic brain injury in mice

Michela Campolo[1†], Emanuela Esposito[1†], Akbar Ahmad[1], Rosanna Di Paola[1], Irene Paterniti[1], Marika Cordaro[1], Giuseppe Bruschetta[1], John L Wallace[2] and Salvatore Cuzzocrea[1,3*]

Abstract

Background: Traumatic brain injury (TBI) induces secondary injury mechanisms, including dynamic interplay between ischemic, inflammatory and cytotoxic processes. We recently reported that administration of ATB-346 (2-(6-methoxynapthalen- 2-yl)-propionic acid 4-thiocarbamoyl-phenyl ester), a hydrogen sulfide-releasing cyclooxygenase inhibitor, showed marked beneficial effects in an animal model of spinal cord injury, significantly enhancing recovery of motor function and reducing the secondary inflammation and tissue injury.

Methods: Here we evaluated the neuroprotective potential of ATB-346, a hydrogen sulfide-releasing derivative of naproxen, using the controlled cortical impact (CCI) injury model in mice, one of the most common models of TBI. Moreover, the aim of the present study was to carefully investigate molecular pathways and subtypes of glial cells involved in the protective effect of ATB-346 on inflammatory reaction associated with an experimental model of TBI. In these studies, TBI was induced in mice by CCI and mice were orally administered ATB-346, naproxen (both at 30 μmol/kg) or vehicle (dimethylsulfoxide:1% carboxymethylcellulose [5:95] suspension) one and six hours after brain trauma and once daily for 10 days.

Results: Results revealed that ATB-346 attenuated TBI-induced brain edema, suppressed TBI-induced neural cell death and improved neurological function. ATB-346 also significantly reduced the severity of inflammation and restored neurotrophic factors that characterized the secondary events of TBI.

Conclusions: These data demonstrate that ATB-346 can be efficacious in a TBI animal model by reducing the secondary inflammation and tissue injury. Therefore, ATB-346 could represent an interesting approach for the management of secondary damage following CNS diseases, counteracting behavioral changes and inflammatory process.

Keywords: Brain trauma, Hydrogen sulfide, Neurotrophic factor, Inflammation, Motor recovery, Infarct area, Infarct volume, Nitrosative stress, Astrogliosis, Neuroprotection

* Correspondence: salvator@unime.it
†Equal contributors
[1]Department of Biological and Environmental Sciences, University of Messina, Viale Ferdinando Stagno D'Alcontres, 31-98166 Messina, Italy
[3]Manchester Biomedical Research Centre, Manchester Royal Infirmary, School of Medicine, University of Manchester, 29 Grafton Street Manchester, M13 9WU Manchester, UK
Full list of author information is available at the end of the article

Background

Traumatic brain injury (TBI) is a growing public health concern worldwide. There are over 1.35 million emergency room visits and 275,000 hospitalizations for nonfatal TBI each year in the United States, and approximately 40% of these individuals suffer from long-term disability due to their injury [1]. The pathophysiology of TBI can be divided into primary and secondary brain injury [2]. Primary injury results from the direct, physical brain trauma with tissue distortion, shearing, vascular injury and cell destruction probably related to rotational acceleration and deceleration inertial forces. Secondary brain injury is related to destructive inflammation and biochemical changes. Secondary injury onsets within minutes of primary injury, may last for several days and contributes to final outcome [3]. Primary and secondary brain injuries induce cerebral edema and bleeding. During secondary neuronal injury, healthy neurons around the injury site progressively degenerate, eventually leading to more serious clinical symptoms. Therefore, secondary neuronal injury plays a key role in the severity of insult and subsequent clinical prognosis.

Non-steroidal anti-inflammatory drugs (NSAIDs) are among the most commonly used anti-inflammatory drugs, but their use is associated with significant, sometimes life-threatening, adverse effects, particularly in the gastrointestinal (GI) tract [4]. Along with nitric oxide (•NO) and carbon monoxide (CO), hydrogen sulfide (H_2S) is regarded as an important gasotransmitter and endogenous neuromodulator, drawing increasing attention in the literature. Traditional neurotransmitters bind and activate membrane receptors, while gasotransmitters can freely diffuse to adjacent cells and directly bind to their target proteins to modify biological functions. Therefore, H_2S is a physiologic gasotransmitter as important as •NO and CO. In the past decade, increasing evidence shows that H_2S plays multiple roles in the CNS under physiological and pathological states. H_2S is produced in various parts of the body including the heart [5], the cardiovascular system [6] and the central nervous system (CNS) [7]. With respect to the CNS, H_2S has been reported to exert neuroprotective and neuromodulatory effects [8,9]. Thus, H_2S has recently been exploited in the design of novel NSAID derivatives that exhibit little, if any, side effects in the GI tract, despite producing suppression of prostaglandin synthesis and reduction of inflammation at least as effectively as the parent NSAID [10]. Recently, beneficial effects of an H_2S-releasing derivative of naproxen have been shown in an animal model of spinal cord injury (SCI), significantly enhancing recovery of motor function, possibly by reducing the secondary inflammation and tissue injury that characterizes this model. The combination of inhibition of cyclooxygenase [11] and delivery of H_2S may offer a promising alternative to existing therapies for traumatic injury [12]. On the basis of these data, H_2S could have an important

role in reducing inflammatory processes and tissue damage post-brain trauma. Therefore, in the current study we evaluated ATB-346, a novel H_2S-releasing derivative of naproxen, for neuroprotective properties in experimental murine TBI using controlled cortical impact injury (CCI), a model of focal brain injury. Moreover, the aim of the present study was to carefully investigate molecular pathways and subtypes of glial cells involved in the protective effect of ATB-346 on inflammatory reaction associated with an experimental model of TBI. In particular, our attention shifts to post-injury recovery of motor function, reduction of infarct area and of brain tissue inflammation after TBI.

Methods

Animals

Male CD1 mice (25 to 30 g, Harlan, Milan, Italy), aged between 10 and 12 weeks, were used for all studies. Mice were housed in individual cages (five per cage) and maintained under a 12:12 hour light/dark cycle at $21 \pm 1°C$ and $50 \pm 5\%$ humidity. Standard laboratory diet and tap water were available *ad libitum*. The study was approved by the University of Messina Review Board for the care of animals. Animal care was in compliance with Italian regulations on protection of animals used for experimental and other scientific purposes (Ministerial Decree 16192) as well as with the Council Regulation (EEC) (Official Journal of the European Union L 358/1 12/18/1986).

Controlled cortical impact experimental traumatic brain injury

TBI was induced in mice by a controlled cortical impactor. The mice were anesthetized under intraperitoneal ketamine and xylazine (2.6/0.16 mg/kg of body weight, respectively). A craniotomy was made in the right hemisphere, encompassing bregma and lambda, and between the sagittal suture and the coronal ridge, with a Micro motor hand piece and drill (UGO Basile SRL, Comerio Varese, Italy). The resulting bone flap was removed and the craniotomy enlarged further with cranial rongeurs (New Adalat Garh, Roras Road, Pakistan). A cortical contusion was produced on the exposed cortex using the controlled impactor device Impact One™ Stereotaxic impactor for CCI (Leica, Milan, Italy). Briefly, the impacting shaft was extended, and the impact tip was centered and lowered over the craniotomy site until it touched the dura mater. Then, the rod was retracted and the impact tip was advanced farther to produce a brain injury of moderate severity for mice (tip diameter: 4 mm; cortical contusion depth: 3 mm; impact velocity: 1.5 m/sec). Immediately after injury, the skin incision was closed with nylon sutures, and 2% lidocaine jelly was applied to the lesion site to minimize any possible discomfort.

Test drugs

ATB-346 (2-(6-methoxynapthalen-2-yl)-propionic acid 4-thiocarbamoyl phenyl ester) is a derivative of naproxen, which includes a H_2S-releasing moiety referred to hereafter as 'TBZ' (4-hydroxythiobenzamide) [13]. ATB-346, TBZ and naproxen were prepared freshly each day as suspensions in dimethylsulfoxide:1% carboxymethylcellulose (5:95).

Prior to beginning these experiments, a pilot study was performed to confirm the equipotency of naproxen and ATB-346 in suppressing cyclooxygenase at the dose selected. At 30 μmol/kg (oral administration), naproxen and ATB-346 equally suppressed gastric (prostaglandin E2) PGE_2 synthesis (by more than 90%) and whole blood thromboxane synthesis (by more than 95%). This level of inhibition was evident within 15 minutes and persisted for at least 12 hours after drug administration. TBZ had no effect on gastric PGE_2 synthesis or whole blood thromboxane synthesis.

Experimental groups

Mice were randomly allocated into one of five groups. In the TBI + vehicle group, mice were subjected to TBI and received the vehicle for TBZ, naproxen and ATB-34 (dimethylsulfoxide:1% carboxymethylcellulose) (orally), at one and six hours after brain trauma (N = 20). The TBZ group was the same as the TBI + vehicle group, but mice were administered TBZ only (30 μmol/kg, orally), at one and six hours after brain trauma (N = 20). The naproxen group was the same as the TBI + vehicle group, but mice were administered naproxen only (30 μmol/kg, orally), at one and six hours after brain trauma (N = 20). The ATB-346 group was the same as the TBI + vehicle group, but mice were administered ATB-346 only (30 μmol/kg, orally), at one and six hours after brain trauma (N = 20). In the sham + vehicle group mice were subjected to identical surgical procedures, except for TBI, and were kept under anesthesia for the duration of the experiment (N = 20).

As described below, mice were sacrificed at 24 hours after TBI in order to evaluate the following parameters: 2,3,5-triphenyltetrazolium chloride (TTC) staining (N = four out of 20 for each group) [14]; histology analysis (N = three out of 20 for each group) and Tumor necrosis factor (TNF)α, Interleukin (IL)-1β, Glial fibrillary acidic protein (GFAP) and Ionized calcium binding adaptor molecule (Iba)1 immunofluorescence (N = three out of 20 for each group) [14]; Western blot analysis (N = five out of 20 for each group) and RT-PCR analysis for *Glial cell-Derived Neurotrophic Factor (GDNF)*, *Nerve Growth Factor (NGF)* and *Vascular Endothelial Growth Factor (VEGF)* levels (N = five out of 20 for each group). In a separate set of experiments, another 10 animals from each group were observed after TBI in order to evaluate the behavioral testing. Several recent results illustrate the importance of initiating therapeutic interventions as soon as possible following TBI, preferably within four hours post-injury, to achieve the best possible neuroprotective effect [15].

Behavioural testing

Mice with TBI display motor and cognitive deficits. Thus, the present behavioural tests involved analyses of motor asymmetry (elevated biased swing test (EBST) and rotarod test). Training for the rotarod test was initiated at one week. Before the CCI injury, whereas no training was required for the EBST. The retard treadmill (Accuscan, Inc., Columbus, Ohio, United States) provided a motor balance and coordination assessment. Data were generated by averaging the scores (total time spent on treadmill divided by five trials) for each animal during training and testing days. Each animal was placed in a neutral position on a cylinder (3 cm and 1 cm diameter for rats and mice, respectively) then the rod was rotated with the speed accelerated linearly from 0 to 24 rpm within 60 seconds, and the time spent on the retard was recorded automatically. The maximum score given to an animal was fixed to 60. For training, animals were given five trials each day and declared having reached the criterion when they scored 60 in three consecutive trials. For testing, animals were given three trials and the average score of these three trials was used as the individual rotarod score. The EBST provided a motor asymmetry parameter and involved handling the animal by its tail and recording the direction of the biased body swings. The EBST consisted of 20 trials with the number of swings ipsilateral and contralateral to the injured hemisphere recorded and expressed in percentage to determine the biased swing activity.

Quantification of infarct volume

Mice were anesthetized with ketamine and decapitated. Their brains were carefully removed. The brains were cut into five coronal slices of 2-mm thickness. Slices were incubated in a 2% solution of TTC at 37°C for 30 minutes and immersion fixed in 10% buffered formalin solution. TTC stains the viable brain tissue red while infracted tissue remains unstained [16,17]. For quantification of infracted area and volumes, the brain slices were photographed using a digital camera (HP Photosmart R707, Milan, Italy) and then image analysis was performed on a personal computer with an image analysis software program (using ImageJ for Windows (Institute of Mental Health, Maryland, USA). To compensate for the effect of brain edema the corrected infarct volume was calculated as previously described in detail [18]:

Corrected infarct area = left hemisphere area - (right hemisphere area - infarct area).

Values are given as mean ± SEM. The corrected total infarct volume was calculated by summing the infarct area in each slice and multiplying it by slice thickness (2 mm).

Tissue processing and histology

Coronal sections of 5-μm thickness were sectioned from the perilesional brain area of each animal and were evaluated by an experienced histopathologist. Damaged neurons were counted and the histopathologic changes of the grey matter were scored on a six-point scale [19]: 0, no lesion observed; 1, grey matter contained one to five eosinophilic neurons; 2, grey matter contained five to 10 eosinophilic neurons; 3, grey matter contained more than 10 eosinophilic neurons; 4, small infarction (less than one third of the grey matter area); 5, moderate infarction (one third to one half of the grey matter area); 6, large infarction (more than half of the grey matter area). The scores from all the sections of each brain were averaged to give a final score for individual mice. All the histological studies were performed in a blinded fashion.

Western blot analyses

Cytosolic and nuclear extracts were prepared as previously described [20], with slight modifications. The ipsilateral hemisphere after injury from each mouse was suspended in extraction Buffer A containing protease inhibitors, homogenized for two minutes, then centrifuged at $1,000 \times g$ for 10 minutes at 4°C. Supernatants contained the cytosolic fraction. The pellets, containing enriched nuclei, were resuspended in Buffer B containing 1% Triton X-100, 150 mM NaCl, 10 mM Tris-HCl pH 7.4, 1 mM, ethylene glycol tetraacetic acid (EGTA), 1 mM, ethylenediaminetetraacetic acid (EDTA), 0.2 mM phenylmethanesulfonylfluoride (PMSF) and protease inhibitors. After centrifugation for 30 minutes at $15,000 \times g$ at 4°C, the supernatants containing the nuclear protein were stored at −80°C for further analysis. The levels of inducible nitric oxide synthase (iNOS), cyclooxygenase (COX)-2, endothelial nitric oxide synthase (eNOS) and IκBα were quantified in cytosolic fractions. NFκBp65 was quantified in nuclear fractions from brain tissue collected 24 hours after TBI. The filters were probed with specific Abs anti-iNOS (1:1,000; BD Biosciences, Milan, Italy), anti-COX-2 (1:1,000; Cayman Chemicals, Tallinn Estonia), anti-eNOS (1:1000; BD Biosciences, Milan, Italy), anti-NFκBp65 (1:500; Santa Cruz Biotechnology, Heidelberg, Germany) and anti-IκBα antibody (1:500; Santa Cruz Biotechnology, Heidelberg, Germany) at 4°C overnight in $1 \times$ PBS, 5% (w/v), non-fat dried milk and 0.1% Tween-20 (PMT). Membranes were incubated with peroxidase-conjugated bovine anti-mouse IgG secondary antibody or peroxidase-conjugated goat anti-rabbit IgG (1:2,000; Jackson ImmunoResearch, West Grove, PA, USA) for one hour at room temperature. To ascertain

that blots were loaded with equal amounts of protein lysates, they were also incubated in the presence of the antibody against β-actin or lamin A/C (1:5,000; Santa Cruz Biotechnology, Heidelberg, Germany). The signals were detected with enhanced a chemiluminescence detection system reagent according to manufacturer's instruction (Super Signal West Pico Chemiluminescent Substrate, Pierce Thermo Scientific, Rockford, IL. USA). The relative expression of the protein bands of IκBα (approximately 37 kDa), NFκB (approximately 65 kDa), eNOS (approximately 140 kDa), iNOS (approximately 130 kDa) and COX-2 (approximately 72 kDa) were quantified by densitometry with Gel Logic 200 PRO software (GE Healthcare, Milwaukee, Wisconsin, USA) and standardized to β-actin and lamin A/C levels. Images of blot signals were imported to analysis software Image Quant TL Software, version 2003 (GE Healthcare, Milwaukee, Wisconsin, USA). A preparation of commercially available molecular weight 10 to 250 kDa was used to define molecular weight positions, and as reference concentrations for each molecular weight.

Reverse transcription polymerase chain reaction

Total RNA, from contused brain tissue at the impact site after injury, was extracted by a modified method [21], using TRIzol™ Reagent (Life Technologies, Milan, Italy) according to the manufacturer's instructions. Reverse transcription was performed by a standard procedure using 2 μg of total RNA. After reverse transcription, 1 μl of reverse transcriptase (RT) products were diluted in 24 μl of PCR mix, to give a final concentration of 50 U ml −1 of Taq DNA polymerase (Life Technologies, Milan, Italy), 10 μm of 5′ and 3′ primers, 10 mM of each deoxynucleotide triphosphates (dNTP), 50 mM MgCl2 and $10 \times$ NH4 buffer. cDNAs underwent 30 cycles for *GDNF, NGF, VEGF* and *β-actin*, each one performed at 94°C for one minute, melting temperature (Tm) °C for 45 seconds and 72°C for 55 seconds (Table 1). After this treatment 10 μl of RT-PCR products were separated by 1.5% agarose gel electrophoresis in Tris/Borate/EDTA (TBE) $0.5 \times$ (Tris-base 0.089 m, boric acid 0.089 m) containing 0.1 μg ml^{-1} of ethidium bromide. Fragments of DNA were seen under ultraviolet light. *β-actin* was used as an internal reference.

Immunofluorescence

After deparaffinization and rehydration, detection of TNFα, IL-1β, GFAP and Iba1 was carried out after boiling in 0.1 M citrate buffer for one minute. Non-specific adsorption was minimized by incubating the section in 2% (volume/volume (vol/vol)) normal goat serum in PBS for 20 minutes. Sections were incubated with mouse monoclonal anti-GFAP (1:100, vol/vol Santa Cruz Biotechnology (Heidelberg, Germany), or with polyclonal rabbit anti-TNFα (1:100, vol/vol Santa Cruz Biotechnology, Heidelberg, Germany), or with rabbit anti-IL-1β (1:100, vol/vol Santa

Table 1 Specific primer sequences

Gene	Forward primer (5′-- > 3′)	Reverse primer (5′-- > 3′)
GDNF	TCA CTG ACT TGG GTT TGG GCT AT	TCA GAC GGC TGT TCT CAC TCC TA
NGF	GCA TCG AGT GAC TTT GGA GC	GTA CGC CGA TCA AAA ACG CA
VEGF	TGG ATG TCT ACC AGC GAA GC	ACA AGG CTC ACA GTG ATT TT
β- actin	CAT GAA GTG CGA CGT TGA CA	CAC ATC TGC TGG AAG GTG GA

Cruz Biotechnology, Heidelberg, Germany) or with mouse monoclonal anti-Iba1 (1:100, vol/vol Santa Cruz Biotechnology, Heidelberg, Germany) antibody in a humidified oxygen and nitrogen chamber for over night at 37°C. Sections were incubated with secondary antibody Fluorescein isothiocyanate (FITC)-conjugated anti-mouse Alexa Fluor-488 antibody (1:2,000 vol/vol Molecular Probes, Monza, Italy) and with TEXAS RED-conjugated anti-rabbit Alexa Fluor-594 antibody (1:1000 in PBS, vol/vol Molecular Probes, Monza, Italy) for one hour at 37°C. For nuclear staining, 2 μg/ml 4′,6′-diamidino-2-phenylindole (DAPI; Hoechst, Frankfurt, Germany) in PBS was added. Sections were observed at 20× magnification using a Leica DM2000 microscope (Leica, Milan, Italy). Optical sections of fluorescence specimens were obtained using a HeNe laser (543 nm), an ultraviolet laser (361 to 365 nm) and an argon laser (458 nm) at a one-minute, two seconds scanning speed with up to eight averages; 1.5 μm sections were obtained using a pinhole of 250. Contrast and brightness were established by examining the most brightly labeled pixels and applying settings that allowed clear visualization of structural details, while keeping the highest pixel intensities close to 200. The same settings were used for all images obtained from the other samples that had been processed in parallel. Digital images were cropped and figure montages prepared using Adobe Photoshop 7.0 (Adobe Systems; Palo Alto, California, United States).

Materials

ATB-346 (2-(6-methoxy-napthalen-2-yl)-propionic acid 4-thiocarbamoyl-phenyl ester), sodium naproxen and TBZ (4-hydroxythiobenzamide) were provided by Antibe Therapeutics Inc. (Toronto, Canada). Unless otherwise stated, all other compounds were obtained from Sigma-Aldrich Company Ltd. (Milan, Italy). All stock solutions were prepared in non-pyrogenic saline (0.9% NaCl; Baxter, Italy) or 10% dimethyl sulfoxide (DMSO).

Statistical evaluation

Data are mean ± SEM. Data were analyzed using Graphpad PRISM V (Graphpad Software Inc., La Jolla, California, United States). Swing activity and time on platform were analyzed using two factor repeated measures analysis of variance (RM ANOVA, group × time). Infarct area, lesion volume and densitometric analysis data were analyzed by ANOVA followed by a Bonferroni *post-hoc* test for multiple comparisons. Histological score and percentage total tissue area were analyzed by Student's t-test. For all comparisons, $P <0.05$ was considered to be significant. In the experiments involving histology or immunohistochemistry, the figures shown are representative of at least three experiments performed on different experimental days on the tissue sections collected from all the animals in each group.

Results

Effect of ATB-346 on IκBα degradation and NFκBp65 translocation

To investigate whether the cellular mechanism through ATB-346 could attenuate inflammatory processes we assessed Western blot analysis of the ipsilateral hemisphere after TBI, using an IκBα and an NFκB-specific antibodies. The results showed a basal expression of IκBα in the brain from sham-mice (Figure 1A, see densitometry analysis A1), while IκBα expression was significantly reduced in mice subject to TBI and TBZ administration, as showed in Figure 1A and 1A1. Naproxen treatment blunted the degradation of IκBα but ATB-346 was able to significantly restore IκBα degradation (Figure 1A, see densitometry analysis A1). Moreover, p65 subunit translocation was increased after TBI and TBZ injection in the nuclear brain homogenates, compared with sham-group. ATB-346 administration significantly reduced the translocation of p65 in nuclei compared to the TBI group (Figure 1B, see densitometry analysis B1).

Effect of ATB-346 on iNOS and COX-2 expression

To determine the role of •NO produced during TBI, iNOS expression was evaluated by Western blot analysis. A significant increase in iNOS expression was observed in the contused area from mice subjected to TBI and TBZ administration (Figure 1C, see densitometry analysis C1). Consequently, naproxen reduced TBI-induced iNOS expression (Figure 1C, see densitometry analysis C1); on the other hand, a significant decrease in iNOS expression was observed after ATB-346 treatment (Figure 1C see densitometry analysis C1). Similarly, COX-2 expression was induced by TBI and TBZ administration compared to the sham group (Figure 1D, see densitometry analysis D1). Both treatments with naproxen and ATB-346 lowered COX-2 expression (Figure 1D, see densitometry analysis D1).

Effect of ATB-346 on TNFα and IL-1β expression in astrocytes after traumatic brain injury

To analyse the activation of astrocytes and cytokines expression, contused brain tissue at the impact site after injury was double-stained with antibodies against GFAP

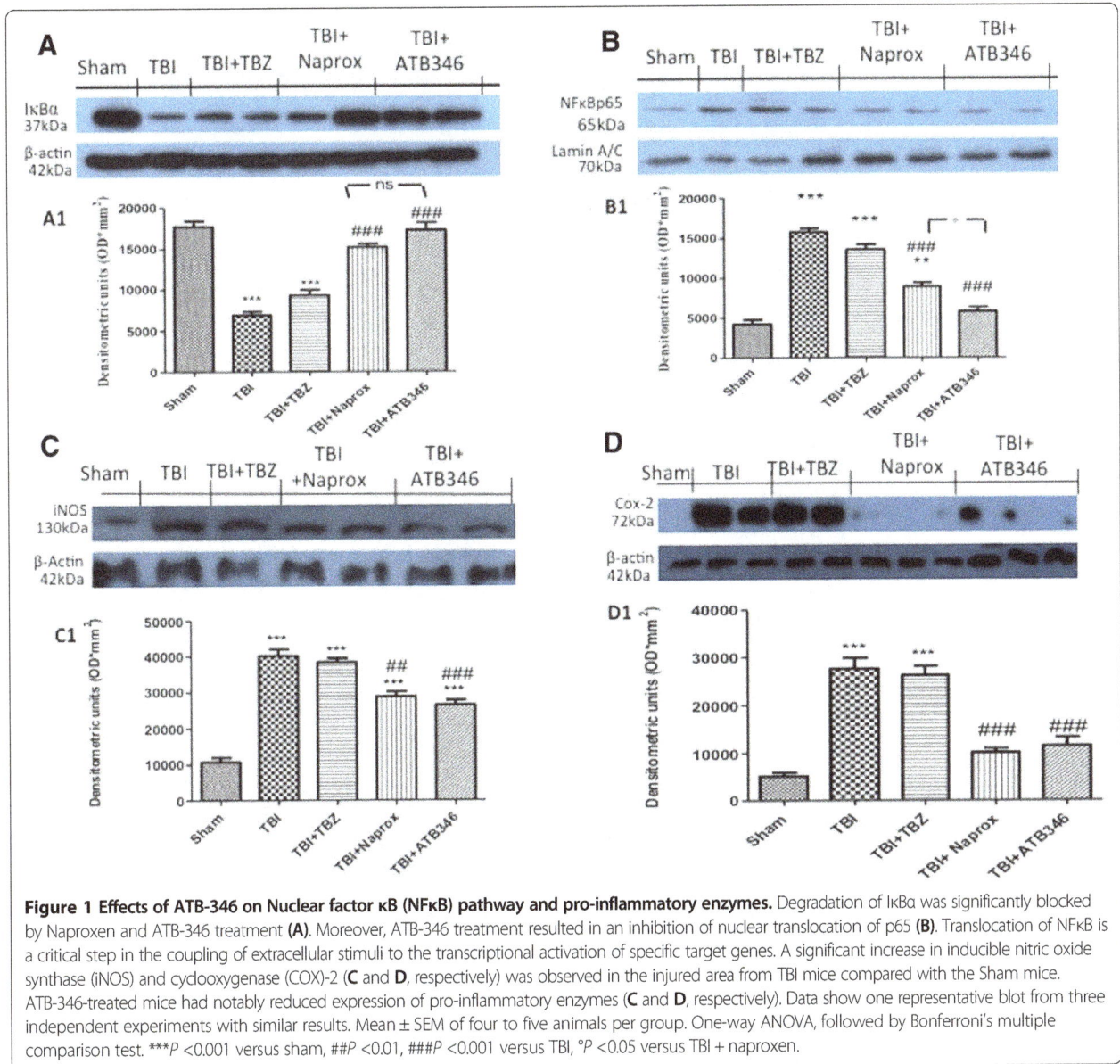

Figure 1 Effects of ATB-346 on Nuclear factor κB (NFκB) pathway and pro-inflammatory enzymes. Degradation of IκBα was significantly blocked by Naproxen and ATB-346 treatment (**A**). Moreover, ATB-346 treatment resulted in an inhibition of nuclear translocation of p65 (**B**). Translocation of NFκB is a critical step in the coupling of extracellular stimuli to the transcriptional activation of specific target genes. A significant increase in inducible nitric oxide synthase (iNOS) and cyclooxygenase (COX)-2 (**C** and **D**, respectively) was observed in the injured area from TBI mice compared with the Sham mice. ATB-346-treated mice had notably reduced expression of pro-inflammatory enzymes (**C** and **D**, respectively). Data show one representative blot from three independent experiments with similar results. Mean ± SEM of four to five animals per group. One-way ANOVA, followed by Bonferroni's multiple comparison test. ***$P < 0.001$ versus sham, ##$P < 0.01$, ###$P < 0.001$ versus TBI, °$P < 0.05$ versus TBI + naproxen.

(green; Figures 2 and 3) and TNFα (red; Figure 2) or IL-1β (red; Figure 3). Brain sections revealed increased astrogliosis (GFAP+ cells) in TBI and TBZ panels. Moreover, a marked co-localization of TNFα in GFAP+ cells was present after TBI and TBZ administration (merged, Figure 2). TNFα and IL-1β expressions were significantly reduced by ATB-346 treatment (TBI + ATB-346 panels; Figures 2 and 3).

Effect of ATB-346 on TNFα and IL-1β expression in microglia after traumatic brain injury

To evaluate the microglia activation and its correlation with cytokines expression, ipsilateral hemisphere to the injury site were double-stained with antibodies against Iba1 (green; Figures 4 and 5) and TNFα (red; Figure 4)

or IL-1β (red; Figure 5). Microglial cells (Iba1- + cells) expressed TNFα and IL-1β in TBI and TBZ panels (Figures 4 and 5, respectively). There was an evident co-localization of TNFα and Iba1 in TBI and TBZ panels (merged, Figure 4). Considerable reductions in cytokines expressions were evident in naproxen panels (Figures 4 and 5, respectively); however, ATB-346 reduced TNFα and IL-1β expressions in microglia (Figures 4 and 5, respectively).

Effect of ATB-346 on mRNA levels of neurotrophic factors

To test whether ATB-346 modulates the levels of the neurotrophic factors, we studied *GDNF* and *NGF* levels in brain tissue using semi-quantitative RT–PCR analysis. A significant decrease in *GDNF* (470 bp) and *NGF* (318 bp) mRNA expression following TBI and TBZ administration

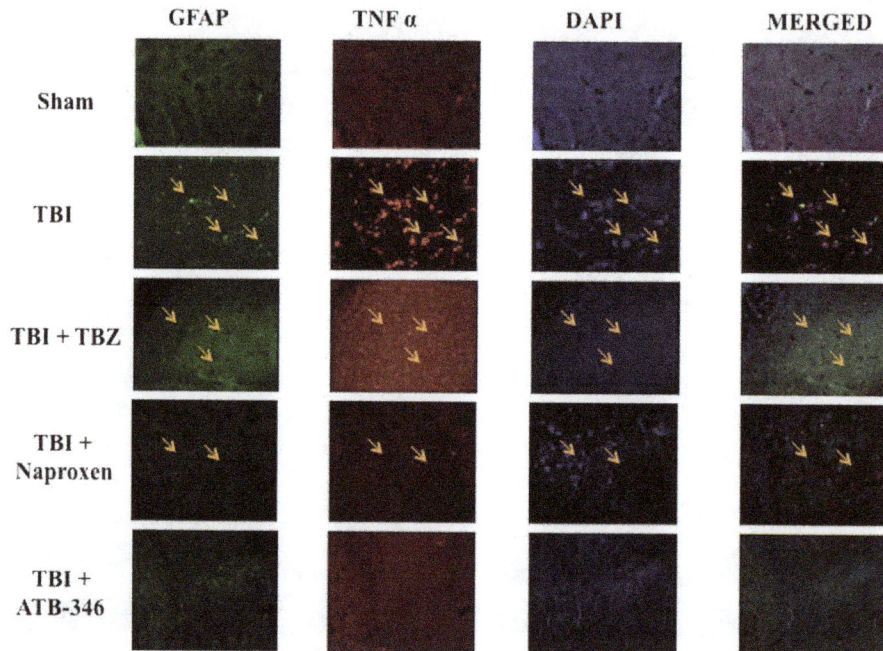

Figure 2 Effects of ATB-346 on tumor necrosis factor (TNF)α expression in glial fibrillary acidic protein (GFAP) positive cells. Brain tissue was double-stained with antibodies against GFAP, green) and TNFα (red). The red spots indicate the co-localizations (merged). Brain sections revealed increased astrogliosis (GFAP+ cells) in TBI and TBZ panels. Considerable GFAP immunoreactivity was present in TBI and TBZ panels. TNFα expression was significantly reduced by ATB-346 treatment (TBI + ATB-346 panels) compared to naproxen treatment (TBI + naproxen panels). All images were digitalized at 600 dpi.

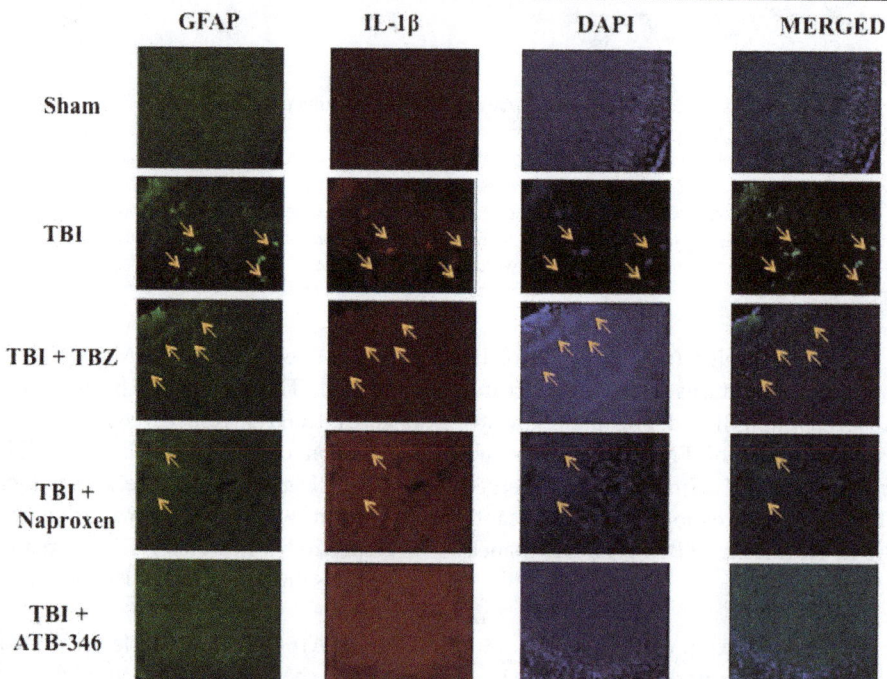

Figure 3 Effects of ATB-346 on interleukin (IL)-1β expression in glial fibrillary acidic protein (GFAP) positive cells. Brain tissue was double-stained with antibodies against GFAP (green) and IL-1β (red). Brain sections revealed increased astrogliosis (GFAP+ cells) in TBI and TBZ panels. Considerable GFAP immunoreactivity was present in TBI and TBZ panels. IL-1β expression was significantly reduced after ATB-346 treatment (TBI + ATB-346 panels) respect to naproxen treatment (TBI + naproxen panels). All images were digitalized at 600 dpi.

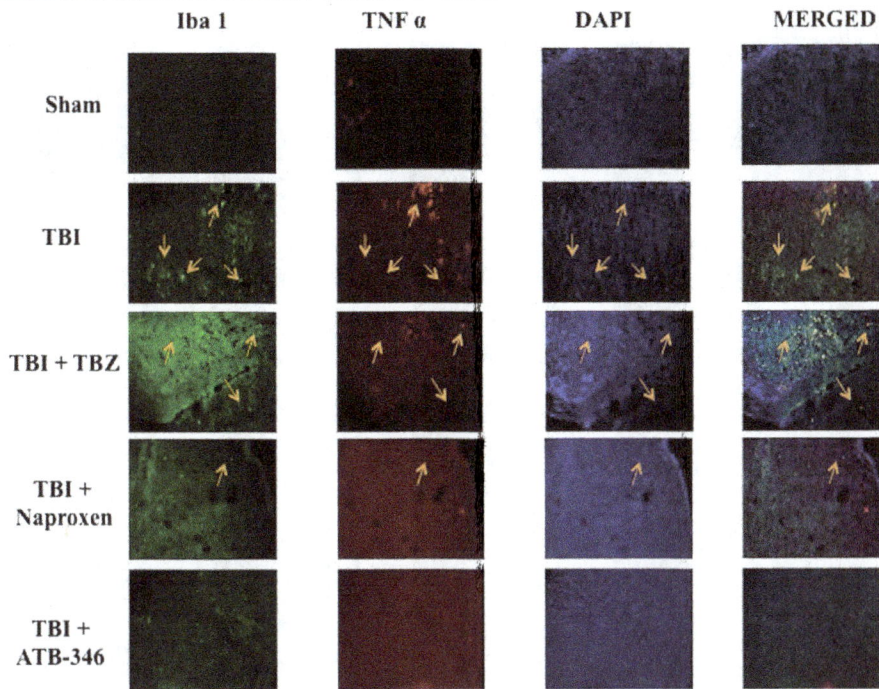

Figure 4 Effects of ATB-346 on tumor necrosis factor (TNF)α in ionized calcium binding adaptor molecule (Iba)1 positive cells. Brain tissue was double-stained with antibodies against Iba1 (green) and TNFα (red). Microglial cells (Iba1+ cells) expressed TNFα in TBI and TBZ panels. A considerable reduction of cytokine expression was present in naproxen panels; however, ATB-346 reduced notably TNFα expressions (TBI + ATB-346 panels). The red spots indicate the co-localizations (merged). All images were digitalized at 600 dpi.

was evident. Moreover, ATB-346 significantly increased mRNA levels of both neurotrophic factors examined (Figure 6A and B respectively, see densitometry analysis A1 and B1 respectively).

Effect of ATB-346 on vascular components after traumatic brain injury

To investigate whether ATB-346 could promote normalization of the impaired neurovascular unit, we observed *VEGF* level and eNOS expression. RT-PCR showed a significant increase in *VEGF* (308 bp) mRNA expression, and ATB-346 significantly increased its level (Figure 6C, see densitometry analysis C1). Moreover, by Western blot analysis we observed a significantly increase in eNOS expression in the TBI group, and ATB-346 upregulated its expression (Figure 6D, see densitometry analysis D1).

Infarct outcome in ATB-346-treated mice after traumatic brain injury

A histological examination of brain sections at the level of the perilesional area, stained 24 hours after injury, revealed significant damage in the TBI and TBI + TBZ groups, such as prominent and thickened blood vessels, ischemic changes and gliosis in the brain parenchyma (Figure 7B and C respectively, see densitometry analysis F) compared to sham mice (Figure 7A, see densitometry analysis F).

Naproxen treatment attenuated the development of inflammation at 24 hours after TBI; ATB-346 significantly reduced the degree of brain injury (Figure 7D and E respectively, see densitometry analysis F).

Brain edema indicates pathology associated with endothelial cell activation and endothelial dysfunction. To evaluate the effect of ATB-346 on brain edema and infarctions in the TBI and TBZ group, we performed TTC staining (Figure 8A). At 24 hours after TBI, ATB-346-treated mice had a significantly smaller infarct area (Figure 8B) and volume (Figure 8C).

Neurological deficits after ATB-346 administration

To investigate the relationship between neurological deficits in the setting of TBI we used two different tests: the EBST and the rotarod test, considered the most sensitive vestibular motor test to assess motor function. The EBST provided a motor asymmetry parameter and involved handling the animal by its tail and recording the direction of the biased body swings. The EBST consisted of 20 trials with the number of swings ipsilateral and contralateral to the ischemic hemisphere recorded and expressed in percentage to determine the biased swing activity. Mice were tested seven days after TBI for both behavioral tests. CCI-injured mice and TBZ-treated mice displayed a range of impairments in locomotor tasks as showed in Figure 8D and E, respectively. Both groups of animals that received

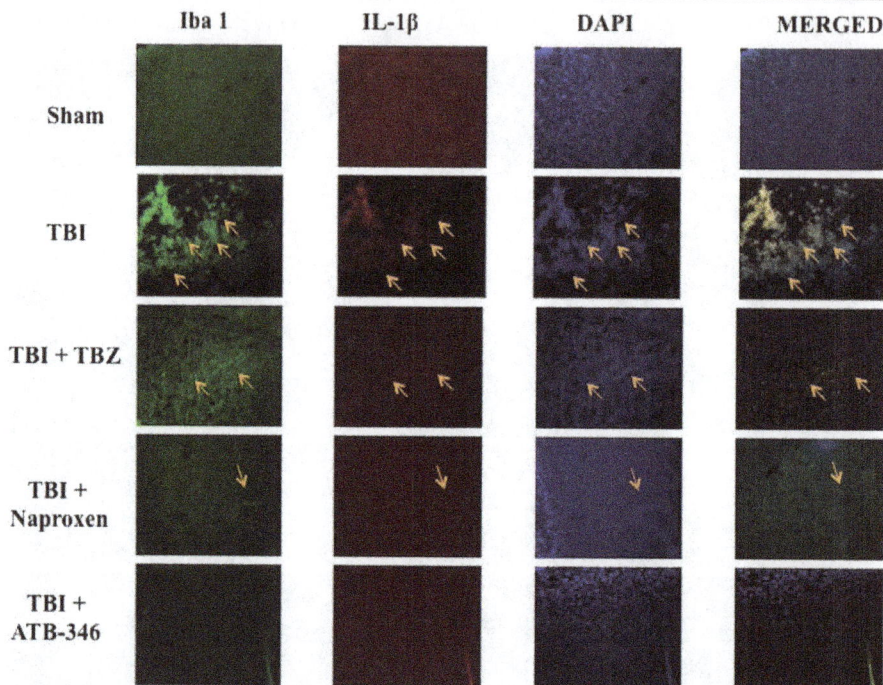

Figure 5 Effects of ATB-346 on interleukin (IL)-1β expression in ionized calcium binding adaptor molecule (Iba)1 positive cells. Brain tissue was double-stained with antibodies against Iba1 (green) and IL-1β (red). Microglial cells (Iba1+ cells) expressed IL-1β in TBI and TBZ panels. A considerable reduction of IL-1β expression was present in naproxen panels; at least, ATB-346 markedly reduced TNFα and IL-1β expressions (ATB-346 panels). The red spots indicate the co-localizations (merged). All images were digitalized at 600 dpi.

naproxen or ATB-346 were significantly less impaired in the EBST and rotarod tests compared with the TBI group (Figure 8D and E, respectively).

Discussion

A number of animal models have been developed to induce brain trauma. Of these the most commonly used are weight-drop injury, fluid percussion injury (FPI) and CCI. The use of TBI models has resulted in an increased understanding of the pathophysiology of TBI, including changes in molecular and cellular pathways and neurobehavioral outcomes. CCI models utilize a pneumatic pistol to laterally deform the exposed dura and provide controlled impact and quantifiable biomechanical parameters. This model produces graded, reproducible brain injury. Dependent on the severity of injury, CCI results in an ipsilateral injury with cortical contusion, hemorrhage and blood-brain barrier disruption. CCI injury reproduces changes reported in clinical head injuries such as cortical contusion, brain edema, subarachnoid hemorrhage, elevated intracerebral pressure, reduced cortical perfusion, decreased cerebral blood flow and neuro-endocrine and metabolic changes [22]. The predominantly focal brain injury caused by CCI makes this model to a useful tool for studying the pathophysiology of the secondary processes induced by focal brain injury. However, there is a lack of brain stem deformation in this model and thus a low mortality rate.

In recent years, H_2S has been recognized as a fundamental signalling molecule that plays important roles in exerting cytoprotective effects in the CNS, since it can protect neurons and glia from oxidative stress [9,23]. H_2S also exert many anti-inflammatory effects, including inhibition of leukocyte-endothelial adherence, reduction of edema formation [24,25] and inhibition of NFκB activation [26]. H_2S is produced endogenously via enzymatic activity, non-enzymatic pathways (such as reduction of thiol-containing molecules), and is also released from intracellular sulfur stores (sulfane sulfur). Cystathionine β-synthase (CBS) is believed to be the critical enzyme that produces H_2S, resulting in the modulation of neurological function. H_2S generated by cystathionine γ-lyase (CSE) was next discovered as an important modulator of vasorelaxation in smooth muscle. They separately coordinate with L-cysteine to produce H_2S, L-serine and ammonium. After the discovery of H_2S as a potential neurological and vasorelaxant signaling molecule, more targets were expected to be found [27,28]. The enhanced beneficial effects of ATB-346 over those of naproxen are most likely attributable to the H_2S release from the former, and may be due to the neuroprotective and anti-inflammatory properties of this gaseous mediator, acting in a complimentary manner to the anti-inflammatory effects associated with inhibition of COX activity. Indeed, the marked reduction of gastrointestinal toxicity of

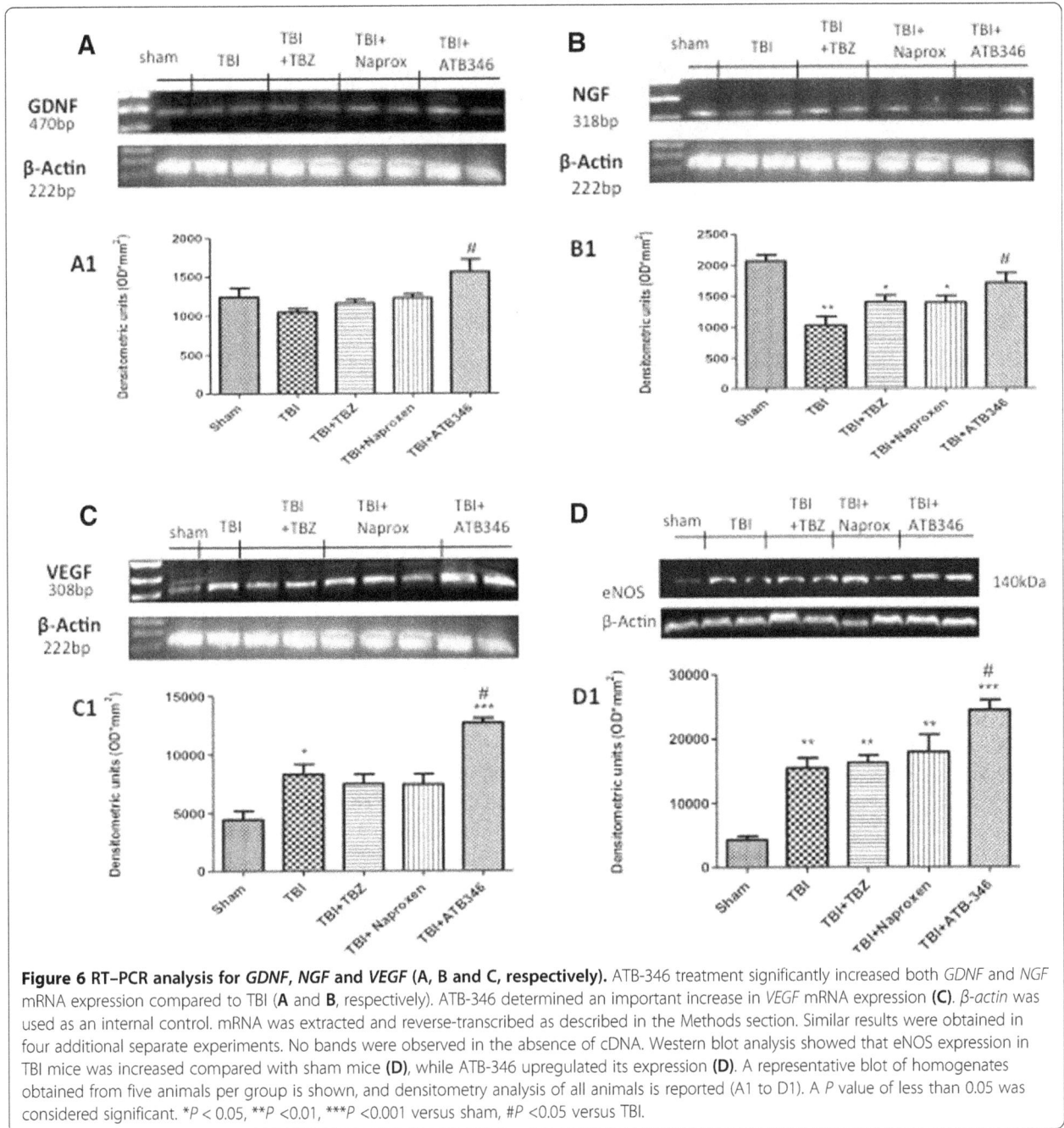

Figure 6 RT–PCR analysis for *GDNF*, *NGF* and *VEGF* (A, B and C, respectively). ATB-346 treatment significantly increased both *GDNF* and *NGF* mRNA expression compared to TBI (**A** and **B**, respectively). ATB-346 determined an important increase in *VEGF* mRNA expression (**C**). *β-actin* was used as an internal control. mRNA was extracted and reverse-transcribed as described in the Methods section. Similar results were obtained in four additional separate experiments. No bands were observed in the absence of cDNA. Western blot analysis showed that eNOS expression in TBI mice was increased compared with sham mice (**D**), while ATB-346 upregulated its expression (**D**). A representative blot of homogenates obtained from five animals per group is shown, and densitometry analysis of all animals is reported (A1 to D1). A *P* value of less than 0.05 was considered significant. *$P < 0.05$, **$P < 0.01$, ***$P < 0.001$ versus sham, #$P < 0.05$ versus TBI.

ATB-346 versus naproxen has been attributed to the mucosal protective and anti-inflammatory effects (for example, inhibition of leukocyte adherence to vascular endothelium) of the H$_2$S released from this drug [29]. We observe a light beneficial effect of TBZ, the H2S-releasing moiety of ATB-346, on several parameters. The release of H$_2$S from TBZ may not be as great as that from an equimolar amount of ATB-346. Previous studies have shown that TBZ alone releases very little H$_2$S, but when covalently linked to another drug, such as an NSAID, considerably more H2S is released [30].

Focal lesions to the brain display a characteristic inflammatory response with infiltration of peripheral immune cells after injury. These cells are believed to be important because they contain and release a multitude of inflammatory mediators associated with increased tissue injury. Neutrophils peak approximately two days post-TBI, and monocytes slightly later [31]. Leukocyte homogenates from post-TBI patients display upregulation of iNOS, COX-2 and nicotinamide adenine dinucleotide phosphate-oxidase; all enzymes involved in producing the damaging neutrophilic oxidative burst

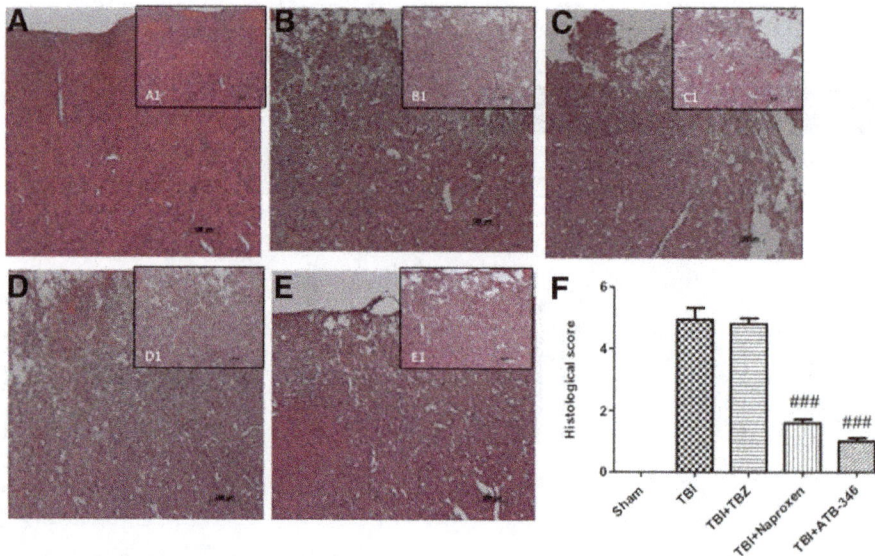

Figure 7 Histological examination of brain sections after 24 hours. Brain sections from TBI mice and TBZ-treated mice (**B** and **C** respectively, see densitometry analysis **F**) demonstrated brain tissue injury and inflammatory cell infiltration. Naproxen treatment did not attenuate completely the development of acute brain injury at one and six hours after TBI (**D**, see densitometry analysis **F**). On the contrary, ATB-346 treatment reduced the degree of brain injury and the inflammatory cells infiltration (**E**, see densitometry analysis **F**). Figure is representative of at least three experiments performed on different experimental days. ###P <0.001 versus TBI.

[32]. To confirm the pathological contributions to brain inflammation, we have demonstrated here expression of COX-2 and iNOS in the injured tissue after TBI, but TBI-induced iNOS and COX-2 expression are significantly lower in injured brains from ATB-346-treated mice.

Post-TBI there is increased infiltration of neutrophils, astrocytosis, edema and both pro- and anti-inflammatory cytokines release. The major pro-inflammatory cytokines released are IL-1β, IL-6 and TNFα. The anti-inflammatory cytokines are IL-10 and transforming growth factor beta. We demonstrate that increased microglial and astrocyte activation is present 24 hours after TBI. Moreover, immunofluorescence staining showed increased TNFα and IL-1β expression in astrocytes and microglia in TBI group. ATB-346 treatment importantly reduced TNFα and IL-1β expression in these glial cells. Apparently, ATB-346 might enhance actual functional neuronal regeneration via inhibiting glial scar formation during TBI.

Neurotrophic factors have well-established roles in survival, differentiation and function of CNS neurons. Exogenous *NGF*, for example, plays a critical role in neuronal plasticity and regenerative potential, as well as the inhibition of neural apoptosis after TBI [33,34]. A study found brain-derived neurotrophic factor,(BDNF) and neurotrophin-3 (NT-3) support the survival of injured CNS neurons *in vitro* and *in vivo*, induce neurite outgrowth and increase the expression of key enzymes for neurotransmitter synthesis [35]. *GDNF* is capable of protecting against hippocampal neuronal death [36],

attenuating brain swelling and reducing the lesion volume [37] after TBI. Our results visibly showed restored *GDNF* and *NGF* levels after ATB-346 treatment, maintaining their protective action.

VEGF, an angiogenic growth and survival factor for endothelial cells that also exhibits neurotrophic and neuroprotective effects, has been implicated in neovascularization that precedes brain tissue repair and nerve regeneration following brain injury and is required to re-establish metabolic support [38]. *VEGF* is upregulated during many pathological events, and it is induced in astrocytes located in and surrounding edematous tissue following brain contusion [39]. Our study showed that ATB-346 significantly increased *VEGF* levels. Thus, it could be hypothesized that ATB-346-facilitated the increase in *VEGF* expression in the lesion area, resulting in the secretion of *VEGF* from synthesizing cells and the restoration of the neurovascular unit.

•NO is a key regulator of cerebral circulation by its contribution to basal vascular tone that in vasculature is mainly derived from eNOS. eNOS is predominantly expressed by vessels endothelial cells and are also located in Purkinje cell bodies in the cerebellar cortex, olfactory bulb, dentate nucleus in granular layer and hippocampal pyramidal cells and astrocytes surrounding the cerebral blood vessels [40]. A recent paper showed that eNOS is central after trauma for the maintenance of blood flow in the injured cortex for at least 24 hours after TBI; this is based on the observation that eNOS knockout mice have lower cerebral blood flow at that

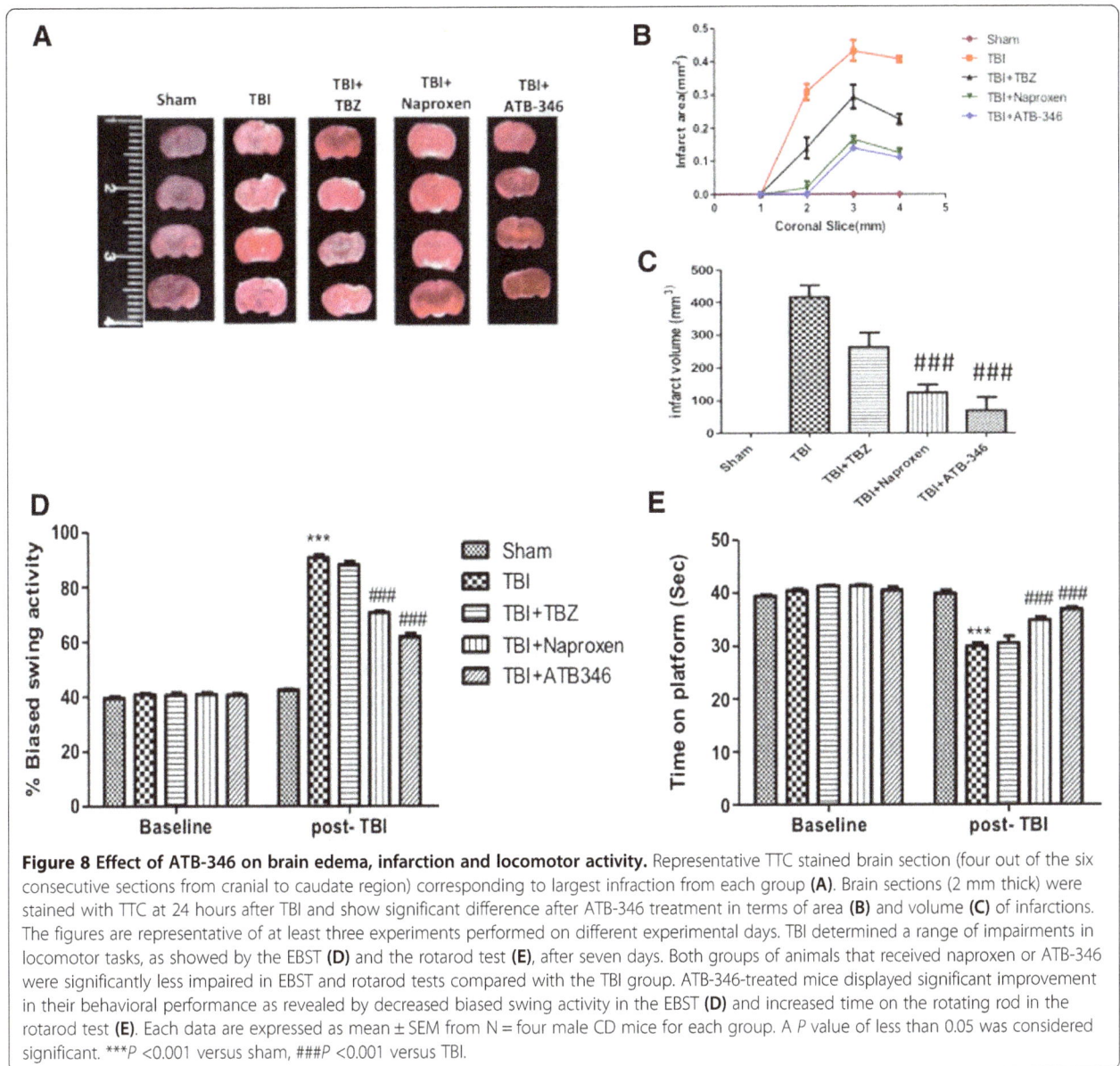

Figure 8 Effect of ATB-346 on brain edema, infarction and locomotor activity. Representative TTC stained brain section (four out of the six consecutive sections from cranial to caudate region) corresponding to largest infraction from each group **(A)**. Brain sections (2 mm thick) were stained with TTC at 24 hours after TBI and show significant difference after ATB-346 treatment in terms of area **(B)** and volume **(C)** of infarctions. The figures are representative of at least three experiments performed on different experimental days. TBI determined a range of impairments in locomotor tasks, as showed by the EBST **(D)** and the rotarod test **(E)**, after seven days. Both groups of animals that received naproxen or ATB-346 were significantly less impaired in EBST and rotarod tests compared with the TBI group. ATB-346-treated mice displayed significant improvement in their behavioral performance as revealed by decreased biased swing activity in the EBST **(D)** and increased time on the rotating rod in the rotarod test **(E)**. Each data are expressed as mean ± SEM from N = four male CD mice for each group. A P value of less than 0.05 was considered significant. ***$P < 0.001$ versus sham, ###$P < 0.001$ versus TBI.

time point compared to wild-type mice [41]. According to this data, our results showed an evident increase in eNOS expression 24 hours after TBI. The increase in eNOS protein may represent either a protective or a reparative response, since it has been reported that eNOS is necessary to counteract posttraumatic cerebral hypoperfusion at 24 hours after CCI-TBI in mice [42]. There is substantial evidence that H$_2$S upregulates •NO production in endothelial cells through the activation of eNOS, inducing angiogenesis and improving functional outcome [43-45]. Therefore, ATB 346 upregulates its expression, increasing functional protein expression and augmentation of cerebral blood flow, also in the brain. Furthermore, treatment with ATB-346 results in a significant reduction in inflammation and it is also accompanied by a detectable

histological improvement of TBI. As shown in our recent paper, ATB-346 can markedly accelerate recovery of motor function in mice subjected to SCI [12]. Here, in a different model of neurotrauma, we confirmed that ATB-346 significantly improved the latency compared to the naproxen group, indicated as a mediator of the mechanism to promote recovery and to enhance the repair mechanism. In the present study, post-TBI administration of ATB-346 not only facilitated functional recovery, but also reduced tissue damage within hours following injection. The ameliorating effect of ATB-346 at tissue level was further corroborated by its ability to reduce the extent of neurodegeneration. The neuroprotective basis for these actions seems to be dependent on the H$_2$S-releasing moiety of ATB-346, as also stated in a recent paper [46].

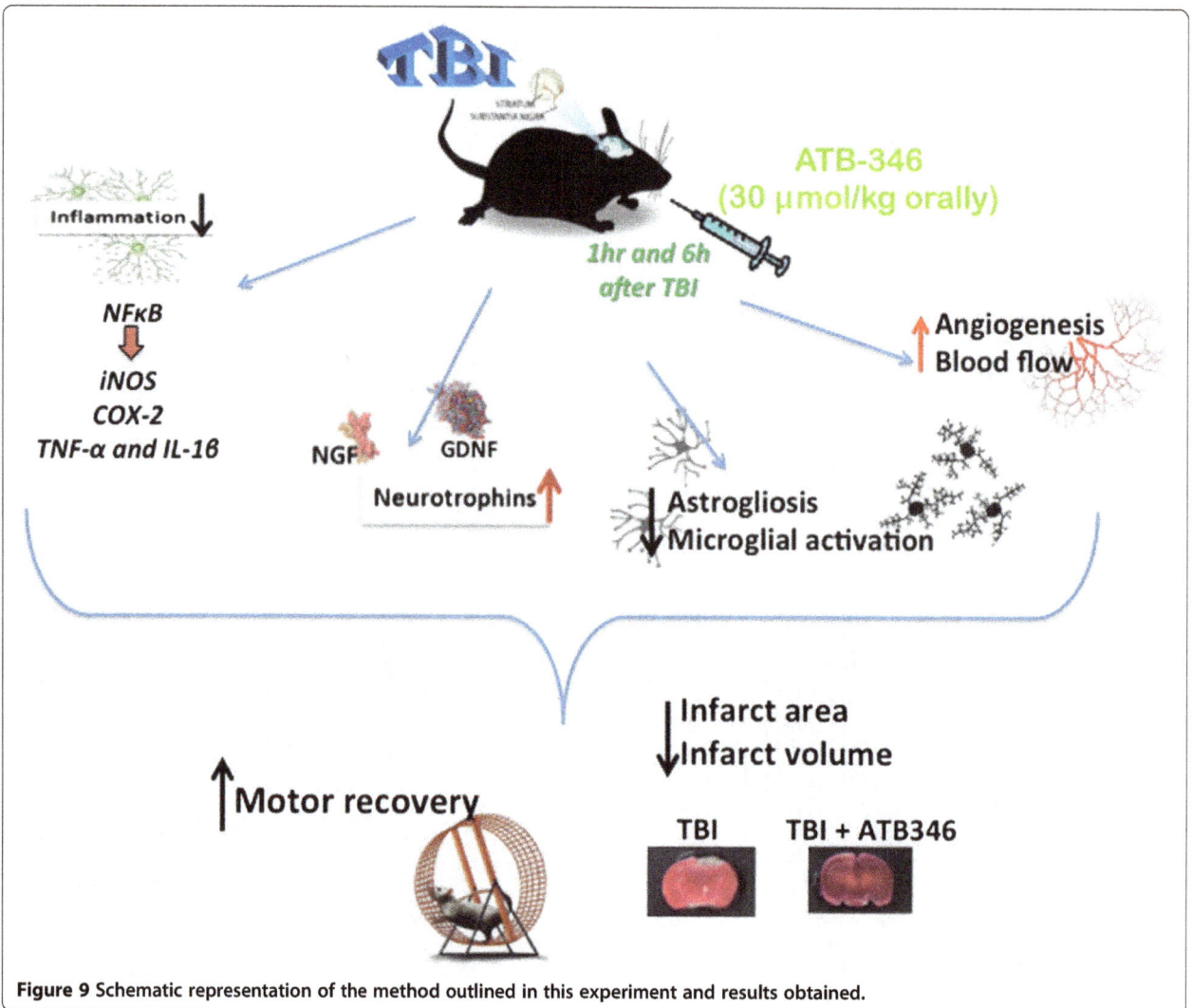

Figure 9 Schematic representation of the method outlined in this experiment and results obtained.

Moreover, the observation that neither naproxen nor TBZ produce the same 'restorative' effect on neurotrophic factors as seen with ATB-346 suggests that both suppression of COX and delivery of H^2S is required to achieve the observed effect. The properties of this compound are summarized in Figure 9. In May 2014 Antibe Therapeutics has announced the submission of a clinical trial application to Health Canada for ATB-346.

Conclusions

The need for developing new therapeutics for TBI treatment and the current lack of specific therapy for this indication underscore the importance of identification and characterization of novel neuroprotective compounds. Released-H_2S may account for the absence of deleterious gastric effects, thus making of ATB-346 a potentially useful therapeutic alternative to traditional naproxen for the management of secondary damage following CNS diseases, counteracting behavioral changes and inflammatory process.

Abbreviations
CCI: Controlled cortical impact; COX: Cyclooxygenase; EBST: Elevated Biased Swing Test; TBZ: 4-hydroxythiobenzamide; DMSO: dimethyl sulfoxide; dNTP: deoxynucleotide triphosphates; EGTA: ethylene glycol tetraacetic acid; EDTA: ethylenediaminetetraacetic acid; iNOS: inducible nitric oxide synthase; NSAIDs: Non-steroidal anti-inflammatory drugs; IL-1β: interleukin 1β; Iba1: ionized calcium binding adaptor molecule 1; TNFα: tumor necrosis factor α; GFAP: glial fibrillary acidic protein; NFκB: Nuclear factor κB.

Competing interests
The authors declare that they have no competing interests.

Authors' contributions
MC and EE performed experiments and prepared the manuscript. AA, RD, RS, MC and GB performed experiments and the biochemical analysis. JLW and SC planned the study, analyzed the results and prepared the manuscript. All authors read and approved the final manuscript.

Acknowledgements

The authors would like to thank Mrs Maria Antonietta Medici for her excellent technical assistance during this study, Mr Francesco Soraci and Mr Giuseppe Mancuso for their secretarial and administrative assistance and Miss Valentina Malvagni for her editorial assistance with the manuscript.

Author details

[1]Department of Biological and Environmental Sciences, University of Messina, Viale Ferdinando Stagno D'Alcontres, 31-98166 Messina, Italy. [2]Inflammation Research Network, University of Calgary, 3330 Hospital Drive NW, Calgary, Alberta T2N 4 N1, Canada. [3]Manchester Biomedical Research Centre, Manchester Royal Infirmary, School of Medicine, University of Manchester, 29 Grafton Street Manchester, M13 9WU Manchester, UK.

References

1. Corrigan JD, Selassie AW, Orman JA: The epidemiology of traumatic brain injury. *J Head Trauma Rehabil* 2010, **25**:72–80.
2. Rosenfeld JV, Maas AI, Bragge P, Morganti-Kossmann MC, Manley GT, Gruen RL: Early management of severe traumatic brain injury. *Lancet* 2012, **380**:1088–1098.
3. Cernak I, Vink R, Zapple DN, Cruz MI, Ahmed F, Chang T, Fricke ST, Faden AI: The pathobiology of moderate diffuse traumatic brain injury as identified using a new experimental model of injury in rats. *Neurobiol Dis* 2004, **17**:29–43.
4. Anisimova IE, Salomatin EM, Pleteneva TV, Popov PI: Toxicity of non-steroid anti-inflammatory drugs. *Sud Med Ekspert* 2004, **47**:37–41.
5. Geng B, Yang J, Qi Y, Zhao J, Pang Y, Du J, Tang C: H2S generated by heart in rat and its effects on cardiac function. *Biochem Biophys Res Commun* 2004, **313**:362–368.
6. Zhao W, Zhang J, Lu Y, Wang R: The vasorelaxant effect of H(2)S as a novel endogenous gaseous K(ATP) channel opener. *EMBO J* 2001, **20**:6008–6016.
7. Warenycia MW, Goodwin LR, Benishin CG, Reiffenstein RJ, Francom DM, Taylor JD, Dieken FP: Acute hydrogen sulfide poisoning. Demonstration of selective uptake of sulfide by the brainstem by measurement of brain sulfide levels. *Biochem Pharmacol* 1989, **38**:973–981.
8. Kimura H: Hydrogen sulfide as a biological mediator. *Antioxid Redox Signal* 2005, **7**:778–780.
9. Kimura H, Shibuya N, Kimura Y: Hydrogen sulfide is a signaling molecule and a cytoprotectant. *Antioxid Redox Signal* 2012, **17**:45–57.
10. Wallace JL: Hydrogen sulfide-releasing anti-inflammatory drugs. *Trends Pharmacol Sci* 2007, **28**:501–505.
11. Morgan K, Stevens EB, Shah B, Cox PJ, Dixon AK, Lee K, Pinnock RD, Hughes J, Richardson PJ, Mizuguchi K, Jackson AP: Beta 3: an additional auxiliary subunit of the voltage-sensitive sodium channel that modulates channel gating with distinct kinetics. *Proc Natl Acad Sci U S A* 2000, **97**:2308–2313.
12. Campolo M, Esposito E, Ahmad A, Di Paola R, Wallace JL, Cuzzocrea S: A hydrogen sulfide-releasing cyclooxygenase inhibitor markedly accelerates recovery from experimental spinal cord injury. *FASEB J* 2013, **27**:4489–4499.
13. Wallace JL, Caliendo G, Santagada V, Cirino G: Markedly reduced toxicity of a hydrogen sulphide-releasing derivative of naproxen (ATB-346). *Br J Pharmacol* 2010, **159**:1236–1246.
14. Salloway S, Sperling R, Gilman S, Fox NC, Blennow K, Raskind M, Sabbagh M, Honig LS, Doody R, Van Dyck CH, Mulnard R, Barakos J, Gregg KM, Liu E, Lieberburg I, Schenk D, Black R, Grundman M, Bapineuzumab 201 Clinical Trial Investigators: A phase 2 multiple ascending dose trial of bapineuzumab in mild to moderate Alzheimer disease. *Neurology* 2009, **73**:2061–2070.
15. Sullivan PG, Sebastian AH, Hall ED: Therapeutic window analysis of the neuroprotective effects of cyclosporine A after traumatic brain injury. *J Neurotrauma* 2011, **28**:311–318.
16. Bederson JB, Pitts LH, Germano SM, Nishimura MC, Davis RL, Bartkowski HM: Evaluation of 2,3,5-triphenyltetrazolium chloride as a stain for detection and quantification of experimental cerebral infarction in rats. *Stroke* 1986, **17**:1304–1308.
17. Schomacher M, Muller HD, Sommer C, Schwab S, Schabitz WR: Endocannabinoids mediate neuroprotection after transient focal cerebral ischemia. *Brain Res* 2008, **1240**:213–220.
18. Schabitz WR, Sommer C, Zoder W, Kiessling M, Schwaninger M, Schwab S: Intravenous brain-derived neurotrophic factor reduces infarct size and counterregulates Bax and Bcl-2 expression after temporary focal cerebral ischemia. *Stroke* 2000, **31**:2212–2217.
19. Kawai T, Akira S: Signaling to NF-kappaB by Toll-like receptors. *Trends Mol Med* 2007, **13**:460–469.
20. Bethea JR, Castro M, Keane RW, Lee TT, Dietrich WD, Yezierski RP: Traumatic spinal cord injury induces nuclear factor-kappaB activation. *J Neurosci* 1998, **18**:3251–3260.
21. Chomczynski P, Sacchi N: Single-step method of RNA isolation by acid guanidinium thiocyanate-phenol-chloroform extraction. *Anal Biochem* 1987, **162**:156–159.
22. Morales DM, Marklund N, Lebold D, Thompson HJ, Pitkanen A, Maxwell WL, Longhi L, Laurer H, Maegele M, Neugebauer E, Graham DI, Stocchetti N, McIntosh TK: Experimental models of traumatic brain injury: do we really need to build a better mousetrap? *Neuroscience* 2005, **136**:971–989.
23. Kimura Y, Kimura H: Hydrogen sulfide protects neurons from oxidative stress. *FASEB J* 2004, **18**:1165–1167.
24. Zanardo RC, Brancaleone V, Distrutti E, Fiorucci S, Cirino G, Wallace JL: Hydrogen sulfide is an endogenous modulator of leukocyte-mediated inflammation. *FASEB J* 2006, **20**:2118–2120.
25. Wallace JL, Caliendo G, Santagada V, Cirino G, Fiorucci S: Gastrointestinal safety and anti-inflammatory effects of a hydrogen sulfide-releasing diclofenac derivative in the rat. *Gastroenterology* 2007, **132**:261–271.
26. Li L, Salto-Tellez M, Tan CH, Whiteman M, Moore PK: GYY4137, a novel hydrogen sulfide-releasing molecule, protects against endotoxic shock in the rat. *Free Radic Biol Med* 2009, **47**:103–113.
27. Polhemus DJ, Lefer DJ: Emergence of hydrogen sulfide as an endogenous gaseous signaling molecule in cardiovascular disease. *Circ Res* 2014, **114**:730–737.
28. Kimura H: Hydrogen sulfide as a neuromodulator. *Mol Neurobiol* 2002, **26**:13–19.
29. Blackler R, Syer S, Bolla M, Ongini E, Wallace JL: Gastrointestinal-sparing effects of novel NSAIDs in rats with compromised mucosal defence. *PLoS One* 2012, **7**:e35196.
30. Wallace JL, Blackler RW, Chan MV, Da Silva GJ, Elsheikh W, Flannigan KL, Gamaniek I, Manko A, Wang L, Motta JP, Buret AG: Anti-inflammatory and cytoprotective actions of hydrogen sulfide: translation to therapeutics. *Antioxid Redox Signal* 2014.
31. Rhodes J: Peripheral immune cells in the pathology of traumatic brain injury? *Curr Opin Crit Care* 2011, **17**:122–130.
32. Liao Y, Liu P, Guo F, Zhang ZY, Zhang Z: Oxidative burst of circulating neutrophils following traumatic brain injury in human. *PLoS One* 2013, **8**:e68963.
33. DeKosky ST, Goss JR, Miller PD, Styren SD, Kochanek PM, Marion D: Upregulation of nerve growth factor following cortical trauma. *Exp Neurol* 1994, **130**:173–177.
34. Goss JR, O'Malley ME, Zou L, Styren SD, Kochanek PM, DeKosky ST: Astrocytes are the major source of nerve growth factor upregulation following traumatic brain injury in the rat. *Exp Neurol* 1998, **149**:301–309.
35. Mocchetti I, Wrathall JR: Neurotrophic factors in central nervous system trauma. *J Neurotrauma* 1995, **12**:853–870.
36. Kim BT, Rao VL, Sailor KA, Bowen KK, Dempsey RJ: Protective effects of glial cell line-derived neurotrophic factor on hippocampal neurons after traumatic brain injury in rats. *J Neurosurg* 2001, **95**:674–679.
37. Hermann DM, Kilic E, Kugler S, Isenmann S, Bahr M: Adenovirus-mediated glial cell line-derived neurotrophic factor (GDNF) expression protects against subsequent cortical cold injury in rats. *Neurobiol Dis* 2001, **8**:964–973.
38. Shore PM, Jackson EK, Wisniewski SR, Clark RS, Adelson PD, Kochanek PM: Vascular endothelial growth factor is increased in cerebrospinal fluid after traumatic brain injury in infants and children. *Neurosurgery* 2004, **54**:605–611. discussion 611–602.
39. Pedersen MO, Larsen A, Pedersen DS, Stoltenberg M, Penkova M: Metallic gold treatment reduces proliferation of inflammatory cells, increases expression of VEGF and FGF, and stimulates cell proliferation in the subventricular zone following experimental traumatic brain injury. *Histol Histopathol* 2009, **24**:573–586.
40. Cui X, Chopp M, Zacharek A, Ning R, Ding X, Roberts C, Chen J: Endothelial nitric oxide synthase regulates white matter changes via the BDNF/TrkB pathway after stroke in mice. *PLoS One* 2013, **8**:e80358.

41. Lundblad C, Grande PO, Bentzer P: **Hemodynamic and histological effects of traumatic brain injury in eNOS-deficient mice.** *J Neurotrauma* 2009, **26:**1953–1962.

42. Hall ED, Wang JA, Miller DM: **Relationship of nitric oxide synthase induction to peroxynitrite-mediated oxidative damage during the first week after experimental traumatic brain injury.** *Exp Neurol* 2012, **238:**176–182.

43. Kondo K, Bhushan S, King AL, Prabhu SD, Hamid T, Koenig S, Murohara T, Predmore BL, Gojon G Sr, Gojon G Jr, Wang R, Karusula N, Nicholson CK, Calvert JW, Lefer DJ: **H(2)S protects against pressure overload-induced heart failure via upregulation of endothelial nitric oxide synthase.** *Circulation* 2013, **127:**1116–1127.

44. Kram L, Grambow E, Mueller-Graf F, Sorg H, Vollmar B: **The anti-thrombotic effect of hydrogen sulfide is partly mediated by an upregulation of nitric oxide synthases.** *Thromb Res* 2013, **132:**e112–e117.

45. Altaany Z, Yang G, Wang R: **Crosstalk between hydrogen sulfide and nitric oxide in endothelial cells.** *J Cell Mol Med* 2013, **17:**879–888.

46. Kamat PK, Kalani A, Givvimani S, Sathnur PB, Tyagi SC, Tyagi N: **Hydrogen sulfide attenuates neurodegeneration and neurovascular dysfunction induced by intracerebral-administered homocysteine in mice.** *Neuroscience* 2013, **252:**302–319.

11

Traumatic brain injury enhances neuroinflammation and lesion volume in caveolin deficient mice

Ingrid R Niesman[1,2], Jan M Schilling[1,2], Lee A Shapiro[3,4], Sarah E Kellerhals[1,2], Jacqueline A Bonds[1,2], Alexander M Kleschevnikov[5], Weihua Cui[1,2,7], April Voong[1,2], Stan Krajewski[6], Sameh S Ali[1,2,8], David M Roth[1,2], Hemal H Patel[1,2], Piyush M Patel[1,2] and Brian P Head[1,2]*

Abstract

Background: Traumatic brain injury (TBI) enhances pro-inflammatory responses, neuronal loss and long-term behavioral deficits. Caveolins (Cavs) are regulators of neuronal and glial survival signaling. Previously we showed that astrocyte and microglial activation is increased in Cav-1 knock-out (KO) mice and that Cav-1 and Cav-3 modulate microglial morphology. We hypothesized that Cavs may regulate cytokine production after TBI.

Methods: Controlled cortical impact (CCI) model of TBI (3 m/second; 1.0 mm depth; parietal cortex) was performed on wild-type (WT; C57Bl/6), Cav-1 KO, and Cav-3 KO mice. Histology and immunofluorescence microscopy (lesion volume, glia activation), behavioral tests (open field, balance beam, wire grip, T-maze), electrophysiology, electron paramagnetic resonance, membrane fractionation, and multiplex assays were performed. Data were analyzed by unpaired t tests or analysis of variance (ANOVA) with *post-hoc* Bonferroni's multiple comparison.

Results: CCI increased cortical and hippocampal injury and decreased expression of MLR-localized synaptic proteins (24 hours), enhanced NADPH oxidase (Nox) activity (24 hours and 1 week), enhanced polysynaptic responses (1 week), and caused hippocampal-dependent learning deficits (3 months). CCI increased brain lesion volume in both Cav-3 and Cav-1 KO mice after 24 hours ($P < 0.0001$, n = 4; one-way ANOVA). Multiplex array revealed a significant increase in expression of IL-1β, IL-9, IL-10, KC (keratinocyte chemoattractant), and monocyte chemoattractant protein 1 (MCP-1) in ipsilateral hemisphere and IL-9, IL-10, IL-17, and macrophage inflammatory protein 1 alpha (MIP-1α) in contralateral hemisphere of WT mice after 4 hours. CCI increased IL-2, IL-6, KC and MCP-1 in ipsilateral and IL-6, IL-9, IL-17 and KC in contralateral hemispheres in Cav-1 KO and increased all 10 cytokines/chemokines in both hemispheres except for IL-17 (ipsilateral) and MIP-1α (contralateral) in Cav-3 KO (versus WT CCI). Cav-3 KO CCI showed increased IL-1β, IL-9, KC, MCP-1, MIP-1α, and granulocyte-macrophage colony-stimulating factor in ipsilateral and IL-1β, IL-2, IL-9, IL-10, and IL-17 in contralateral hemispheres ($P = 0.0005$, n = 6; two-way ANOVA) compared to Cav-1 KO CCI.

Conclusion: CCI caused astrocyte and microglial activation and hippocampal neuronal injury. Cav-1 and Cav-3 KO exhibited enhanced lesion volume and cytokine/chemokine production after CCI. These findings suggest that Cav isoforms may regulate neuroinflammatory responses and neuroprotection following TBI.

* Correspondence: bhead@ucsd.edu
[1]Veterans Affairs San Diego Healthcare System, 3350 La Jolla Village Drive, San Diego, CA 92161, USA
[2]Department of Anesthesiology, University of California, San Diego, La Jolla, CA 92093, USA
Full list of author information is available at the end of the article

Background

Traumatic brain injury (TBI) is the leading cause of morbidity and mortality among young people in the Western world. Patients with TBI sustain long-term neurological, cognitive and behavioral deficits leading to a greater requirement for institutional and long-term care. Despite intensive investigative efforts, there is a paucity of interventions designed to reduce morbidity and mortality associated with TBI [1].

Immediately following TBI, there is a substantial excess release of neurotransmitters such as glutamate and signaling nucleotides such as adenosine. Excessive glutamate leads to hyperactivation of N-methyl-D-aspartate receptor (NMDAR) and subsequent excitotoxic neuronal injury. Recent data indicate that hyperactivation of glutamate receptors is short lived (< 1 hour), and there is a substantial reduction in NMDAR expression and signaling within 48 hours of injury [2,3]. Signaling pathways and molecules that are normally associated with neuronal survival (such as BDNF, TrkR, Src, ERK, cAMP and CREB) are reduced for several weeks following TBI [2,4,5]. In addition to glutamate release and neuronal loss, TBI can also produce astro- and microgliosis and enhance the production of proinflammatory cytokines [6-9]. This increased cytokine production can result in alterations in synaptic connections that can lead to additional neuronal loss. The latter effect can contribute to post-traumatic epilepsy (PTE) and long-term behavioral dysfunction with few therapies readily available [10-13].

Membrane/lipid rafts (MLRs) are discrete regions of the plasma membrane enriched in cholesterol, glycosphingolipids and sphingomyelin, and the cholesterol binding and scaffolding protein caveolin (Cav). Three isoforms exist, with Cav-1 and Cav-2 usually co-expressed in a wide variety of tissues, while Cav-3 is canonically expressed in striated muscle [14]. All three isoforms have been described in the central nervous system (CNS) [15-17]. Cav-1 participates in the inflammatory response to the endotoxin lipopolysaccharide through toll-like receptor 4 (TLR4) and through negative regulation of endothelial nitric oxide synthase (eNOS) [18]. Cav-3, normally associated with striated muscles, is not well studied in the CNS. We have recently shown that astrogliosis and microgliosis is increased in the brains of young Cav-1 knock-out (KO) mice [19], and that Cav-1 and Cav-3 modulate microglia morphology [20]. It is therefore conceivable that Cav-1 and Cav-3 might play an important role in the neuroinflammatory response in the brain following controlled cortical impact (CCI). To address this hypothesis, we first performed a variety of assays on wild-type (WT) mice with and without CCI (that is, histological, biochemical, electrophysiological, and by electron paramagnetic resonance (EPR)) to demonstrate establishment of the TBI model. We next conducted CCI and measured the neuroinflammatory response in the brains of WT, Cav-1 KO and Cav-3 KO mice subjected to CCI.

Materials and methods

Animal care

All animals were treated in compliance with the Guide for the Care and Use of Laboratory Animals (National Academy of Science, Washington, DC, USA). All animal-use protocols were approved by the Veterans Administration San Diego Healthcare System Institutional Animal Care and Use Committee (IACUC, San Diego, California, USA) prior to performed procedures. C57BL/6 WT and Cav-1 KO mice were purchased from Jackson Laboratories (Bar Harbor, ME, USA) and Cav-3 KO mice were a kind gift from Drs Ishikawa (Professor, Cardiovascular Research Institute, Yokohama City University School of Medicine, Yokohama, Japan) and Hagiwara (Professor, National Institute of Neuroscience, Kodaira, Tokyo, Japan) [21].

Reagents

The following primary antibodies were used for Western blot (WB) and immunofluorescence microscopy (IF) analysis: Abcam (1 Kendall Square, Suite B2304, Cambridge, MA 02139-1517, USA) - $A_{2A}AR$ #ab79714, β_3-tubulin #ab11314, Cav-3 #ab2912, MAP2 #ab32454; BD Transduction Labs (2350 Qume Drive, San Jose, CA 95131, USA) - NR2B #610417, TrkB #610102; Cell Signaling (3 Trask Lane, Danvers, MA, 01923, USA) - AMPAR #2460 s, Cav-1 #3267, NR1 #4204, NR2A #4205, PSD-95 #2507; Epitomics (863 Mitten Road, Suite 103, Burlingame, CA, 94010-1303, USA) - LDLR #1956-1, LRP-1 #2703-1; Imgenex (11175 Flintkote Ave, Suite E, San Diego, CA, 92121, USA) - GAPDH #IMG-5019A-1; Millipore (290 Concord Road, Billerica, MA, 01821, USA) - GFAP AB5541; Santa Cruz (10410 Finnell Street, Dallas, TX, 75220, USA) - A_1AR sc-28995, A_3AR sc-12938, TLR4 sc-30002, goat anti-mouse IgG-HRP sc-2031, goat anti-rabbit IgG-HRP, sc-2030 goat anti-rat IgG-HRP sc-2006; Stressgen (4243 Glanford Avenue, Victoria, BC, Canada) - HSP90 #SPA835; WAKO (1-2 Doshomachi 3-Chome, Chuo-Ku, Osaka, 540-8605, Japan) - Iba1 WB #016-20001, IF #019-19741; Molecular Probes (3175 Staley Road, Grand Island, NY, 14072, USA) - goat anti-rabbit-488 IgG (H + L) #A11008, goat anti-mouse-594 IgG (H + L) #A11005.

Controlled cortical impact model of traumatic brain injury

CCI was performed as described previously [22]. Briefly, isoflurane (2% vol/vol) anesthetized mice were fixed into a stereotactic frame, maintaining basal temperature (37°C) throughout the procedure. A burr hole was made approximately 5 mm anterior to posterior (0 to –5 A-P) from the bregmatic suture and 4 mm laterally from the sagittal suture over the right hemisphere. Craniotomies were made with a portable drill over the right parietotemporal cortex and the bone flap was removed. Using a stereotaxic impactor (Impact One™; myNeuoLab.com), a 3-mm tip was accelerated down to a 1 mm depth at a speed of 3 m/second with an 85 ms dwell time.

Histology (n = 4/group) and immunofluorescence (n = 3/group)

For histology, animals were transcardially perfused with 4% paraformaldehyde in 0.1 M PO_4 buffer then stored in the same buffer for 24 hours and processed for paraffin embedding. Serial sections through the hippocampus (two 5-μm sections per slide, 100 μm apart) were stained with Masson's trichrome. Digital virtual slides obtained with Aperio Scanscope CS-1 scanner were used for extensive computer assisted morphometry in a Spectrum image analysis system (Aperio Technology Inc., 1700 Leider Lane, Buffalo Grove, IL, 60089, USA). Scanscope software and associated algorithms were applied for measurements of lesion volume and the count of dead or viable neurons in the impact zone, penumbra and relevant area of the contralateral hemisphere control (internal control) as described by Krajewska and colleagues [23]. Whole brains were perfused with 4% paraformaldehyde, cryoprotected with 30% sucrose and frozen for cryostat sectioning in optimal cutting temperature embedding media. Free floating sections (50 μm) were washed in phosphate-buffered saline, blocked and incubated overnight with primary antibodies followed by species-specific secondary antibodies. Species-specific fluroconjugated Alexa® (3175 Staley Road, Grand Island, NY, 14072, USA) secondary antibodies were used at a 1:500 dilution with DAPI in 10% goat blocking solution. Sections were incubated for 1 to 2 hours at room temperature, gently rotating. We have previously characterized and optimized our immunofluorescence protocols for GFAP (glial fibrillary acidic protein), Iba1 (ionized calcium-binding adapter molecule 1) and MAP2 (microtubule associated protein 2) as previously described [19,20,24,25]. Incubation with 10% goat and no primary antibodies, with and without secondary antibodies, served as controls samples for these experiments. Coverslips or brain sections were mounted with an anti-fade solution and imaged; when appropriate, matched exposures were obtained. All other images were exposure and saturation optimized. All quantitation was done using NIH Image J.

Cognitive and motor tests (n = 20/group)

Male mice (2 to 3 months old) were subjected to CCI and monitored for an additional 3 months followed by a behavioral battery. Open field activity allows assessment of basic activity and general behavior/anxiety of the mouse. Locomotion was recorded and analyzed by a computerized video tracking system (Noldus XT 7.1, 1503 Edwards Ferry Road, Suite 310, Leesburg, VA, 201276, USA). Animals were habituated to the testing room; spontaneous locomotion was assessed in a white plexiglass open field box (41 × 41 × 34 cm enclosures) for 10 minutes. Recorded parameters were distance moved (cm), velocity (cm/second), and time spent in the center of the arena represented by 50% of the total arena (seconds). The wire grip test tests the ability of mice to hang on a metal rail [26]. The metal wire is situated 40 cm from the ground and a soft surface is placed below the wire to prevent physical trauma to the mice. Latency to fall was timed and the test was repeated three times with an inter-trial interval of 30 seconds. The highest latency to fall was multiplied with the body weight to present the holding impulse (seconds × g). In the beam-walking test, mice traverse an elevated narrow beam to reach a platform. The protocol described here measures foot slips while crossing the beam. The apparatus was custom made according to a published protocol of Carter and colleagues [27] with the height of the apparatus set at 50 cm. Continuous alternating T-maze test was used to assess the cognitive ability of the CCI mice; this enclosed apparatus is in the form of a T placed horizontally. Animals are started from the base of the T and allowed to choose one of the goal arms abutting the other end of the stem. Two trials are given in quick succession; on the second trial the rodent tends to choose the arm not visited before, reflecting memory of the first choice, termed as 'spontaneous alternation'. We assessed this tendency in a test with 14 possible alternations according to plans and a protocol from a previously published method [28,29].

Electrophysiology (n = 4/group)

Transverse hippocampal slices were prepared as previously described [30]. Mice were anesthetized with isoflurane before decapitation. The brain was quickly removed and immersed for 2 minutes in ice-cold artificial cerebrospinal fluid (ACSF) containing 119 mM NaCl, 2.5 mM KCl, 2.5 mM $CaCl_2$, 1.3 mM $MgSO_4$, 1 mM NaH_2PO_4, 26 mM $NaHCO_3$, 10 mM glucose, osmolarity 310 mOsm, continuously bubbled with carbogen (95% O_2-5% CO_2), pH 7.4. The hippocampus was extracted and cut in ice cold ACSF with a vibratome (Leica 1000, 1700 Leider Lane, Buffalo Grove, IL, 60089, USA) into 350 μm slices, which were allowed to recover in oxygenated ACSF at 35°C for 30 minutes, and then at room temperature for at least 1 hour prior to experimental recordings.

A slice was transferred into the submerged recording chamber and superfused with ACSF at a constant rate of 1.0 ml/minute at 32°C. To prevent de-oxygenation of ACSF in the recording chamber, the surface was continuously blown over by carbogen warmed to 32°C. Recording electrodes were made of borosilicate glass capillaries

(1B150F, World Precision Instruments, Sarasota, FL, USA) and filled with ACSF (resistance 0.3 to 0.5 MΩ). Monopolar stimulating electrodes were made of Pt/Ir wires of diameter 25.4 µm (PTT0110, World Precision Instruments) and had 100 µm long exposed tips. The stimulating and recording electrodes were inserted under visual control perpendicular to the slice surface into the CA1 stratum radiatum 80 to 100 µm from the pyramidal layer, at a distance of 300 to 350 µm apart from each other. The magnitude of monosynaptic responses was evaluated as initial slope of field excitatory postsynaptic potential at latencies 0.1 to 0.9 ms, and the magnitude of polysynaptic responses as the averaged amplitude at latencies 12 to 45 ms after the stimulus. Testing stimuli (duration 100 µs, currents 60 to 80 µA) evoked field responses with amplitudes of 70 to 80% of maximum. Long-term potentiation was induced by tetanizations consisting of a single train of stimuli: 1 second at 100 Hz.

Superoxide measurements in synaptosomes by electron paramagnetic resonance (n = 3/group)

Brain NADPH oxidase (Nox) activity was assayed by detecting superoxide radical in synaptosomal isolations using EPR spin trapping spectroscopy according to a previously published protocol [31]. Synaptosomal protein (0.2 to 0.5 mg) was mixed with 70 mM 5-(diethylphosphoryl)-5-methyl-1-pyrroline-N-oxide (Axxora, San Diego, CA, USA) and combinations of the substrates/inhibitors was loaded into a 50 µl glass capillary and introduced into the EPR cavity of a MiniScope MS300 Benchtop spectrometer (Louis-Bleriot-Str. 5, D-12487, Berlin, Germany) at a constant temperature of 37°C. Time evolution of the EPR spectra was recorded over 11 minutes from triggering Nox activity by adding appropriate combinations of substrates. For correlative analysis, the signals were quantified over the acquisition time of approximately 6 minutes (that is, the area under oxidative burst curves and normalized by the protein concentration). EPR conditions were as follows: microwave power, 5 mW; modulation amplitude, 2 G; modulation frequency, 100 kHz; MW frequency, 9.49 kHz; sweep width, 150 G centered at 3349.0 G; scan rate, 7.5 G/s and each spectrum was the average of 2 scans.

Cell culture

Primary cells were isolated using a Papain dissociation kit (#3150; Worthington Chemicals, Lakewood, NJ, USA) as previously described [20,24,25]. Cultures were obtained from post-natal day 3 mouse pups. Mixed glia were separated from neurons according to manufacturer's instructions and grown to confluence in T-75 flasks in Dulbecco's modified Eagle's medium with 10% fetal bovine serum.

Sucrose density fractionation and Western blot (n = 4/group)

Mouse cortex (50 to 100 mg) was homogenized using a carbonate lysis buffer (500 mM sodium carbonate, pH 11.0) containing protease and phosphatase inhibitors. Lysates were sonicated (three cycles for 15 seconds on ice). Protein was quantified by Bradford assay and normalized to 1 mg/ml. Sucrose was dissolved in MES buffered saline (25 mM MES (2-(N-morpholino)ethanesulfonic acid) and 150 mM NaCl, pH 6.5) buffer to prepare 80%, 35% and 5% solutions [25]. Sucrose gradients were prepared by adding 1 ml 80% sucrose followed by 1 ml sonicated sample with brief vortexing followed by 6 ml 35% sucrose followed by 4 ml 5% sucrose. Gradients were spun in an ultracentrifuge using an SW-41 rotor at 39 krpm at 4°C for 3 hours. Fractions (1 ml) were collected from the top of each tube starting at 4 ml to 12 ml. CCI samples were run as individual fractions and f4-6 (buoyant fractions; BF) and f10-12 (heavy fractions; HF) combined for WB. Samples were run on 10% or 4 to 12% bis-tris gels. After transfer to polyvinylidene fluoride membranes, samples were incubated with blocking buffer (3% bovine serum albumin in 20 mM Tris buffered saline containing 1% Tween) for 30 minutes and then incubated overnight with primary antibodies (in blocking buffer) at 4°C. Next day, membranes were washed (3 × 15 minute washes) and re-incubated with species-specific secondary antibodies conjugated to horseradish peroxidase from Santa Cruz at 1:5000 dilution in blocking buffer for 1 hour at room temperature. After extensive washing (4 to 5 × 15 minute washes) membranes were incubated with enhanced chemiluminescence reagent (Amersham Biosciences, PO Box 117, Rockford, IL, 61105, USA) and imaged with the UVP BioSpectrum Imaging System (UVP, 2066 W. 11th Street, Upland, CA, 91786 and saved as .tif files. Densitometric analysis was measured as previously described [25].

MAGPIX cytokine multiplex assay (n = 6/group)

CCI or sham was performed on the WT, Cav-1 KO and Cav-3 KO mice (2 to 3 months old) and cytokine multiplex assay was performed on the cortex 4 hours post-CCI. Cortices were harvested and frozen 4 hours post-CCI separately from each hemisphere in liquid nitrogen. Frozen tissue was homogenized following the manufacturer's instructions and 25 µl undiluted homogenate was added to 25 µl assay buffer. Magnetic beads (bead size = 6.45 µm) coated with specific antibodies (RCYTOMAG-80 K-PMX) were added to this solution and the reaction was incubated at 4°C for 24 hours. The beads were washed and incubated with 24 µl biotinylated detection antibody at room temperature for 2 hours. Completing the reaction, 25 µl streptavidin–phycoerythrin conjugate compound was added and allowed to incubate for 30 minutes at room temperature. Beads were washed and incubated with 150 μl sheath fluid for 5 minutes. Concentration of the samples was determined by Bio-Plex Manager version 5.0, after fluorescent capture, and MAGPIX xPONENT software (Millipore, 290 Concord Road, Billerica, MA, 01821, USA [32]. The assays were run in triplicate to confirm the results. Samples were normalized to total protein concentration. Samples were analyzed for the following: IL-1α, IL-1β, IL-2, IL-4, IL-5, IL-6, IL-10, IL-12p70, IL-13, IL-17, IL-18, IFNγ, induced protein 10, chemokine C-C motif ligand (CCL)2 (previously known as monocyte chemoattractant protein 1; MCP-1), CCL3 (previously known as macrophage inflammatory protein 1 alpha; MIP-1α), CCL5 (also known as Regulated upon Activation Normal T-cell Expressed; RANTES), TNFα, vascular endothelial growth factor, eotaxin, growth related oncogene KC (keratinocyte chemoattractant) (CXCL1), leptin, granulocyte colony-stimulating factor, and granulocyte-macrophage colony-stimulating factor (GMCSF).

Statistical analysis

All data were analyzed by unpaired t tests or analysis of variance (ANOVA) with *post-hoc* Bonferroni's multiple comparison or Student Neuman Keuls test as appropriate. Significance was set at $P < 0.05$. All data are presented as mean ± SEM. All statistical analysis was performed using Prism 6 (GraphPad Software, Inc., 7825 Fay Avenue, Suite 230, La Jolla, CA, 92037.

Results

Verification of a controlled cortical impact model of traumatic brain injury shows neuronal damage after 24 hours

To assess cortical and hippocampal damage after CCI, serial coronal sections of the brain were prepared and stained with Masson's trichrome. Figure 1A (2 hours post-CCI) and Figure 1C (24 hours post-CCI) are coronal sections showing cortical lesions. The inserts (boxed areas) are representative of the underlying hippocampal regions (a and b). Neuronal injury was analyzed for dying neurons by Aperio ScanScope imaging and Spectrum analysis algorithm packages as described by Krajewska and colleagues [22], with dead neurons indicated by red/brown coloring superimposed. The results showed minimal hippocampal cell death at 2 hours post-CCI (n = 4) in either ipsilateral or contralateral hemispheres but considerable cell death in CA1 and CA3 is evident at 24 hours post-CCI (n = 4) (Figure 1C-a). Sucrose density fractionation revealed that MLR localization of synaptic proteins and receptors (PSD-95, TrkB, NR2B) and Cav-1 was still intact 2 hours post-CCI (Figure 1B), but there was a drastic reduction after 24 hours (Figure 1D). These results show that there is CA1 neuronal cell death 24 hours post-CCI and a

loss in MLR-localized pro-survival and pro-growth synaptic components.

Hippocampal-dependent learning is decreased 3 months post-controlled cortical impact

Behavioral analysis revealed no significant difference between CCI (n = 20) and sham (n = 20) for open field distance (cm) moved (CCI versus sham: 6,413 ± 217 versus 6,479 ± 216; $P = 0.793$), velocity (cm/second) (CCI versus sham: 12.88 ± 0.49 versus 13.56 ± 0.34; $P = 0.41$) or time spent in the center of the arena (seconds) (CCI versus sham: 46.9 ± 6.8 versus 41.12 ± 3.25; $P = 0.61$) (Figure 1E). Furthermore no significant difference was seen in foot slips on the balance beam (CCI versus sham: 1.5 ± 0.2 versus 1.4 ± 0.3; $P = 0.56$) or the holding impulse (seconds x grams) in the wire grip test (CCI versus sham: 1,606 ± 146 versus 1,450 ± 110; $P = 0.4$). However, a significant difference between groups was recorded in the alternations made (% alternations) in the continuous alternating T-maze (CCI versus sham: 59.6 ± 3.7 versus 71.8 ± 3.0; $P = 0.028$) (Figure 1F). Taken together, the results suggest that no gross difference between groups was present in read outs of basic activity, general behavior/anxiety and neuromuscular function, yet there was a difference in hippocampal dependent 'spontaneous alternations', suggesting that the hippocampal injury detected histologically in Figure 1C and the subcellular biochemical changes seen in Figure 1D may contribute to the hippocampal-dependent behavioral changes.

Controlled cortical impact model of traumatic brain injury enhances polysynaptic responses in isolated hippocampal slices at 1 week

Electrophysiological changes were assessed in hippocampal slices isolated from contralateral (n = 4) and ipsilateral (n = 4) hemispheres. No changes in long-term potentiation of monosynaptic responses were observed (Figure 2A,B). However, changes in the response shape were more pronounced in the ipsilateral (CCI) versus the contralateral slices. Thus, the averaged amplitude of the field potentials at 14 to 45 ms that represent mostly polysynaptic responses were considerably greater in the ipsilateral versus contralateral slices from CCI brains (Figure 2A,C). The observed increase in polysynaptic responses in the CCI hippocampal hemisphere is an indicator of increased pro-epileptic activity, and this neurophysiological change could be an important component that contributed to the behavioral change observed in Figure 1F.

Controlled cortical impact model of traumatic brain injury exhibits enhanced NADPH oxidase activity

To test if injury-induced neuronal loss and the subsequent neuroinflammation in our current TBI model are associated with Nox activation, Nox activity was assessed

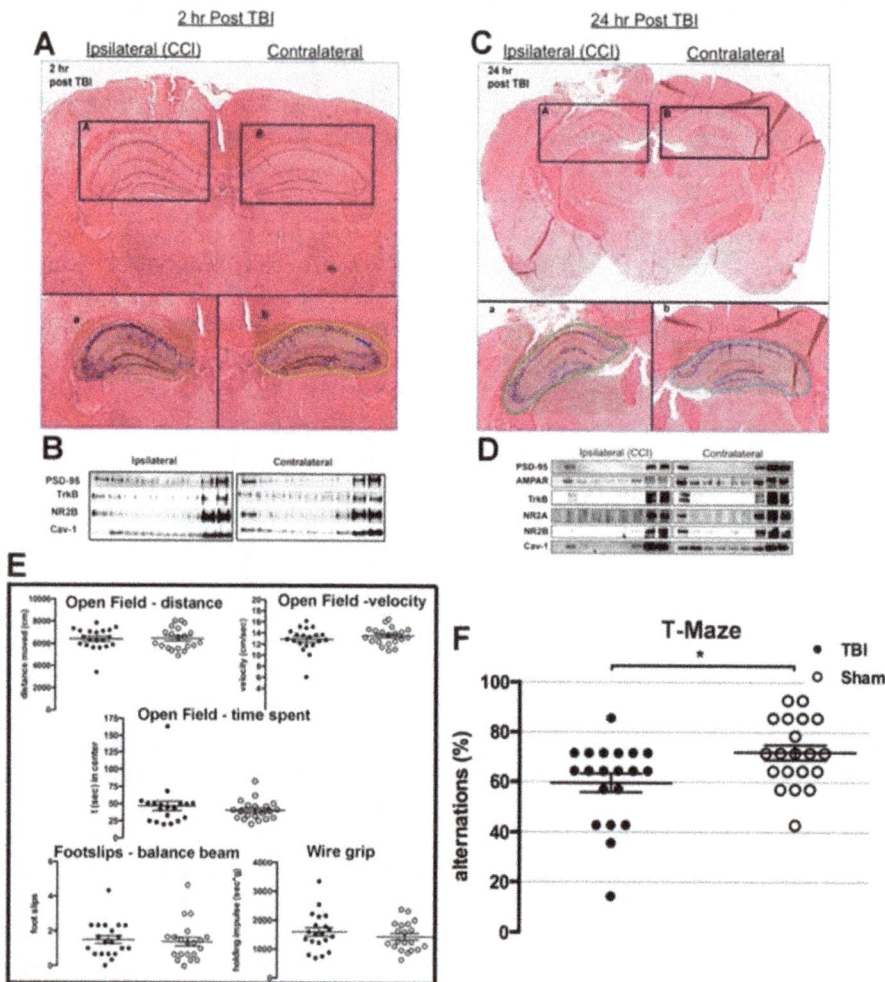

Figure 1 Controlled cortical impact (CCI) is a viable model of murine traumatic brain injury (TBI). (A) Trichrome stained paraffin section 2 hours post-CCI with both ipsilateral and contralateral hemispheres. Bottom panels (a) and (b) are the enlargements of the hippocampal area outlined. **(B)** Sucrose density fractionation (SDF) to purify membrane/lipid rafts (MLRs) from ispilateral and contralateral hemispheres. Buoyant fractions contain the cholesterol and sphingolipid enriched MLR, while heavy fractions contain non-MLR cellular components. Western blot of SDF purification of MLR from ipsilateral and contralateral hemispheres 2 hours post-CCI. **(C)** Trichrome stained paraffin section 24 hours post-CCI shows considerable damage to ipsilateral cortex and underlying hippocampus. Bottom panels (a) and (b) are the enlargements of the hippocampal area outlined. **(D)** Western blot of SDF purification of MLR from ipsilateral and contralateral hemispheres 24 hours post-CCI. **(E)** Behavior battery tests performed 3 months post-CCI: open field (distance, velocity, time spent), footslips and wire grip. **(F)** T-maze alternation behavioral test on sham and CCI groups after 3 months.

24 hours (n = 3) and 1 week (n = 3) post-CCI by EPR (Figure 2D,E). TBI mice exhibited enhanced Nox-derived superoxide generation 24 hours and 1 week after CCI in both contralateral and ipsilateral hemispheres. Interestingly, increased Nox activity in the contralateral side indicates that 'global' brain inflammation was induced 1 week post-CCI.

Caveolin knock-out animals have altered expression of membrane/lipid raft localized neuronal and glial proteins
WT, Cav-1 KO and Cav-3 KO mouse cortex were homogenized and processed for sucrose density fractionation to

analyze neuronal and glial proteins (Figure 3). BF (consisting of fractions 4 to 6) and HF (consisting of fractions 10 to 12) were used for WB. PSD-95, NR2A, NR2B, and TrkB were all reduced in both BF and HF from Cav-1 KO brains, results akin to our previously published work [19]. BF from Cav-3 KO brains showed increased expression of PSD-95, NR2B, NR1A, and TrkB (Figure 3A) compared to Cav-1 KO, yet the pattern-recognition receptor TLR4 was nearly lost in HF from Cav-3 KO brains and decreased in Cav-1 KO (Figure 3B).

Adenosine receptors exhibited differential expression patterns among the three groups (Figure 3B). WT brains

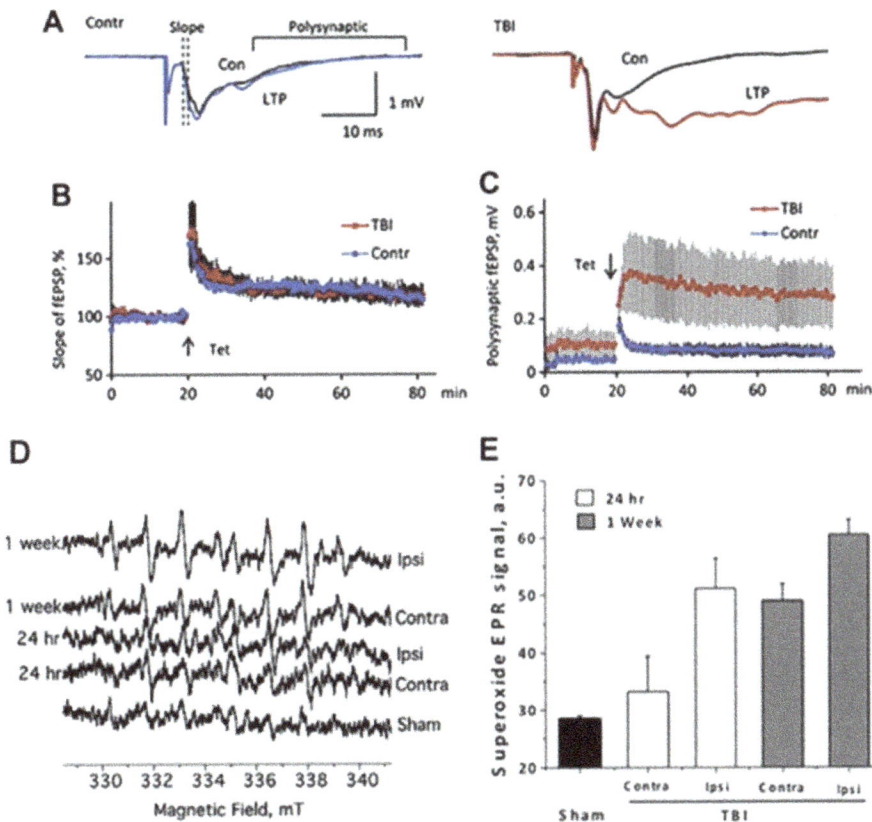

Figure 2 Electrophysiological properties of the commissural-collateral input in the CA1 region of the hippocampus at 1 week post-traumatic brain injury (TBI). (A) Representative responses in slices from the contralateral (Contra; left) and the TBI (controlled cortical impact (CCI), right) hippocampus before and after the tetanus. (B) Long-term potentiation (LTP) of monosynaptic responses after CCI. (C) Changes of polysynaptic response (averaged amplitude at latencies 12 to 45 ms after the stimulus). (D) Enhanced NADPH oxidase (Nox) activity in both ipsilateral and contralateral hemispheres 24 hours and 1 week post-TBI as shown by increased superoxide electron paramagnetic resonance (EPR) signal amplitude relative to sham animals. (E) Isolated synaptosomes from the ipsilateral side exhibited greater Nox activity, which increased 1 week post-CCI. Con, control; Contra, contralateral; fEPSP, field excitatory postsynaptic potential; Ispi, ipsilateral.

showed limited BF localization of $A_{2A}R$, an inflammation promoting subtype of adenosine receptors. Interestingly, $A_{2A}R$ expression was enhanced in both Cav KO brains, with Cav-3 KO displaying the highest BF-localized expression. The anti-inflammatory A_1AR and A_3AR isoforms were only detected in HF for all groups. Cav-1 and Cav-3 KO mice expressed less A_1AR and A_3AR compared to WT.

Because Cavs are cholesterol binding proteins, and lipoprotein receptors LRP-1 and LDL-R subcellularly localize to MLR [33,34], we assessed the expression of these receptors (Figure 3C). Both Cav-1 KO and Cav-3 KO showed decreased expression of LRP-1, with the same ratio of BF to HF. There was little detection of LDL-R in BF from WT, Cav-1 and Cav-3 KO, yet Cav-3 KO showed the least expression compared to Cav-1 KO and WT. The KO phenotype was confirmed by WB for Cav-1 KO and Cav-3 KO hippocampi.

Caveolin knock-out animals have altered resident central nervous system cell populations

Primary mixed glial cultures were isolated from WT, Cav-1 KO and Cav-3 KO on postnatal day 3 to match passage and days in vitro. WB analysis (Figure 4A) and IF (immunofluorescence microscopy) (Figure 4B) indicate that Cav-1 KO and Cav-3 KO have increased number of Iba1 positive cells and decreased GFAP positive cells compared to WT, with Cav-3 KO cells showing the greatest reduction in GFAP positive cells as indicated by IF (Figure 4B, right image). To confirm these findings, age-matched hippocampi were examined by IF for Iba1 (microglia), GFAP (astrocytes) (Figure 4C) and MAP2 (neuronal dendrites) (Figure 4D). Cav-1 KO brains exhibit slightly increased Iba1 positive microglia and GFAP positive staining in CA1 and dentate gyrus (DG) compared to WT, similar to previously reported findings from our group [19]. Hippocampi from Cav-3 KO brains

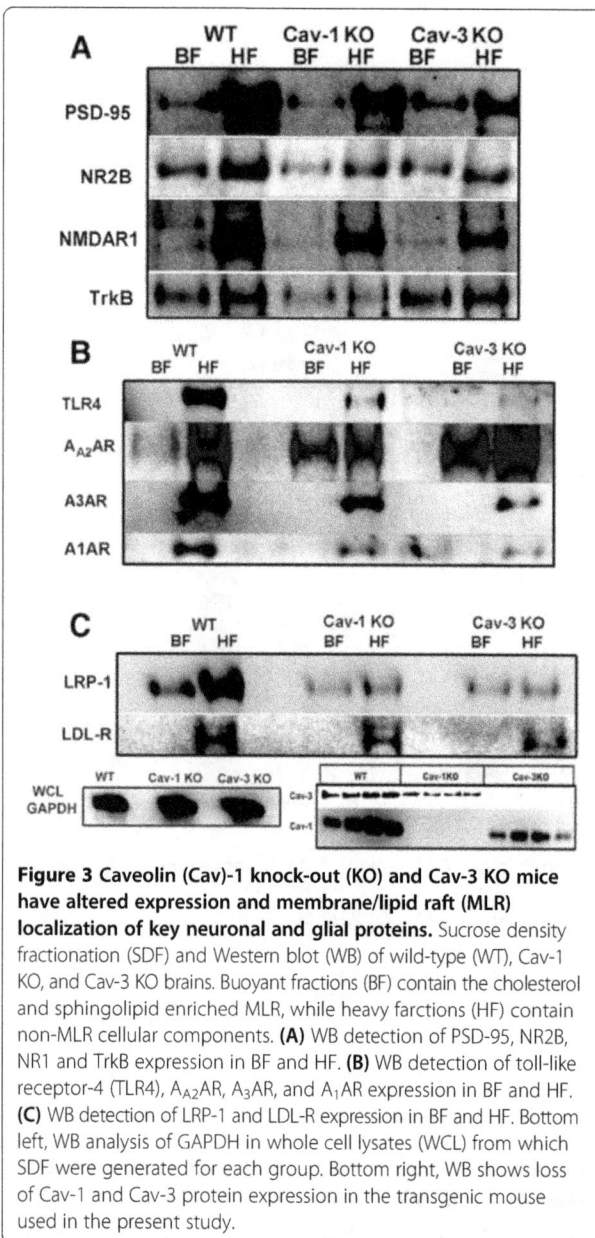

Figure 3 Caveolin (Cav)-1 knock-out (KO) and Cav-3 KO mice have altered expression and membrane/lipid raft (MLR) localization of key neuronal and glial proteins. Sucrose density fractionation (SDF) and Western blot (WB) of wild-type (WT), Cav-1 KO, and Cav-3 KO brains. Buoyant fractions (BF) contain the cholesterol and sphingolipid enriched MLR, while heavy farctions (HF) contain non-MLR cellular components. **(A)** WB detection of PSD-95, NR2B, NR1 and TrkB expression in BF and HF. **(B)** WB detection of toll-like receptor-4 (TLR4), $A_{A2}AR$, A_3AR, and A_1AR expression in BF and HF. **(C)** WB detection of LRP-1 and LDL-R expression in BF and HF. Bottom left, WB analysis of GAPDH in whole cell lysates (WCL) from which SDF were generated for each group. Bottom right, WB shows loss of Cav-1 and Cav-3 protein expression in the transgenic mouse used in the present study.

displayed less GFAP positive cells in the CA1 and DG compared to both WT and Cav-1 KO. WT MAP2 labeling of CA1 pyramidal neurons shows a typical pattern of normally arranged neuronal cell layer and aligned processes in the molecular layer of the DG. Cav-1 KO showed less MAP2 positive neurites, which is consistent with our previous findings [19], yet Cav-3 KO exhibited greater MAP2 staining compared to Cav-1 KO and WT (Figure 4D). Quantitation of the IF images are shown in Figure 4E: Cav-3 KO showed increased Iba1 positive cells ($P < 0.01$, n = 3) compared to WT or Cav-1, less GFAP positive cells ($P < 0.01$, n = 3) compared to WT and Cav-1 KO, and increased MAP2 positive neurites ($P < 0.01$, n = 3) compared to WT and Cav-1 KO. Basal hippocampi from

WT, Cav-1 and Cav-3 KO were analyzed by WB for Iba1, GFAP and neuronal specific β_3-tubulin to assess the cell-specific protein expression pattern (Figure 4F). Iba1 was significantly reduced ($P < 0.001$) in Cav-1 KO and significantly elevated in Cav-3 KO ($P = 0.04$). GFAP was significantly reduced ($P = 0.01$) and β_3-tubulin was elevated ($P = 0.004$) in Cav-3 KO, findings consistent with IF data.

Caveolin-1 knock-out and Caveolin-3 knock-out mice exhibit larger lesion volume 24 hours post-controlled cortical impact compared to wild-type mice

To assess brain injury after CCI, serial coronal sections of the brain were prepared and stained with Masson's trichrome and lesion volume was quantitated as previously described [22]. Both Cav-1 (n = 4; 11.9 ± 1.2 mm^3) and Cav-3 KO (n = 4; 15.1 ± 2.2 mm^3) had a significantly larger lesion volume compared WT (n = 4; 7.5 ± 0.8 mm^3) and sham (n = 4; 0.8 ± 0.4 mm^3) ($P < 0.0001$, Figure 5) 24 hours post-CCI.

Controlled cortical impact enhances pro-inflammatory cytokines and chemokines in caveolin-1 knock-out and caveolin-3 knock-out mice at 4 hours post-impact

Brain homogenates from WT, Cav-1 KO and Cav-3 KO mice were analyzed for 23 different cytokine/chemokines to assess the inflammatory response in our CCI model. Of the 23 analytes, 10 exhibited significantly different expression patterns among the three groups (Table 1). Sham data from all three groups (WT, Cav-1 KO and Cav-3 KO; n = 6/group) revealed no significant difference in the analytes measured. Of note, many of the measured cytokines from sham (n = 6) samples were below the level of detection, in contrast to the CCI (n = 6) samples which all yielded measurable amounts. Following CCI, both ipsilateral and contralateral hemispheres from Cav-1 (n = 6) and Cav-3 KO (n = 6) exhibited significant elevation in IL-1β, IL-2, IL-6, IL-9, IL-10, IL-17, KC, MCP-1, MIP-1α, and GMCSF compared to the respective transgenic sham corresponding hemispheres (that is, ipsilateral and contralateral) ($P = 0.0005$, two-way ANOVA, Table 1). For WT alone, CCI significantly enhanced IL-1β, IL-9, IL-10, KC, and MCP-1 in ipsilateral hemisphere and IL-9, IL-10, IL-17, and MIP-1α in contralateral versus corresponding sham hemisphere. For Cav-1 KO, CCI significantly elevated IL-1β, IL-2, IL-6, IL-9, IL-10, IL-17, KC, and MCP-1 versus ipsilateral Cav-1 KO sham and significantly increased all 10 cytokines/chemokines versus contralateral Cav-1 KO sham. When compared to WT CCI corresponding hemisphere, Cav-1 CCI increased IL-2, IL-6, KC and MCP-1 in ipsilateral and IL-6, IL-9, IL-17 and KC in contralateral. For Cav-3 KO, all 10 cytokines/chemokines were significantly elevated in both ipsilateral and contralateral versus Cav-3 KO corresponding sham hemispheres.

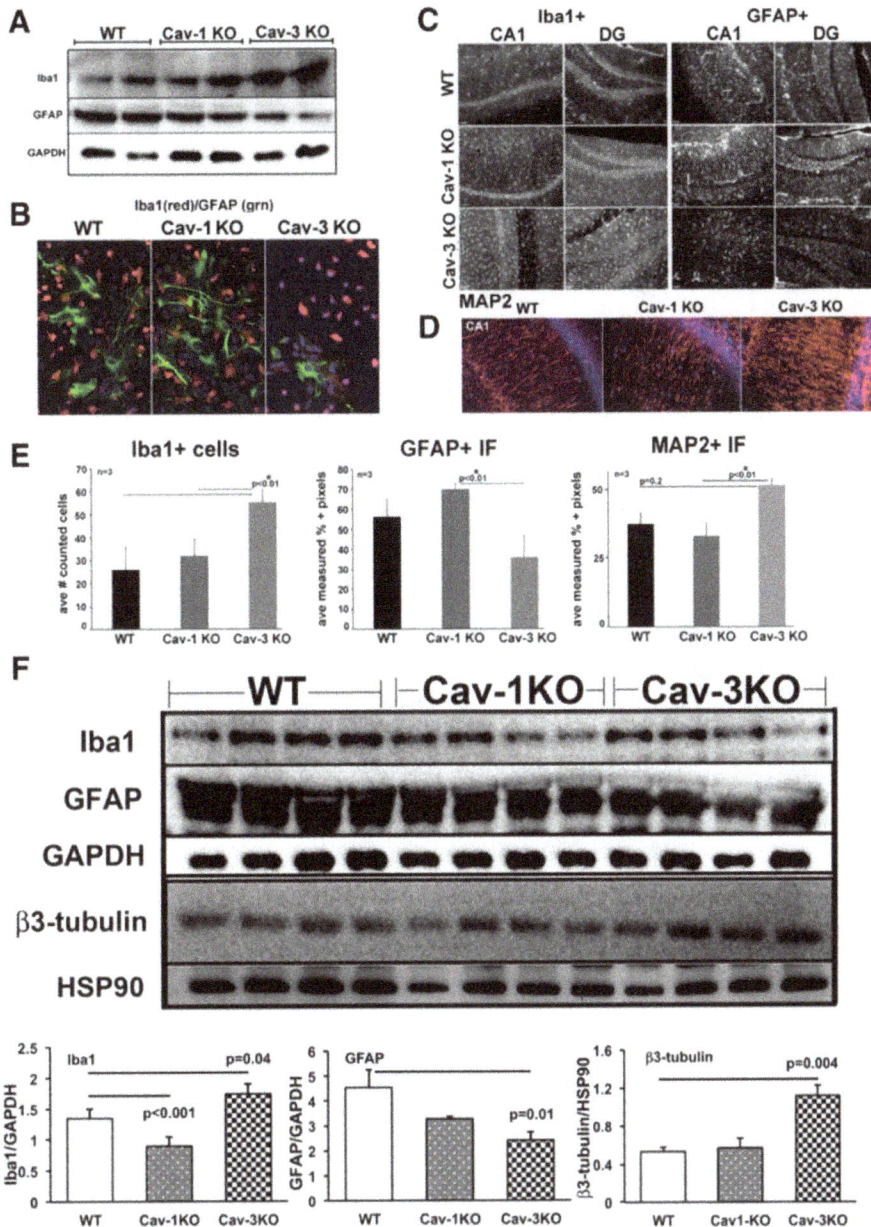

Figure 4 Caveolin (Cav)-1 knock-out (KO) and Cav-3 KO mice have different microglial and astrocyte populations. Primary mixed glia were cultured from brains from wild-type (WT), Cav-1 KO and Cav-3 KO postnatal day 3 pups. **(A)** Western blot (WB) analysis of GFAP (glial fibrillary acidic protein) and Iba1 (ionized calcium-binding adapter molecule 1) in primary mixed glia cultures normalized to GAPDH. **(B)** Immunofluorescence microscopy of GFAP (green) and Iba1 (red) in primary mixed glia cultures. Nuclei were stained with DAPI. **(C)** Sections of hippocampal CA1 and dentate gyrus (DG) regions from WT, Cav-1 KO and Cav-3 KO mice labeled with Iba1 (left) and GFAP (right). **(D)** Sections of hippocampal CA1 region with the neuronal dendritic marker MAP2 (microtubule associated protein 2). **(E)** Quantitation of cell numbers from n = 3 animals. A statistically significant increase in Iba1 cells is found in Cav-3 KO mice compared to WT ($P < 0.01$, left graph). A significant decrease in GFAP labeling is found in Cav-3 KO mice compared to Cav-1 KO ($P < 0.01$, middle graph), and a trending decrease when compared to WT (not significant). A statistically significant increase in MAP2 labeling is also detected in Cav-3 KO versus Cav-1 KO ($P < 0.01$, right graph). Data displayed as mean ± SEM. **(F)** Bottom panels are quantitative WB analysis of Iba1, GFAP and β_3-tubulin from mouse hippocampi. Statistically significant increased expression of Iba1 and β_3-tubulin and decreased GFAP expression was detected in Cav-3 KO mice. Conversely, decreased Iba1 expression was observed in Cav-1 KO.

When compared to WT CCI, Cav-3 CCI displayed a significant increase in all 10 cytokines/chemokines in both hemispheres except for IL-17 (ipsilateral) and MIP-1α (contralateral). When compared to Cav-1 KO CCI, Cav-3 KO CCI had a significant increase in IL-1β, IL-9, KC, MCP-1, MIP-1α, and GMCSF in the ipsilateral hemisphere and IL-1β, IL-2, IL-9, IL-10, and IL-17 in the contralateral hemisphere.

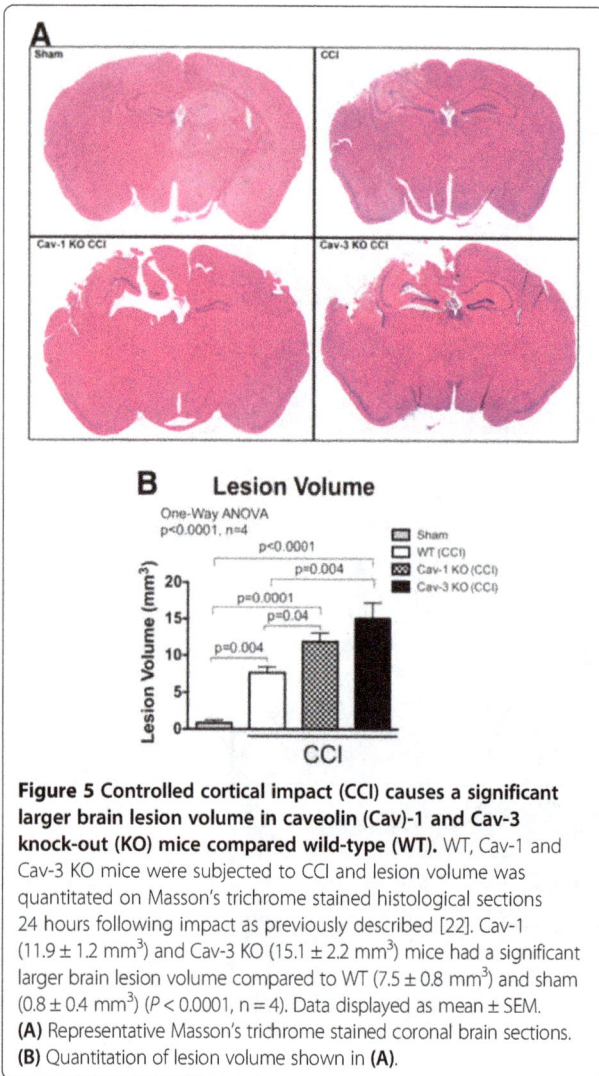

Figure 5 Controlled cortical impact (CCI) causes a significant larger brain lesion volume in caveolin (Cav)-1 and Cav-3 knock-out (KO) mice compared wild-type (WT). WT, Cav-1 and Cav-3 KO mice were subjected to CCI and lesion volume was quantitated on Masson's trichrome stained histological sections 24 hours following impact as previously described [22]. Cav-1 (11.9 ± 1.2 mm³) and Cav-3 KO (15.1 ± 2.2 mm³) mice had a significant larger brain lesion volume compared to WT (7.5 ± 0.8 mm³) and sham (0.8 ± 0.4 mm³) ($P < 0.0001$, n = 4). Data displayed as mean ± SEM. **(A)** Representative Masson's trichrome stained coronal brain sections. **(B)** Quantitation of lesion volume shown in **(A)**.

Discussion

The current findings are the first to demonstrate that loss of Cav isoforms produces isoform-specific effects on inflammation in a CCI model of TBI. The objective of the present study was to quantitatively assess neuroinflammation in the brain of Cav-1 KO and Cav-3 KO mice early after CCI. Many previously published studies have evaluated downstream signaling proteins involved in the induction of cytokines/chemokines after injury [35,36], but none have directly investigated the role of Cav and MLR-localized receptors and associated downstream signaling mediators on TBI-induced inflammatory responses. The loss of Cav-1, specifically, has been found to result in increased ischemic damage following transient middle cerebral artery occusion [37]. One possible mechanism for increased injury is a lack of eNOS inhibition by Cav-1 leading to increased metalloproteinase activity and blood–brain barrier degradation [38]. Because both microglia and astrocytes express Cav-1

and Cav-3, it is critical to understand how these proteins regulate receptor signaling, and secondary messengers such as NO, to induce or repress inflammation following CNS injury. Moreover, Cav-1 KO mice have previously been shown to exhibit enhanced anxiety and impaired spatial memory, demonstrating an important role for Cav-1 in normal neurological phenotype [39]. Although it has yet to be determined which cell type contributes to these behavioral abnormalities, our previous work that demonstrates a reduction in MLR and MLR-localized synaptic proteins accompanied with reduced hippocampal synapses does indicate in part that loss of Cav-1 causes cellular morphological changes essential for normal brain physiology regardless of the cell type [19].

Using a well-characterized CCI model of TBI, we detected glial reactivity in the ipsilateral hemisphere 4 hours post-injury and hippocampal neuronal death 24 hours post-injury. Behavioral studies revealed cognitive deficits in working memory, as determined by T-maze, 3 months post-injury with no motor deficits. Not surprisingly, the damage was not limited to the hippocampus, as extensive parietal cortical damage was also evident by 4 hours, which included enhanced neuroinflammation as indicated by the significantly elevated cytokine production in the ipsilateral cortex.

TBI can produce epileptogenesis, a neuropathological change that is frequently associated with depression, anxiety disorders and side effects from anti-epileptic treatments [40]. PTE is a significant complication for the returning Veteran population with estimates that approximately 34% of returning Veterans who experienced moderate to severe head trauma are at risk for developing PTE. The findings from the current study show an increase in polysynaptic responses in the CCI hippocampal hemisphere, an indicator of increased pro-epileptic activity. Such a finding is a potential indicator of increased pro-epileptic activity because aberrant circuit formation is believed to be involved in epileptogenesis [41,42]. Therefore, these results (that is, enhanced polysynaptic responses) could be an important factor contributing to the post-TBI death of hippocampal neurons and development of epilepsy.

Another putative mechanism involved in the development of PTE is enhanced generation of reactive oxygen species [43], as seen in the current study (Figure 2D,E). Previous studies have shown Nox activation leads to increased neurotoxic activation of microglia [44]. Gene array studies have shown that changes in synaptic plasticity, glial proliferation and inflammatory reactivity occur before initial seizures manifest [45,46]. Anti-epileptic drugs, as a prophylactic intervention administered soon after TBI, have shown some efficacy in preventing early seizures (< 1 week), but are ineffective in preventing later, more devastating episodes of seizures [47]. Therefore,

Table 1 Multiplex array reveals brain changes in certain cytokines, chemokines, and growth factors after CCI

	Ipsilateral						Contralateral					
	WT		Cav-1 KO		Cav-3 KO		WT		Cav-1 KO		Cav-3 KO	
	Sham	TBI	Sham	TBI	Sham	TBI	Sham	TBI	Sham	TBI	Sham	TBI
IL-1β	0.072±0.004	0.83±0.06*	0.06±0.005	1.4±0.3*	0.07±0.007	2.5±0.4*#	0.08±0.01	0.59±0.07	0.06±0.005	1.05±0.13*	0.07±0.01	2.3±0.2*#^
IL-2	011±0.002	0.36±0.03	0.11±0.005	0.7±0.07*#	013±0.004	0.96±0.15#	0.11±0.01	0.22±0.05	0.12±0.004	0.6±0.1*	0.13±0.01	0.9±0.1*#^
IL-6	0.04±0.006	2.0±0.4	0.03±0.007	30.9±3.9*#	0.03±0.003	42.2±7.1*#	0.03±0.005	0.58±0.06	0.02±0.001	14.2±3.9*#δ	0.02±0.005	7.5±1.3*#
IL-9	0.69±0.03	9.6±0.4*	0.6±0.06	15.1±1.5*	0.8±0.09	23.3±3.3*#^	0.79±0.19	7.4±1.3*	0.8±0.03	13.6±2.2*#	0.7±0.06	21.0±1.5*#^
IL-10	0.034±0.003	1.0±0.08*	0.04±0.003	1.5±0.2*	0.06±0.002	2.0±0.3*#	0.046±0.012	0.62±0.08*	0.04±0.001	1.03±0.17*	0.05±0.01	1.8±0.1*#^
IL-17	0.0009±0.0003	0.22±0.02	0.002±0.0003	0.3±0.04*	0.003±0.0001	0.4±0.1*	0.0014±0.0005	0.13±0.03*	0.001±0.0002	0.3±0.05*#	0.003±0.001	0.4±0.04*#^
KC	0054±0.01	6.3±1.2*	0.05±0.006	31.8±3.1*#	0.05±0.005	49.1±7.7*#^	0.027±0.009	1.6±0.2	0.02±0.001	9.5±1.8#	0.03±0.01	11.0±2.5*#
MCP-1	0.051±0.004	7.0±2.2*	0.05±0.009	19.4±1.5*#	0.05±0.004	39.4±6.3*#^	0.042±0.009	1.9±0.2	0.04±0.004	5.6±1.2*	0.07±0.01	8.6±1.9*#
MIP-1α	0.031±0.004	2.0±0.07	0.02±0.008	6.7±0.6	0.03±0.003	20.1±4.8*#^	0.022±0.006	1.6±0.2*	0.01±0.002	2.0±0.6*	0.02±0.01	2.4±0.3*
GMCSF	NA	0.84±0.2	NA	1.9±0.6	0.2±0.03	3.4±0.6*#^	0.14±0.05	0.7±0.2	0.11±0.01	2.0±0.4*#	0.3±0.04	2.5±0.3*#

Four hours post-CCI, contralateral and ipsilateral hemispheres were analyzed with the MAGPIX Cytokine Multiplex Assay for IL-1β, IL-2, IL-6, IL-9, IL-10, IL-17, KC (keratinocyte chemoattractant), monocyte chemoattractant protein 1 (MCP-1), macrophage inflammatory protein 1 alpha (MIP-1α), and granulocyte-macrophage colony-stimulating factor (GMCSF). Data (n = 6 mice/group) represent mean ± SEM. $P < 0.05$ or less were considered statistically significant. *$P < 0.05$ versus sham hemisphere, #$P < 0.05$ versus caveolin (Cav)-1 knock-out (KO) TBI hemisphere, ^$P < 0.05$ versus wild-type (WT) traumatic brain injury (TBI) hemisphere, δ$P < 0.05$ versus Cav-3 KO TBI hemisphere. NA, not available (below detection).

more efficacious interventions that attenuate these initial key changes may alter the course of PTE development and potentially reverse the long-term cognitive changes that result from TBI.

We have previously shown a role for Cavs as regulators of neuronal survival [19,24,25] and microglia activation [20]. In an attempt to understand the potential role of Cavs in mediating the early inflammatory responses after TBI, 23 cytokines were measured 4 hours post-injury. Interestingly, 10 analytes were significantly elevated in both hemispheres of brains from either Cav-1 KO or Cav-3 KO mice. Common pro-inflammatory cytokines/chemokines, including IL-1β, IL-2, IL-6, IL-9, IL-10, IL-17, KC, MCP-1, MIP-1α, and GMCSF were upregulated in both Cav KO mice, yet only IL-6, KC, MCP-1, and MIP-1α were significantly elevated with CCI compared to the contralateral Cav. MCP-1 (CCL2) was significantly increased in the contralateral and ipsilateral hemisphere of both Cav KO mice; these results are in agreement with previously published work that demonstrated increased expression in a pilocarpine model of status epilepticus [48]. Persistently elevated expression of MCP-1 in both Cav KO mice indicates a disruption in the normal signaling and trafficking of the MCP-1/CCR2 (MCP-1 receptor) complex, an interesting finding considering that previous work showed that MCP-1 KO mice have attenuated lesion size and less astrogliosis following TBI [49]. Other studies have shown that Cav-1 plays a prominent role in astrocytic responses to MCP-1 by mediation of cellular signaling transduction through caveolae-localized CCR2 [50,51]. Therefore, interventions that increase Cav expression and restore normal CCR2 expression and function may be a potential therapeutic target. As a final Cav-mediated chemokine example from the multiplex analysis, MIP-1α (CCL3), a ligand for CCR5 (MIP-1α receptor), is significantly elevated after CCI in the ipsilateral hemisphere. Although many groups have found increased expression of MIP-1α following induced status epilepticus models, the role for MIP-1α, either protective or inflammatory, is still under debate [52].

Various G-protein coupled receptors that are regulated by Cav, such as adenosine receptors, are involved in the complex process of microglia or astrocyte activation [53-56]. The data from the current study demonstrated reduced expression of adenosine A_1AR and the anti-inflammatory A_3AR in both Cav-1 KO and Cav-3 KO brains. Evidence exists that the loss of A_1AR (A_1AR KO mice) results in an increased risk for epileptogenesis [57,58]. Because the current data show a reduction in A_1AR expression in Cav KO mice, loss of Cav isoforms due to injury (as shown in Figure 1D) may render the brain more susceptible to physiological changes (Figure 2C) and subsequent seizure development.

$A_{2A}AR$ sits at the intersection of multiple control points for the development of neuropathology and neuropsychiatric conditions (reviewed in [59,60]). Activation of $A_{2A}AR$ can negatively affect the functionality of A_1AR [61], resulting in an enhanced inflammatory state. Additional evidence suggests that $A_{2A}AR$ activation plays a major regulatory role in microglia-dependent neurotrophin release and subsequent microglia proliferation during neuroinflammation [62]. The present findings demonstrate that both Cav KO mice have increased MLR localization of the pro-inflammatory $A_{2A}AR$ compared to WT (Figure 3B). After injury, local adenosine concentrations greatly increase activating plasmalemmal localized $A_{2A}AR$ receptors in microglia [7,63]. The present finding that Cav KO mice exhibit increased MLR-localized $A_{2A}AR$ basally may in part explain the elevated cytokine/chemokine production in the brains of these mice both with and without CCI.

Cholesterol is a key component of MLR and for maintaining synaptic integrity. Because synaptic loss is one of the dynamic changes associated with the latency period for development of PTE [64-67], changes in cholesterol homeostasis and MLR integrity may in part contribute to the etiology of PTE. Lipoprotein receptors are key players in cholesterol homeostasis [68], and two important lipoprotein receptors in the brain, LRP-1 and LDL-R, are subcellularly localized to MLR [33,34]. Because Cav KO mice have reduced expression of LRP-1 and to a lesser extent LDL-R compared to WT (Figure 3C), events that cause decreased Cav expression in the brain (age or injury) may reduce cholesterol transport from glia to neurons and therefore increase the risk for synaptic loss, intercellular events we are presently investigating [19].

Conclusions

We have demonstrated for the first time that loss of Cav isoforms results in enhanced cytokine/chemokine production following TBI. The present study extends previously published results showing the neuropathology of Cav-1 KO mice, and shows for the first time that loss of Cav-3 significantly enhances cytokine/chemokine production in the setting of TBI. The extent of injury and inflammation was considerably greater in the Cav-1 KO and Cav-3 KO mice. Some degree of inflammation is clearly necessary for neuroregeneration and brain repair after TBI. Modulation of the inflammatory response, rather than its suppression, may be necessary. To that end, our data are consistent with the premise that modulation of Cav-1 and Cav-3 levels in a cell-type-specific manner (neurons, astrocytes and microglia) might afford novel therapeutic options for the treatment of TBI.

Abbreviations

ACSF: artificial cerebrospinal fluid; ANOVA: analysis of variance; BF: buoyant fractions; Cav: caveolin; CCI: controlled cortical impact; CCL: chemokine C-C motif ligand; CNS: central nervous system; DG: dentate gyrus; DMEM: Dulbecco's modified Eagle's medium; eNOS: endothelial nitric oxide synthase; EPR: electron paramagnetic resonance; GFAP: (glial fibrillary acidic protein); GMCSF: granulocyte-macrophage colony-stimulating factor; HF: heavy fractions; Iba1: ionized calcium-binding adapter molecule 1; IF: immunofluorescence microscopy; IFN: interferon; IL: interleukin; KC: keratinocyte chemoattractant; KO: knock-out; MAP2: microtubule associated protein; MCP-1: monocyte chemoattractant protein 1; MIP-1α: macrophage inflammatory protein 1 alpha; MLR: membrane/lipid raft; NMDAR: N-methyl-D-aspartate receptor; Nox: NADPH oxidase; PTE: post-traumatic epilepsy; TBI: traumatic brain injury; TNF: tumor necrosis factor; TLR4: toll-like receptor 4; WB: Western blot; WT: wild-type.

Competing interests

The authors declare that they have no competing interests.

Authors' contributions

IRN performed cell culture, biochemistry experiments (WB and IF), and participated in the draft of the manuscript. JMS assisted in behavioral analysis and participated in the draft of the manuscript. LAS performed cytokine array and assisted in analysis. SK and JAB performed CCI experiments. AK conducted electrophysiology experiments. WC assisted in CCI experiments and histology. AV performed behavioral studies. JAB and SK assisted in establishment of CCI model. SSA conducted EPR experiments and analysis. DMR participated in draft of the manuscript. HHP participated in the draft of the manuscript. PMP participated in establishment of CCI model and the draft of the manuscript. BPH participated in establishment of CCI model, study design, data analysis, and draft of the manuscript. All authors read and approved the final manuscript.

Authors' information

Work in the authors' laboratories is supported by Veteran Affairs Merit Award from the Department of Veterans Affairs BX001225 (B. P. Head), BX000783 (D. M. Roth), and BX001963 (H. H. Patel), National Institutes of Health, Bethesda, MD, U.S.A., NS073653 (B. P. Head) and HL091071 and HL107200 (H. H. Patel), Department of Defense W81XWH-10-0847 (S. Krajewski).

Acknowledgements

The authors wish to thank Khurshed Katki for technical assistance with the MAGPIX multiplex assay and Yue (Pauline) Hu for performing brain dissections.

Author details

[1]Veterans Affairs San Diego Healthcare System, 3350 La Jolla Village Drive, San Diego, CA 92161, USA. [2]Department of Anesthesiology, University of California, San Diego, La Jolla, CA 92093, USA. [3]Neuroscience Research Institute, Scott & White Hospital, Central Texas Veterans Health System, Temple, TX, USA. [4]Department of Surgery, Department of Neurosurgery, Department of Neuroscience and Experimental Therapeutics, College of Medicine, Texas A&M Health Science Center, Temple, TX, USA. [5]Department of Neurosciences, University of California, San Diego, 9500 Gilman Drive, La Jolla, CA 92093, USA. [6]Sanford-Burnham Medical Research Institute, La Jolla, CA, USA. [7]Department of Anesthesiology, Beijing Tiantan Hospital, Capital Medical University, Beijing, China. [8]Center for Aging and Associated Diseases, Helmy Institute of Medical Sciences, Zewail City of Science and Technology, Giza, Egypt.

References

1. Narayan RK, Michel ME, Ansell B, Baethmann A, Biegon A, Bracken MB, Bullock MR, Choi SC, Clifton GL, Contant CF, Coplin WM, Dietrich WD, Ghajar J, Grady SM, Grossman RG, Hall ED, Heetderks W, Hovda DA, Jallo J, Katz RL, Knoller N, Kochanek PM, Maas AI, Majde J, Marion DW, Marmarou A, Marshall LF, McIntosh TK, Miller E, Mohberg N, et al: Clinical trials in head injury. J Neurotrauma 2002, 19:503–557.
2. Atkins CM, Falo MC, Alonso OF, Bramlett HM, Dietrich WD: Deficits in ERK and CREB activation in the hippocampus after traumatic brain injury. Neurosci Lett 2009, 459:52–56.
3. Biegon A, Fry PA, Paden CM, Alexandrovich A, Tsenter J, Shohami E: Dynamic changes in N-methyl-D-aspartate receptors after closed head injury in mice: implications for treatment of neurological and cognitive deficits. Proc Natl Acad Sci U S A 2004, 101:5117–5122.
4. Conte V, Raghupathi R, Watson DJ, Fujimoto S, Royo NC, Marklund N, Stocchetti N, McIntosh TK: TrkB gene transfer does not alter hippocampal neuronal loss and cognitive deficits following traumatic brain injury in mice. Restor Neurol Neurosci 2008, 26:45–56.
5. Hicks RR, Zhang L, Dhillon HS, Prasad MR, Seroogy KB: Expression of trkB mRNA is altered in rat hippocampus after experimental brain trauma. Brain Res Mol Brain Res 1998, 59:264–268.
6. Brambilla R, Cottini L, Fumagalli M, Ceruti S, Abbracchio MP: Blockade of A2A adenosine receptors prevents basic fibroblast growth factor-induced reactive astrogliosis in rat striatal primary astrocytes. Glia 2003, 43:190–194.
7. Orr AG, Orr AL, Li XJ, Gross RE, Traynelis SF: Adenosine A(2A) receptor mediates microglial process retraction. Nat Neurosci 2009, 12:872–878.
8. Talley Watts L, Sprague S, Zheng W, Garling RJ, Jimenez D, Digicaylioglu M, Lechleiter J: Purinergic 2Y1 receptor stimulation decreases cerebral edema and reactive gliosis in a traumatic brain injury model. J Neurotrauma 2013, 30:55–66.
9. Bachstetter AD, Rowe RK, Kaneko M, Goulding D, Lifshitz J, Van Eldik LJ: The p38alpha MAPK regulates microglial responsiveness to diffuse traumatic brain injury. J Neurosci 2013, 33:6143–6153.
10. Frey LC: Epidemiology of posttraumatic epilepsy: a critical review. Epilepsia 2003, 44(Suppl 10):11–17.
11. Annegers JF, Hauser WA, Coan SP, Rocca WA: A population-based study of seizures after traumatic brain injuries. N Engl J Med 1998, 338:20–24.
12. Beghi E: Overview of studies to prevent posttraumatic epilepsy. Epilepsia 2003, 44(Suppl 10):21–26.
13. Goodrich GS, Kabakov AY, Hameed MQ, Dhamne SC, Rosenberg PA, Rotenberg A: Ceftriaxone treatment after traumatic brain injury restores expression of the glutamate transporter GLT-1, reduces regional gliosis, and reduces posttraumatic seizures in the rat. J Neurotrauma 2013, 30:1434–1441.
14. Chidlow JH Jr, Sessa WC: Caveolae, caveolins, and cavins: complex control of cellular signalling and inflammation. Cardiovasc Res 2010, 86:219–225.
15. Shin T, Kim H, Jin JK, Moon C, Ahn M, Tanuma N, Matsumoto Y: Expression of caveolin-1, -2, and -3 in the spinal cords of Lewis rats with experimental autoimmune encephalomyelitis. J Neuroimmunol 2005, 165:11–20.
16. Silva WI, Maldonado HM, Velazquez G, Garcia JO, Gonzalez FA: Caveolins in glial cell model systems: from detection to significance. J Neurochem 2007, 103(Suppl 1):101–112.
17. Stern CM, Mermelstein PG: Caveolin regulation of neuronal intracellular signaling. Cell Mol Life Sci 2010, 67:3785–3795.
18. Mirza MK, Yuan J, Gao XP, Garrean S, Brovkovych V, Malik AB, Tiruppathi C, Zhao YY: Caveolin-1 deficiency dampens toll-like receptor 4 signaling through eNOS activation. Am J Pathol 2010, 176:2344–2351.
19. Head BP, Peart JN, Panneerselvam M, Yokoyama T, Pearn ML, Niesman IR, Bonds JA, Schilling JM, Miyanohara A, Headrick J, Ali SS, Roth DM, Patel PM, Patel HH: Loss of caveolin-1 accelerates neurodegeneration and aging. PLoS One 2010, 5:e15697.
20. Niesman IR, Zemke N, Fridolfsson HN, Haushalter KJ, Levy K, Grove A, Schnoor R, Finley JC, Patel PM, Roth DM, Head BP, Patel HH: Caveolin isoform switching as a molecular, structural, and metabolic regulator of microglia. Mol Cell Neurosci 2013, 56:283–297.
21. Hagiwara Y, Sasaoka T, Araishi K, Imamura M, Yorifuji H, Nonaka I, Ozawa E, Kikuchi T: Caveolin-3 deficiency causes muscle degeneration in mice. Hum Mol Genet 2000, 9:3047–3054.
22. Krajewska M, You Z, Rong J, Kress C, Huang X, Yang J, Kyoda T, Leyva R, Banares S, Hu Y, Sze CH, Whalen MJ, Salmena L, Hakem R, Head BP, Reed JC, Krajewski S: Neuronal deletion of caspase 8 protects against brain injury in mouse models of controlled cortical impact and kainic acid-induced excitotoxicity. PLoS One 2011, 6:e24341.
23. Krajewska M, Smith LH, Rong J, Huang X, Hyer ML, Zeps N, Iacopetta B, Linke SP, Olson AH, Reed JC, Krajewski S: Image analysis algorithms for immunohistochemical assessment of cell death events and fibrosis in tissue sections. J Histochem Cytochem 2009, 57:649–663.
24. Head BP, Patel HH, Tsutsumi YM, Hu Y, Mejia T, Mora RC, Insel PA, Roth DM, Drummond JC, Patel PM: Caveolin-1 expression is essential for N-methyl-D-aspartate receptor-mediated Src and extracellular signal-regulated kinase 1/2 activation and protection of primary neurons from ischemic cell death. FASEB J 2008, 22:828–840.
25. Head BP, Hu Y, Finley JC, Saldana MD, Bonds JA, Miyanohara A, Niesman IR, Ali SS, Murray F, Insel PA, Roth DM, Patel HH, Patel PM: Neuron-targeted

caveolin-1 protein enhances signaling and promotes arborization of primary neurons. *J Biol Chem* 2011, **286:**33310–33321.

26. Paylor R, Nguyen M, Crawley JN, Patrick J, Beaudet A, Orr-Urtreger A: **Alpha7 nicotinic receptor subunits are not necessary for hippocampal-dependent learning or sensorimotor gating: a behavioral characterization of Acra7-deficient mice.** *Learn Mem* 1998, **5:**302–316.

27. Carter RJ, Morton J, Dunnett SB: **Motor coordination and balance in rodents.** *Curr Protoc Neurosci* 2001, **Chapter 8:**Unit 8.12.

28. Deacon RM, Rawlins JN: **T-maze alternation in the rodent.** *Nat Protoc* 2006, **1:**7–12.

29. Sharma S, Rakoczy S, Brown-Borg H: **Assessment of spatial memory in mice.** *Life Sci* 2010, **87:**521–536.

30. Kleschevnikov AM, Belichenko PV, Faizi M, Jacobs LF, Htun K, Shamloo M, Mobley WC: **Deficits in cognition and synaptic plasticity in a mouse model of down syndrome ameliorated by GABAB receptor antagonists.** *J Neurosci* 2012, **32:**9217–9227.

31. Ali SS, Young JW, Wallace CK, Gresack J, Jeste DV, Geyer MA, Dugan LL, Risbrough VB: **Initial evidence linking synaptic superoxide production with poor short-term memory in aged mice.** *Brain Res* 2011, **1368:**65–70.

32. Mukherjee S, Katki K, Arisi GM, Foresti ML, Shapiro LA: **Early TBI-induced cytokine alterations are similarly detected by two distinct methods of multiplex assay.** *Front Mol Neurosci* 2011, **4:**21.

33. Truong TQ, Aubin D, Bourgeois P, Falstrault L, Brissette L: **Opposite effect of caveolin-1 in the metabolism of high-density and low-density lipoproteins.** *Biochim Biophys Acta* 2006, **1761:**24–36.

34. Wu L, Gonias SL: **The low-density lipoprotein receptor-related protein-1 associates transiently with lipid rafts.** *J Cell biochem* 2005, **96:**1021–1033.

35. Neary JT, Kang Y, Tran M, Feld J: **Traumatic injury activates protein kinase B/Akt in cultured astrocytes: role of extracellular ATP and P2 purinergic receptors.** *J Neurotrauma* 2005, **22:**491–500.

36. Huang T, Solano J, He D, Loutfi M, Dietrich WD, Kuluz JW: **Traumatic injury activates MAP kinases in astrocytes: mechanisms of hypothermia and hyperthermia.** *J Neurotrauma* 2009, **26:**1535–1545.

37. Jasmin JF, Rengo G, Lymperopoulos A, Gupta R, Eaton GJ, Quann K, Gonzales DM, Mercier I, Koch WJ, Lisanti MP: **Caveolin-1 deficiency exacerbates cardiac dysfunction and reduces survival in mice with myocardial infarction.** *Am J Physiol Heart Circ Physiol* 2011, **300:**H1274–H1281.

38. Gu Y, Zheng G, Xu M, Li Y, Chen X, Zhu W, Tong Y, Chung SK, Liu KJ, Shen J: **Caveolin-1 regulates nitric oxide-mediated matrix metalloproteinases activity and blood–brain barrier permeability in focal cerebral ischemia and reperfusion injury.** *J Neurochem* 2012, **120:**147–156.

39. Gioiosa L, Raggi C, Ricceri L, Jasmin JF, Frank PG, Capozza F, Lisanti MP, Alleva E, Sargiacomo M, Laviola G: **Altered emotionality, spatial memory and cholinergic function in caveolin-1 knock-out mice.** *Behav Brain Res* 2008, **188:**255–262.

40. Adewuya AO, Oseni SB: **Impact of psychiatric morbidity on parent-rated quality of life in Nigerian adolescents with epilepsy.** *Epilepsy Behav* 2005, **7:**497–501.

41. Duchowny M, Jayakar P, Levin B: **Aberrant neural circuits in malformations of cortical development and focal epilepsy.** *Neurology* 2000, **55:**423–428.

42. Babb TL, Ying Z, Mikuni N, Nishiyama K, Drazba J, Bingaman W, Wyllie E, Wyllie CJ, Yacubova K: **Brain plasticity and cellular mechanisms of epileptogenesis in human and experimental cortical dysplasia.** *Epilepsia* 2000, **41**(Suppl 6):S76–S81.

43. Kim JH, Jang BG, Choi BY, Kim HS, Sohn M, Chung TN, Choi HC, Song HK, Suh SW: **Post-treatment of an NADPH oxidase inhibitor prevents seizure-induced neuronal death.** *Brain Res* 2013, **1499:**163–172.

44. Cheret C, Gervais A, Lelli A, Colin C, Amar L, Ravassard P, Mallet J, Cumano A, Krause KH, Mallat M: **Neurotoxic activation of microglia is promoted by a nox1-dependent NADPH oxidase.** *J Neurosci* 2008, **28:**12039–12051.

45. Pitkanen A, Lukasiuk K: **Molecular and cellular basis of epileptogenesis in symptomatic epilepsy.** *Epilepsy Behav* 2009, **14**(Suppl 1):16–25.

46. Pitkanen A, Lukasiuk K: **Mechanisms of epileptogenesis and potential treatment targets.** *Lancet Neurol* 2011, **10:**173–186.

47. Schierhout G, Roberts I: **Anti-epileptic drugs for preventing seizures following acute traumatic brain injury.** *Cochrane Database Syst Rev* 2001, **4:**CD000173.

48. Foresti ML, Arisi GM, Katki K, Montanez A, Sanchez RM, Shapiro LA: **Chemokine CCL2 and its receptor CCR2 are increased in the hippocampus following pilocarpine-induced status epilepticus.** *J Neuroinflammation* 2009, **6:**40.

49. Semple BD, Bye N, Rancan M, Ziebell JM, Morganti-Kossmann MC: **Role of CCL2 (MCP-1) in traumatic brain injury (TBI): evidence from severe TBI patients and CCL2–/– mice.** *J Cerebral Blood Flow Metabol* 2010, **30:**769–782.

50. Andjelkovic AV, Song L, Dzenko KA, Cong H, Pachter JS: **Functional expression of CCR2 by human fetal astrocytes.** *J Neurosci Res* 2002, **70:**219–231.

51. Ge S, Pachter JS: **Caveolin-1 knockdown by small interfering RNA suppresses responses to the chemokine monocyte chemoattractant protein-1 by human astrocytes.** *J Biol Chem* 2004, **279:**6688–6695.

52. Guzik-Kornacka A, Sliwa A, Plucinska G, Lukasiuk K: **Status epilepticus evokes prolonged increase in the expression of CCL3 and CCL4 mRNA and protein in the rat brain.** *Acta Neurobiolog Experimental* 2011, **71:**193–207.

53. Patel HH, Murray F, Insel PA: **G-protein-coupled receptor-signaling components in membrane raft and caveolae microdomains.** *Handb Exp Pharmacol* 2008, **186:**167–184.

54. Hasko G, Pacher P, Vizi ES, Illes P: **Adenosine receptor signaling in the brain immune system.** *Trends Pharmacol Sci* 2005, **26:**511–516.

55. Fields RD, Burnstock G: **Purinergic signalling in neuron-glia interactions.** *Nat Rev Neurosci* 2006, **7:**423–436.

56. Boison D, Chen JF, Fredholm BB: **Adenosine signaling and function in glial cells.** *Cell Death Differ* 2010, **17:**1071–1082.

57. Fedele DE, Li T, Lan JQ, Fredholm BB, Boison D: **Adenosine A1 receptors are crucial in keeping an epileptic focus localized.** *Exp Neurol* 2006, **200:**184–190.

58. Kochanek PM, Vagni VA, Janesko KL, Washington CB, Crumrine PK, Garman RH, Jenkins LW, Clark RS, Homanics GE, Dixon CE, Schnermann J, Jackson EK: **Adenosine A1 receptor knockout mice develop lethal status epilepticus after experimental traumatic brain injury.** *J Cerebral Blood Flow Metabol* 2006, **26:**565–575.

59. Ribeiro JA, Sebastiao AM, de Mendonca A: **Adenosine receptors in the nervous system: pathophysiological implications.** *Prog Neurobiol* 2002, **68:**377–392.

60. Shen HY, Chen JF: **Adenosine A(2A) receptors in psychopharmacology: modulators of behavior, mood and cognition.** *Curr Neuropharmacol* 2009, **7:**195–206.

61. Dixon AK, Widdowson L, Richardson PJ: **Desensitisation of the adenosine A1 receptor by the A2A receptor in the rat striatum.** *J Neurochem* 1997, **69:**315–321.

62. Gomes C, Ferreira R, George J, Sanches R, Rodrigues DI, Goncalves N, Cunha RA: **Activation of microglial cells triggers a release of brain-derived neurotrophic factor (BDNF) inducing their proliferation in an adenosine A2A receptor-dependent manner: A2A receptor blockade prevents BDNF release and proliferation of microglia.** *J Neuroinflammation* 2013, **10:**16.

63. Di Virgilio F, Ceruti S, Bramanti P, Abbracchio MP: **Purinergic signalling in inflammation of the central nervous system.** *Trends Neurosci* 2009, **32:**79–87.

64. Heverin M, Engel T, Meaney S, Jimenez-Mateos EM, Al-Saudi R, Henshall DC: **Bi-lateral changes to hippocampal cholesterol levels during epileptogenesis and in chronic epilepsy following focal-onset status epilepticus in mice.** *Brain Res* 2012, **1480:**81–90.

65. Biagini G, Marinelli C, Panuccio G, Puia G, Avoli M: **Glia-neuron interactions: neurosteroids and epileptogenesis.** In *Jasper's Basic mechanisms of the epilepsies.* 4th edition. Edited by Noebels JL, Avoli M, Rogawski MA, Olsen RW, Delgado-Escueta AV. Bethesda MD: National Center for Biotechnology Information (US); 2012. http://www.ncbi.nlm.nih.gov/books/NBK98132/.

66. Adibhatla RM, Hatcher JF: **Altered lipid metabolism in brain injury and disorders.** *Subcell Biochem* 2008, **49:**241–268.

67. Diaz-Arrastia R, Gong Y, Fair S, Scott KD, Garcia MC, Carlile MC, Agostini MA, Van Ness PC: **Increased risk of late posttraumatic seizures associated with inheritance of APOE epsilon4 allele.** *Arch Neurol* 2003, **60:**818–822.

68. Spuch C, Ortolano S, Navarro C: **LRP-1 and LRP-2 receptors function in the membrane neuron: trafficking mechanisms and proteolytic processing in Alzheimer's disease.** *Front Physiol* 2012, **3:**269.

12

Long noncoding RNA MALAT1 in exosomes drives regenerative function and modulates inflammation-linked networks following traumatic brain injury

Niketa A. Patel[1,2*†], Lauren Daly Moss[3†], Jea-Young Lee[3†], Naoki Tajiri[3,4], Sandra Acosta[3], Charles Hudson[1], Sajan Parag[2], Denise R. Cooper[1,2], Cesario V. Borlongan[3,5*] and Paula C. Bickford[1,3,5*] (iD)

Abstract

Background: Neuroinflammation is a common therapeutic target for traumatic brain injury (TBI) due to its contribution to delayed secondary cell death and has the potential to occur for years after the initial insult. Exosomes from adipose-derived stem cells (hASCs) containing the long noncoding RNA MALAT1 are a novel, cell-free regenerative approach to long-term recovery after traumatic brain injury (TBI) that have the potential to modulate inflammation at the genomic level. The long noncoding RNA MALAT1 has been shown to be an important component of the secretome of hASCs.

Methods: We isolated exosomes from hASC containing or depleted of MALAT1. The hASC-derived exosomes were then administered intravenously to rats following a mild controlled cortical impact (CCI). We followed the rats with behavior, in vivo imaging, histology, and RNA sequencing (RNA Seq).

Results: Using in vivo imaging, we show that exosomes migrate into the spleen within 1 h following administration and enter the brain several hours later following TBI. Significant recovery of function on motor behavior as well as a reduction in cortical brain injury was observed after TBI in rats treated with exosomes. Treatment with either exosomes depleted of MALAT1 or conditioned media depleted of exosomes showed limited regenerative effects, demonstrating the importance of MALAT1 in exosome-mediated recovery. Analysis of the brain and spleen transcriptome using RNA Seq showed MALAT1-dependent modulation of inflammation-related pathways, cell cycle, cell death, and regenerative molecular pathways. Importantly, our data demonstrates that MALAT1 regulates expression of other noncoding RNAs including snoRNAs.

Conclusion: We demonstrate that MALAT1 in hASC-derived exosomes modulates multiple therapeutic targets, including inflammation, and has tremendous therapeutic potential for treatment of TBI.

* Correspondence: Niketa.Patel@va.gov; npatel@health.usf.edu;
cborlong@health.usf.edu; pbickfor@health.usf.edu
†Niketa A. Patel, Lauren Daly Moss and Jea-Young Lee contributed equally to this work.
[1]James A Haley Veterans Hospital, Research Service, Tampa, FL, USA
[3]Department of Neurosurgery and Brain Repair, University of South Florida Morsani College of Medicine, Tampa, FL, USA
Full list of author information is available at the end of the article

Background

Approximately two million Americans suffer from traumatic brain injury (TBI) annually, accounting for 30% of all injury-related fatalities [1, 2]. Currently, treatment options for TBI consist predominantly of rehabilitation and symptom management. Thus, there is an urgent need for novel treatments to prevent or slow the progression of secondary injury in TBI. Due to its contribution to secondary cell death, which can occur years after the initial insult, neuroinflammation is a common target for prospective TBI therapeutics [3–8]. Recruitment of macrophages into the area of brain damage is an important aspect of secondary injury, and numerous approaches have been explored to intervene in this process [9–12]. One of the organs important in the flux of monocytes and T cells into the peripheral circulation following injury is the spleen, and it has been demonstrated that the intact spleen is important for the neuroprotective action of multipotent adult progenitor cells after several models of brain insult [13–16].

The neuroprotective capacity of mesenchymal stem cells (MSCs) derived from adipose tissue has garnered great interest in regenerative medicine. Human adipose-derived stem cells (hASCs) manifest a secretome that is capable of modulating the environment of the host. Among these secreted molecules, small membrane-bound vesicles known as exosomes have gained particular interest due to their diverse cargo including cellular proteins, mRNA, and noncoding RNAs, as well as their ability to evade immune rejection by the host and modify immune responses [17]. Compelling evidence suggests that exosomes play an important role in cell-to-cell communication, and rats or mice treated with exosomes have demonstrated improved functional recovery after models of stroke and TBI [18–20]. These MSC-derived extracellular vesicles are also thought to modulate immune function as part of their mechanism of prevention of injury following TBI [21].

Long noncoding RNA (lncRNA) are important regulators of gene expression and have been shown to mediate several pathways such as cell cycle, proliferation as well as apoptosis, and immune modulation. Additionally, they are involved in epigenetic regulation, transcription, and translation as well as alternative splicing of genes. Aberrant expression of lncRNAs is associated with human diseases [22–25]. Of the cargo secreted in exosomes, lncRNA metastasis-associated lung adenocarcinoma transcript 1 (MALAT1) controls key biological processes such as cellular proliferation and differentiation and is thought to have a special role in regeneration after injury [26–28]. We previously used the secretome (collected as conditioned media) of hASC as treatment and showed that it promotes repair following TBI [26]. MALAT1 is part of the cargo secreted by hASC [29], and our in vitro studies using the HT22 cell line demonstrated that MALAT1 promotes survival and proliferation [27]. Here, we sought to examine the use of hASC-derived exosomes as a novel, cell-free regenerative approach to injury recovery in an in vivo model of TBI. We identify the cellular processes crucial to recovery that are specifically mediated by MALAT1. Importantly, we also elucidate the genomic impact exosome treatment using RNA sequencing (RNA Seq) transcriptome analysis. Our results show that MALAT1 in hASC-derived exosomes is therapeutically beneficial after TBI.

Methods

Exosome isolation and collection from ASCs

hASC (Zenbio, catalog #ASC-F) were trypsinized, and cell pellets were collected in 100 μL Nucleofector® kit (Lonza, catalog #VPE-1001) and combined with pMAX GFP (2 μg). The cell/DNA solution was transferred to a cuvette, and the program initiated (0.34 kV, 960 μF). Medium (500 μL) was added immediately, and cells were gently transferred to 100-mm plates and allowed to grow for 48 h. To deplete MALAT from hASC exosomes, we used MALAT1 antisense oligonucleotide (ASO; ID 39524 ASO from Ionis Pharmaceuticals), validated for specificity and designed for efficient uptake by cells. The ASOs were added to hASC and incubated for 48 h. The expression levels of MALAT1 were verified in the exosomes using human MALAT1 primers in qPCR. Exosomes were isolated from conditioned media (CM) and verified that exosomes contain GFP as previously described by our lab [27, 29]. Briefly, CM derived from hASC was collected after 48 h and centrifuged at $3000g$ for 15 min to remove dead cells. ExoQuick™ (System Biosciences, Catalog #EXOTC-50A-1) reagent was added to the CM and incubated overnight at 4 °C along with XenoLight 1,1-dioctadecyl-3,3,3,3-tetramethylindotricbocyanine iodide (DiR) (catalog #125964; Caliper Life Sciences). Following centrifugation at $1500g$ for 30 min, the pellet was further processed. ExoCap™ (JSR Life Sciences, Catalog #EX-COM) composite reagent containing magnetic beads for CD9, CD63, and CD81 was used to purify exosomes. Exosomes were eluted from beads using 500 μL of the manufacturer's elution buffer. Buffer was then exchanged by Ambicon columns. Nanoparticle tracking analysis from NanoSight (NTA3.1, Build 3.1.46 RRID SCR-014239) was used to analyze peak diameter and concentration of exosomes obtained from 10^6 hASC. Analysis showed exosome size to be 89 ± 7 nm.

Animal model and surgical procedures

The University of South Florida Institutional Animal Care and Use Committee (IACUC) approved all experimental procedures with animals. All rats were housed under normal conditions (20 °C, 50% relative humidity, and a 12-h light/dark cycle). All studies were performed by personnel blinded to the treatment condition.

A total of 79 Fisher 344 male rats were subjected to either TBI by controlled cortical impact or sham surgery. The rats were randomly distributed into the following groups: surgery with no TBI (sham control C, $N = 11$), TBI with unconditioned media as vehicle (T; $N = 20$), TBI treated with exosomes (TE, $N = 18$), TBI treated with exosomes depleted of MALAT1 (TEdM, $N = 20$), and TBI with injection of conditioned media depleted of exosomes (TdCM; $N = 7$). Deep anesthesia was administered to all rats undergoing TBI surgery using 1–2% isoflurane in nitrous oxide/oxygen (69%/30%) and was maintained using a gas mask. TBI-induced animals were fixed in a stereotaxic frame (David Kopf Instruments). The TBI procedure was performed as previously described [26]. Briefly, the skull was exposed by a midline incision, coordinates of + 0.2 mm anterior and + 0.2 mm lateral to the midline were found, and craniotomy was performed; the brain was then impacted at the frontoparietal cortex with a velocity of 6.0 m/s reaching a depth of 0.5 mm (mild TBI) below the dura matter layer and a dwell time of 150 ms. Body temperature of the animals was maintained within normal limits by a computer-operated thermal pad and rectal thermometer. All animals were closely monitored postoperatively and analgesic ketoprofen was administered prior to surgery and as needed thereafter. Rats were maintained on regular rodent diet throughout the experiment.

Intravenous administration of exosomes and CM

Three hours after TBI induction, rats were anesthetized using 1–2% isoflurane in nitrous oxide/oxygen (69%/30%) and were maintained using a gas mask. Intravenous injections through the jugular vein were then performed and divided as follows: TBI-Veh (T) received 500-μl unconditioned media, TBI animals with exosomes depleted conditioned media (TdCM) received 500-μl conditioned media depleted of exosomes, TBI animals with exosomes (TE) received exosomes (100 μg in 500 μl of sterile saline), and TBI animals with exosomes depleted of MALAT1 (TEdM) received exosomes (100 μg in 500 μl of sterile saline). Sham animals did not receive any injection, and animals receiving unconditioned media were used as control groups. To evaluate the migration of the transplanted exosomes, exosomes were incubated with DiR during isolation.

XenoLight DiR for in vivo and ex vivo biodistribution imaging procedures

To visualize DiR fluorescence emitted from the injected exosomes in vivo, animal's abdomens were shaved to avoid light scattering and anesthetized in a chamber with 3.0% isoflurane. Animals were then transferred from the chamber to the IVIS Spectrum 200 Imaging System (Xenogen), and the isoflurane level was maintained at 1–2% throughout image acquisition. The biodistribution of DiR-labeled exosomes were monitored in vivo at 1, 4, 12, 24, 48, and 72 h and again at 11 days post-surgery and transplantation. Images were also obtained of ex vivo organs including the brain, liver, lungs, and spleen after 1, 3, 7, and 11 days post-surgery and transplantation. Full-body imaging was performed ventrally at all time points, and a second set of images were obtained for the head region using a higher magnification. The parameters used throughout the experiment were as follows: exposure time = auto; lamp voltage = high; F/stop = 2; binning = 8; excitation filter = 745 nm; emission filter = 800 nm; field of view = D (for whole body), C (for ex vivo organs), or B (for head region). All captured images were analyzed using Living Image Software 4.0 (Xenogen RRID:SCR_014247). To analyze the change in DiR fluorescence intensity, identical regions of interest (ROIs) were placed on the abdomen and head area for all animals. The same ROI was also placed on the control animal as the background reference. Background efficiency was subtracted from each of the individual animal's efficiency and presented as an average radiant efficiency (photons per second per square centimeter per steridian divided by microwatts per square centimeter).

Behavioral testing

Each rat was subjected to a series of behavioral tests to assess motor and neurological performance of animals, at baseline before surgery and post TBI at days 0, 3, and 7.

Elevated body swing test (EBST)

EBST is a measure of asymmetrical motor behavior that does not require animal training or drug injection [30]. The rats were held, in the vertical axis, 1 in. from the base of its tail and then elevated to an inch above the surface on which it has been resting. The frequency and direction of the swing behavior were recorded for 20 tail elevations. A swing was counted when the head of the rat moved 10° from the vertical axis to either side. A score of 10 indicates no bias. The higher number of swings made to one side was added per group and divided by the n, giving us the average number of biased swings per treatment group.

Forelimb akinesia

Before and after TBI surgery, rats from all groups were evaluated for forelimb akinesia [31]. Ipsilateral and contralateral forepaw strength and motility were scored by two experimentally blinded evaluators using the following forelimb akinesia scale. On a scale of 1 to 3, 1 is normal, 2 is impaired, and 3 is severely impaired. Scores were tallied for each individual animal, and then, mean scores for treatment groups were used for analyses.

Paw grasp

Before and after TBI surgery, grip strength of rats from all groups was evaluated. An abnormal grip is indicative of impaired neuromuscular function. In this test, rats were held by their bodies against a pole. Both ipsilateral and contralateral paw grip strength were scored by two experimentally masked evaluators using the following grip strength scale. On a scale of 1 to 3, 1 is normal, 2 is impaired, and 3 is severely impaired. Scores were tallied for each individual animal, and then, mean scores for treatment groups were used for analyses.

Brain and organ harvesting, fixation, and sectioning

Under deep anesthesia, rats were sacrificed on days 1, 3, 7, and 11 following TBI for protein analysis, RNA sequencing, and/or immunohistochemical investigations. Briefly, animals were perfused through the ascending aorta with 200 ml of cold PBS, followed by 200 ml of 4% paraformaldehyde in phosphate buffer (PB). The brains, spleen, lungs, and liver were removed and post-fixed in the same fixative for 24 h, followed by 30% sucrose in PB until completely sunk. Series of coronal sections were cut at a thickness of 40 um with a cryostat and stored at − 20 °C. Six coronal sections between the anterior edge and posterior edge of the impacted area were collected and processed for GFP expression in exosome-injected animals.

Measurement of impact and peri-impact area: Nissl staining analysis

Serial sections corresponding to the same group of animals were stained with Nissl (Thermo Fisher Scientific Cat# N21483 RRID:AB_2572212) for impact and peri-impact calculations. Six coronal sections between the anterior edge and posterior edge of the impacted area were collected and processed for Nissl staining from each brain perfused at day 11 after TBI. Sections were cut at a thickness of 40 μm by a cryostat. Coronal tissue sections were randomly selected for measurement of impact and peri-impact area. Brain sections were examined using a light microscope (Olympus) and Keyence microscope. The impact area was outlined and measured in each of the six slices and quantified by a computer-assisted image analysis system (NIH Image RRID:SCR_003070). To measure the peri-impact area, we examined the same six sections through the impact zone and placed four 20× fields along the edge of the impact core. Each 20× image was then analyzed for the number of live neurons with Nissl staining (see Fig. 1f for example). Impact and peri-impact area was then expressed as a percentage of the ipsilateral hemisphere compared with the contralateral hemisphere.

RNA sequencing: RNA quality control

RNA was isolated from the brains (area near impact site) and spleens of rats at day 7 following TBI in the sham surgery—control (C), TBI with vehicle (T), TBI treated with exosomes (TE), and TBI treated with MALAT1-depleted exosomes (TEdM) groups. Four rats from each group were randomly chosen and pooled to maximize biological diversity and sent for RNA Seq (Ocean Ridge Biosciences). Eight total RNA samples (four rat spleen tissue and four rat brain tissue) were submitted to Ocean Ridge Biosciences for RNA sequencing. RNA was quantified by O.D. measurement and assessed for quality on a 1% agarose–2% formaldehyde RNA quality control (QC) gel. The RNA was then digested with RNase-free DNase I (Epicentre; Part # D9905K) and re-purified on RNeasy MinElute columns (Qiagen; Part # 74204) using an alternative high ethanol protocol to preserve low molecular weight (LMW) RNAs. The newly purified RNA samples were then quantified by O.D. measurement.

Library preparation

Ribosomal RNA was depleted from 1 μg of DNA-free total RNA using the Ribo-Zero Gold rRNA Removal Kit for Human/Mouse/Rat (Illumina, part number MRZG126). Template DNA molecules suitable for cluster generation were then prepared from the rRNA-depleted samples using the ScriptSeq V2 RNA-Seq Library Prep Kit (Illumina, part number SSV21124). The quality and size distribution of the amplified libraries were determined by chip-based capillary electrophoresis on an Agilent 2100 Bioanalyzer. Libraries were quantified using the KAPA Library Quantification Kit (Kapa Biosystems, Boston, MA).

Sequencing

The libraries were pooled at equimolar concentrations and diluted prior to loading onto the flow cell of the Illumina cBot cluster station. The libraries were extended and bridge amplified to create sequence clusters using the Illumina HiSeq PE Cluster Kit v4 and sequenced on an Illumina HiSeq Flow Cell v4 with 50-bp paired-end reads plus index read using the Illumina HiSeq SBS Kit v4. Real-time image analysis and base calling were performed on the instrument using the HiSeq Sequencing Control Software version 2.2.58. All samples had a minimum of 43,303,826 passed-filter single-end reads. The sequences aligned at an average of 72% ± 2% (SD) efficiency to the reference genome.

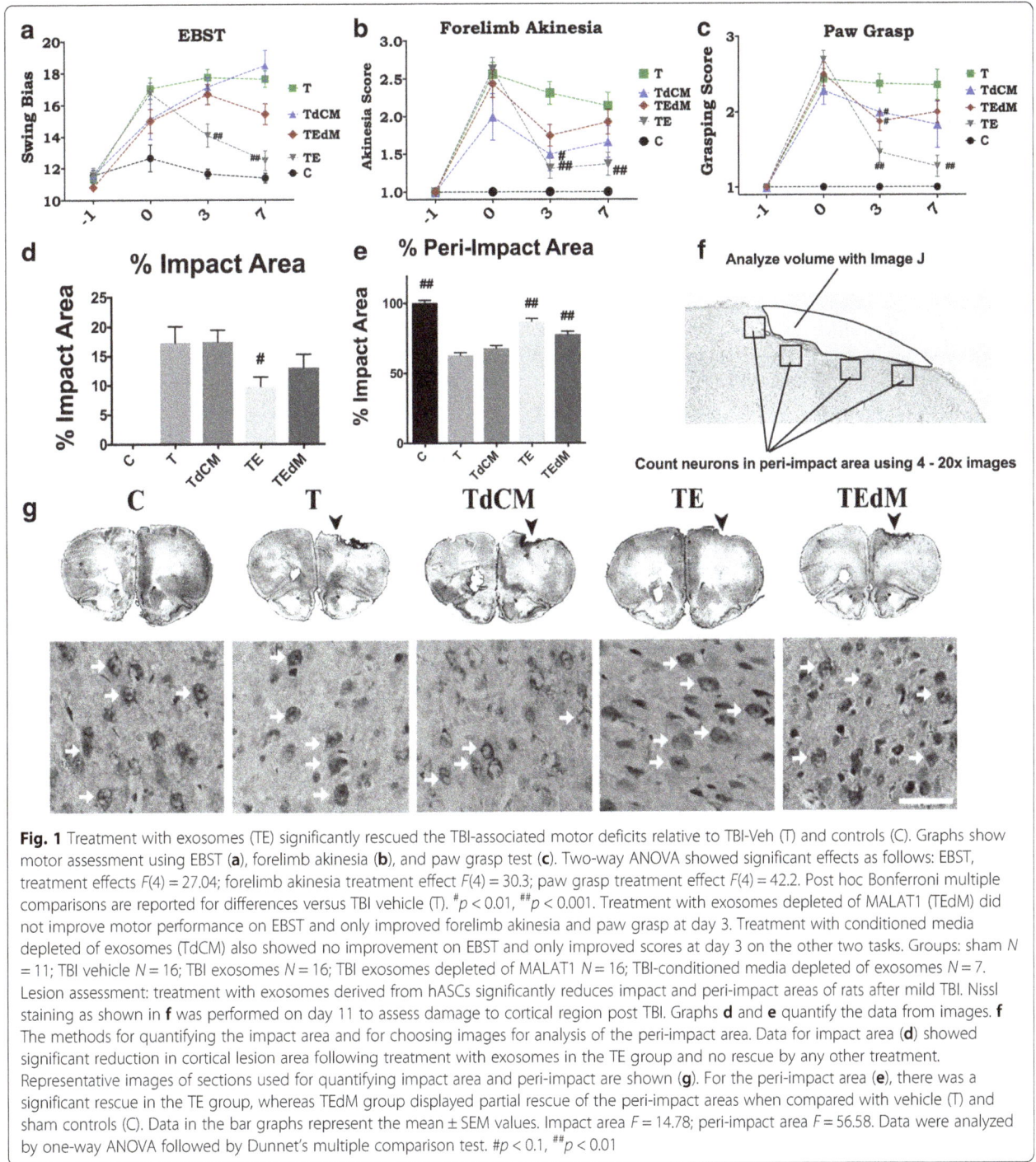

Fig. 1 Treatment with exosomes (TE) significantly rescued the TBI-associated motor deficits relative to TBI-Veh (T) and controls (C). Graphs show motor assessment using EBST (**a**), forelimb akinesia (**b**), and paw grasp test (**c**). Two-way ANOVA showed significant effects as follows: EBST, treatment effects $F(4) = 27.04$; forelimb akinesia treatment effect $F(4) = 30.3$; paw grasp treatment effect $F(4) = 42.2$. Post hoc Bonferroni multiple comparisons are reported for differences versus TBI vehicle (T). $^{#}p < 0.01$, $^{##}p < 0.001$. Treatment with exosomes depleted of MALAT1 (TEdM) did not improve motor performance on EBST and only improved forelimb akinesia and paw grasp at day 3. Treatment with conditioned media depleted of exosomes (TdCM) also showed no improvement on EBST and only improved scores at day 3 on the other two tasks. Groups: sham $N = 11$; TBI vehicle $N = 16$; TBI exosomes $N = 16$; TBI exosomes depleted of MALAT1 $N = 16$; TBI-conditioned media depleted of exosomes $N = 7$. Lesion assessment: treatment with exosomes derived from hASCs significantly reduces impact and peri-impact areas of rats after mild TBI. Nissl staining as shown in **f** was performed on day 11 to assess damage to cortical region post TBI. Graphs **d** and **e** quantify the data from images. **f** The methods for quantifying the impact area and for choosing images for analysis of the peri-impact area. Data for impact area (**d**) showed significant reduction in cortical lesion area following treatment with exosomes in the TE group and no rescue by any other treatment. Representative images of sections used for quantifying impact area and peri-impact are shown (**g**). For the peri-impact area (**e**), there was a significant rescue in the TE group, whereas TEdM group displayed partial rescue of the peri-impact areas when compared with vehicle (T) and sham controls (C). Data in the bar graphs represent the mean ± SEM values. Impact area $F = 14.78$; peri-impact area $F = 56.58$. Data were analyzed by one-way ANOVA followed by Dunnet's multiple comparison test. #$p < 0.1$, ##$p < 0.01$

Alignment to genome

Sequence alignment was performed using TopHat v1.4.1 (RRID SCR-013035) with the following settings:

tophat -p 2 -o [OUTPUT FOLDER] –library-type fr-secondstrand –r [Dx] –mate-std-dev [Ds] [rn5 BOW-TIE GENOME INDEX] [FASTQ 1] [FATSQ 2]

where Dx and Ds represent sample-specific values for the mean and standard deviation, respectively, of the inner distance between reads, as determined by non-gapped alignment to rat mRNA. rn5 BOWTIE GENOME INDEX was built from the soft-masked genome sequence. In practice FASTQ files for each sample were split into multiple FASTQs having 4 million reads each in order to accelerate processing.

ncRNA counting and annotation

The number of reads aligning to each ncRNA feature were counted using BEDtools v2.16.2 (RRID SCR-006646) with the following settings: bedtools multicov -bams C80R4ANXX_s8illumina12index_4_SL134409.fastq_05.-bam -bed rnacentral_active_v3_rat-mouse-human.gff C80R4ANXX_s8illumina12index_4_SL134409.fastq_05/counts.txt.

In practice, FASTQ files for each sample were split into multiple FASTQs having 4 million reads each in order to accelerate processing. For each sample, the resulting BAM files were merged as well as the count files. For all ncRNAs having at least one read aligned, annotations were added using RNAcentral's RESTful API. The RPKM values were filtered to retain a list of ncRNAs with an RPKM equivalent to 50 mapped reads in one or more samples. The threshold of 50 mapped reads per ncRNA is considered the Reliable Quantification Threshold, since the RPKM values for a ncRNA represented by 50 reads should be reproducible in technical replicates. To avoid reporting large fold changes due to random variation of counts from low abundance ncRNA, RPKM values equivalent to a count of <= 10 reads per ncRNA were replaced in the following way. First, for each sample, the RPKM value equivalent to 10 reads/ncRNA was calculated (assuming a median ncRNA length of 0.122 kb). These RPKMs were then averaged across all the samples in the experiment, and this average value was used for replacement.

Fold change calculations

The filtered RPKM data for 19,058 detectable rat genes (RPKM values > Reliable Quantification Threshold (RQT) in at least one sample) were used to calculate the fold changes for TBI exosome/TBI vehicle, TBI exosome MALAT1/TBI exosome, and TBI vehicle/no TBI independently for the spleen and brain samples. Fold changes are expressed as the negative reciprocal in tables and for additional analysis. The splicing index was calculated based on the following formula: exon RPKM/gene RPKM.

Hierarchical clustering

Similarly, the same RPKM data for all 19,058 detectable rat genes were used for hierarchical clustering analysis by Cluster 3.0 software[4] (RRID SCR-013505). Genes were log-2 transformed and median centered prior to hierarchical clustering. Hierarchical clustering was conducted on genes and samples using centered correlation as the similarity metric and average linkage as the clustering method. The intensity scale shown is arbitrary.

Real-time qPCR using SYBR green

Total RNA as described above for RNA Seq was used for validation. One microliter of cDNA was amplified by real-time quantitative PCR using Maxima SYBR Green/Rox qPCR master mix (Thermo Scientific) in an ABI ViiA7 sequence detection system (PE Applied

Biosystems) to quantify the relative levels of the transcripts in the samples. The primers were GAPDH sense primer 5′- TGACGTGCCGCCTGGAGAAAC -3′ and antisense 5′- CCGGCATCGAAGGTGGAAGAG -3′; human MALAT1 sense 5′ CTTCCCTAGGGGAT TTCAGG 3′ and antisense 5′ GCCCACAGGAACAA GTCCTA 3′; rat MALAT1 sense 5′ TGCAGTGTG CCAATGTTTCG 3′ and antisense 5′ GGCCAGCTG CAAACATTCAA 3′; U1snRNA sense 5′ TCCC AGGGCGAGGCTTATCCATT 3′ and antisense 5′ GAACGCAGTCCCCCACTACCACAAAT 3′.

Real-time PCR was then performed in triplicate on samples. The plate setup included a no template control, no RNA control, no reverse transcriptase control, and no amplification control. After primer concentrations were optimized to give the desired standard curve and a single melt curve, relative quotient (RQ) was determined using the $\Delta\Delta C_T$ method with U6snRNA or GAPDH as the endogenous control and no TBI sample as the calibrator sample. Experiments were repeated four times.

For absolute quantification, a standard curve was generated for each gene in every assay. Briefly, 100 to 0.4 ng of RNA were reverse transcribed as described above. The resulting cDNA was used to obtain a standard curve correlating the amounts with the threshold cycle number (C_t values). A linear relationship ($r^2 > 0.96$) was obtained for each gene. Real-time PCR was then performed on samples and standards in triplicates. The plate setup also included a standard series, no template control, no RNA control, no reverse transcriptase control, and no amplification control. The dissociation curve was analyzed for each sample. Absolute quantification of mRNA expression levels for MALAT1 or GFP was calculated by normalizing the values to GAPDH.

Results

Exosome treatment improves motor impairment and reduces lesion volume in a MALAT1-dependent manner

Fisher 344 male rats were subjected to either TBI by controlled cortical impact (CCI) injury model or no TBI (sham surgery only, control group) and treated with hASC-derived exosomes 3 h after surgery. Surgery is described in the "Methods" section. The rats were randomly distributed into the following groups: surgery with no TBI (sham control C, $N = 11$), TBI with unconditioned media as vehicle (T; $N = 20$), TBI treated with exosomes (TE, $N = 18$), TBI treated with exosomes depleted of MALAT1 (TEdM, $N = 20$), and TBI with injection of conditioned media depleted of exosomes (TdCM). TdCM-treated animals were included to delineate the effect of the exosomes from other biomolecules of the secretome and because our previous study had demonstrated that conditioned media harvested from hASCs was an effective treatment post TBI [26]. Each rat was subjected to a series of behavioral tests including elevated body swing test (EBST), forelimb akinesia, and paw grasp to reveal motor and neurological performance of animals, before injury and after TBI on days 0, 1, 3, and 7.

The EBST records the number of lateral swings to one side or the other and defines a swing bias to one side as a motor defect. A score of 10 equals no bias, and higher scores indicate asymmetry. EBST revealed that rats subjected to TBI exhibited heightened swing bias and therefore significant asymmetry in motor activity after injury. TBI (T) animals displayed no recovery when tested on days 3 and 7, whereas significant recovery of motor symmetry was detected in TBI exosome-treated rats (TE) (two-way ANOVA followed by Tukey's post hoc, $p < 0.01$ versus TBI-Veh; Fig. 1a). Treatment with either conditioned media depleted of exosomes (TdCM) or exosomes depleted of MALAT1 (TEdM) did not affect recovery of the animals, and scores for these groups were not significantly different from the TBI-vehicle (T) group).

The forelimb akinesia test indicated an apparent loss of motor strength in TBI rats after injury when compared with sham controls. TBI-Veh (T) animals retained impairment through day 7 and did not display any significant amelioration of forelimb akinesia. TBI animals treated with exosomes (TE) recovered by day 3 (Fig. 1b), whereas TBI animals treated with conditioned media depleted of exosomes (TdCM) had only modest recovery after day 3, but not day 7.

Assessment of paw grasp function is indicative of TBI-associated loss of strength and was apparent in all animals subjected to injury. After day 3 post TBI, TBI exosome-treated (TE) animals scored significantly better on the paw grasp test compared to TBI-vehicle-treated (T) animals. The animals in the conditioned media depleted of exosomes and the exosomes depleted of MALAT1 groups again showed a modest improvement at day 3 that was not maintained at day 7 (Fig. 1c). Results show only the cohort treated with exosomes maintained this significant treatment effect on the paw grasp assessment demonstrating continued recovery of strength for the exosome-treated group compared to TBI sham treatment (two-way ANOVA followed by Tukey's post hoc, $p < 0.001$).

We performed Nissl staining to quantify the lesion volumes and surrounding damage after TBI in the peri-impact area. Administration of exosomes was found to significantly reduce both the impact (Fig. 1d) and peri-impact (Fig. 1e) area of TBI-associated injury in the ipsilateral hemisphere. Exosomes depleted of MALAT1 (TEdM) had moderate improvement in peri-impact measures, but not in impact area (Fig. 1d, e). Treatment with conditioned media depleted of exosomes did not show recovery in either the impact or the peri-impact

area after TBI injury. Examples of images used for analysis are shown in Fig. 1g, as well as examples of images used to quantify the live neurons in the peri-impact area.

Imaging of exosomes in vivo shows distribution primarily to the abdomen and head regions

We determined the biodistribution of XenoLight DiR-labeled exosomes in vivo in rats with CCI treated with exosomes and exosomes depleted of MALAT1. Exosomes were administered through the jugular vein of TBI animals 3 h after injury, and their biodistribution was tracked at time points 1, 4, 12, 24, 48, and 72 h and 11 days after surgery (Fig. 2). Minimal DiR signal was detected in both the head and body regions of the sham control animals as expected which provided a reference value throughout the analysis. Within the first hour of transplantation, no noticeable signal was observed in the head region of either treatment groups, whereas a high level of fluorescent signal was present in the abdomen of both TBI groups treated with either exosomes (TE) or exosomes deleted of MALAT1 (TEdM) animals. Fluorescent signal slightly increased after 4 h for both groups in both the head and abdomen regions of the animals. At the 12-h time point, the signal in the head region had increased from the previous time points and continued to increase at 24 h where it seemed to plateau through 48 and 72 h until decreasing on day 11 after transplantation. The abdomen region instead displayed the opposite trend and showed a gradually decreasing DiR signal after 4 h that continued to decline at the 12-, 24-, 48-, and 72-h time points with the lowest radiant efficiency observed on day 11. Quantitative analysis confirmed these observations, as shown in Fig. 2a, b. Throughout all the data points, the group treated with exosomes depleted of MALAT1 showed a slightly higher average radiant efficiency while following the same trend as exosome-treated animals, but this did not achieve significance.

Imaging of exosomes ex vivo in organs shows localization primarily to the spleen and brain

Next, we determined the biodistribution of XenoLight DiR-labeled exosomes ex vivo in organs of rats with CCI treated with exosomes and exosomes depleted of MALAT1 when administered as described above for in vivo imaging. A separate cohort was examined, and each organ including the brain, lungs, liver, and spleen was imaged ex vivo at 1 h and at 3, 7, and 11 days following TBI (Fig. 3a–e). One hour after administration, the highest signal was observed in the spleen whereas the liver and the lungs showed lower signal intensity and there was no signal observed in the brain. Interestingly, there was higher signal for the exosomes depleted of MALAT1 (TEdM) in the liver at 1 h suggesting a higher rate of

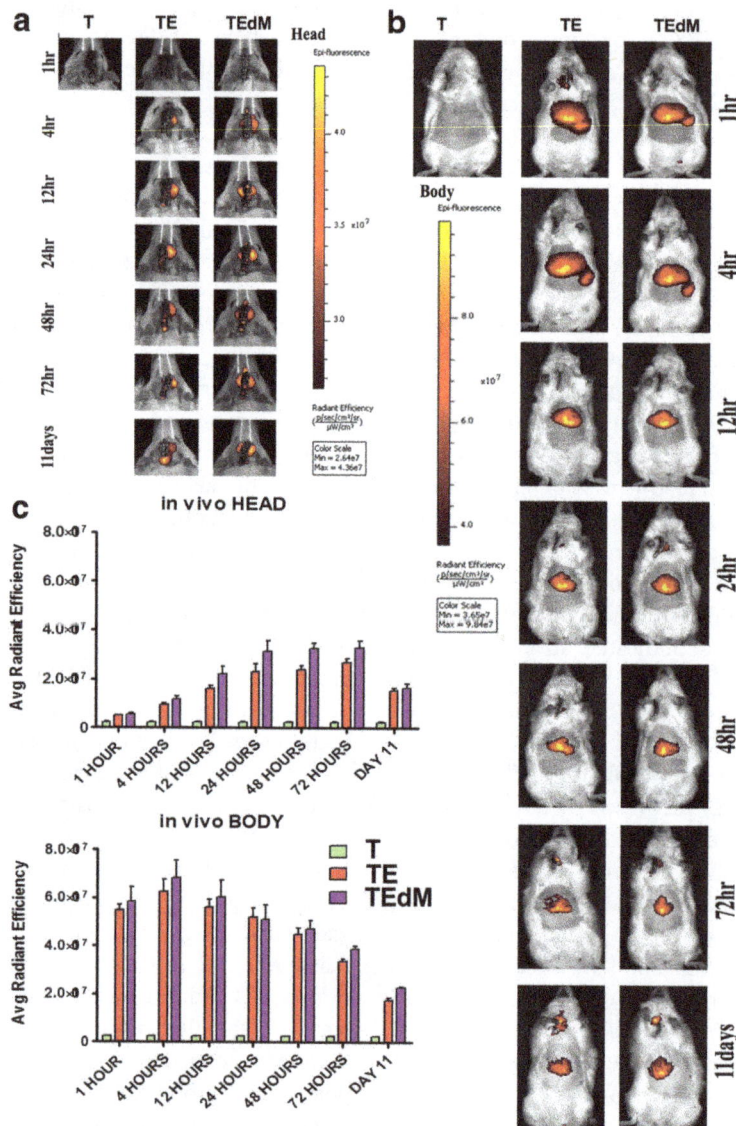

Fig. 2 In vivo biodistribution of DiR-labeled exosomes after TBI (**a**, **b**). Imaging revealed exosomes migrated robustly to the spleen and liver at 1 and 4 h after transplantation before gradually decreasing. Exosomes also migrated to the impact site of the brain 4 h after transplantation and steadily increased through 72 h relative to sham controls. Graphs in **c** show radiant efficiency is expressed as photons per second per square centimeter per steridian divided by microwatts per square centimeter(((p/s)/ ⟦ cm) ^ 2/sr)/(μW/ ⟦ cm) ^ 2)). Data in bargraphs represent the mean ± SEM values N = 3 per group

clearance initially. At day 3, a reduction in signal was observed in the spleen and liver and this continued over time. Signal intensity in the brain, however, increased on day 3 and continued to increase through day 7.

RNA sequencing transcriptome analysis identifies cellular processes crucial to recovery that are specifically mediated by MALAT1

To gain insight into genomic changes following CCI and its treatment with hASC-derived exosomes, we performed RNA sequencing. Transcriptome analysis provides valuable knowledge of genomic changes

following brain injury and the response to treatment with exosomes. We isolated RNA from the brains, specifically an area near the impact site, and the spleens of rats at day 7 following TBI in the sham surgery—control (C), TBI with vehicle (T), TBI treated with exosomes (TE), and TBI treated with MALAT1-depleted exosomes (TEdM) groups. Four rats of each group were randomly chosen and pooled to maximize biological diversity and sent for RNA Seq (Ocean Ridge Biosciences). The percent of mapped reads to total genome over total read across all sequencing was 96 ± 0.7%.

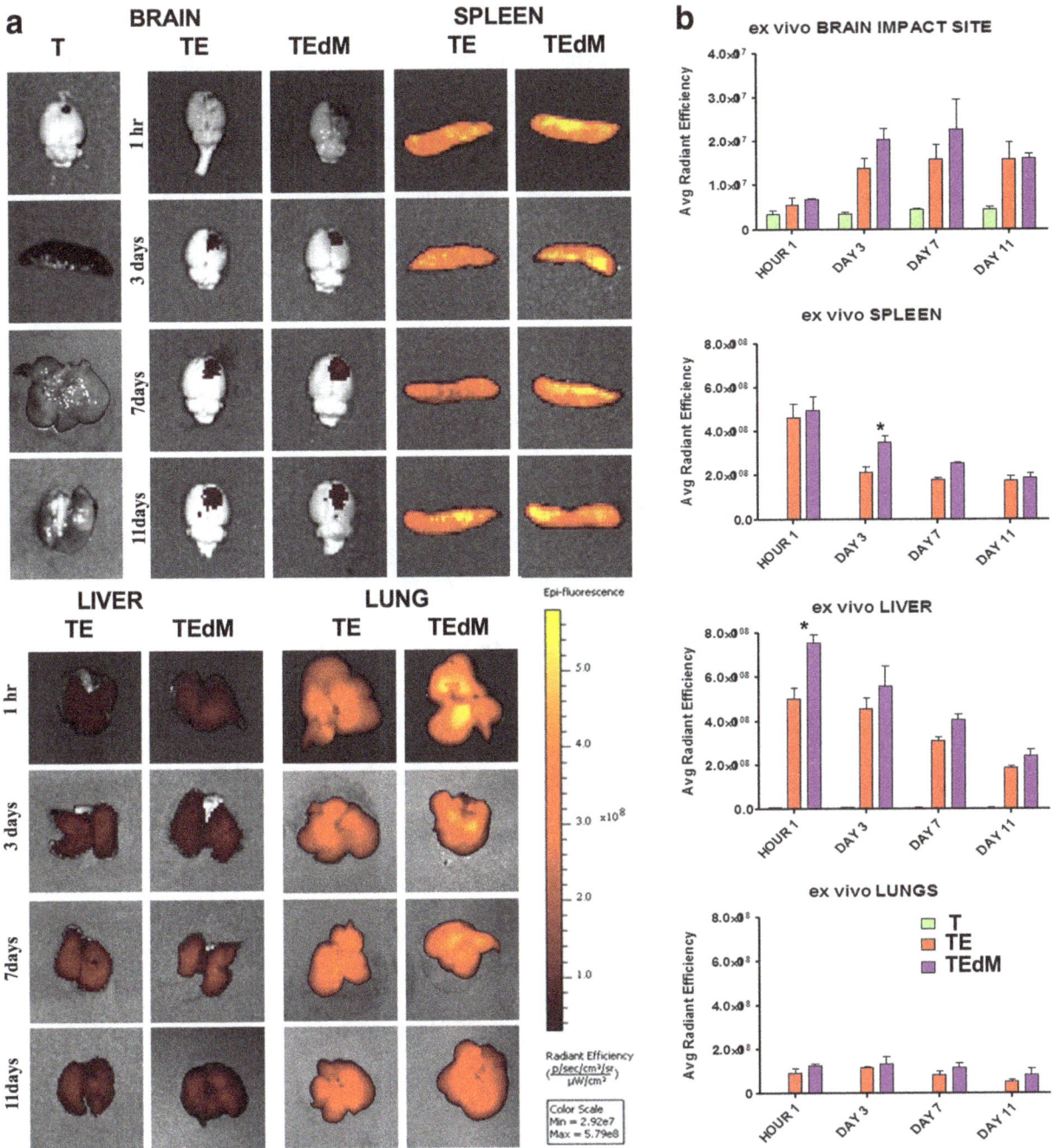

Fig. 3 Ex vivo biodistribution of DiR-labeled exosomes after TBI. **a** Imaging revealed exosomes migrating to the spleen, liver, and lungs 1 h after transplantation and migrating to the impact site of the brain on day 3 after TBI relative to sham controls. Ex vivo analysis shows the fluorescent signal intensity was highest in the spleen and liver 1 h after transplantation and gradually declined through day 11, whereas the lungs slightly increased at day 3 before declining through days 7 and 11. The brain impact site showed no apparent signal when compared to TBI-sham treatment animals 1 h after exosome transplantation, but increased by day 3 where the signal remained through day 7 and only TEdM radiant efficiency declined by day 11. **b** Radiant efficiency is expressed as photons per second per square centimeter per steridian divided by microwatts per square centimeter$((p/s)/[cm]^2/sr)/(\mu W/[cm]^2))$. Data represent the mean ± SEM values $N = 3$ per group

We performed hierarchical clustering of the entire RNA Seq transcriptome data in order to evaluate the relationship between gene expression profiles in the brain or spleen with respect to the different treatments, i.e., no TBI sham surgery control (C), TBI treated with vehicle (T), TBI treated with exosomes (TE), and TBI treated with exosomes depleted of MALAT1 (TEdM). The same RPKM data for all 19,058 detectable genes

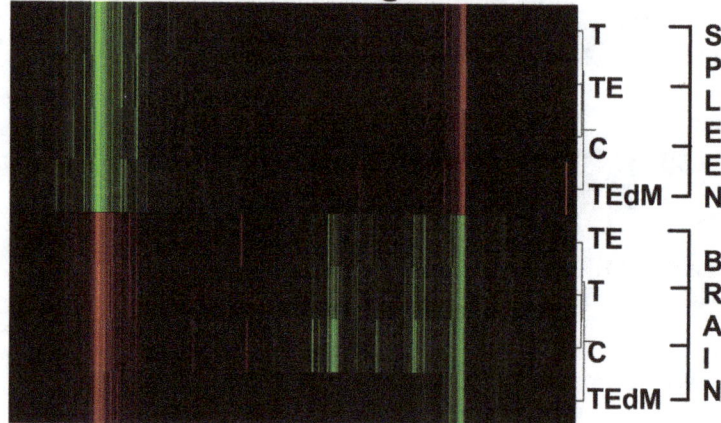

were used for hierarchical clustering analysis by Cluster 3.0 software. Genes were log-2 transformed and median centered prior to hierarchical clustering. Hierarchical clustering (Fig. 4a) was conducted on genes and samples using centered correlation as the similarity metric and average linkage as the clustering method. Figure 4b shows the hierarchical clustering conducted for ncRNAs as described above for gene expression. Each color-bar unit in both hierarchical clustering represents a difference of one log 2 unit in RPKM value. Zero (0) is the median RPKM value across all samples. Heat maps with row dendograms are shown to visualize the result of the hierarchical clustering calculation. This depicts the distance or similarity between rows and which nodes in each row belongs to, as a result of clustering. For both the brain and spleen, the results of the clustering heat map show groups of genes or ncRNAs whose expression is affected by TBI and the exosome treatments. Principal component analysis showed similar distinction between groups (data not shown).

RNA Seq of the brain and spleen transcriptome identifies genes affected by TBI and treatment with exosomes

We further analyzed the highly enriched genes for the spleen and brain. The results (above Fig. 4a, b) indicated specific sets of genes that were affected by TBI that were distinct between the spleen and brain as expected based on cell type and cell-specific markers. Based on fold changes, the top genes affected by TBI and treatment with exosomes in the spleen were enzymes such as prancreatic α-amylase, prancreatic α-amylase precursor, phospholipase A2, caroxypeptidase B precursor, bile

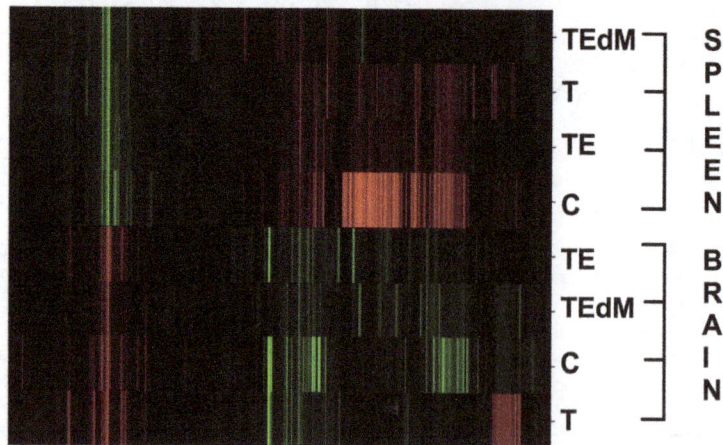

Fig. 4 Hierarchical heat map of gene expression of (**a**) coding genes or (**b**) noncoding RNA from the RNA Seq dataset. The gene clustering from the spleen is on the top, and brain is the lower half of the dendrograms. For both **a** and **b**, RPKM data from 19,058 detectable rat genes were used in analysis by hierarchical clustering with Gene Cluster 3.0. RPKMs were log-2-transformed and adjusted by centering genes using the median. Clustering was performed on genes and arrays using centered correlation as distance measure and average linkage as method. Data shows clusters of genes or noncoding RNA that are affected by TBI and restored towards the no TBI pattern with exosome treatment

salt-activated lipase precursor, chymotrypsinogen B precursor, carboxypeptidase A2 precursor, and anionic trypsin 1 which were elevated after TBI and reduced with exosome treatment. Further, in the spleen, genes that were upregulated following TBI were related to GO categories of enzyme inhibitor activity, defense response, platelet alpha granule lumen, and protein-DNA complexes. In the brain, our RNA Seq data revealed previously undescribed transcripts ENSRNOG00000047520, ENSRNOG00000049727, ENSRNOG00000050024, and ENSRNOG00000046742 whose levels changed with TBI and exosome treatment. Additionally, genes in the brain that were upregulated following TBI were related to immune responses, cellular response to stress, aging, and DNA damage. The splicing index of genes in the spleen that were predominantly changed with TBI and exosome treatment were *Tbcd, Chmp1a, Cnst, Lphn1, Zfp560, Mrpl23, Emc4, Zfp329*. The splicing index of genes in the brain that were predominantly changed with TBI and exosomes treatment were *Rps6ka3, Nrtk3, Nap1l1, Eif4g1, Fsd1, Trim44, Dst, Rps15, Fkbp2, Rabgap1l*.

Gene expression patterns following treatment with hASC exosomes

Of most interest to this study are gene changes that fit the pattern observed with both behavioral testing and lesion area analysis. This expression pattern changes shown following TBI are lessened with exosome treatment but not by treatment with exosomes depleted of MALAT1. The genes that fit this pattern of gene expression responses were labeled (+ 1; up with TBI (T), down with TBI + exosomes (TE), and up with TBI + MALAT-depleted exosomes (TEdM)) or the opposite pattern (− 1; down with TBI (T), up with TBI+ exosomes (TE), and down with TBI + MALAT-depleted exosomes (TEdM)). The data was further filtered for a minimum of twofold gene expression change compared with TBI and analyzed using Ingenuity Pathway Analysis (IPA) for both the brain and the spleen separately. The IPA bioinformatics package identifies regulatory nodes (upstream regulators) based upon the fold change values of dataset to predict a relationship of these nodes to drive the detected changes in gene expression. In this manner, the top upstream regulators that fit the pattern + 1 and − 1 are listed for the brain and spleen in Table 1. Only values with a significant -log (*p* value) were included in the tables and if the Z score indicates a predicted significant up- or downregulation within each pattern than it is also noted in the table. Canonical pathways identified as significant are listed in Table 2.

Brain mRNA changes

For the pattern + 1, several of the predominant predicted upstream nodal regulators from the IPA analysis are

related to inflammatory pathways, IL1β, IFNG, etc. which is in agreement with the literature on TBI alone. To illustrate this graphically, Fig. 5 shows top upstream regulatory networks in the C vs. T comparison. There is a strong predicted upstream activation of inflammatory regulators such as IL1β, IFNG, TLR2, IL27, and CD40 (indicated in orange). Also illustrated in this figure are the actual gene expression changes driving the predictions, which show significant overlap in the nodal networks depicted. Furthermore, CTF1 was also predicted to be an upstream regulator by this analysis, which is consistent with its role in other brain injury models and inflammation. In addition, there were changes in CTNNB1: the gene for beta catenin which is an important regulator for the WNT pathway, WNT is known to be involved in neural repair pathways and neurogenesis, and is also related to SOX15 which is discussed further below. This pathway is downregulated with TBI, and the extent of down regulation is lessened following treatment with exosomes as reflected in the color of the regulator moving from a darker orange to a lighter color. The right side of the figure illustrates the overlay of the pattern of gene expression and predictions for the nodal regulation in the TBI treated with exosomes group. All of the inflammatory nodes such as IL1ß, IFNG, CD40, and IL27 show no predicted upregulation from control which is indicated by the lack of color, and demonstrates that the exosomes significantly lower the pro-inflammatory gene expression patterns observed with injury. This is driven by decreased gene expression of pro-inflammatory genes PTX3, MMP9, POMC, and CD80 in this dataset which is shown by the green color. Not shown in this figure is the network of these upstream regulators for the third aspect of this pattern which is C vs. TdM comparison; when exosomes depleted in MALAT1 are given after TBI, the network of gene expression and predicted upstream regulators is an almost identical pattern to the C vs. T network shown here. This is in agreement with the pattern of behavioral and histological changes presented above.

The predicted upstream regulators for the pattern − 1 with (gene expression going down with TBI) are related to transcription regulators such as SOX15, RFX3, and TCF7L1 as well as ubiquitin and HSP70 (Table 1, different functional groups depicted by colors). This suggests that there is a decline in transcriptional activation in regenerative pathways as illustrated by changes in SOX15 expression, which is part of the WNT/β-catenin pathway involved in cellular proliferation and stem cell proliferation.

For canonical pathways identified again the + 1 pattern shows the highest *p* value of overlap with no significant canonical pathways identified in the brain for the − 1 pattern. Canonical pathways that are increased with TBI and responsive to the exosome treatment also include

Table 1 Upstream regulators

Pattern +1	Pattern -1
BRAIN	
IL1B *	TNNI1
IFNG*	PIH1D3
CSF2*	SOX15
TLR2*	mir-194
P38 MAPK*	LNX2
STAT3	RFX3
CTNNB1	SFPQ
IL27*	OXT
NFkB (complex)*	SIX1
TNF*	Ubiquitin
TAGLN	HEY2
Immunoglobulin	TCF7L1
S100A4	UPF2
STAT1	ADRB2
Jnk	COMMD3-BMI1
CTF1	Hsp70
Mek	PAX5
STAT	
NFKBIA	
MAPK8*	
CNTF	
SPLEEN	
CDKN1A#	CACNG8
E2F4	KRT18
RABL6*	CYP1A1
CSF2*	CAV1
PTGER2*	EFNA4
EP400*	EFNA3
CCND1*	EFNA5
E2F3*	ADCY6
Irgm1#	NAB1
ABCB6#	CYP1A2
BNIP3L#	PTPN1
E2f*	CYP1B1
FOXM1*	EFNA2
ERBB2*	GATA4
let-7#	RREB1
E2F1*	EOMES
E2F7	SLC12A2
GATA1*	TBX5
KLF1	FOXN3
NUPR1#	PTGDS

Inflammation, Apoptosis, Transcription, cardiovascular, RNA processing, metabolism

Asterisk indicates a positive Z score indicating a predicted activation
Number sign indicates a negative Z score

Table 2 Canonical pathways

Brain

Pattern 1

Pancreatic adenocarcinoma signaling

Role of CHK proteins in cell cycle checkpoint control

T helper cell differentiation

Cyclins and cell cycle regulation

Th1 pathway

Bladder cancer signaling

Inhibition of angiogenesis by TSP1

Dopamine receptor signaling

ILK signaling

B cell development

Cell cycle regulation by BTG family proteins

Inhibition of matrix metalloproteases

Thyroid cancer signaling

HIF1α signaling

Crosstalk between dendritic cells and natural killer cells

Th1 and Th2 activation pathway

Role of JAK family kinases in IL-6-type cytokine signaling

Role of JAK1 and JAK3 in γc cytokine signaling

Role of Oct4 in mammalian embryonic stem cell pluripotency

Autoimmune thyroid disease signaling

Spleen

Pattern 1

Heme biosynthesis II

Mitotic roles of polo-like kinase

Heme biosynthesis from uroporphyrinogen-III I

Tetrapyrrole biosynthesis II

Estrogen-mediated S-phase entry

GADD45 signaling

Cell cycle: G2/M DNA damage checkpoint regulation

Cyclins and cell cycle regulation

dTMP de novo biosynthesis

Cell cycle control of chromosomal replication

DNA damage-induced 14-3-3σ signaling

Rapoport-Luebering glycolytic shunt

Pyrimidine deoxyribonucleotides de novo biosynthesis I

ATM signaling

Antiproliferative role of TOB in T cell signaling

Role of CHK proteins in cell cycle checkpoint control

Cell cycle: G1/S checkpoint regulation

Cell cycle regulation by BTG family proteins

Asparagine biosynthesis I

γ-Glutamyl cycle

Pattern − 1

cAMP-mediated signaling

G-Protein coupled receptor signaling

Serine biosynthesis

Superpathway of serine and glycine biosynthesis I

LPS/IL-1-mediated inhibition of RXR function

Protein kinase A signaling

Cardiac hypertrophy signaling

Fatty acid activation

nNOS signaling in skeletal muscle cells

Corticotropin releasing hormone signaling

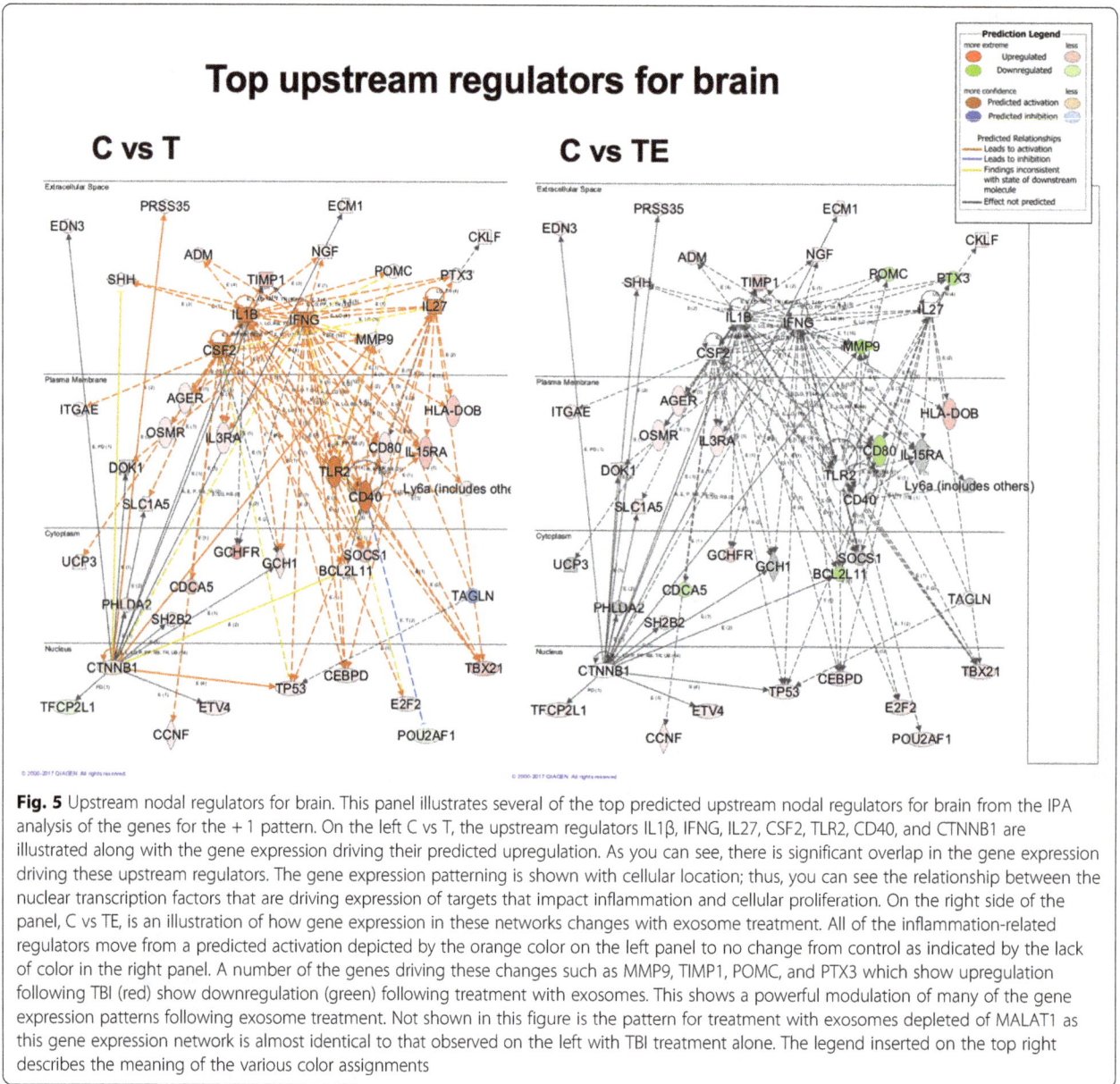

Fig. 5 Upstream nodal regulators for brain. This panel illustrates several of the top predicted upstream nodal regulators for brain from the IPA analysis of the genes for the + 1 pattern. On the left C vs T, the upstream regulators IL1β, IFNG, IL27, CSF2, TLR2, CD40, and CTNNB1 are illustrated along with the gene expression driving their predicted upregulation. As you can see, there is significant overlap in the gene expression driving these upstream regulators. The gene expression patterning is shown with cellular location; thus, you can see the relationship between the nuclear transcription factors that are driving expression of targets that impact inflammation and cellular proliferation. On the right side of the panel, C vs TE, is an illustration of how gene expression in these networks changes with exosome treatment. All of the inflammation-related regulators move from a predicted activation depicted by the orange color on the left panel to no change from control as indicated by the lack of color in the right panel. A number of the genes driving these changes such as MMP9, TIMP1, POMC, and PTX3 which show upregulation following TBI (red) show downregulation (green) following treatment with exosomes. This shows a powerful modulation of many of the gene expression patterns following exosome treatment. Not shown in this figure is the pattern for treatment with exosomes depleted of MALAT1 as this gene expression network is almost identical to that observed on the left with TBI treatment alone. The legend inserted on the top right describes the meaning of the various color assignments

inflammatory pathways. Cell cycle and cancer-related pathways are further noted, most likely changing due to cell death and injury caused by CCI (Table 2).

Spleen mRNA expression

We also examined gene expression in the spleen as our data shows predominant localization of exosomes to the spleen. This finding was important, as a significant body of literature has demonstrated that intravenous treatments with exogenous cell therapies and other treatments such as conditioned media from stem cells involve the spleen. Our data presented here shows the presence of exosomes in the spleen at an early time point following injection, prior to the exosomes being observed in the brain. Table 1 shows the top ranking

predicted upstream regulators based upon p value of overlap, and if there was a significant Z score for predicted activation or inhibition. For the + 1 pattern of expression that increases with TBI, there was a predicted inhibition of CDKN1A suggesting a decrease in cellular proliferation. This is supported by changes in other proliferation-related pathways like CCND1, which is a cell cycle regulator related to both AMPK and PTEN bioenergetics pathways as well as inflammation pathways like IL8 and ILK. Many of the predicted upstream regulators are nuclear transcription factors influencing many aspects of cellular function including cellular proliferation, cell cycle control, and DNA damage. This again is likely a reflection of the response to the brain injury effecting other organ systems.

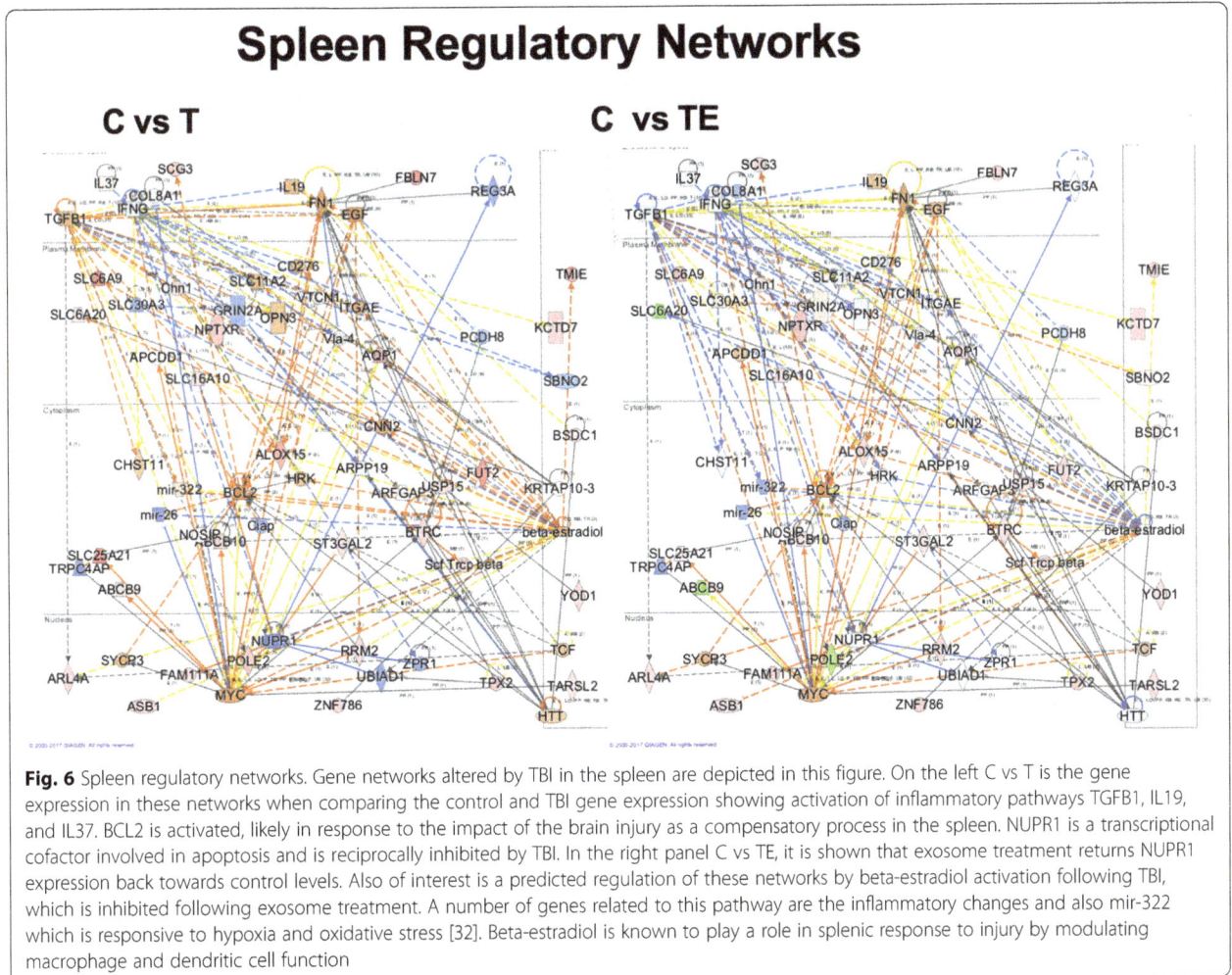

Fig. 6 Spleen regulatory networks. Gene networks altered by TBI in the spleen are depicted in this figure. On the left C vs T is the gene expression in these networks when comparing the control and TBI gene expression showing activation of inflammatory pathways TGFB1, IL19, and IL37. BCL2 is activated, likely in response to the impact of the brain injury as a compensatory process in the spleen. NUPR1 is a transcriptional cofactor involved in apoptosis and is reciprocally inhibited by TBI. In the right panel C vs TE, it is shown that exosome treatment returns NUPR1 expression back towards control levels. Also of interest is a predicted regulation of these networks by beta-estradiol activation following TBI, which is inhibited following exosome treatment. A number of genes related to this pathway are the inflammatory changes and also mir-322 which is responsive to hypoxia and oxidative stress [32]. Beta-estradiol is known to play a role in splenic response to injury by modulating macrophage and dendritic cell function

To explore the regulatory networks of genes affected in the spleen in response to the + 1 pattern of expression, we merged two of the top networks identified in IPA and this is illustrated in Fig. 6. The left panel shows these network changes along with predicted nodes in addition to relationships with canonical pathways. Again, as in the brain, a number of inflammation-related pathways including TGFβ and INFG are altered with TBI. Also shown are a number of changes to pathways related to the transcriptional regulators MYC and NUPPR1. The predicted inhibition of NUPPR1 with TBI is mitigated with the exosome treatment as shown in the right panel and might be related to an increase in POLE2 in the exosome-treated group. Also of interest is a predicted regulation of these networks by beta-estradiol activation following TBI which is inhibited following exosome treatment (Fig. 6). A number of genes related to this pathway are involved in inflammatory responses and cellular stress, such as mir-322 which is responsive to hypoxia and oxidative stress [32]. Beta-estradiol is known to play a role in splenic response to injury [33–36] by

modulating macrophage and dendritic cell function, thus are consistent with effects of estradiol in other injury models. It is important to note that this does not necessarily mean that estradiol is driving this alteration in our dataset; it simply means that estradiol alters splenic inflammatory markers in the same way as what is observed in our dataset. Several investigations have suggested that estradiol reduces MALAT1 [37–39]; thus, a predicted inhibition of estradiol by exosome treatment may reflect increased action of MALAT1. Further studies are needed to elucidate an interaction of exosome treatment with estradiol.

The expression of genes in the – 1 pattern demonstrated inhibition of several aspects of splenic function including the ephrins A2, 3, 4, and 5, which regulate interaction with hematopoiesis [40]. While these processes are more related to ephrin A1, for our study, ephrin A2 is of particular interest as it plays an important role in monocyte adhesion and transendothelial migration via integrins. In a report by Konda et al., an increase in ephrin A2 stimulated monocyte

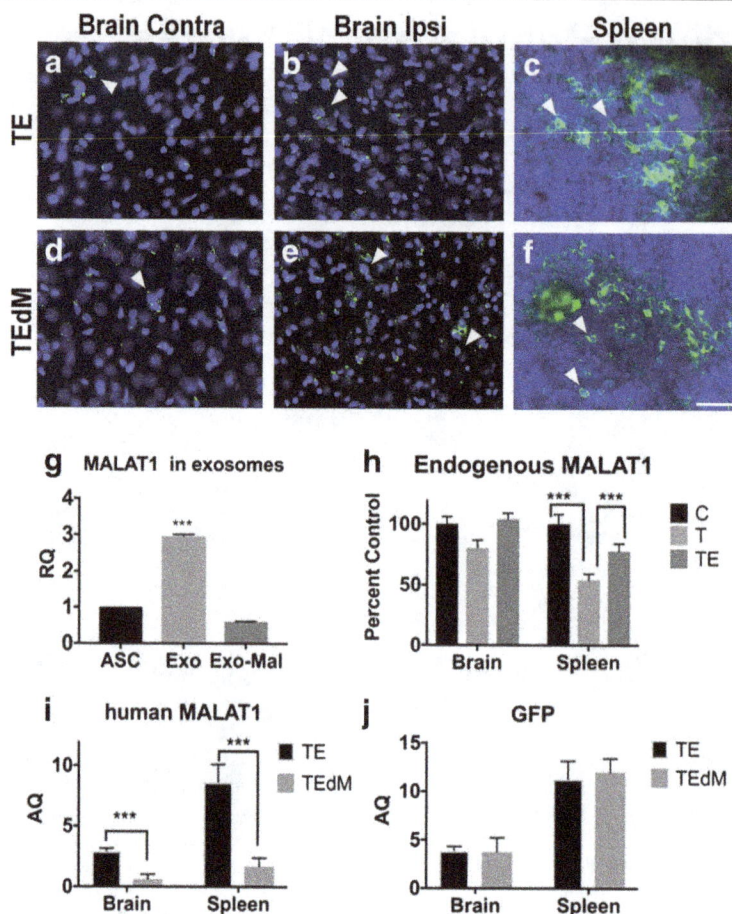

Fig. 7 Localization of exosomes and validation of MALAT1 and GFP levels. Localization of exosomes and MALAT1 to the brain and spleen. Confocal imaging of exosome-positive expression of GFP in the brain and spleen of TBI rats. Images reveal migration of exosomes to both the contralateral and ipsilateral cortical region of the TBI-impacted brains near the impact site (**a, b, d, e**) and the spleen (**c, f**) of TE and TEdM rats as shown by detecting GFP expression (green) in cells with DAPI-positive staining (blue) 11 days after transplantation. White arrows indicate cells with exosomes. There was higher migration to the ipsilateral cortex near the impact site than that observed in the contralateral cortex which agrees with our ex vivo imaging data in Fig. 3. Scale bar in **f** equals 50 μm. **g** MALAT1 expression was measured in hASC-isolated exosomes and isolated exosomes with MALAT1 knockdown. Relative to the MALAT1 level in hASC, there is an increase in MALAT1 in the secreted exosomes, and this was knocked down significantly with the antisense oligonucleotide treatment. The results were analyzed with two-tailed Student's t test using PRISM4 statistical analysis software (GraphPad, San Diego, CA). A level of $p < 0.05$ was considered statistically significant. ***$p < 0.001$. **h** Endogenous MALAT1 levels in rat brain and spleen decrease with TBI: Following TBI and treatment with hASC exosomes, the levels of MALAT1 within the rat brain and spleen were analyzed by PCR using rat-specific primers. RNA was extracted and samples were pooled from four rats each from the no TBI, TBI treated with vehicle, and TBI treated with exosomes. Graph represents percent control with no TBI group designated as 100%. The experiment was repeated five times. The results were analyzed with two-tailed Student's t test using PRISM4 statistical analysis software (GraphPad, San Diego, CA). A level of $p < 0.05$ was considered statistically significant. ***$p < 0.001$ highly significant between control (no TBI) and TBI with vehicle treatment and between TBI and TBI treated with hASC exosomes for MALAT1. **i** Verification that hASC exosomes were taken up by the brain and spleen: SYBR Green real-time qPCR using human MALAT1 primers and **j** GFP primers was performed for absolute quantification. GAPDH served as control. For absolute quantification, a standard curve was generated for each gene in every assay. Absolute quantification of mRNA expression levels for MALAT1 and GFP was calculated by normalizing the values to GAPDH. The experiments were repeated four times with similar results. The results were analyzed with two-tailed Student's t test using PRISM4 statistical analysis software (GraphPad, San Diego, CA). A level of $p < 0.05$ was considered statistically significant. ***$p < 0.0001$ highly significant between TBI treated with hASC exosomes and TBI treated with MALAT1-depleted (M1 aso) exosomes for MALAT1. The levels of GFP did not change with depletion of MALAT1

infiltration and sequestration into the red pulp of the spleen via an interaction with integrin and additional undetermined molecular pathways [41]. The release of monocytes from the red pulp of the spleen is a known consequence of injury [42]; therefore, we would predict that inhibition of ephrin A2 would be consistent with release of monocytes from the splenic red pulp into the bloodstream. As presented, this predicted loss of the inhibition of ephrins is seen following treatment with exosomes, but treatment with exosomes depleted of MALAT1 showed similar results to those observed for rats that received TBI with no treatment. This is a potentially interesting finding, and although at this point we cannot make a direct correlation between this predicted change in ephrin A2 regulation following TBI and treatment with exosomes, it is consistent with the observed behavioral and histological improvement with the exosome treatment. As previously discussed, one possible role of the spleen in TBI and other brain insults is the release of monocytes into circulation, which participate in the secondary insult at the site of injury.

Validation of RNA Seq results of gene expression

Confocal microscopy confirmed positive localization of GFP-labeled exosomes within both the contralateral and ipsilateral brain regions as well as in the spleen (Fig. 7a–f). The GFP signal was more robust in the ipsilateral hemisphere compared to the contralateral and was located mainly in close proximity to the impacted area. This may be the result of a breakdown of the blood-brain barrier at the site of injury. To further validate that exosomes were taken up by the brain and spleen, RNA isolated from either the brain or the spleen was reverse transcribed to cDNA and used in quantitative SYBR Green

real-time qPCR using primers for rat and human MALAT1. Our results show that endogenous rat MALAT1 is depleted in the spleen and the cortex near the injury site following injury and increased with exosome treatment. Further, exosomes not depleted of MALAT1 were shown to deliver human MALAT1 to the brain and spleen (Fig.7g, h). These results show that exosomes are efficiently taken by the brain and spleen.

To validate our results from RNA Seq, we used quantitative SYBR Green real-time qPCR to determine levels of the genes altered in both the spleen and the brain following TBI with and without exosome treatment. Figure 8 shows validation of spleen expression of PLAg2, TNFα, E2F4, and RABL6 and brain cortex expression of IL1β, TNFa, IFNG, and IL10. These genes showed significant fold changes in RNA Seq data and are components of the predicted networks. Although the pattern of expression for IL10 is not consistent with the overall predicted changes in inflammatory networks, it does replicate the data in the RNA Seq dataset. Our qPCR results show expression of these genes that are in agreement with the RNA Seq data.

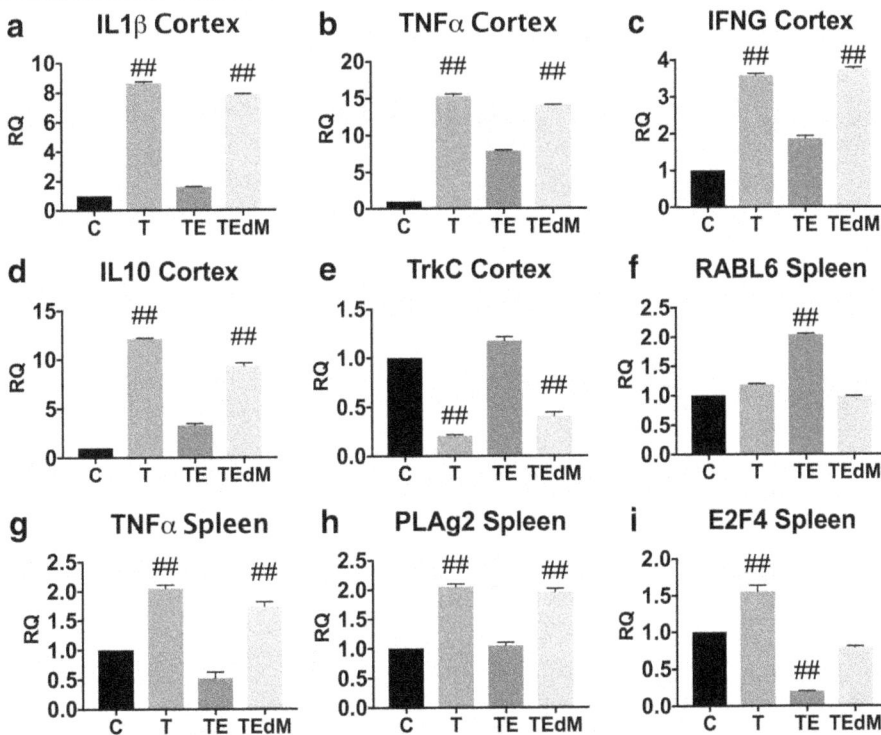

Fig. 8 a–i Validation of RNA Seq data using qPCR. Real-time qPCR validation of representative genes identified by RNA Seq data in the cortex and spleen that are affected by TBI and treatment with exosomes. All assays were run in triplicate, and data is expressed as the mean ± SEM. Data for each gene was analyzed by one-way ANOVA followed by Dunnet's multiple comparison test. $^{\#\#}p < 0.01$ indicates that group was different from control. ANOVA for each graph are IL1ß cortex ($F(3, 8) = 16,008$); TNFα cortex ($F(3, 8) = 5989$); IFNG cortex ($F(3, 8) = 1784$); TrkC cortex ($F(3, 8) = 814$); IL10 cortex ($F(3, 8) = 2980$); RABL6 spleen ($F(3, 8) = 4640$); TNFα spleen ($F(3, 8) = 286$); E2F4 spleen ($F(3, 8) = 516$); PLAg2 spleen ($F(3, 8) = 451$)

Table 3 Changes in noncoding RNA miRNA

Brain + 1	C vs T	C vs TE	C vs TEdM	Spleen + 1	C vs T	C vs TE	C vs TEdM
rno-miR-429	346.52	26.50	208.76	rno-miR-451-3p	3.70	− 1.15	4.82
rno-miR-200b-5p	99.01	7.42	127.07	rno-miR-1949	1.78	− 1.05	1.45
rno-miR-183-5p	59.14	6.56	122.37	rno-miR-6216	1.38	− 1.22	1.30
rno-miR-182	56.38	1.00	43.57	rno-miR-17-5p	1.51	− 1.13	1.52
rno-miR-96-5p	48.13	1.00	61.72	rno-miR-144-5p	3.85	2.01	4.19
rno-miR-6216	2.67	− 1.04	2.82	rno-miR-484	1.52	− 1.10	1.88
rno-miR-1193-3p	1.34	1.03	1.20	rno-miR-132-3p	2.07	1.01	1.83
rno-miR-218a-2-3p	1.24	1.07	1.30	rno-miR-702-3p	4.89	2.44	3.59
				rno-miR-409a-5p	1.85	1.04	1.84
				rno-miR-92a-3p	1.33	− 1.08	1.29
				rno-miR-339-5p	1.39	− 1.07	1.30
				rno-miR-93-5p	1.53	1.07	1.74
				rno-miR-361-5p	1.30	− 1.01	1.50
				rno-miR-31a-5p	1.18	− 1.13	1.30
				rno-miR-21-3p	1.29	− 1.07	1.31
				rno-miR-423-5p	1.19	− 1.10	1.26
				rno-miR-210-3p	1.35	1.11	1.45
				rno-miR-532-3p	1.25	1.11	1.26
				rno-miR-103-3p	1.18	− 1.01	1.24
				rno-miR-6319	1.39	1.12	1.27
				rno-miR-378a-5p	1.10	1.05	1.17
				rno-miR-342-3p	1.06	− 1.05	1.09
Brain −1				**Spleen −1**			
rno-miR-154-5p	− 1.48	−1.17	− 1.32	rno-miR-708-3p	− 10.9	1.69	− 1.39
rno-miR-7b	− 1.65	−1.04	− 1.80	rno-miR-6329	− 3.33	− 1.07	− 1.57
rno-miR-665	− 2.57	−1.11	− 1.69	rno-miR-148b-5p	− 1.22	1.14	− 1.10
rno-miR-487b-3p	− 1.38	1.32	− 1.54	rno-miR-212-5p	− 1.44	− 1.09	− 2.17
rno-miR-672-3p	− 1.77	1.09	− 1.41	rno-miR-181a-1-3p	− 1.55	1.23	− 1.16
rno-miR-10a-5p	− 1.47	1.29	− 1.29	rno-miR-1843b-5p	− 1.79	1.07	− 1.37
rno-miR-770-5p	− 1.53	1.12	− 1.60	rno-miR-10a-5p	− 1.49	1.16	− 1.22
rno-miR-666-5p	− 1.29	1.24	− 1.32	rno-miR-379-5p	− 1.92	− 1.01	− 1.32
rno-miR-29c-3p	− 1.52	1.07	− 1.22	rno-miR-411-5p	− 1.66	− 1.12	− 2.09
rno-miR-3594-3p	− 1.61	− 1.04	− 1.37	rno-miR-192-5p	− 1.72	1.01	− 1.80
rno-miR-485-3p	− 1.41	− 1.13	− 1.32	rno-let-7f-5p	− 1.58	1.12	− 1.20
rno-miR-139-3p	− 1.45	1.02	− 1.27	rno-miR-1b	− 1.53	1.14	− 1.37
rno-miR-139-5p	− 1.54	− 1.09	− 1.41	rno-miR-148a-3p	− 1.40	− 1.10	− 1.20
rno-miR-668	− 1.19	1.12	− 1.20	rno-miR-126a-5p	− 1.46	1.09	− 1.47
rno-miR-342-5p	− 1.15	1.10	− 1.11	rno-miR-28-5p	− 1.39	1.08	− 1.30
rno-miR-344a-3p	− 1.18	1.01	− 1.21	rno-miR-204-5p	− 1.47	1.00	− 1.20
rno-miR-330-3p	− 1.30	− 1.05	− 1.19	rno-miR-181c-3p	− 1.67	− 1.14	− 1.42
rno-miR-1843a-3p	− 1.13	1.01	− 1.16	rno-miR-3068-3p	− 1.58	− 1.08	− 1.24
rno-miR-328a-3p	− 1.18	− 1.08	− 1.18	rno-miR-30c-5p	− 1.41	1.03	− 1.15
				rno-miR-27a-3p	− 1.16	1.06	− 1.21

Table 3 Changes in noncoding RNA miRNA *(Continued)*

					rno-miR-139-5p	− 1.33	− 1.07	− 1.24
					rno-miR-140-5p	− 1.30	1.06	− 1.25
					rno-miR-337-5p	− 1.42	− 1.05	− 1.34
					rno-miR-30a-5p	− 1.16	1.03	− 1.08
					rno-miR-150-5p	− 1.29	− 1.10	− 1.16
					rno-miR-147	− 1.12	1.04	− 1.09
					rno-miR-30e-5p	− 1.24	− 1.08	− 1.14

ncRNA including snoRNA, snRNA

Brain + 1		C vsT	C vs TE	C vs TEdM	Brain − 1		C vsT	C vs TE	C vs TEdM
snRNA	U6	1.57	1.00	1.37	snoRNA	SNORD42	− 1.90	− 1.24	− 1.82
snoRNA	SNORD24	1.28	1.11	1.38	lncRNA	PVT1 3	− 1.98	− 1.34	− 2.18
snoRNA	SNORD60	1.25	1.00	1.22	snoRNA	SNORA28	− 1.29	− 1.07	− 1.97
snRNA	U6	1.09	1.00	1.06	rRNA	Rnr2	− 1.25	− 1.07	− 1.23
snoRNA	ACEA U3	1.64	1.05	1.59	rRNA	Rnr2	− 1.09	− 1.10	− 1.29
snoRNA	SNORA62	1.51	− 1.04	1.27	lncRNA	RMST 2	− 1.19	− 1.06	− 1.13
snoRNA	SNORA73	1.39	− 1.24	1.30					
snoRNA	SNORD62	1.76	− 1.21	1.32					
snoRNA	SNORD15	3.17	1.38	3.12					
snoRNA	SNORA38	1.06	− 1.00	1.06					
Spleen + 1					Spleen − 1				
snoRNA	SNORD74	1.85	− 1.39	1.52	snoRNA	SNORA41	− 3.84	− 1.14	− 1.85
snRNA	U6	1.67	− 1.27	1.67	snoRNA	SNORD33	− 3.68	− 1.64	− 3.91
snoRNA	SNORD75	1.68	− 1.03	1.50	snoRNA	SNORA54	− 3.49	1.06	− 1.98
scRNA		1.32	− 1.23	1.14	snoRNA	SNORD21	− 3.48	− 1.48	− 3.88
lncRNA	LOC100909539	1.37	− 1.06	1.48	snoRNA	SNORA71	− 2.94	− 1.55	− 3.67
misc_RNA		1.31	1.10	1.42	vault_RNA	Vault	− 2.93	− 1.49	− 5.34
lncRNA	Bc1	1.15	1.04	1.25	snoRNA	SNORA11	− 2.71	− 1.08	− 2.24

Noncoding RNA levels change with injury and exosome treatment in a MALAT1-dependent manner

Long noncoding RNAs promote epigenetic modifications and regulate gene expression by direct interaction with pre-mRNA of genes or by acting as scaffolding to tether a complex of micro RNAs to promote transcription of genes. There is an emerging appreciation for its ability to not only interact with other noncoding RNAs but also promote transcription of these noncoding RNAs. Among the noncoding RNAs (ncRNAs) detected in the brain and spleen, a large number are associated with tRNA, rRNA, and small nuclear RNAs (snRNAs) whose function is constitutive in transcription and translation processes. Our study points to two primary classes of ncRNAs that are directly affected by the exosomes containing MALAT1: the microRNAs (miR) and the small nucleolar RNAs (snoRNAs).

miRNAs regulate gene expression by directly binding to their target mRNA. Our RNA Seq data identified miR-200b, miR-200a, miR-183, miR-182, miR-96, and miR-451a as being significantly upregulated four- to eightfold in the brain with TBI (Table 3). These miRNAs were previously shown to regulate apoptosis in various diseases [43–52]. Significantly, treatment with exosomes downregulated their expression; however, MALAT1-depleted exosomes did not have a significant effect on the expression of these miRNAs. When the RNA Seq data of the brain is sorted and analyzed by the + 1 pattern described above, we note that miR-96-5p, miR-182, miR-183-5p, miR-200b-5p, miR-429, mir-6216, miR-1193-3p, and miR-218a-2-3p increase following TBI, decreased by exosome treatment, and the reversal is not seen with MALAT1-deficient exosomes. miR200b-3p and miR-182-5p are increased following TBI in the brain, the latter of which is directly modulated by MALAT1. Both of these miRNAs also show a reduction following treatment with exosomes, but not exosomes depleted of MALAT1, opening the possibility that MALAT1 in exosomes may be responsible for the shift in pattern. A second set of miRNAs include miR-487b-3p, miR-672-3p, miR-10a-5p, miR-770-5p, miR-666-5p, miR-29c-3p, miR-139-3p, miR-668, miR-344a-3p, and miR1843a-3p that follow the – 1 pattern such that they decrease following TBI, increased by exosome treatment, and the reversal is not seen with MALAT1-deficient exosomes. Of the miRNAs whose expression changes with injury and exosome treatment, miR10a-5p follows the – 1 pattern in the brain and the spleen. miR10a-5p is extensively studied for its role in the development and regulation of TOP mRNAs [53]. miR10a-5p promotes expression of ribosomal proteins, elongation factors, and other proteins associated with translation apparatus, thereby influencing global protein synthesis. miR10a-5p expression is increased in stem cells and in our experiments, making it possible that miR10a-5p is part of the exosomal cargo, which is transferred both to the brain and spleen, and has a predominant role in enhancing the response to injury and aiding the recovery upon treatment with exosomes.

SnoRNAs function as sequence-specific guides to direct site-specific nucleoside modifications for other noncoding RNAs such as rRNA and snRNA. A select few snoRNAs are shown to interact with mRNA and regulate its splicing [54–56]. Recent breakthroughs have predicted the interaction of lncRNAs with snoRNAs [57]; however, their association are not shown in vivo. SnoRNAs are transcribed as nuclease products from genes. Our data shows, for the first time, that a long noncoding RNA MALAT1 regulates the expression of snoRNAs in the brain. Notably, SNORA31, SNORD33, SNORD64, SNORA18, SNORA17, SNORD44, SNORD47, SNORD28, SNORD113, SNORD62, SNORA29, and SNORD2 were upregulated two- to fourfold with exosome treatment following TBI; MALAT1-depleted exosomes did not increase the levels of these snoRNAs (Table 3). Brain-specific snoRNAs in mice MBI48 and MBI52 were shown to promote memory and learning [58, 59]. While lncRNAs are known to have a role in pre-mRNA splicing, mRNA editing, and mRNA stability control, this is the first evidence showing that lncRNA MALAT1 regulates the expression and transcription of brain snoRNAs.

Discussion

In summary, we have demonstrated that exosomes secreted from hASCs have a beneficial role in modulating pathology following mild TBI, particularly those containing MALAT1. Our results have shown an attenuation in TBI-induced motor deficits as well as decreased cortical damage at both the impact and peri-impact level after administration of exosome treatment that is dependent on MALAT1. Our previous in vitro study using HT22 cells demonstrated that MALAT1 has a role in neuroprotection in vitro. Indeed, we showed that hASC-derived exosomes

increase neuronal survival and proliferation in vitro in the context of several models of injury and this activity is lost when the exosomes are depleted of MALAT1 [27]. These results suggest that intravenous administration of exosomes generated from hASCs may represent a novel therapeutic approach for treatment of TBI. This is consistent with the report that MALAT1 regulates pathology following ischemic injuries [28]. To distinguish the actions of subcomponents of conditioned media, we treated rats with CM that did not contain exosomes and found it had a reduced effect on most measures when compared to exosome treatment. However, there was still some effect seen from CM depleted of exosomes. The difference between the exosome treatment and the CM depleted of exosomes suggests the cargo found within the exosome is important for providing significant neuroprotection and promoting regeneration after injury. Secondly, the effect shown with CM treatment, even depleted of exosomes, suggests the possibility that the CM maintains valuable secreted factors.

Exosomes are known to hold a plethora of biological molecules in its complex cargo including proteins, lipids, mRNAs, and miRNAs capable of interacting with surrounding cells in order to modify the host environment [60]. Exosomes generated from MSCs have been shown to significantly increase brain angiogenesis and neurogenesis as well as reduce neuroinflammation; however, the specific molecular constituents driving regeneration were not identified in most studies [20]. It is thought that RNA cargo plays an important role in the cell-to-cell communication driving neuroprotection, making it a key component in promoting the recovery seen following injury. Our study demonstrates that lncRNA MALAT1 is a critical component of the hASC exosomes and drives the recovery process. Many single molecular pathway approaches have shown little or no promise in clinical trials [61], and this emphasizes a need for combination therapies to tackle the complexity of secondary neurological injury post TBI. Treatment with exosomes is considered to be a multi-targeted approach as they are able to seek and modulate multiple targets and enforce a neuroprotective environment, providing further promise for their use as a therapeutic approach.

In this study, we demonstrate for the first time the in vivo and ex vivo biodistribution of intravenous DIR-labeled exosomes derived from hASCs. It is well known that when administering cell therapy intravenously, the cells migrate to multiple organs and here we show exosomes migrating to the same organ sites, with some differences in time course and degree of migration. Most importantly, we found that the exosomes are observed in the spleen and liver area within 1 h of IV treatment when observed both in vivo and ex vivo, followed by a decrease in radiance efficiencies over time. Though migration to the liver probably serves as a filtering and elimination process, the migration of the exosomes to the spleen implicates a probable immune interaction. It has been shown that injury induces the release of immune cells from the spleen with consequent infiltration into the brain [62] and that this is a significant aspect of the secondary insult following TBI as discussed in the introduction. It has been shown that blocking entry of inflammatory monocytes into the brain can significantly reduce the observed damage and offers recovery of cognitive function [9]. The spleen is one source of peripheral macrophages and monocytes, and it is possible that treatment with exosomes inhibits the release of these immune cells into circulation. This in turn lessens the infiltration into the brain through the disrupted BBB and prevents the contribution of peripheral immune cells to the secondary injury. This was supported by the observed inhibition of ephrin family gene expression following TBI as a predicted upstream regulator in the spleen following injury. This inhibition was modulated by exosome treatment but not by treatment with exosomes depleted of MALAT1. Ephrins are regulators of transendothelial migration of monocyte/macrophages and have been shown to play a role in monocyte adhesion in the red pulp of the spleen [41]. Thus, a decrease with TBI could be reflective of a migration of monocytes into the circulation. Therefore, the observed migration of the exosomes to the spleen immediately after administration could be an important aspect of the mechanism of action that elicits the improvement in both cellular and functional recovery as seen here post TBI. Future studies can look deeper into this potential mechanism of action and the role of MALAT1 at the level of the spleen.

Exosomes were also observed in the brain, albeit with a much lower degree of signal and with a different time course than that observed for the spleen. Exosomes were primarily observed around the site of injury. The BBB is known to be disrupted by TBI [63] peaking at 4–6 h and 2–3 days after injury [64] and therefore may explain one factor for the observed delayed localization of exosomes. Alternatively, it is also possible that there is expression of chemokine or signaling molecules that would attract the exosomes to the area of injury. At this time, we do not know if the primary site for the therapeutic effect of the exosomes is at the level of the spleen or the brain, and it is likely that both play some role. It has been shown that hASC-derived exosomes like those studied here have direct neuroprotective effect on neuronal cells [27] and this is another area of future investigation.

RNA Seq is a robust method to evaluate the effect of TBI at the genomic level. We have identified genes and pathways that are affected by TBI as well as the genomic influences of exosome treatment. Our study has demonstrated that treatment with exosomes post TBI significantly improves the outcome by modulating gene networks. The knowledge of specific genes and pathways as well as the influence of noncoding RNA in exosome treatment post TBI is crucial to develop an understanding of the multitude of events that occur simultaneously to promote healing. Our data indicates that not only genes involved in survival are affected but also those genes that are involved in the inflammatory and immune response to injury. The cargo carried by the exosomes is pivotal in cell-cell communication and influences the response to injury and recovery. Exosomes from hASC contain not only lncRNA MALAT1 but also additional lncRNAs and proteins [29]. Our study specifically focused on the role of MALAT1; however, as shown in the data, other ncRNAs or proteins carried in the exosomes may also aid in the recovery process. Further studies are being undertaken to delineate additional players and the complex interactions between lncRNAs and other RNA and proteins.

The above results demonstrate that the lncRNA MALAT1 regulates expression of mRNA and ncRNA involved in the inflammatory response, apoptosis and cell survival, signal transduction by MAPK pathways, and transcription of genes. There is also an emerging appreciation for the ability of lncRNA to not only interact with other ncRNAs but also promote transcription of these ncRNAs. Our data demonstrates for the first time that a lncRNA promotes expression of snoRNAs. Our dataset contains a tremendous amount of information on novel and known genes in the brain and spleen that were not previously recognized. This RNA Seq data provides a valuable tool to elucidate additional genes and ncRNAs in the brain and spleen and provides a robust biological system to validate its findings.

Conclusions

Taken together, our data demonstrate that hASC-derived exosomes containing MALAT1 have a beneficial effect on function and pathology following a CCI injury. Importantly, we show that the lncRNA MALAT1 affects not only mRNA expression but also expression of noncoding RNA. Thus, the action of the exosomes is multifold and impacts a number of cell survival, inflammatory, and regulatory pathways in both the spleen and the brain. As exosomes show tremendous promise as therapeutics, understanding the importance of the cargo of the exosomes is critical for understanding their mechanism of action as well as determining how to identify the exosomes with the most potential for benefit.

Abbreviations
BBB: Blood-brain barrier; CCI: Controlled cortical impact; CDC: Center for Disease Control; EBST: Elevated body swing; GFAP: Glial fibrillary acid protein; GFP: Green fluorescent protein; hASC: Human adipose-derived stem cell;

lncRNA: Long noncoding RNA; MALAT1: Metastasis-associated lung adenocarcinoma transcript 1; miRNA: Micro RNA; mRNA: Messenger RNA; MSC: Mesenchymal stem cell; ncRNA: Noncoding RNA; RNA: Ribonucleic acid; SGZ: Subgranular zone; SVZ: Subventricular zone; TBI: Traumatic brain injury

Acknowledgements
This work was supported by the VA Medical Research Service; however, this work does not reflect the view or opinion of the James A. Haley VA Hospital nor the US Government. We thank Ionis Pharmaceuticals for MALAT1 antisense oligonucleotides.

Funding
This work was supported by a grant from USF to PCB and CB and VAMR grant I01BX003421 to PCB and VAMR grant 821-MR-EN-20606 to NAP.

Authors' contributions
NAP, PCB, CVB, and DRC designed the experiments. NAP, PCB, CVB, LD, JYL, NT, SP, and CH carried out the experiments. NAP, PCB, CVB, LD, and JYL analyzed and interpreted the data and wrote the manuscript. All authors read and approved the final manuscript.

Consent for publication
Not applicable

Competing interests
PCB, CVB, DRC, and NAP have IP related to this manuscript. The authors declare that they have no competing interests.

Author details
[1]James A Haley Veterans Hospital, Research Service, Tampa, FL, USA. [2]Department of Molecular Medicine, University of South Florida Morsani College of Medicine, 12901 Bruce B Downs Blvd, Tampa, FL 33612, USA. [3]Department of Neurosurgery and Brain Repair, University of South Florida Morsani College of Medicine, Tampa, FL, USA. [4]Present address: Department of Neurophysiology & Brain Science, Graduate School of Medical Sciences & Medical School, Nagoya City University, 1 Kawasumi, Mizuho-cho, Mizuho-ku, Nagoya, Aichi 467-8601, Japan. [5]USF Health Center of Excellence for Aging and Brain Repair MDC-78, 12901 Bruce B Downs, Blvd, Tampa, FL 33612, USA.

References
1. Dams-O'Connor K, Cuthbert JP, Whyte J, Corrigan JD, Faul M, Harrison-Felix C. Traumatic brain injury among older adults at level I and II trauma centers. J Neurotrauma. 2013;30(24):2001–13.
2. Leo P, McCrea M. Epidemiology. In: Laskowitz D, Grant G, editors. Translational research in traumatic brain injury. Boca Raton: Taylor and Francis Group, LLC; 2016.
3. McKee AC, Daneshvar DH. The neuropathology of traumatic brain injury. Handb Clin Neurol. 2015;127:45–66.
4. Levin H, Smith D. Traumatic brain injury: networks and neuropathology. Lancet Neurol. 2013;12(1):15–6.
5. Blennow K, Hardy J, Zetterberg H. The neuropathology and neurobiology of traumatic brain injury. Neuron. 2012;76(5):886–99.
6. Magnuson J, Leonessa F, Ling GS. Neuropathology of explosive blast traumatic brain injury. Curr Neurol Neurosci Rep. 2012;12(5):570–9.
7. Acosta SA, Tajiri N, Shinozuka K, Ishikawa H, Grimmig B, Diamond DM, Sanberg PR, Bickford PC, Kaneko Y, Borlongan CV. Long-term upregulation of inflammation and suppression of cell proliferation in the brain of adult rats exposed to traumatic brain injury using the controlled cortical impact model. PLoS One. 2013;8(1):e53376.
8. Johnson VE, Stewart JE, Begbie FD, Trojanowski JQ, Smith DH, Stewart W. Inflammation and white matter degeneration persist for years after a single traumatic brain injury. Brain. 2013;136(Pt 1):28–42.
9. Morganti JM, Jopson TD, Liu S, Riparip LK, Guandique CK, Gupta N, Ferguson AR, Rosi S. CCR2 antagonism alters brain macrophage polarization and ameliorates cognitive dysfunction induced by traumatic brain injury. J Neurosci. 2015;35(2):748–60.
10. Saiwai H, Kumamaru H, Ohkawa Y, Kubota K, Kobayakawa K, Yamada H, Yokomizo T, Iwamoto Y, Okada S. Ly6C+ Ly6G- Myeloid-derived suppressor cells play a critical role in the resolution of acute inflammation and the subsequent tissue repair process after spinal cord injury. J Neurochem. 2013; 125(1):74–88.
11. Semple BD, Bye N, Ziebell JM, Morganti-Kossmann MC. Deficiency of the chemokine receptor CXCR2 attenuates neutrophil infiltration and cortical damage following closed head injury. Neurobiol Dis. 2010;40(2): 394–403.
12. Semple BD, Bye N, Rancan M, Ziebell JM, Morganti-Kossmann MC. Role of CCL2 (MCP-1) in traumatic brain injury (TBI): evidence from severe TBI patients and CCL2–/– mice. J Cereb Blood Flow Metab. 2010;30(4):769–82.
13. Vendrame M, Gemma C, de MD, Collier L, Bickford PC, Sanberg CD, Sanberg PR, Pennypacker KR, Willing AE. Anti-inflammatory effects of human cord blood cells in a rat model of stroke. Stem Cells Dev. 2005;14(5):595–604.
14. Walker PA, Shah SK, Jimenez F, Gerber MH, Xue H, Cutrone R, Hamilton JA, Mays RW, Deans R, Pati S, et al. Intravenous multipotent adult progenitor cell therapy for traumatic brain injury: preserving the blood brain barrier via an interaction with splenocytes. ExpNeurol. 2010;225(2):341–52.
15. Walker PA, Bedi SS, Shah SK, Jimenez F, Xue H, Hamilton JA, Smith P, Thomas CP, Mays RW, Pati S, et al. Intravenous multipotent adult progenitor cell therapy after traumatic brain injury: modulation of the resident microglia population. J Neuroinflammation. 2012;9:228.
16. Walker PA, Shah SK, Jimenez F, Aroom KR, Harting MT, Cox CS Jr. Bone marrow-derived stromal cell therapy for traumatic brain injury is neuroprotective via stimulation of non-neurologic organ systems. Surgery. 2012;152(5):790–3.
17. Gupta A, Pulliam L. Exosomes as mediators of neuroinflammation. J Neuroinflammation. 2014;11:68.
18. Ge X, Han Z, Chen F, Wang H, Zhang B, Jiang R, Lei P, Zhang J. MiR-21 alleviates secondary blood-brain barrier damage after traumatic brain injury in rats. Brain Res. 2015;1603:150–7.
19. Xin H, Li Y, Cui Y, Yang JJ, Zhang ZG, Chopp M. Systemic administration of exosomes released from mesenchymal stromal cells promote functional recovery and neurovascular plasticity after stroke in rats. J Cereb Blood Flow Metab. 2013;33(11):1711–5.
20. Zhang Y, Chopp M, Meng Y, Katakowski M, Xin H, Mahmood A, Xiong Y. Effect of exosomes derived from multipluripotent mesenchymal stromal cells on functional recovery and neurovascular plasticity in rats after traumatic brain injury. J Neurosurg. 2015;122(4):856–67.
21. Kim DK, Nishida H, An SY, Shetty AK, Bartosh TJ, Prockop DJ. Chromatographically isolated CD63+CD81+ extracellular vesicles from mesenchymal stromal cells rescue cognitive impairments after TBI. Proc Natl Acad Sci U S A. 2016;113(1):170–5.
22. Zhu M, Chen Q, Liu X, Sun Q, Zhao X, Deng R, Wang Y, Huang J, Xu M, Yan J, et al. lncRNA H19/miR-675 axis represses prostate cancer metastasis by targeting TGFBI. FEBS J. 2014;281(16):3766–75.
23. Zhao Q, Li T, Qi J, Liu J, Qin C. The miR-545/374a cluster encoded in the Ftx lncRNA is overexpressed in HBV-related hepatocellular carcinoma and promotes tumorigenesis and tumor progression. PLoS One. 2014;9(10):e109782.
24. Schmidt LH, Gorlich D, Spieker T, Rohde C, Schuler M, Mohr M, Humberg J, Sauer T, Thoenissen NH, Huge A, et al. Prognostic impact of Bcl-2 depends on tumor histology and expression of MALAT-1 lncRNA in non-small-cell lung cancer. J Thorac Oncol. 2014;9(9):1294–304.
25. Qin X, Yao J, Geng P, Fu X, Xue J, Zhang Z. LncRNA TSLC1-AS1 is a novel tumor suppressor in glioma. Int J Clin Exp Pathol. 2014;7(6):3065–72.
26. Tajiri N, Acosta SA, Shahaduzzaman M, Ishikawa H, Shinozuka K, Pabon M, Hernandez-Ontiveros D, Kim DW, Metcalf C, Staples M, et al. Intravenous transplants of human adipose-derived stem cell protect the brain from traumatic brain injury-induced neurodegeneration and motor and cognitive impairments: cell graft

biodistribution and soluble factors in young and aged rats. J Neurosci. 2014;34(1):313–26.

27. El Bassit G, Patel RS, Carter G, Shibu V, Patel AA, Song S, Murr M, Cooper DR, Bickford PC, Patel NA. MALAT1 in human adipose stem cells modulates survival and alternative splicing of PKCdeltaII in HT22 cells. Endocrinology. 2017;158(1):183–95.

28. Zhang X, Tang X, Liu K, Hamblin MH, Yin KJ. Long noncoding RNA Malat1 regulates cerebrovascular pathologies in ischemic stroke. J Neurosci. 2017; 37(7):1797–806.

29. Patel RS, Carter G, El Bassit G, Patel AA, Cooper DR, Murr M, Patel NA. Adipose-derived stem cells from lean and obese humans show depot specific differences in their stem cell markers, exosome contents and senescence: role of protein kinase C delta (PKCdelta) in adipose stem cell niche. Stem Cell Investig. 2016;3:2.

30. Borlongan CV, Sanberg PR. Elevated body swing test: a new behavioral parameter for rats with 6-hydroxydopamine-induced hemiparkinsonism. J Neurosci. 1995;15(7 Pt 2):5372–8.

31. Borlongan CV, Hida H, Nishino H. Early assessment of motor dysfunctions aids in successful occlusion of the middle cerebral artery. Neuroreport. 1998; 9(16):3615–21.

32. Zeng Y, Liu H, Kang K, Wang Z, Hui G, Zhang X, Zhong J, Peng W, Ramchandran R, Usha Raj J, et al. Hypoxia inducible factor-1 mediates expression of miR-322: potential role in proliferation and migration of pulmonary arterial smooth muscle cells. Sci Rep. 2015;5:12098.

33. Kawasaki T, Choudhry MA, Suzuki T, Schwacha MG, Bland KI, Chaudry IH. 17beta-Estradiol's salutary effects on splenic dendritic cell functions following trauma-hemorrhage are mediated via estrogen receptor-alpha. Mol Immunol. 2008;45(2):376–85.

34. Bruce-Keller AJ, Dimayuga FO, Reed JL, Wang C, Angers R, Wilson ME, Dimayuga VM, Scheff SW. Gender and estrogen manipulation do not affect traumatic brain injury in mice. JNeurotrauma. 2007;24(1):203–15.

35. Suzuki T, Shimizu T, Yu HP, Hsieh YC, Choudhry MA, Bland KI, Chaudry IH. Estrogen receptor-alpha predominantly mediates the salutary effects of 17beta-estradiol on splenic macrophages following trauma-hemorrhage. Am J Physiol Cell Physiol. 2007;293(3):C978–84.

36. Hildebrand F, Hubbard WJ, Choudhry MA, Thobe BM, Pape HC, Chaudry IH. Are the protective effects of 17beta-estradiol on splenic macrophages and splenocytes after trauma-hemorrhage mediated via estrogen-receptor (ER)-alpha or ER-beta? J Leukoc Biol. 2006;79(6): 1173–80.

37. Aiello A, Bacci L, Re A, Ripoli C, Pierconti F, Pinto F, Masetti R, Grassi C, Gaetano C, Bassi PF, et al. MALAT1 and HOTAIR long non-coding RNAs play opposite role in estrogen-mediated transcriptional regulation in prostate cancer cells. Sci Rep. 2016;6:38414.

38. Fang D, Yang H, Lin J, Teng Y, Jiang Y, Chen J, Li Y. 17beta-estradiol regulates cell proliferation, colony formation, migration, invasion and promotes apoptosis by upregulating miR-9 and thus degrades MALAT-1 in osteosarcoma cell MG-63 in an estrogen receptor-independent manner. Biochem Biophys Res Commun. 2015;457(4): 500–6.

39. Zhao Z, Chen C, Liu Y, Wu C. 17beta-Estradiol treatment inhibits breast cell proliferation, migration and invasion by decreasing MALAT-1 RNA level. Biochem Biophys Res Commun. 2014;445(2):388–93.

40. Ting MJ, Day BW, Spanevello MD, Boyd AW. Activation of ephrin A proteins influences hematopoietic stem cell adhesion and trafficking patterns. Exp Hematol. 2010;38(11):1087–98.

41. Konda N, Saeki N, Nishino S, Ogawa K. Truncated EphA2 likely potentiates cell adhesion via integrins as well as infiltration and/or lodgment of a monocyte/macrophage cell line in the red pulp and marginal zone of the mouse spleen, where ephrin-A1 is prominently expressed in the vasculature. Histochem Cell Biol. 2017;147(3):317–39.

42. Swirski FK, Nahrendorf M, Etzrodt M, Wildgruber M, Cortez-Retamozo V, Panizzi P, Figueiredo JL, Kohler RH, Chudnovskiy A, Waterman P, et al. Identification of splenic reservoir monocytes and their deployment to inflammatory sites. Science. 2009;325(5940):612–6.

43. Guo Y, Liu H, Zhang H, Shang C, Song Y. miR-96 regulates FOXO1-mediated cell apoptosis in bladder cancer. Oncol Lett. 2012;4(3):561–5.

44. Tian Y, Nan Y, Han L, Zhang A, Wang G, Jia Z, Hao J, Pu P, Zhong Y, Kang C. MicroRNA miR-451 downregulates the PI3K/AKT pathway through CAB39 in human glioma. Int J Oncol. 2012;40(4):1105–12.

45. Xu XM, Qian JC, Deng ZL, Cai Z, Tang T, Wang P, Zhang KH, Cai JP. Expression of miR-21, miR-31, miR-96 and miR-135b is correlated with the clinical parameters of colorectal cancer. Oncol Lett. 2012;4(2):339–45.

46. Zhu W, Xu H, Zhu D, Zhi H, Wang T, Wang J, Jiang B, Shu Y, Liu P. miR-200bc/429 cluster modulates multidrug resistance of human cancer cell lines by targeting BCL2 and XIAP. Cancer Chemother Pharmacol. 2012;69(3):723–31.

47. Du ZW, Ma LX, Phillips C, Zhang SC. miR-200 and miR-96 families repress neural induction from human embryonic stem cells. Development. 2013; 140(12):2611–8.

48. Fendler A, Jung M, Stephan C, Erbersdobler A, Jung K, Yousef GM. The antiapoptotic function of miR-96 in prostate cancer by inhibition of FOXO1. PLoS One. 2013;8(11):e80807.

49. Li HP, Zeng XC, Zhang B, Long JT, Zhou B, Tan GS, Zeng WX, Chen W, Yang JY. miR-451 inhibits cell proliferation in human hepatocellular carcinoma through direct suppression of IKK-beta. Carcinogenesis. 2013;34(11):2443–51.

50. Lewis A, Felice C, Kumagai T, Lai C, Singh K, Jeffery RR, Feakins R, Giannoulatou E, Armuzzi A, Jawad N, et al. The miR-200 family is increased in dysplastic lesions in ulcerative colitis patients. PLoS One. 2017;12(3): e0173664.

51. Magenta A, Ciarapica R, Capogrossi MC. The emerging role of miR-200 family in cardiovascular diseases. Circ Res. 2017;120(9):1399–402.

52. Majer A, Caligiuri KA, Gale KK, Niu Y, Phillipson CS, Booth TF, Booth SA. Induction of multiple miR-200/182 members in the brains of mice are associated with acute herpes simplex virus 1 encephalitis. PLoS One. 2017; 12(1):e0169081.

53. Lund AH. miR-10 in development and cancer. Cell Death Differ. 2010;17(2):209–14.

54. de Turris V, Di Leva G, Caldarola S, Loreni F, Amaldi F, Bozzoni I. TOP promoter elements control the relative ratio of intron-encoded snoRNA versus spliced mRNA biosynthesis. J Mol Biol. 2004;344(2):383–94.

55. Kishore S, Stamm S. Regulation of alternative splicing by snoRNAs. Cold Spring Harb Symp Quant Biol. 2006;71:329–34.

56. Bazeley PS, Shepelev V, Talebizadeh Z, Butler MG, Fedorova L, Filatov V, Fedorov A. snoTARGET shows that human orphan snoRNA targets locate close to alternative splice junctions. Gene. 2008;408(1–2):172–9.

57. Chaudhry MA. Small nucleolar RNA host genes and long non-coding RNA responses in directly irradiated and bystander cells. Cancer Biother Radiopharm. 2014;29(3):135–41.

58. Kishore S, Khanna A, Zhang Z, Hui J, Balwierz PJ, Stefan M, Beach C, Nicholls RD, Zavolan M, Stamm S. The snoRNA MBII-52 (SNORD 115) is processed into smaller RNAs and regulates alternative splicing. Hum Mol Genet. 2010; 19(7):1153–64.

59. Kishore S, Stamm S. The snoRNA HBII-52 regulates alternative splicing of the serotonin receptor 2C. Science. 2006;311(5758):230–2.

60. Vlassov AV, Magdaleno S, Setterquist R, Conrad R. Exosomes: current knowledge of their composition, biological functions, and diagnostic and therapeutic potentials. Biochim Biophys Acta. 2012;1820(7):940–8.

61. McConeghy KW, Hatton J, Hughes L, Cook AM. A review of neuroprotection pharmacology and therapies in patients with acute traumatic brain injury. CNS Drugs. 2012;26(7):613–36.

62. Stewart IB, McKenzie DC. The human spleen during physiological stress. Sports Med. 2002;32(6):361–9.

63. Baldwin SA, Fugaccia I, Brown DR, Brown LV, Scheff SW. Blood-brain barrier breach following cortical contusion in the rat. J Neurosurg. 1996;85(3):476–81.

64. Baskaya MK, Rao AM, Dogan A, Donaldson D, Dempsey RJ. The biphasic opening of the blood-brain barrier in the cortex and hippocampus after traumatic brain injury in rats. Neurosci Lett. 1997;226(1):33–6.

13

Time-dependent effects of CX3CR1 in a mouse model of mild traumatic brain injury

Heidi Y. Febinger[1,6], Hannah E. Thomasy[1,2], Maria N. Pavlova[1], Kristyn M. Ringgold[1], Paulien R. Barf[1], Amrita M. George[1], Jenna N. Grillo[1,3], Adam D. Bachstetter[4], Jenny A. Garcia[5], Astrid E. Cardona[5], Mark R. Opp[1] and Carmelina Gemma[1*]

Abstract

Background: Neuroinflammation is an important secondary mechanism that is a key mediator of the long-term consequences of neuronal injury that occur in traumatic brain injury (TBI). Microglia are highly plastic cells with dual roles in neuronal injury and recovery. Recent studies suggest that the chemokine fractalkine (CX3CL1, *FKN*) mediates neural/microglial interactions via its sole receptor CX3CR1. CX3CL1/CX3CR1 signaling modulates microglia activation, and depending upon the type and time of injury, either protects or exacerbates neurological diseases.

Methods: In this study, mice deficient in CX3CR1 were subjected to mild controlled cortical impact injury (CCI), a model of TBI. We evaluated the effects of genetic deletion of CX3CR1 on histopathology, cell death/survival, microglia activation, and cognitive function for 30 days post-injury.

Results: During the acute post-injury period (24 h–15 days), motor deficits, cell death, and neuronal cell loss were more profound in injured wild-type than in $CX3CR1^{-/-}$ mice. In contrast, during the chronic period of 30 days post-TBI, injured $CX3CR1^{-/-}$ mice exhibited greater cognitive dysfunction and increased neuronal death than wild-type mice. The protective and deleterious effects of CX3CR1 were associated with changes in microglia phenotypes; during the acute phase $CX3CR1^{-/-}$ mice showed a predominant anti-inflammatory M2 microglial response, with increased expression of Ym1, CD206, and TGFβ. In contrast, increased M1 phenotypic microglia markers, Marco, and CD68 were predominant at 30 days post-TBI.

Conclusion: Collectively, these novel data demonstrate a time-dependent role for CX3CL1/CX3CR1 signaling after TBI and suggest that the acute and chronic responses to mild TBI are modulated in part by distinct microglia phenotypes.

Keywords: CX3CR1, TBI, Microglia, Cognitive function, Cytokines

Background

Traumatic brain injury (TBI) is a serious public health problem in the United States. Mild TBI is rarely recognized in a timely manner because symptoms often do not manifest for some time after the injury. However, the consequences of mild TBI can be long lasting. The pathophysiology of TBI is complex, in part because multiple pathways are involved in the primary and secondary injuries that result from the insult.

A consensus based on recent evidence considers neuroinflammation as an important secondary mechanism

that plays a role in delaying injury after TBI [1–3]. Dysregulated and uncontrolled microglial activation may be a key component of chronic neuroinflammatory processes. Recent studies suggest that the chemokine fractalkine (CX3CL1, *FKN*) mediates neural/microglial interactions via its sole receptor CX3CR1. Indeed, deleting CX3CR1 [4] exacerbates microglial neurotoxicity induced by systemic inflammation in rodent models of Parkinson's disease and amyotrophic lateral sclerosis [5]. In addition, $CX3CR1^{-/-}$ microglia exacerbate cell-autonomous microglial neurotoxicity induced by lipopolysaccharide (LPS), suggesting that fractalkine signaling is important for limiting microglia toxicity [5, 6]. CX3CL1 also protects against excitotoxicity through the activation of the ERK1/2 and PI3K/Akt pathways [7, 8]. However, the role of FKN/

* Correspondence: cgemma@u.washington.edu
[1]Department of Anesthesiology and Pain Medicine, University of Washington, BOX # 359724, Seattle, WA 98001, USA
Full list of author information is available at the end of the article

CX3CR1 signaling in neurodegenerative disease is an intricate and highly debated research topic that is becoming even more complicated as new studies reveal seemingly discordant results. It appears that FKN/CX3CR1 signaling plays a direct role in neurodegeneration and/or neuroprotection depending upon the CNS insult. Both beneficial and detrimental effects of CX3CR1 deficiency are associated with microglia activation [9–11]. Data from some models of chronic neuronal injury suggest that CX3CR1 is protective because the absence of this receptor increases microglia activity and is associated with less favorable outcome [8, 12–16]. For instance, in a model of Alzheimer's disease (AD), CX3CR1-deficient microglia from mice overexpressing hTau have increased hyperphosphorylated tau and more toxicity, as has been observed in other animal's disease models [5, 17–20]. On the other hand, in 3x-Tg AD mice, which reproduces both Aβ and tau pathologies, deleting CX3CR1 prevents neuronal loss and microglial migration without affecting amyloid deposition [21]. Finally, other reports indicate that CX3CR1 deficiency attenuates amyloid deposition in AD mouse models characterized by extensive plaque deposition [18, 22].

The complex CX3CL1/CX3CR1 signaling pathway is further complicated by its functional role in acute injuries. Results from some acute injury models suggest that CX3CR1 is detrimental because its absence is associated with a favorable outcome. For instance, in a model of cerebral ischemia and spinal cord injury, CX3CR1$^{-/-}$ mice showed neuroprotection and improved functional recovery [23–26]. These observations suggest that CX3CR1 may play different roles in neuronal injury depending on the type of injury and on the post-injury time point assessed (chronic vs acute). CX3CL1 levels increase in the cerebrospinal fluid and in the brain of patients with head trauma, and increased CX3CL1/CX3CR1 is associated with better clinical outcome [27, 28]. However, few preclinical studies of TBI focus on the CX3CL1/CX3CR1 system. Determining a role for CX3CL1/CX3CR1 signaling in outcomes after mild TBI during the acute and chronic phase is a goal of the present study.

We now know that the microglia assume diverse phenotypes in response to specific microenvironmental signals. Although there is a spectrum of different microglial types, there are two major microglia phenotypes characterized by a molecular signature of gene expression: the "classical" inflammatory state (M1) and the "alternative" activation state (M2). M1 microglia are generally considered pro-inflammatory whereas M2 microglia are generally anti-inflammatory [29–34]. In the healthy young brain, M1 and M2 microglia exist in a state of dynamic equilibrium. Following an injury, there is a shift into an M1 phenotype that exacerbates tissue injury or into an M2 phenotype that promotes CNS repair, depending on the local signals in the lesion's microenvironment [35].

In this study, we demonstrate that lack of CX3CL1/CX3CR1 signaling in the brain leads to delayed neuronal damage and neurologic and cognitive impairment after TBI that is associated with a switch in microglia phenotype. Our data suggest a time-dependent effect of CX3CR1 on modulating brain injury and suggests a potential unique therapeutic window for treating TBI neuroinflammation.

Materials and methods

Animals

All experiments were conducted in accordance with the National Institute of Health Guide on Care and Use of Laboratory Animals and were approved by the Institutional Animal Care and Use Committee of the University of Washington. CX3CR1$^{-/-}$ (CX3CR1$^{GFP/GFP}$) mice were obtained from The Jackson Laboratory (Bar Harbor, Maine) and a colony established at the University of Washington. A total of 180 3-month-old male CX3CR1$^{-/-}$ and littermate CX3CR1$^{+/+}$ (wild-type) mice were used in these experiments. Mice were group-housed in environmentally controlled conditions (12:12 h light-to-dark cycle at 21 ± 1 °C) and provided with food and water ad libitum. After surgery, animals were single-housed.

Traumatic brain injury

Adult mice were anesthetized with isoflurane (induced at 4 %, maintained at 1.25–1.5 %) and placed in a stereotaxic frame equipped with a heating pad to maintain body temperature. A midline incision was made, fascia removed, and a 5-mm diameter craniotomy was made over the left parietal cortex between the lambda and bregma. The bone flap was removed and the integrity of the underlying dura assessed. TBI was induced using a controlled cortical impact (CCI) device (Leica Impact One, Richmond, IL, USA) equipped with an electrically driven 3-mm diameter metal piston controlled by a linear velocity displacement transducer. Impact velocity was set at 5.0 m/s, with a dwell time of 100 ms, and a depth of 0.5 mm from the dura. Previous studies have reported that these parameters produce a mild injury [36, 37]. A 5-mm disk created from a polystyrene weighing boat was glued to the skull over the craniotomy, and the incision closed with sutures. Mice were kept on a heating pad and allowed to recover until ambulatory before being returned to their home cages. Sham (uninjured control) animals received identical anesthesia and craniotomy but were not subjected to CCI brain injury.

Tissue collection and processing

For immunohistochemistry studies, animals were anesthetized with isofluorane and transcardially perfused with ice-cold phosphate-buffered saline (PBS), followed by 4 % paraformaldehyde in PBS. The brains were postfixed in

4 % paraformaldehyde for 24 h, after which they were transferred to a 30 % sucrose in PBS for at least 16 h at 4 °C. Coronal sections of the left hemisphere were made at 40 μm using a cryostat (Leica CM1950) and stored in cryoprotectant at 4 °C. Animals used for protein assessment were euthanized by rapid decapitation. Brain regions of interest were dissected and rapidly frozen in liquid nitrogen before storage at −80 °C. Subsequently, both the hippocampi and the sections of cortex were homogenized using an electric tissue homogenizer in 1:10 weight-to-volume ratio of ice-cold RIPA buffer (Millipore; Billerica, MA, USA) containing protease inhibitors and EDTA (Pierce; Rockford, IL, USA). Following homogenization, sample lysates were centrifuged at 10,000×g at 4 °C for 15 min and the supernatant collected.

Biochemical endpoints

Enzyme-linked immunosorbent assay (ELISA)

The total protein in each sample was determined using the bicinchoninc acid method (BCA; Pierce Biotechnology, Inc.).

Analysis of gene expression by qRT-PCR

Dissected cortex tissues from adult male mice were stored at −80 °C, and total RNA was isolated with RNeasy Lipid Tissue Mini Kit (QIAGEN, catalog # 74804) with on-column DNase treatment (QIAGEN, catalog # 79254) according to the manufacturer's protocol. RNA quantity and quality were determined using A260/A280 readings by a NanoDrop (ThermoScientific) spectrophotometer. Reverse transcription (RT) was performed using High Capacity cDNA Reverse Transcription Kit Assay (Applied Biosystems, catalog # 4368814) following the manufacturer's protocol. "No template" and "no RT" controls were included in all assays.

RT-PCR was performed using the TaqMan Gene Expression Assay (Applied Biosystems, catalog # 4331182) according to the manufacturer's instructions on a 7300 Real Time PCR System (Applied Biosystems). The following TaqMan probes were used: Il-1β (Mm00434228_m1), Cd86 (Mm0444543_m1), Fcgr1 (Mm0438874_m1), Tgfb1 (Mm01178820_m1), Arg1 (Mm00475988_m1), Nos2 (iNOS), (Mm00440502_m1), and 18S (Mm03928 990_g1). Relative gene expression was calculated by $2^{-\Delta\Delta CT}$ method.

Immunohistochemistry

Except where indicated, staining was done on 40-μm free-floating sections of a one-in-six series through the entire hippocampus and cortex. Tissue was blocked in 10 % normal serum from the species in which the secondary antibody was raised, with the addition of 0.1 % Triton X-100. Primary antibodies were diluted in 3 % normal serum with

0.1 % Triton X-100, and tissue incubated overnight at 4 °C. Biotinylated secondary antibodies were diluted in 3 % normal serum with 0.1 % Triton X-100 and were incubated for 2 h at room temperature. Enzyme detection was done using avidin-biotin substrate (ABC kit, Vector Laboratories, Burlingame, CA, USA) followed by color development in diaminobenzidine solution (Sigma-Aldrich, St. Louis, MO, USA). Antibodies and dilutions were as follows: rat CD11b (Serotec, Raleigh, NC, USA; 1:500); mouse CD68 (Serotec; 1:200); rabbit YM1 (Stem cell technology, Vancouver, BC, Canada; 1:400); rat Marco (Serotec; 1:500); mouse NeuN (Millipore, Temecula, CA, USA; 1:1000). After incubation for 24–48 h with appropriate primary and biotinylated secondary antibodies, tissue was treated with Vectastain ABC reagent (Vector Labs) and visualized with DAB reaction (Sigma-Aldrich). *Controls included omitting primary or secondary antibodies.*

Fluoro-Jade B staining

Fluoro-Jade B staining was performed according to Kubova et al. [38]. Briefly, 40-μm coronal free-floating sections were washed three times for 10 min with 0.1 M phosphate buffer saline (PBS), mounted on glass slides, and dried overnight at 37 °C. The sections were then incubated in chloroform-ethanol (1:1) for 1 h. Next, tissue was rehydrated in absolute ethanol (3 min), 70 % ethanol (2 min), distilled water (2 min), incubated in 0.06 % $KMnO_4$ for 15 min, rinsed in distilled water (2 min), and incubated for 30 min in a solution containing 0.001 % Fluoro-Jade B (Histo-Chem, Jefferson, AR, USA) and 0.1 % acetic acid. Sections were then rinsed in distilled water, dehydrated in a series of xylene and coverslipped.

Stereological analysis

All cell counts were obtained using the Optical Fractionator method of unbiased stereological counting techniques [39]. An Olympus BX-51 microscope and the Stereo Investigator software (MBF Bioscience, Colchester, VT, USA) were used to obtain cell counts on sections systematically sampled throughout the entire hippocampus and parietal cortex as described earlier [40]. Neuroanatomical borders of the hilus of the dentate gyrus were outlined, and counting was confined to these areas. The virtual grid (175 × 175) and counting frame (100 × 100) were optimized to count at least 200 cells per animal with error coefficients less than 0.07. Outlines of the anatomical structures were made using a 10×/0.45 objective, and cell quantification was done with a 60×/1.40 objective.

Isolation of mononuclear cells and flow cytometry

Perfused brains were dissected from mice 15 and 30 days post-TBI, mononuclear cells separated over discontinuous 70/30 % percoll gradients as previously described

[41, 42], and cellular pellets resuspended in cell staining buffer (Biolegend, San Diego, CA, USA). Blood for single stained controls was collected from the submandibular vein and RBCs depleted by hypotonic lysis and washed in staining buffer. Isolated cells were incubated on ice for 5 min with anti-mouse CD16/CD32 (clone 2.4G2; BD Pharmingen) to block Fc fragment receptor (FcR)s and then incubated on ice for 30 min with a mix of fluorochrome-conjugated anti-mouse Abs; CD45-APC-Cy7 or APC (Clone 30-F11, BD Pharmingen), CD11b-APC or PerCP-Cy5.5 (Clone M1/70), CD11c-PeCy7 (Clone N418, eBioscience), Ly6G-PE (Clone 1A8, Biolegend), and I-A/I-E-PerCP or Pacific Blue (Mouse MHC-II Clone M5/114.15.2). After washes, cells were resuspended in 2 % paraformaldehyde and analyzed in a LSR-II (BD Biosciences, Franklin Lakes, NJ, USA). To quantify the proportion of resident and infiltrating myeloid cells undergoing cell proliferation, CNS mononuclear cells were stained first with cell surface markers, fixed with 4 % PFA for 30 min and then incubated at RT for 10 min in permeabilization buffer (eBioscience). Cells were then stained with Ki67-V450 (Clone B56) in permeabilization buffer for 20 min, washed, resuspended in 2 % PFA, and acquired on an LSR-II [43].

Behavioral analysis
Composite neuroscore
Evaluation of neuromotor impairment following CCI was performed by using a 28-point composite neuroscore. In brief, mice were evaluated by an investigator blinded to the injury status (sham, TBI) of the animal. Scoring for each animal ranged from 0 (severely impaired) to 4 (normal strength or function) for each of the following modalities: (1) left and (2) right forelimb flexion during suspension by the tail; (3) left and (4) right hind limb flexion with the forelimbs remaining on a flat surface as the hind limbs are lifted by the tail; (5) ability to resist lateral pulsation to the left and (6) right; and (7) ability to stand on an inclined plane in the left, (8) right, and (9) vertical position. In addition, the ability of mice to stand on an inclined plane for at least 5 s in each of three directions (facing up, left, and right) was determined. The angle was increased in 2.5° increments starting at 40°; the maximal angle was noted and compared with pre-injury (baseline) values. A score was then assigned based on the decrease from baseline angle in degrees, where 4 = 0° change, 3 = 2.5° change, 2 = 5° change, 1 = 7.5° change, and 0 = 10° change or greater. Each of the three directions was scored separately, after which a mean was calculated, giving a maximum score of 4 for the inclined plane. The scores for (7), (8), and (9) were averaged, and a composite neurological motor score (0–28) was calculated by summation of individual test scores. Neuromotor function was assessed in both injured and sham-operated animals, and baseline composite neuromotor scores were calculated from values obtained 24 h prior to injury.

Open-field and elevated plus maze
The open-field and elevated plus maze were used to determine general activity levels and to measure anxiety-like behavior. Animals were monitored under moderate lighting for 15 min in a 40-cm^2 open field using video tracking software (ANY-Maze, Stoelting, IL, USA). General activity was evaluated by determining the total of distance traveled. Anxiety-like behavior was assessed based on the pattern of exploration in the open field (center versus periphery). Anxiety-like behavior was also assessed using the elevated plus maze. Our elevated plus maze consists of two well-lit open arms (35 cm) facing each other and two enclosed arms (30.5 cm) also facing each other. Each arm is attached to a common center platform (4.5 cm^2), and the entire apparatus was elevated 40 cm off the floor. The mice were placed in the center platform and allowed to explore for 5 min. Video tracking software (ANY-Maze) measured movement and time spent in each section.

Rota-rod
Mice were tested for overall balance, motor coordination, and motor learning on an accelerating rota-rod apparatus (Ugo Basile, Italy). The center rotor is a 3-cm diameter cylinder, and rotation started at 4 rpm and accelerated to 40 rpm within a 5-min period. Mice were tested for the time spent on the rotor during each of four trials with a 30-min inter-trial interval, and time to fall off the rotor was the outcome measured.

Morris water maze
The Morris hidden platform water maze (MWM) consisted of a circular pool (1.38 m diameter) filled with room temperature water containing non-toxic opaque paint with an escape platform (10 cm diameter) hidden 3 cm beneath the surface. Each mouse was placed in the pool in a pseudorandom order and given 60 s to locate the escape platform. When the mouse found the platform, or if it failed to find the platform within 60 s, it was placed on the platform and left for 30 s. Each mouse was given four trials per day for 7 days with 1-h inter-trial interval between trials. Sessions were recorded, and the time to find the platform (escape latency), the total distance traveled, and swim speed were determined by video tracking software (ANY-Maze). After each session, mice were towel-dried and placed in a cage on a heating pad until dry, after which they were returned to their home cage. On day 8 post-training, all mice were subjected to one probe trial in which the platform was

removed and each animal had 60 s to search the pool for the platform.

Statistical analysis

Statistical analyses comparing two genotypes, two manipulations (sham and TBI), and two time points (15 and 30 days post-injury) were done using a one-way analysis of variance (ANOVA) or two-way ANOVA with post hoc multiple comparison analysis (Tukey-Kramer or Bonferroni post hoc test). Repeated measures ANOVA followed by Bonferroni post hoc comparisons were used to analyze rota-rod data. Flow cytometry data are presented as number of cells or percentage of specific cell populations. Differences between groups were analyzed using ANOVA or an unpaired t test with GraphPad Prism software (San Diego, CA, USA). P values are shown in the data (*) when $P < 0.05$. Statistical analysis was done in the GraphPad Prism software.

Results

Mild TBI impairs neuromotor function

Prior to surgery, there were no differences in composite neuroscores between WT and CX3CR1$^{-/-}$ mice. The brain-injured WT mice had lower composite neuroscores at 24 h, 7, and 15 days post-surgery than sham WT mice (Fig. 1). By 30 days post-surgery, composite neuroscores for the brain-injured WT and sham WT mice did not differ, indicating recovery of neuromotor function. Composite neuroscores for the brain-injured WT mice were significantly lower than those of brain-injured CX3CR1$^{-/-}$ mice at 24 h post-injury but not at 7 or 15 days post-injury. Composite neuroscores for the brain-injured CX3CR1$^{-/-}$ mice did not differ from those of sham CX3CR1$^{-/-}$ mice at any time point, indicating that CX3CR1 deficiency is neuroprotective.

Mild TBI does not affect spontaneous locomotor activity or cause excessive anxiety but impairs motor learning and cognitive function

Separate groups of animals ($n = 10$/group) were evaluated in open-field, elevated plus maze, rota-rod, and Morris water maze 30 days post-TBI.

To examine spontaneous locomotor activity in response to a novel environment, all mice were tested in the open-field behavioral task. The open-field task monitors activity in a brightly lit, novel environment. Spontaneous locomotor activity was assessed as the total amount of distance traveled in the chamber. In addition, anxiety levels can be measured in the open-field task through assessment of the distances traveled in the center versus perimeter of the chamber. This task exploits the natural tendency of mice to avoid open areas.

In the open-field task, there were no genotype differences in distance traveled. WT mice subjected to TBI

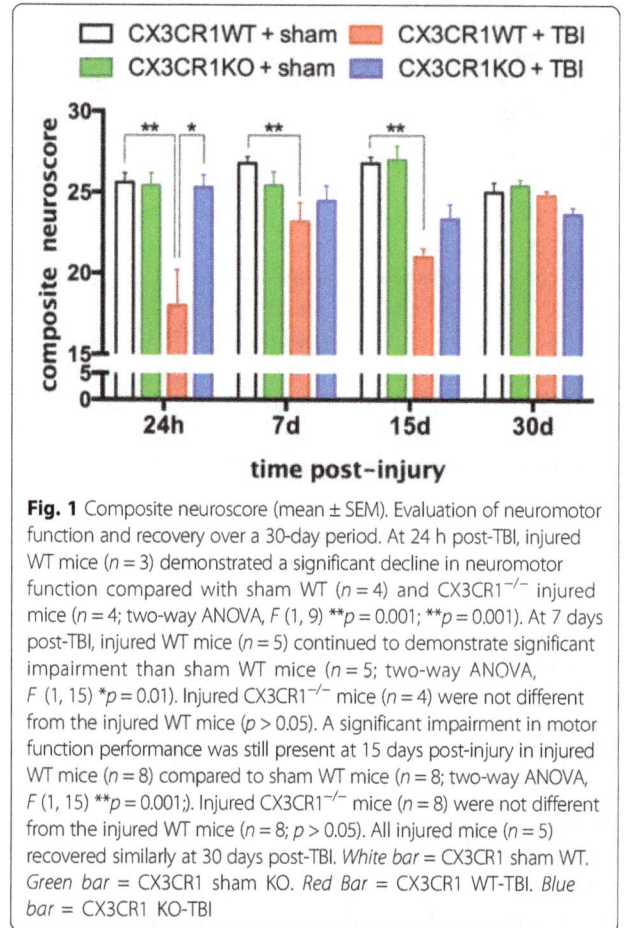

Fig. 1 Composite neuroscore (mean ± SEM). Evaluation of neuromotor function and recovery over a 30-day period. At 24 h post-TBI, injured WT mice ($n = 3$) demonstrated a significant decline in neuromotor function compared with sham WT ($n = 4$) and CX3CR1$^{-/-}$ injured mice ($n = 4$; two-way ANOVA, $F (1, 9)$ **$p = 0.001$; **$p = 0.001$). At 7 days post-TBI, injured WT mice ($n = 5$) continued to demonstrate significant impairment than sham WT mice ($n = 5$; two-way ANOVA, $F (1, 15)$ *$p = 0.01$). Injured CX3CR1$^{-/-}$ mice ($n = 4$) were not different from the injured WT mice ($p > 0.05$). A significant impairment in motor function performance was still present at 15 days post-injury in injured WT mice ($n = 8$) compared to sham WT mice ($n = 8$; two-way ANOVA, $F (1, 15)$ **$p = 0.001$;). Injured CX3CR1$^{-/-}$ mice ($n = 8$) were not different from the injured WT mice ($n = 8$; $p > 0.05$). All injured mice ($n = 5$) recovered similarly at 30 days post-TBI. *White bar* = CX3CR1 sham WT. *Green bar* = CX3CR1 sham KO. *Red Bar* = CX3CR1 WT-TBI. *Blue bar* = CX3CR1 KO-TBI

spent less time in the perimeter zone of the open-field chamber than did CX3CR1$^{-/-}$-injured (TBI) mice (two-way ANOVA **$p = 0.01$; Fig. 2a). A modest, yet statistically significant difference in total distance traveled was revealed between sham and TBI groups for both genotypes; however, no difference was observed between WT-TBI and CX3CR1$^{-/-}$ TBI mice. No difference was revealed between genotypes and/or injury groups in the elevated plus maze task (data not shown).

After open-field and elevated plus maze assessments, the same mice were also tested for coordination and motor skill acquisition using an accelerating rota-rod during each of four trials per day on two consecutive days (Fig. 2b). The amount of time an animal stays on the rota-rod is an indicator of its general level of balance and coordination. In general, mice improve their performance over time with training, which is an indicator of motor learning. Sham wild-type mice performed significantly better than sham CX3CR1$^{-/-}$ mice, during the 2 days of training (Fig. 2b), confirming our previous finding of motor learning deficits in CX3CR1$^{-/-}$ mice [40]. No differences were observed among injury groups during the first day of training. On the second day of training (trials 5–8), sham WT mice remained on the rotor for longer

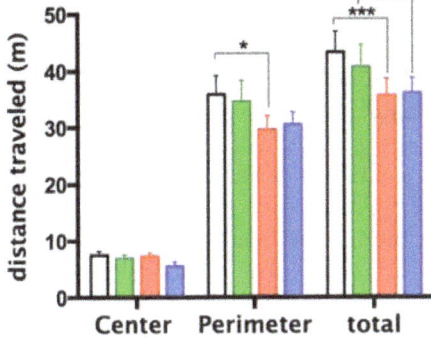

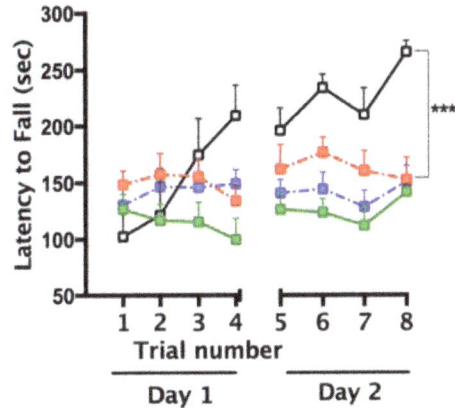

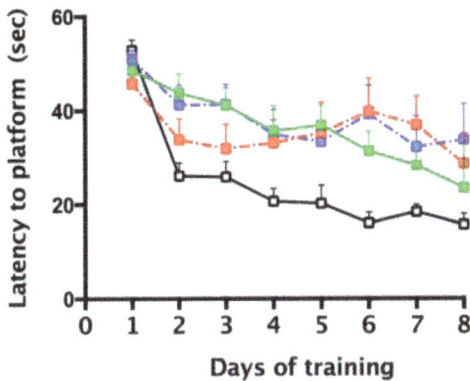

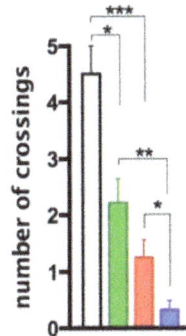

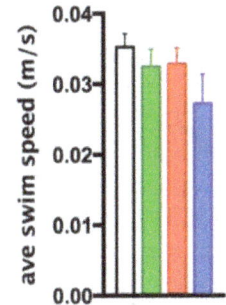

□ CX3CR1 WT + sham   ■ CX3CR1 KO + sham   ■ CX3CR1 WT + TBI   ■ CX3CR1 KO + TBI

Fig. 2 Evaluation of behavioral analysis 30 days post-TBI. **a** In the open-field task, all mice traveled the same distance in the center zone compared to the perimeter zone. CX3CR1 WT-TBI spent less time in the perimeter zone of the open-field chamber compared to CX3CR1 KO-TBI (two-way ANOVA ($F = 3$, 72, **$p = 0.01$). Total distance traveled in the chamber was significantly different between CX3CR1 sham WT and CX3CR1 sham KO mice. Two-way ANOVA ($F = 1$, 36, **$p = 0.001$) and between shams and TBI groups two-way ANOVA ($F = 1$, 36, **$p = 0.001$). CX3CR1 sham WT ($n = 10$ *white bar*), CX3CR1 sham KO ($n = 10$ *green bar*), CX3CR1 WT-TBI ($n = 10$ *red bar*), and CX3CR1 KO-TBI ($n = 10$ *blue bar*) mice. **b** Rota-rod. CX3CR1 sham WT mice performed significantly better than CX3CR1 sham KO mice, over the 2 days of training (repeated measures ANOVA, *$p = 0.5$). No difference between injured groups was observed in the learning ability in the rota-rod task during the first day of training. On the second day of training (trials 5–8), CX3CR1 sham WT mice learned the rota-rod task as demonstrated by their ability to remain on the rod for longer periods compared to CX3CR1 WT-TBI (**$p = 0.01$). CX3CR1 KO-TBI mice showed a significantly worse performance than CX3CR1 WT-TBI wild-type (*$p = 0.5$). Neither the CX3CR1 KO-TBI nor the CX3CR1 WT-TBI mice showed significant improvement in motor coordination with training when compared to sham WT. CX3CR1 sham WT ($n = 10$; *white open square*). CX3CR1 WT-TBI ($n = 10$; *red square*). CX3CR1 sham KO ($n = 10$; *green square*). CX3CR1 KO-TBI ($n = 10$; *blue squares*). **c–e** Morris water maze. **c** Mean latency to escape from a pool to a hidden platform across training days. All groups spent more time in learning to find the platform compared to sham WT. CX3CR1 sham WT ($n = 8$; *white bar*). CX3CR1 WT-TBI ($n = 9$; *red square*). CX3CR1 sham KO ($n = 8$; *green square*). CX3CR1 KO-TBI ($n = 9$; *blue squares*). **d** A probe test was performed on day 8 to determine the number of pseudo platform crossings in the target quadrant. All TBI groups crossed less number of time the target quadrant zone when compared to CX3CR1 sham WT. CX3CR1 KO-TBI mice crossed the target quadrant less number of time than CX3CR1 sham KO and CX3CR1 WT-TBI. **e** No difference was observed in the average swim speed between groups. CX3CR1 sham WT ($n = 8$; *white bar*). CX3CR1 WT-TBI ($n = 9$; *red square*). CX3CR1 sham KO ($n = 8$; *green square*). CX3CR1 KO-TBI ($n = 9$; *blue squares*). All data are presented as mean ± SEM $p < 0.01$

periods. Injured CX3CR1$^{-/-}$ mice performed worse than injured WT. However, the motor impairment of injured CX3CR1$^{-/-}$ mice was similar to that one observed in sham CX3CR1$^{-/-}$, likely due to the baseline (floor) effect associated with CX3CR1 deficiency. Neither injured CX3CR1$^{-/-}$ mice nor injured WT mice significantly

improved motor coordination on the second day of training when compared to day 1 of training; (Fig. 2b; repeated measures ANOVA, $p < 0.0001$).

Spatial learning was evaluated using the Morris water maze (MWM) task as previously described [40]. As previously shown, the escape latency (time to find the platform) of sham CX3CR1$^{-/-}$ mice during training was longer than that of sham WT mice (Fig. 2c). All mice subjected to TBI, irrespective of genotype, took longer to find the platform during training as compared to sham WT mice. During the probe trial (day 8), the number of target platform crossings was decreased in injured mice irrespective of genotype as compared to sham WT mice. Injured CX3CR1$^{-/-}$ mice performed worse than injured WT and sham mice (Fig. 2d). A similar trend was observed in the time that each group spent in the platform zone (data not shown). There was no difference in the average swim speed among groups (Fig. 2e).

TBI-induced neuronal cell death and survival

We used Fluoro-Jade B and NeuN staining to determine the impact of mild TBI on neuronal cell death and survival in the cortex during the transition from the acute to chronic post-traumatic period, days 15 and 30 post-TBI. Stereological analyses revealed increased numbers of degenerating neurons (Fluoro-Jade B$^+$ cells) in the cortex of WT mice 15 days post-TBI as compared to CX3CR1$^{-/-}$ mice (Fig. 3a; two way ANOVA, $p = 0.0001$; Bonferroni post hoc $p = 0.01$). By 30 days post-injury, however, the number of degenerating neurons in injured CX3CR1$^{-/-}$ mice was greater than in injured WT mice (Fig. 3, $p = 0.001$). Stereological quantification revealed that the number of Fluoro-Jade B$^+$ cells in CX3CR1$^{-/-}$ mice increased from day 15 to 30 post-TBI, suggesting delayed cell degeneration in these animals (CX3CR1$^{-/-}$-TBI—15 vs 30 days, $p < 0.01$). Microscope visualization did not reveal any Fluoro-Jade B$^+$ cells in sham animals irrespective of genotype (nd).

Neuronal survival was determined by the stereological quantification of NeuN$^+$ cells (Fig. 3b). At 15 days post-TBI time point, we analyzed tissue from all groups of animals (CX3CR1 sham KO, CX3CR1 sham WT, CX3CR1 KO-TBI, CX3CR1 WT-TBI). However, at 30 days, only tissue from injured TBI animals was analyzed. Neuronal cell loss was apparent after TBI in WT mice and CX3CR1$^{-/-}$ mice (Fig. 3b). In WT mice, there were fewer NeuN$^+$ cells 15 days post-TBI than at 30 days post-TBI. In contrast, there were more NeuN$^+$ cells in CX3CR1$^{-/-}$ mice 15 days post-TBI than at 30 days post-TBI, indicating neuronal cell loss over time. Comparison of genotypes indicated significant differences in numbers of NeuN$^+$ cells such that there were more NeuN$^+$ cells in CX3CR1$^{-/-}$ mice 15 days post-TBI and more NeuN$^+$ cells in WT mice 30 days post-TBI. Collectively, these data demonstrate that CX3CR1 exacerbates cell loss during the acute phase post-TBI (number of neurons is greater in CX3CR1$^{-/-}$ mice 15 days post-TBI than in WT mice) and protects cells during the chronic phase post-TBI (number of neurons is less in CX3CR1$^{-/-}$ mice than WT mice 30 days post-TBI).

CX3CR1 deficiency correlates with increased microglial proliferation and does not modulate the trafficking of hematogenous myeloid cells to the brain after TBI

Because TBI involves infiltration of peripheral blood monocytes into the brain [44], we first isolated mononuclear cells from WT and CX3CR1$^{-/-}$ mice at 15 or 30 days post-TBI and analyzed them with flow cytometry (Fig. 4a). Total brain mononuclear cells were counted and compared among groups (Fig. 4b; Table 1). After TBI in WT mice, there was an increase in overall

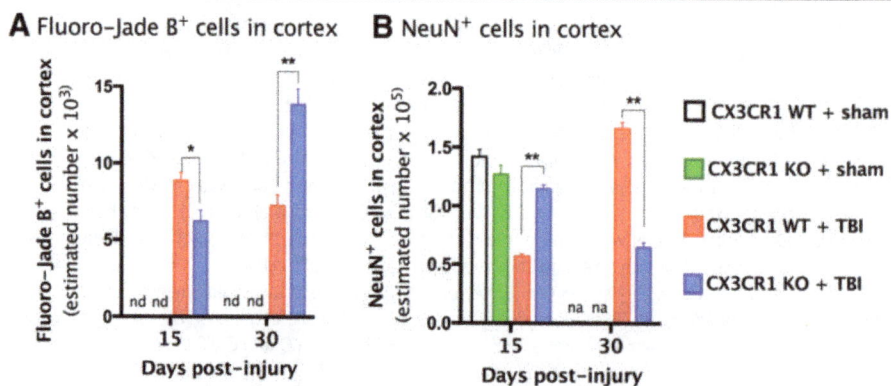

Fig. 3 Quantification of neuronal loss at 15 and 30 days post-TBI. *Left* panel **(a)**: unbiased stereology quantification showed a significant decrease in the number of Fluoro-Jade B$^+$ cells in the ipsilateral cortex ($F = 1, 10$; *$p = 0.001$) of CX3CR1 KO-TBI mice ($n = 3$; *blue bar*) at 15 days post-TBI, when compared to CX3CR1 WT-TBI ($n = 3$; *red bar*). CX3CR1 sham WT (not detected), CX3CR1 sham KO (not detected). Fifteen days post-TBI, the decrease in the number of Fluoro-Jade B$^+$ cells in CX3CR1 KO-TBI mice was associated with a significant increase in the number of NeuN$^+$ cells (*right pane* **(b)**; $n = 3$) compared to CX3CR1 WT-TBI ($n = 3$ **$p = 0.001$). Thirty days post-TBI CX3CR1 KO mice showed increased number of Fluoro-Jade B$^+$ cells ($n = 3$; *$p = 0.01$) which was associated with decreased NeuN immunoreactivity ($n = 5$; **$p = 0.001$; mean ± SE (*WT vs CX3CR1$^{-/-}$ ± 15 vs 30 days). CX3CR1 sham WT (*white bar*), CX3CR1 sham KO (*green bar*), CX3CR1 WT-TBI (*red bar*), and CX3CR1 KO-TBI (*blue bar*). At 30 days, the number of NeuN$^+$ cells was not determined (nd). Two-way ANOVA performed across genotype, treatment, and time point revealed a significant difference in the number of Fluoro-Jade and NeuN$^+$ cells when compared between 15 and 30 days post-injury

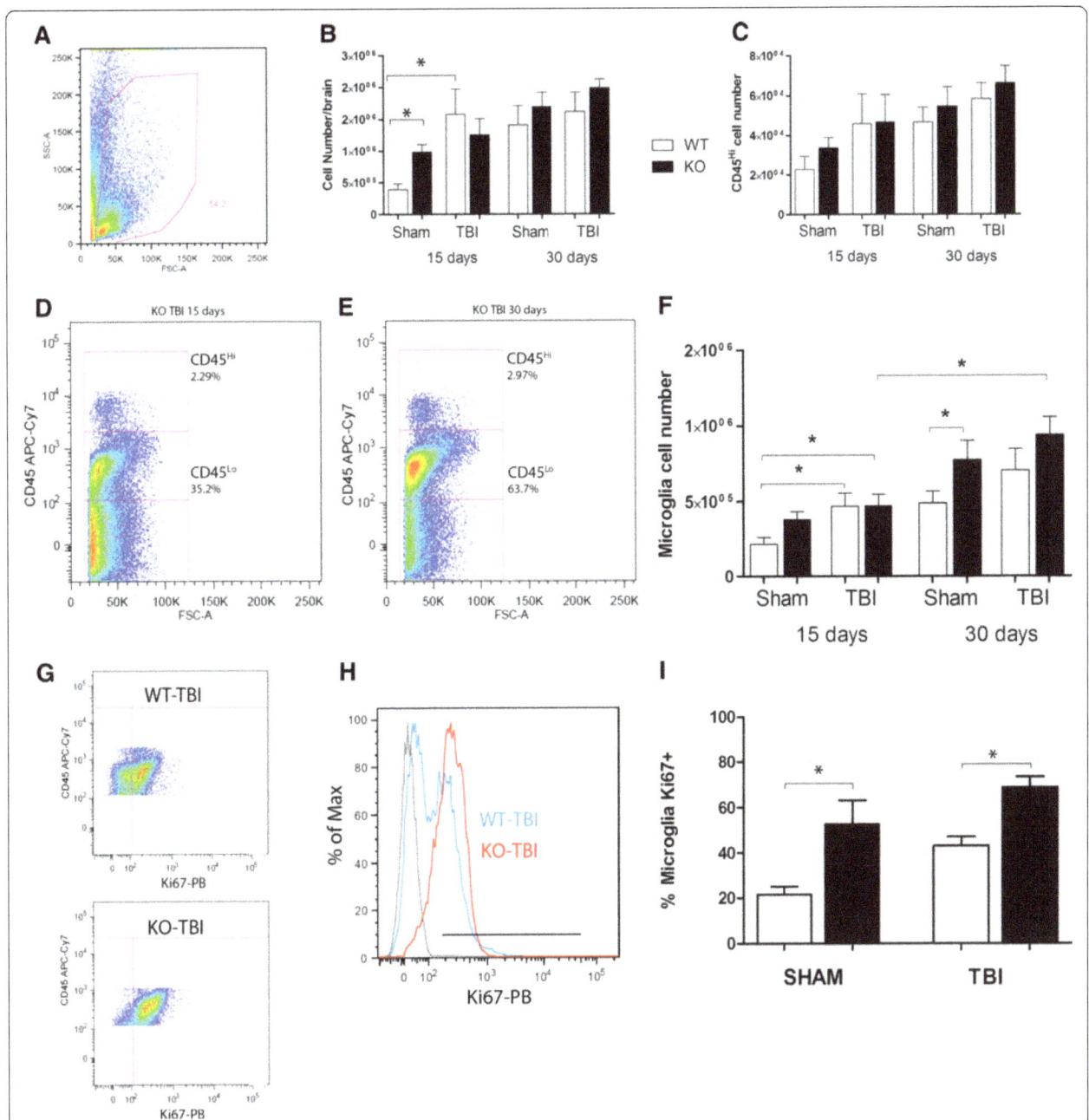

Fig. 4 Increased microglial reaction after TBI. CX3CR1$^{+/+}$ (WT; *white bar*) and CX3CR1$^{-/-}$ (KO, *black bar*) brain leukocytes were analyzed by flow cytometry, and total cellularity, numbers of blood derived infiltrating cells, and CD45^{Low} microglial cells were compared. **a–c** After TBI, a significant increase in the overall cellularity was observed when comparing all groups at 15 days (*$P < 0.05$ comparing sham WT versus WT-TBI 15 days post-TBI), and these changes were sustained 30 days post-TBI. CD45^{High} hematogenous population did not show statistical significance among injured WT and KO mice. **d–f** There was a significant increase in microglial cell number at 15 days post-TBI in WT mice when compared to sham WT group. CX3CR1 KO-TBI group also showed a significant increase in microglia number when comparing 15 and 30 days post-TBI, although effects were also seen in the sham-treated KO group. **g–i** Staining for Ki67 in representative sample of WT-TBI (**g** *upper panel*) and KO-TBI (**g** *lower panel*) groups and also presented in histogram (**h**) with *gray line* showing the isotype controls, WT-TBI Ki67 intensity in *blue line*, and KO-TBI in *red*. Data were quantified (**i**) revealing that in the absence of CX3CR1, microglial cells exhibit a higher proliferative capacity (*$P < 0.05$)

cellularity 15 days post-TBI when compared to the sham group (Fig. 4b, *$P < 0.05$). CX3CR1-KO mice showed a slight increase in overall cellularity at 15 days post-TBI but not statistically significant from the sham group. However, there were no significant differences between injured WT and CX3CR1$^{-/-}$ mice in the CD45^{High} hematogenous population (Fig. 4c), suggesting that overall the contribution of blood-derived cells

Table 1 Total microglia cell numbers in the brain tissue. Microglia cell numbers in sham WT, sham KO, WT-TBI, and KO-TBI at 15 and 30 days post-TBI as plotted in Fig. 4b. Total microglia cell numbers in the brain tissue. Microglia cell numbers in sham WT, sham KO, WT-TBI, and KO-TBI at 15 and 30 days post-TBI as plotted in Fig. 4f

	15 days				30 days			
	Sham WT	Sham KO	WT-TBI	KO-TBI	Sham WT	Sham KO	WT-TBI	KO-TBI
Total cell numbers in the brain tissue after TBI (Fig. 4b)								
Mean	390,777	984,242	1.581×10^6	1.255×10^6	1.408×10^6	1.697×10^6	1.617×10^6	1.986×10^6
Standard error	90,972	120,144	389,298	254,594	302,104	222,274	301,655	137,642
n	6	6	6	6	8	7	9	8
Microglia cell numbers in the brain tissue after TBI (Fig. 4f)								
Mean	216,305	377,880	468,937	471,776	487,667	885,237	701,797	862,206
Standard error	46,031	56,377	84,401	73,242	79,322	156,709	142,253	128,469
n	6	6	6	6	8	7	9	8

to the inflammatory process is not altered in CX3CR1$^{-/-}$ mice. Further analysis of the CD45^{High} population was performed using CD11b to identify all myeloid cells, CD11c for dendritic cells (DCs), Ly6G to mark neutrophils, and CD3 to identify T cells. The results did not reveal differences between sham and TBI groups in T cells or infiltrating myeloid cells, including monocytes/macrophages (CD11b$^+$CD11c$^-$), myeloid derived DCs (CD11b$^+$CD11c$^+$), conventional DCs (CD11b$^-$CD11c$^+$), or neutrophils (CD11b$^+$Ly6G$^+$) (data not shown). Comparison of the CD45^{Low} microglia population between WT (Fig. 4d) and CX3CR1$^{-/-}$ mice (Fig. 4e) reveals a significant increase in both groups when compared to sham controls at 15 and 30 days post-TBI (Fig. 4f). Figure 4d–e shows representative plots, actual numbers are shown on Fig. 4f; (Table 1). There is a significant effect of the sham procedure in the microglia response in CX3CR1-KO mice that is particularly evident at day 30 and significant between the sham WT and sham KO groups. We and others have evidence that the microglia in these mice are more prone to activation in setting of LPS injection, EAE, and MPTP challenge among other models. However, TBI does have a slight effect toward an increased number of microglia at day 30 although not statistically significant. To assess differences in the proliferation of the CNS-resident microglial population, we performed flow cytometry on cells stained with the proliferation marker Ki67 on sham controls and TBI-induced WT mice (Fig. 4g) and CX3CR1$^{-/-}$ mice (Fig. 4h) 30 days after injury (Fig. 4g–i). CX3CR1$^{-/-}$ mice exhibited a higher proportion of Ki67+ microglia (Fig. 4i) irrespective of injury. This result highlights the importance of CX3CR1 in controlling microglial proliferation even under conditions of skull exposure without CCI because microglial proliferation in naïve (unmanipulated) CX3CR1$^{-/-}$ mice is similar to that of WT mice [43]. Collectively, these results suggest that CX3CR1 plays an

important role in inhibiting the microglia reaction in this model of TBI.

Impact of mild TBI on microglia phenotypes

To determine whether the protective and neurotoxic effects of CX3CR1 signaling following mild TBI were due to activation of different microglia phenotypes, we quantified microglia immunoreactivity in cortical sections obtained from mice 15 and 30 days post-TBI. We first analyzed CD11b, a marker common to all microglia phenotypes, and found there were more CD11b$^+$ cells in CX3CR1$^{-/-}$ mice than in WT mice 15 days post-TBI. By 30 days post-TBI, the number of CD11b$^+$ cells increased to the same extent in WT and in CX3CR1$^{-/-}$ mice (Fig. 5 a, b). We performed immunostaining for both sham groups, CX3CR1 KO and WT. CD11b staining intensity showed similar intensity in the cortex of KO and sham WT animals, and it appeared to be lower compared to TBI groups. Therefore, we did not perform stereological analysis for sham animals.

Then, we immunostained cortical tissues for markers associated with M2 microglial and M1 microglial activation phenotype and at 7, 15, and 30 days post-TBI (YM1 chitinase 3-like 3; CD206 mannose receptor; CD68 Marco). At 7 days post-TBI, the expression of the M2a markers YM1 and CD206 increased in the cortex of brain-injured CX3CR1$^{-/-}$ mice, but not brain-injured WT mice (Fig. 6a–h showing M2 expression in the cortex). YM1 and CD206 were not detected in the brains of sham animals of either genotype (Fig. 6d, h). No M2 markers were detected at 15 or 30 days post-TBI. We then used qRT-PCR to determine M2-TGFβ-associated gene expression at 7 days post-TBI. Sham CX3CR1$^{-/-}$ mice had decreased TGFβ mRNA levels ($p < 0.001$) compared to sham WT mice (Fig. 6i). Seven days post-TBI, TGFβ mRNA significantly increased in injured CX3CR1$^{-/-}$ mice as compared to sham CX3CR1$^{-/-}$ ($p < 0.001$). No difference was

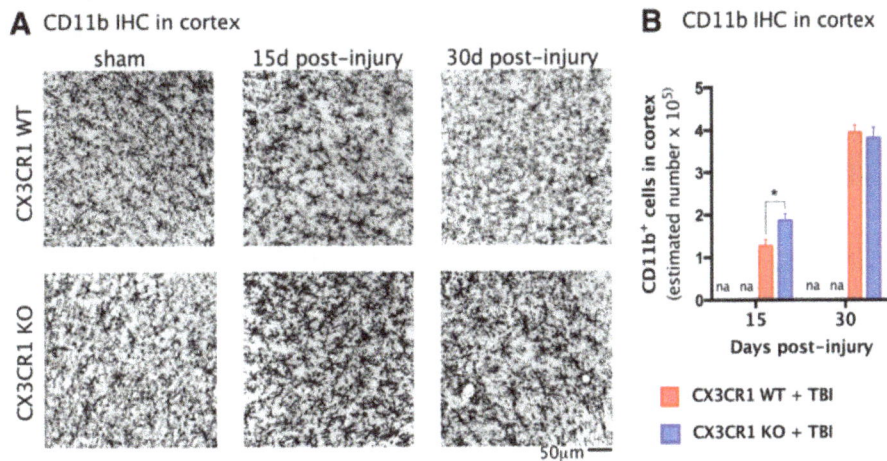

Fig. 5 Stereological quantification of CD11B$^+$ cells in the cortex at 15 and 30 days post-injury. **a** ×10 magnification micrographs of CD11B staining in the cortex in the vicinity of the lesion. *Upper panel* shows the staining's intensity in CX3CR1 sham WT and CX3CR1 WT-TBI at 15 and 30 days post-injury. *Lower panels* show the staining's intensity in CX3CR1 sham KO and CX3CR1 KO-TBI at 15 and 30 days post-injury. **b** The cortical expression of CD11b$^+$ cells was significantly increased in CX3CR1 KO-TBI ($n = 6$) mice compared to CX3CR1 WT-TBI mice ($n = 5$) at 15 days post-TBI (*$p = 0.05$). Two-way ANOVA revealed that the number of CD11b$^+$ cells increased in the cortex from day 15–30 post-TBI to the same extent in CX3CR1 WT-TBI and in CX3CR1 KO-TBI mice ($^{++}p = 0.001$). Staining in sham animals was not determined (nd). CX3CR1 sham WT (*white bar*), CX3CR1 sham KO (*green bar*), CX3CR1 WT-TBI (*red bar*), CX3CR1 KO-TBI (*blue bar*)

observed between injured CX3CR1$^{-/-}$ and injured WT mice. We also analyzed gene expression of iNOS and IL-1β at 7 days post-TBI. Levels of mRNA for iNOS and IL-1 were significantly greater in sham CX3CR1$^{-/-}$ mice than sham WT mice (Fig. 6i, $p < 0.001$). In contrast, iNOS and IL-1 significantly decreased in injured CX3CR1$^{-/-}$ mice compared to injured WT mice. Furthermore, iNOS and IL-1 mRNA levels in injured CX3CR1$^{-/-}$ mice were significantly decreased compared to sham CX3CR1$^{-/-}$ mice (see Table 2). Finally, we analyzed M1 and M2-associated protein expression of IL-1β, IL-6, and IL-4, respectively, in CX3CR1$^{-/-}$ and WT mice at 15 days post-TBI. Figure 7 shows that IL-1 and IL-6 increased in WT mice subjected to TBI, whereas IL-4 increased in CX3CR1$^{-/-}$ mice. M1 marker Marco was analyzed at 30 days post-TBI, and M1 marker CD68 was analyzed at 15 and 30 days post-TBI (Fig. 8). The time course and anatomical expression of Marco was different between WT and CX3CR1$^{-/-}$. In WT mice, Marco was expressed in the hippocampus (but not in the cortex) at 7, 15, and 30 days post-TBI, while in CX3CR1$^{-/-}$ mice, Marco expression was only evident at 30 days post-TBI; thus we only quantified Marco at 30 days in hippocampus. Thirty days post-TBI, Marco was highly expressed in injured CX3CR1$^{-/-}$ mice (Fig. 8a–c). CD68, a specific marker of phagocytic microglia, was decreased at 15 days post-TBI in CX3CR1$^{-/-}$ mice relative to WT mice, but by 30 days post-injury, there were no significant differences between genotypes (Fig. 8d, e).

Discussion

Results of this study demonstrate for the first time that CX3CR1 modulates responses to mild TBI in a time-dependent manner. During the acute post-traumatic period (24 h–15 days), neuronal cell loss is greater in the brain-injured WT than in the brain-injured CX3CR1$^{-/-}$ mice. In contrast, during the chronic phase (30 days post-injury), lack of CX3CR1 exacerbates neuronal damage. The acute post-TBI phase in CX3CR1$^{-/-}$ mice is associated with a protective M2 microglia phenotype as evidenced by upregulation of YM1 and CD206 and increased TGFβ, IL-4, and IL-10. Concurrently with the M2 microglia phenotype during this acute post-traumatic period, responses of CX3CR1$^{-/-}$ mice to TBI include a reduction in M1 microglia phenotype markers, such as iNOS and IL-1β. During the chronic post-injury phase, the brains of injured CX3CR1$^{-/-}$ mice show a profound inflammatory response compared to brains of injured WT mice. This post-traumatic chronic response in mice lacking CX3CR1 is characterized by an inflammatory M1 microglia phenotype, as evidenced by upregulation of Marco, CD68, and the inflammatory cytokines IL-1β and IL-6.

One interpretation for the decrease in TGFβ and IL-4 in the sham KO mice is that lack of CX3CR1 leads to a decrease in the M2-type responses in favor of M1-type responses (increased IL-1β). However, future work will be necessary to test this interpretation and to determine if the polarization of M1-type over M2 type responses is cell autonomous or involves a paracrine signaling mechanism.

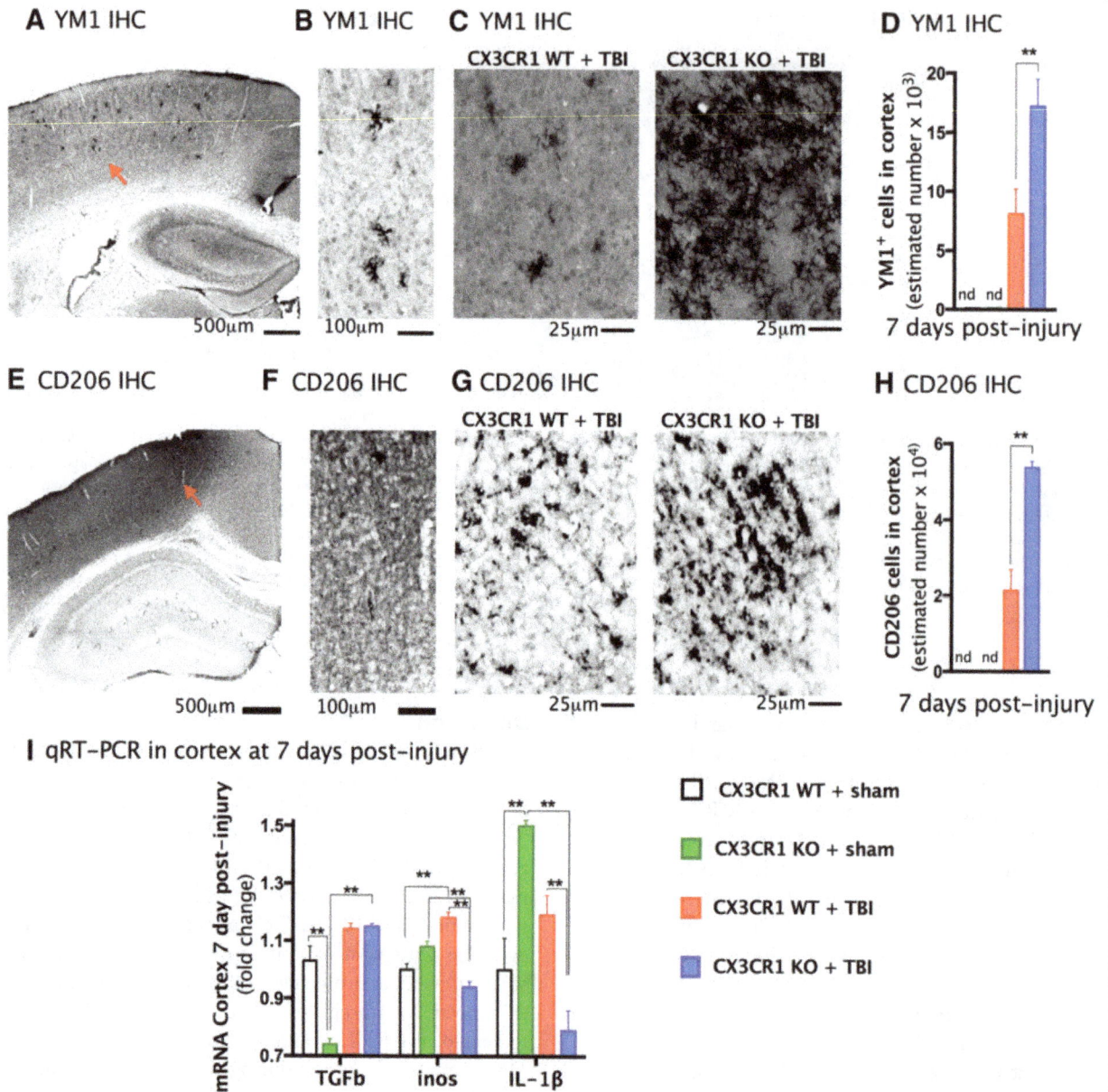

Fig. 6 Immunostaining, stereological quantification, and qPCR analysis of M2 and M1 polarization markers in cortex at 7 days post-TBI. **a–d** YM1 shows a strong increase in staining in the CX3CR1 KO-TBI compared to CX3CR1 WT-TBI at 7 days post-injury. **a** Micrograph at ×4 magnification showing YM1 staining in the proximity of the lesion area in CX3CR1 KO-TBI mice. **b** Higher magnification (×10) of the area indicated by the *red arrow* in (**a**). **c** Higher magnification (×20) of the area in the proximity of the lesion of CX3CR1 WT-TBI and CX3CR1 KO-TBI showing in more detail microglial YM1 morphology. **d** Unbiased stereology revealed a significant increase in the number of YM1 and CD2O6+ cells (*right panel*) in the cortex of CX3CR1 KO-TBI mice (*n* = 3) compared to CX3CR1 WT-TBI (*n* = 4). **e–h** CD206 shows a strong increase in staining in the CX3CR1 KO-TBI compared to CX3CR1 WT-TBI at 7 days post-injury. **e** Micrograph at ×4 magnification showing CD206 staining in the proximity of the lesion area in CX3CR1 KO-TBI mice. **f** Higher magnification (×10) of the area indicated by the *red arrow* in (**a**). **g** Higher magnification (×20) of the area in the proximity of the lesion of CX3CR1 WT-TBI and CX3CR1 KO-TBI showing in more detail microglial CD206 morphology. **h** Unbiased stereology revealed a significant increase in the number of CD2O6+ cells in the cortex of CX3CR1 KO-TBI mice compared to CX3CR1 WT-TBI. YM1 and CD206 were not detected in sham mice (**$p < 0.001$). **i** Relative mRNA levels of M2 marker TGFβ were significantly lower in sham CX3CR1 sham KO (*n* = 5) compared to CX3CR1 sham WT (*n* = 5). Following TBI, the expression of TGFβ significantly increased in CX3CR1 KO mice compared to sham (*n* = 5; **$p < 0.001$) but was not different compared to CX3CR1 WT-TBI (*n* = 5). M1 markers iNOS (*middle panel*) and IL-1β (*right panel*) were similar in the cortex of CX3CR1 sham KO (*n* = 5) compared to CX3CR1 sham WT (*n* = 5). Following injury, iNOS and IL-1β mRNA levels in CX3CR1 KO-TBI (*n* = 5) were significantly decreased compared to CX3CR1 WT-TBI (*n* = 5). **$p < 0.001$). CX3CR1 sham WT (*white bar*), CX3CR1 sham KO (*green bar*), CX3CR1 WT-TBI (*red bar*), and CX3CR1 KO-TBI (*blue bar*)

Table 2 CT, ΔCT, and fold change. TGFβ, iNOS, and IL-1β raw numbers as plotted in Fig. 6g. Numbers are expressed as CT, ΔCT, and fold change (means and standard deviations) normalized against wild-type sham

Treatment	Genotype	Gene	CT (mean ± SD)	ΔCT (mean ± SD)	Fold change (mean ± SD)
Sham	WT	TGFβ	25.368 ± 0.31	12.429 ± 0.31	1.000 ± 0.20
	KO		25.751 ± 0.23	12.775 ± 0.26	0.782 ± 0.14
TBI	WT		25.268 ± 0.03	12.255 ± 0.11	1.107 ± 0.08
	KO		25.451 ± 0.32	12.451 ± 0.33	1.154 ± 0.06
Sham	WT	iNOS	29.156 ± 0.11	16.558 ± 0.11	1.000 ± 0.07
	KO		29.037 ± 0.12	16.450 ± 0.14	1.080 ± 0.11
TBI	WT		28.802 ± 0.24	16.335 ± 0.29	1.187 ± 0.13
	KO		29.168 ± 0.06	16.654 ± 0.08	0.933 ± 0.09
Sham	WT	IL-1β	28.340 ± 1.01	16.747 ± 099	1.000 ± 0.60
	KO		29.705 ± 1.73	17.109 ± 1.72	1.521 ± 0.17
TBI	WT		28.903 ± 0.93	16.435 ± 0.90	1.191 ± 0.57
	KO		29.259 ± 0.80	16.715 ± 0.80	0.968 ± 0.51

The predominant M1 response in injured CX3CR1$^{-/-}$ brain is associated with poorer performance in the Morris water maze. We previously demonstrated that lack of CX3CR1 impairs motor and cognitive function [40]. We now show that lack of CX3CR1 during the chronic phase of mild brain injury exacerbates this already impaired cognitive function. However, it is important to take in consideration that both RT-PCR and ELISA data have been obtained from whole brain tissue, not from extracted microglia; therefore, we cannot determine with absolute certainty the cellular source of these signals. Furthermore, it has to be noted that although the statistical analysis indicated significant difference between CX3CR1 WT-TBI and CX3CR1 KO-TBI in mRNA levels for TGFβ, iNOS, and IL1, the physiological significance

of such changes may be questionable and bigger changes may be observed at earlier time points.

Collectively, these observations demonstrate that CX3CR1 is both neuroprotective and neurotoxic in brain injury depending on the time post-injury. Importantly, these findings suggest that antagonizing the CX3CL1/CX3CR1 pathway during a critical period after mild TBI may reprogram the brain inflammatory environment from detrimental to beneficial, favoring endogenous neuroprotective or neurorestorative mechanisms. Furthermore, results from this study provide important new knowledge that is relevant to the differential roles of the CX3CL1/CX3CR1 pathway that have been described in a number of pathologies.

Our findings are in agreement with several reports demonstrating in other models that CX3CR1 drives inflammatory responses during the acute period following CNS injury. For instance, in focal cerebral ischemia, Dénes et al. [24] reported reduced damage to the blood-brain barrier, which correlated with a protected phenotype, reduced ischemic volume, fewer apoptotic cells, and better performance in the behavioral test of adhesive tape removal. Similarly, CX3CR1$^{-/-}$ mice are protected from the middle cerebral artery occlusion, with smaller infarct size at early time points after injury, which is associated with an M2 microglial phenotype [26]. In a model of spinal cord injury, CX3CR1$^{-/-}$ mice had more favorable outcome 5 days post-injury, with neuroprotection and functional recovery, than WT control mice [23]. The improved recovery after traumatic spinal cord injury is associated with reduced recruitment of monocytes/macrophages to the site of injury. Collectively, these studies underscore a role for CX3CR1 signaling in response to CNS injury and suggest that mechanisms by which CX3CR1 promotes neuroprotection during the acute phase of brain injury include a protective microglia phenotype and reduced monocyte/macrophage recruitment.

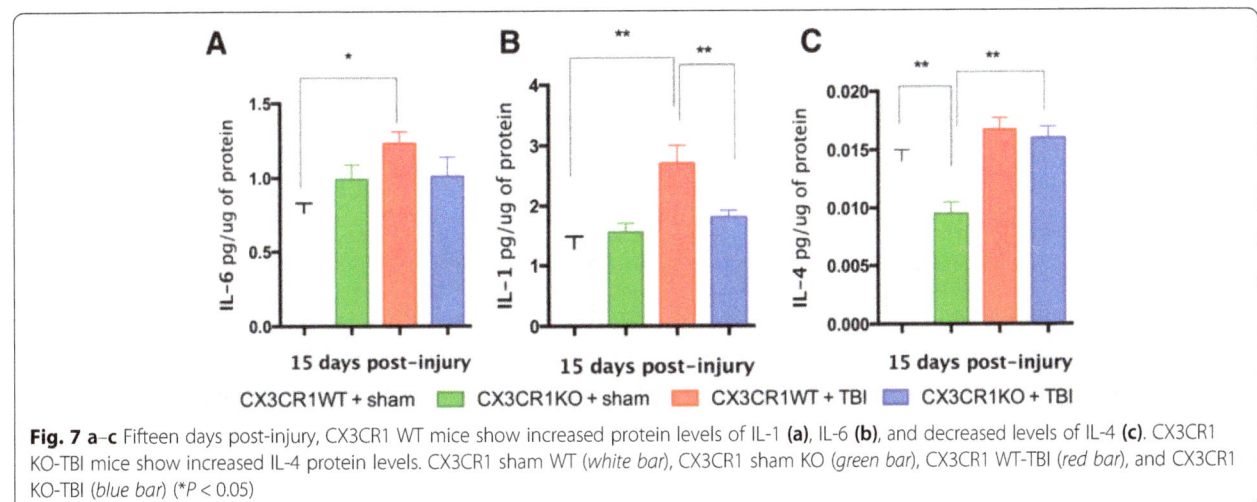

Fig. 7 a–c Fifteen days post-injury, CX3CR1 WT mice show increased protein levels of IL-1 (**a**), IL-6 (**b**), and decreased levels of IL-4 (**c**). CX3CR1 KO-TBI mice show increased IL-4 protein levels. CX3CR1 sham WT (*white bar*), CX3CR1 sham KO (*green bar*), CX3CR1 WT-TBI (*red bar*), and CX3CR1 KO-TBI (*blue bar*) (*P < 0.05)

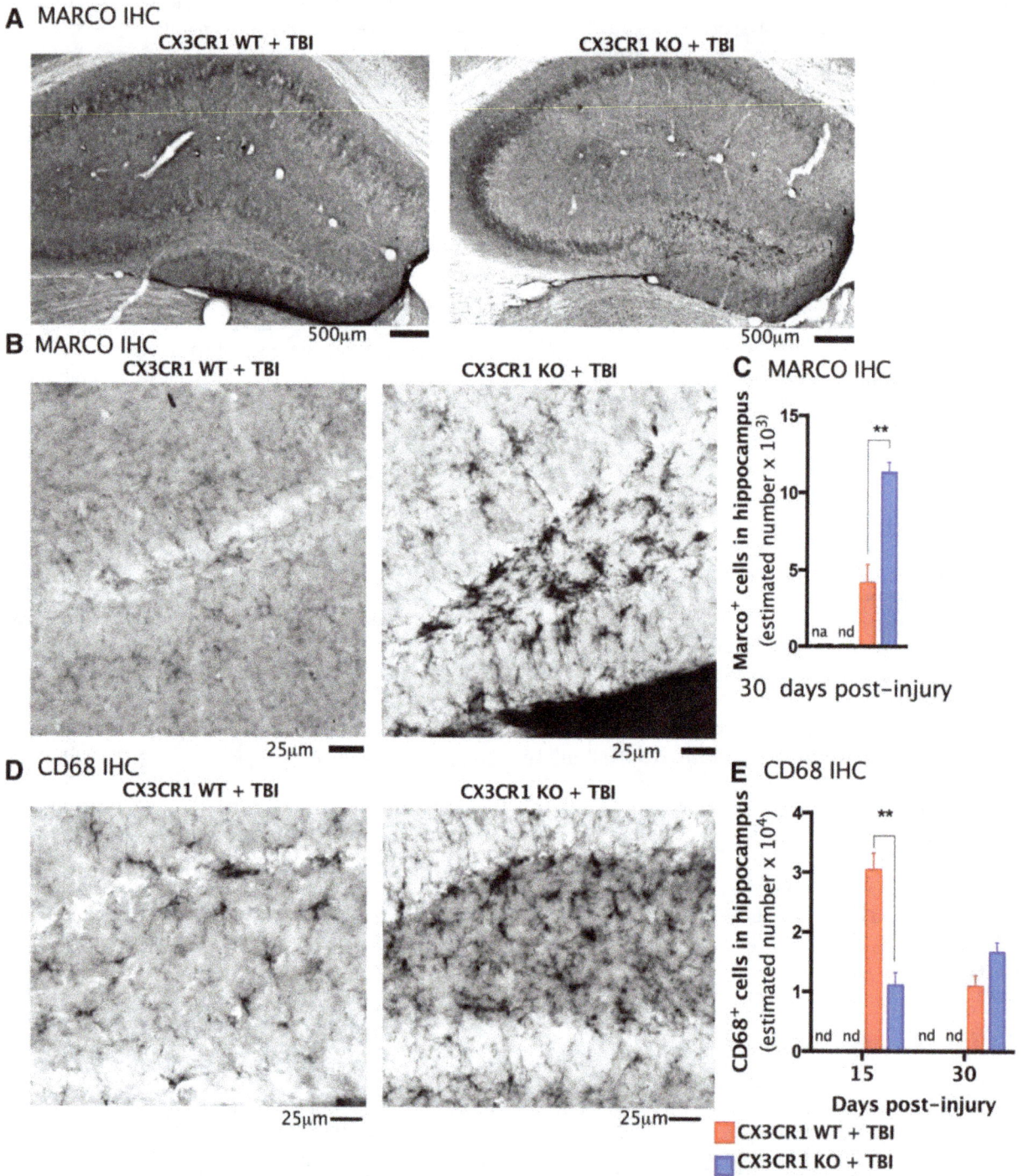

Fig. 8 Immunostaining and stereological quantification for M1 polarization markers in hippocampus at 30 days post-TBI. **a** Micrograph at ×4 magnification showing Marco staining at 30 days post-TBI in the dentate gyrus of CX3CR1 WT-TBI and CX3CR1 KO-TBI mice. **b** Higher magnification (×20) of the dentate gyrus of CX3CR1 WT-TBI and CX3CR1 KO-TBI showing in the hippocampus show a strong increase in staining in the CX3CR1 KO-TBI compared to CX3CR1 WT-TBI at 30 days. **c** Unbiased stereology quantification of Marco revealed a significant increase in the number of Marco+ cells in the hippocampus of CX3CR1 KO-TBI compared to CX3CR1 WT-TBI ($p < 0.001$). **d** Micrograph at ×20 magnification of the dentate gyrus of CX3CR1 WT-TBI and CX3CR1 KO-TBI showing in the hippocampus show a strong increase in CD68 staining in the CX3CR1 KO-TBI compared to CX3CR1 WT-TBI at 30 days post-TBI. **e** Time course of CD68 expression at 15 and 30 days post-injury. Stereological quantification of CD68+ cells revealed a significant decrease in CX3CR1 KO-TBI mice compared to CX3CR1 WT-TBI at 15 days post-TBI. Although the difference did not reach statistical significance, at 30 days post-TBI, expression of CD68 was higher in CX3CR1 KO-TBI mice compared to wild-type (**$p < 0.001$)

Our data indicate that CD68, a specific marker of phagocytic microglia, is decreased at 15 days post-trauma in CX3CR1$^{-/-}$ mice and, in this present study, tends to increase by 30 days post-injury. Although microglial phagocytosis of dead or dying neurons can be beneficial by preventing the release of pro-inflammatory molecules, under some conditions, such as inflammation, microglia also phagocytize viable neurons, thus contributing to cell death [45]. Intraventricular infusion of mesenchymal stem cells after TBI induces early and lasting acquisition of a protective M2 microglial phenotype that is associated with reduced CD68 immunoreactivity [46]. Based on these observations, we hypothesize that the reduced phagocytic activity in CX3CR1$^{-/-}$ mice could be beneficial to neurons and perhaps explain neuroprotection at 15 days post-trauma on these animals. On the other hand, increased phagocytosis 30 days post-TBI could be detrimental and increase neuronal death. However, CD68 immunoreactivity may not necessarily correlate with phagocytosis [47, 48]. For example, microglia that are phagocytizing apoptotic cells in physiological conditions in the hippocampus do not express CD68 [47, 48]. Experiments to specifically address this issue remain to be conducted. Nevertheless, our data show that a transient protective M2 microglia phenotype with decreased CD68 phagocytic activity manifests early after mild TBI in CX3CR1$^{-/-}$ mice.

The dramatic shift during the chronic phase of brain injury in CX3CR1$^{-/-}$ mice limits the recruitment of M2 microglia and switches the balance toward the M1 phenotype, which contributes to excessive inflammatory responses and exacerbated neuronal damage. Although a shift in microglia phenotype between the acute and chronic phase of TBI has recently been reported [49], we extend these observations by identifying CX3CR1 as a possible regulator of this microglia/macrophage phenotype switch following mild TBI. It is important to note however, that the transition between M1 and M2 microglia phenotypes is not all or none, and several intermediate microglia phenotypes with overlapping features have been described during the shift between alternatively activated phenotypes. Indeed, recently Morganti et al. [50] using CX3CR1$^{GFP/+}$ CCR2$^{RFP/+}$ reporter mice have demonstrated a broad spectrum of M1-M2 polarization mRNA gene expression following TBI, with changes occurring primarily during the first 48 h. Importantly, they reported that there was not a clear delineation of an exclusive M1, M2a, or M2c phenotype. Several factors could explain differences between our study and that of Morganti et al.; ours is a model of mild TBI model, and our M1 and M2 analysis was based on both gene expression and immunohistochemical assessment, whereas the Morganti study only reported on gene expression.

Although our data do not provide information as to precisely how CX3CR1 dictates the recruitment of M1/M2 microglia during acute or chronic stages of the disease, there likely are multiple mechanisms that regulate the neuroprotective vs. neurotoxic effects of microglia after mild TBI. Relative expression of CX3CR1 defines two phenotypically distinct monocyte subsets. Monocytes of the Ly6C^{high}/CX3CR1^{low} subset express CCR2, a chemokine receptor that facilitates recruitment of inflammatory monocytes to the site of injury. Conversely, monocytes of the subset Ly6C^{low}/CX3CR1^{high} are CCR2 deficient and are dependent on CX3CR1 for recruitment [51–53]. CX3CR1$^+$ monocytes may differentiate from Ly6C^{high} monocytes in tissue and thus may not require CX3CR1 for recruitment [54, 55]. These distinct monocyte populations are associated with tissue pathology and repair. For example, in a model of myocardial infarction, tissue repair requires recruitment of Ly6C^{high} and then Ly6C^{low} monocytes [53]. Ly6C^{high} monocytes are proteolitic, degrade injured tissue, and give rise to M1 macrophages in vivo [35, 56]. Other reports demonstrate that the Ly6C^{low}/CX3CR1^{high} monocyte subset is associated with beneficial effects as this population is capable of tissue healing [53].

In experimental models of spinal cord injury and focal cerebral ischemia, tissue damage is attenuated and function recovers earlier following injury in CX3CR1-deficient mice, effects attributed to reduced recruitment and/or activation of microglia/macrophages [23, 24, 57, 58]. Inhibiting CX3CR1 at early time points in a model of ischemic brain injury protects neurological function and reduces neuropathology by decreasing CD11b$^+$/Ly6C^{low}/iNOS$^+$ monocyte recruitment, microglia proliferation, and leukocyte infiltration [58]. Similarly, Donnelly et al. [23] showed that abolishing CX3CR1 reduces accumulation of CD11b$^+$/Ly6C^{low}/iNOS$^+$ monocytes, which confers neuroprotection and promotes recovery of function at early time points after spinal cord injury. These benefits are associated with suppressed inflammatory signaling in microglia and microglia-derived macrophages.

In our model of mild focal TBI, we did not detect differences in leukocyte infiltration from the periphery between wild-type and CX3CR1-deficient mice. Lack of differences between CX3CR1-deficient and wild-type mice could be due to the post-TBI time point analyzed and/or the mild TBI induced in this study. However, based on these aforementioned observations and our data, we hypothesize that after focal TBI, CX3CR1 plays a fundamental role in dictating the timing of recruitment of inflammatory monocyte populations relative to the protective monocyte populations, which results in a detrimental and protective microglia phenotype, respectively. Our results may reconcile data obtained from a number of pathologies with respect to whether CX3CR1 is protective or neurotoxic. Taken together, our data suggest that CX3CR1 may be an ideal target for therapeutic intervention in the acute post-traumatic period to delay secondary brain damage.

Competing interests

The authors declare that they have no competing interests.

Authors' contributions

HYF performed all animal surgeries and wrote the first draft of the manuscript. HKT assisted with the immunostaining and stereological analysis. MNP maintained and genotyped the mouse colony and performed the qRT-PCR experiments. KMR carried out the ELISA for IL-1, IL-4, and IL-6. PRB assisted with the cardiac perfusion and animal surgeries. AMG and JNG assisted with the immunohistochemistry experiments. ADB assisted in the performance and analysis of qRT-PCR. JG assisted with the flow cytometry experiments. AEC designed, performed, and analyzed all flow cytometry experiments. MRO assisted with the experimental design and manuscript preparation and provided the basis for the development of the experimental design. CG conceived and designed the entire study, carried out behavioral experiments, stereological analysis, analyzed data, and assisted with manuscript preparation. All authors read and approved the final manuscript.

Acknowledgements

This study was supported by the Department of Anesthesiology and Pain Medicine of the University of Washington and by NIH SC1GM095426.

Author details

[1]Department of Anesthesiology and Pain Medicine, University of Washington, BOX # 359724, Seattle, WA 98001, USA. [2]Neuroscience Graduate Program, University of Washington, Seattle, WA 98104, USA. [3]Department of Biology, University of Washington, Seattle, WA 98104, USA. [4]Sanders-Brown Center on Aging, University of Kentucky, Lexington, KY 40536, USA. [5]Department of Biology and South Texas Center for Emerging Infectious Diseases, University of Texas at San Antonio, San Antonio, TX 78249, USA. [6]Present address: Interdepartmental Program in Neuroscience, University of Utah School of Medicine, Salt Lake City, Utah, USA.

References

1. Ramlackhansingh AF, Brooks DJ, Greenwood RJ, Bose SK, Turkheimer FE, Kinnunen KM, et al. Inflammation after trauma: microglial activation and traumatic brain injury. Ann Neurol. 2011;70(3):374–83.
2. Giunta B, Obregon D, Velisetty R, Sanberg PR, Borlongan CV, Tan J. The immunology of traumatic brain injury: a prime target for Alzheimer's disease prevention. J Neuroinflammation. 2012;9:185.
3. Hernandez-Ontiveros DG, Tajiri N, Acosta S, Giunta B, Tan J, Borlongan CV. Microglia activation as a biomarker for traumatic brain injury. Front Neurol. 2013;4:30.
4. Jung S, Aliberti J, Graemmel P, Sunshine MJ, Kreutzberg GW, Sher A, et al. Analysis of fractalkine receptor CX(3)CR1 function by targeted deletion and green fluorescent protein reporter gene insertion. Mol Cell Biol. 2000;20(11):4106–14.
5. Cardona AE, Pioro EP, Sasse ME, Kostenko V, Cardona SM, Dijkstra IM, et al. Control of microglial neurotoxicity by the fractalkine receptor. Nat Neurosci. 2006;9(7):917–24.
6. Mizuno T, Kawanokuchi J, Numata K, Suzumura A. Production and neuroprotective functions of fractalkine in the central nervous system. Brain Res. 2003;979(1–2):65–70.
7. Limatola C, Lauro C, Catalano M, Ciotti MT, Bertollini C, Di AS, et al. Chemokine CX3CL1 protects rat hippocampal neurons against glutamate-mediated excitotoxicity. J Neuroimmunol. 2005;166(1–2):19–28.
8. Meucci O, Fatatis A, Simen AA, Miller RJ. Expression of CX3CR1 chemokine receptors on neurons and their role in neuronal survival. Proc Natl Acad Sci U S A. 2000;97(14):8075–80.
9. Frank-Cannon TC, Alto LT, McAlpine FE, Tansey MG. Does neuroinflammation fan the flame in neurodegenerative diseases? Mol Neurodegener. 2009;4:47.
10. Wyss-Coray T, Mucke L. Inflammation in neurodegenerative disease—a double-edged sword. Neuron. 2002;35(3):419–32.
11. Cameron B, Landreth GE. Inflammation, microglia, and Alzheimer's disease. Neurobiol Dis. 2010;37(3):503–9.
12. Yoshida H, Imaizumi T, Fujimoto K, Matsuo N, Kimura K, Cui X, et al. Synergistic stimulation, by tumor necrosis factor-alpha and interferon-gamma, of fractalkine expression in human astrocytes. Neurosci Lett. 2001;303(2):132–6.
13. Nishiyori A, Minami M, Ohtani Y, Takami S, Yamamoto J, Kawaguchi N, et al. Localization of fractalkine and CX3CR1 mRNAs in rat brain: does fractalkine play a role in signaling from neuron to microglia? FEBS Lett. 1998;429(2):167–72.
14. Harrison JK, Jiang Y, Chen S, Xia Y, Maciejewski D, McNamara RK, et al. Role for neuronally derived fractalkine in mediating interactions between neurons and CX3CR1-expressing microglia. Proc Natl Acad Sci U S A. 1998;95(18):10896–901.
15. Pan Y, Lloyd C, Zhou H, Dolich S, Deeds J, Gonzalo JA, et al. Neurotactin, a membrane-anchored chemokine upregulated in brain inflammation. Nature. 1997;387(6633):611–7.
16. Hatori K, Nagai A, Heisel R, Ryu JK, Kim SU. Fractalkine and fractalkine receptors in human neurons and glial cells. J Neurosci Res. 2002;69(3):418–26.
17. Bhaskar K, Konerth M, Kokiko-Cochran ON, Cardona A, Ransohoff RM, Lamb BT. Regulation of tau pathology by the microglial fractalkine receptor. Neuron. 2010;68(1):19–31.
18. Lee S, Varvel NH, Konerth ME, Xu G, Cardona AE, Ransohoff RM, et al. CX3CR1 Deficiency alters microglial activation and reduces beta-amyloid deposition in two Alzheimer's disease mouse models. Am J Pathol. 2010;177(5):2549–62.
19. Ransohoff RM, Liu L, Cardona AE. Chemokines and chemokine receptors: multipurpose players in neuroinflammation. Int Rev Neurobiol. 2007;82:187–204.
20. Cho SH, Sun B, Zhou Y, Kauppinen TM, Halabisky B, Wes P, et al. CX3CR1 protein signaling modulates microglial activation and protects against plaque-independent cognitive deficits in a mouse model of Alzheimer disease. J Biol Chem. 2011;286(37):32713–22.
21. Fuhrmann M, Bittner T, Jung CK, Burgold S, Page RM, Mitteregger G, et al. Microglial Cx3cr1 knockout prevents neuron loss in a mouse model of Alzheimer's disease. Nat Neurosci. 2010;13(4):411–3.
22. Liu Z, Condello C, Schain A, Harb R, Grutzendler J. CX3CR1 in microglia regulates brain amyloid deposition through selective protofibrillar amyloid-beta phagocytosis. J Neurosci. 2010;30(50):17091–101.
23. Donnelly DJ, Longbrake EE, Shawler TM, Kigerl KA, Lai W, Tovar CA, et al. Deficient CX3CR1 signaling promotes recovery after mouse spinal cord injury by limiting the recruitment and activation of Ly6Clo/iNOS+ macrophages. J Neurosci. 2011;31(27):9910–22.
24. Denes A, Ferenczi S, Halasz J, Kornyei Z, Kovacs KJ. Role of CX3CR1 (fractalkine receptor) in brain damage and inflammation induced by focal cerebral ischemia in mouse. J Cereb Blood Flow Metab. 2008;28(10):1707–21.
25. Cipriani R, Villa P, Chece G, Lauro C, Paladini A, Micotti E, et al. CX3CL1 is neuroprotective in permanent focal cerebral ischemia in rodents. J Neurosci. 2011;31(45):16327–35.
26. Fumagalli S, Perego C, Ortolano F, de Simoni MG. CX3CR1 deficiency induces an early protective inflammatory environment in ischemic mice. Glia. 2013;61(6):827–42.
27. Rancan M, Bye N, Otto VI, Trentz O, Kossmann T, Frentzel S, et al. The chemokine fractalkine in patients with severe traumatic brain injury and a mouse model of closed head injury. J Cereb Blood Flow Metab. 2004;24(10):1110–8.
28. Gaetani P, Pisano P, Solinas G, Colombo P, Destro A, Levi D, et al. Immunohistochemical expression of the chemokine fractalkine and its receptor in the human brain cortex after severe traumatic brain injury and brain hemorrhage. J Neurosurg Sci. 2013;57(1):55–62.
29. Chhor V, Le CT, Lebon S, Ore MV, Celador IL, Josserand J, et al. Characterization of phenotype markers and neuronotoxic potential of polarised primary microglia in vitro. Brain Behav Immun. 2013;32:70–85.
30. Lynch MA. The multifaceted profile of activated microglia. Mol Neurobiol. 2009;40(2):139–56.
31. Colton CA. Heterogeneity of microglial activation in the innate immune response in the brain. J Neuroimmune Pharmacol. 2009;4(4):399–418.
32. Colton CA, Mott RT, Sharpe H, Xu Q, Van Nostrand WE, Vitek MP. Expression profiles for macrophage alternative activation genes in AD and in mouse models of AD. J Neuroinflammation. 2006;3:27.
33. Gordon S. Alternative activation of macrophages. Nat Rev Immunol. 2003;3(1):23–35.

34. Mantovani A, Sica A, Sozzani S, Allavena P, Vecchi A, Locati M. The chemokine system in diverse forms of macrophage activation and polarization. Trends Immunol. 2004;25(12):677–86.

35. Kigerl KA, Gensel JC, Ankeny DP, Alexander JK, Donnelly DJ, Popovich PG. Identification of two distinct macrophage subsets with divergent effects causing either neurotoxicity or regeneration in the injured mouse spinal cord. J Neurosci. 2009;29(43):13435–44.

36. Washington PM, Forcelli PA, Wilkins T, Zapple DN, Parsadanian M, Burns MP. The effect of injury severity on behavior: a phenotypic study of cognitive and emotional deficits after mild, moderate, and severe controlled cortical impact injury in mice. J Neurotrauma. 2012;29(13):2283–96.

37. Bolkvadze T, Pitkanen A. Development of post-traumatic epilepsy after controlled cortical impact and lateral fluid-percussion-induced brain injury in the mouse. J Neurotrauma. 2012;29(5):789–812.

38. Kubova H, Druga R, Lukasiuk K, Suchomelova L, Haugvicova R, Jirmanova I, et al. Status epilepticus causes necrotic damage in the mediodorsal nucleus of the thalamus in immature rats. J Neurosci. 2001;21(10):3593–9.

39. West MJ, Slomianka L, Gundersen HJ. Unbiased stereological estimation of the total number of neurons in thesubdivisions of the rat hippocampus using the optical fractionator. Anat Rec. 1991;231(4):482–97.

40. Rogers JT, Morganti JM, Bachstetter AD, Hudson CE, Peters MM, Grimmig BA, et al. CX3CR1 deficiency leads to impairment of hippocampal cognitive function and synaptic plasticity. J Neurosci. 2011;31(45):16241–50.

41. Mizutani M, Pino PA, Saederup N, Charo IF, Ransohoff RM, Cardona AE. The fractalkine receptor but not CCR2 is present on microglia from embryonic development throughout adulthood. J Immunol. 2012;188(1):29–36.

42. Pino PA, Cardona AE. Isolation of brain and spinal cord mononuclear cells using percoll gradients. J Vis Exp. 2011. doi:10.3791/2348.

43. Garcia JA, Pino PA, Mizutani M, Cardona SM, Charo IF, Ransohoff RM, et al. Regulation of adaptive immunity by the fractalkine receptor during autoimmune inflammation. J Immunol. 2013;191(3):1063–72.

44. Woodcock T, Morganti-Kossmann MC. The role of markers of inflammation in traumatic brain injury. Front Neurol. 2013;4:18.

45. Neher JJ, Neniskyte U, Brown GC. Primary phagocytosis of neurons by inflamed microglia: potential roles in neurodegeneration. Front Pharmacol. 2012;3:27.

46. Zanier ER, Pischiutta F, Riganti L, Marchesi F, Turola E, Fumagalli S, et al. Bone marrow mesenchymal stromal cells drive protective M2 microglia polarization after brain trauma. Neurotherapeutics. 2014;11(3):679–95.

47. Sierra A, Encinas JM, Deudero JJ, Chancey JH, Enikolopov G, Overstreet-Wadiche LS, et al. Microglia shape adult hippocampal neurogenesis through apoptosis-coupled phagocytosis. Cell Stem Cell. 2010;7(4):483–95.

48. Sierra A, Abiega O, Shahraz A, Neumann H. Janus-faced microglia: beneficial and detrimental consequences of microglial phagocytosis. Front Cell Neurosci. 2013;7:6.

49. Wang G, Zhang J, Hu X, Zhang L, Mao L, Jiang X, et al. Microglia/macrophage polarization dynamics in white matter after traumatic brain injury. J Cereb Blood Flow Metab. 2013;33(12):1864–74.

50. Morganti JM, Jopson TD, Liu S, Riparip LK, Guandique CK, Gupta N, et al. CCR2 antagonism alters brain macrophage polarization and ameliorates cognitive dysfunction induced by traumatic brain injury. J Neurosci. 2015;35(2):748–60.

51. Geissmann F, Jung S, Littman DR. Blood monocytes consist of two principal subsets with distinct migratory properties. Immunity. 2003;19(1):71–82.

52. Combadiere C, Potteaux S, Rodero M, Simon T, Pezard A, Esposito B, et al. Combined inhibition of CCL2, CX3CR1, and CCR5 abrogates Ly6C(hi) and Ly6C(lo) monocytosis and almost abolishes atherosclerosis in hypercholesterolemic mice. Circulation. 2008;117(13):1649–57.

53. Nahrendorf M, Swirski FK, Aikawa E, Stangenberg L, Wurdinger T, Figueiredo JL, et al. The healing myocardium sequentially mobilizes two monocyte subsets with divergent and complementary functions. J Exp Med. 2007;204(12):3037–47.

54. Thawer SG, Mawhinney L, Chadwick K, de Chickera SN, Weaver LC, Brown A, et al. Temporal changes in monocyte and macrophage subsets and microglial macrophages following spinal cord injury in the Lys-Egfp-ki mouse model. J Neuroimmunol. 2013;261(1–2):7–20.

55. Arnold L, Henry A, Poron F, Baba-Amer Y, van Rooijen N, Plonquet A, et al. Inflammatory monocytes recruited after skeletal muscle injury switch into antiinflammatory macrophages to support myogenesis. J Exp Med. 2007;204(5):1057–69.

56. Lin SL, Castano AP, Nowlin BT, Lupher Jr ML, Duffield JS. Bone marrow Ly6Chigh monocytes are selectively recruited to injured kidney and differentiate into functionally distinct populations. J Immunol. 2009;183(10):6733–43.

57. Lesnik P, Haskell CA, Charo IF. Decreased atherosclerosis in CX3CR1−/− mice reveals a role for fractalkine in atherogenesis. J Clin Invest. 2003;111(3):333–40.

58. Tang Z, Gan Y, Liu Q, Yin JX, Liu Q, Shi J, et al. CX3CR1 deficiency suppresses activation and neurotoxicity of microglia/macrophage in experimental ischemic stroke. J Neuroinflammation. 2014;11:26.

14

Co-grafting of neural stem cells with olfactory ensheathing cells promotes neuronal restoration in traumatic brain injury with an anti-inflammatory mechanism

Su-Juan Liu[1], Yu Zou[2], Visar Belegu[3], Long-Yun Lv[4], Na Lin[4], Ting-Yong Wang[4], John W McDonald[3], Xue Zhou[1], Qing-Jie Xia[2*] and Ting-Hua Wang[1,2,4*]

Abstract

Background: We sought to investigate the effects of co-grafting neural stem cells (NSCs) with olfactory ensheathing cells (OECs) on neurological behavior in rats subjected to traumatic brain injury (TBI) and explore underlying molecular mechanisms.

Methods: TBI was established by percussion device made through a weight drop (50 g) from a 30 cm height. Cultured NSCs and OECs isolated from rats were labeled by Hoechst 33342 (blue) and chloromethyl-benzamidodialkyl carbocyanine (CM-DiI) (red), respectively. Then, NSCs and/or OECs, separately or combined, were transplanted into the area surrounding the injury site. Fourteen days after transplantation, neurological severity score (NSS) were recorded. The brain tissue was harvested and processed for immunocytochemistry, terminal deoxynucleotidyl transferase-mediated dUTP nick end labeling (TUNEL), and reverse transcription-polymerase chain reaction (RT-PCR).

Results: Significant neurological function improvement was observed in the three transplant groups, compared to the TBI group, and co-transplantation gave rise to the best improvement. Morphological evaluation showed that the number of neurons in cortex from combination implantation was more than for other groups (P <0.05); conversely, the number of apoptotic cells showed a significant decrease by TUNEL staining. Transplanted NSCs and OECs could survive and migrate in the brain, and the number of neurons differentiating from NSCs in the co-transplantation group was significantly greater than in the NSCs group. At the molecular level, the expressions of IL-6 and BAD in the co-graft group were found to be down regulated significantly, when compared to either the NSC or OEC alone groups.

Conclusion: The present study demonstrates for the first time the optimal effects of co-grafting NSCs and OECs as a new strategy for the treatment of TBI via an anti-inflammation mechanism.

Keywords: Neural stem cells (NSCs), Olfactory en sheathing cells (OECs), Traumatic brain injury (TBI), Anti-inflammation

Background

Traumatic brain injury (TBI) occurs as a result of direct mechanical insult to the brain, and induces degeneration and death in the central nervous system (CNS) [1,2]. TBI is prevalent especially in male adolescents and adults, and severely affects the quality of peoples' lives.

Based on an epidemiological study in eastern China, traffic accidents, a blow or penetrating injury to the head, and falls from a high place were the primary causes of TBI, and their percentages were 60.9%, 13.4%, and 13.1%, respectively [3]. Among these, traffic accidents were the major cause for TBI in all age groups except for those over 75 years of age. For all patients, although 77.3% had good recovery, there was still a 10.8% mortality; 2.6% remained in a persistent vegetative state, 2.2% had severe disability, and 7.2% had moderate disability [4]. Much of this unfavorable outcome was due to secondary brain damage that occurred in the hours,

* Correspondence: 193374073@qq.com; tinghua_neuron@263.net
[2]Institute of Neurological Disease, Translational Neuroscience Center, West China Hospital, Sichuan University, Chengdu, Sichuan 610041, China
[1]Department of Histology, Embryology and Neurobiology, West China School of Preclinical and Forensic Medicine, Sichuan University, Chengdu, Sichuan 610041, China
Full list of author information is available at the end of the article

days, and weeks after the primary insult [5]. Secondary cerebral injury was associated with impaired cerebral metabolism, hypoxia, and ischemia, which resulted in a complex, potentially irreversible pathophysiologic cascade of events. Currently, few interventions have been shown to be efficacious for the treatment of TBI in clinical trials [6], and it is therefore necessary to develop new therapeutic interventions for the clinical treatment of TBI.

Neural stem cells (NSCs) are characterized by their capacity for self-renewal and ability to differentiate into target cells [7]. It has been shown that transplanted NSCs can survive, differentiate into neurons and/or glia, and attenuate motor dysfunction after TBI [8,9]. These exciting advances in the stem cell field have boosted efforts to explore their therapeutic potential to ameliorate TBI deficits and efforts to elucidate their underlying molecular mechanism of action. However, the survival and differentiation of NSCs and their effect in traumatic brain is limited, and some new ways are needed to resolve these problems.

Olfactory en sheathing cells (OECs), as unique glial cells in the olfactory bulb and olfactory nerve, have properties of Schwann cells in promoting and assisting growth of axons [10-12]. Use of OECs in preclinical models of transplantation has been increasing in recent years. OECs not only promote long-distance regeneration of descending supraspinal and ascending propriospinal axons within both cord stumps of transected adult mammalian spinal cord [13], but can also successfully improve functional and structural recovery [14]. Importantly, OECs can act as bridges [15], and then release several cytokines that could promote neuronal survival and neurite outgrowth following injury. Therefore, OECs transplants might be considered as a supporting strategy for NSCs survival and for enhancing NSCs effects for lasting functional recovery in a traumatic milieu in the adult mammalian CNS.

In the present study, we aimed to investigate functional improvement and associated anti-inflammatory mechanisms involving the cytokines IL-1 and IL-6 following a combination graft of NSCs and OECs in TBI rats. The study could suggest new strategies for co-grafting of NSCs and OECs to promote functional recovery of TBI rats, and could elucidate underlying mechanisms. The results could be useful for the treatment of patients with TBI in future clinical trials.

Methods
Cell culture, characterization, and transplantation
NSCs were obtained from hippocampus of rat embryos [16]. They were cultured in a standard medium containing a mixture of Dulbecco's modified Eagle's medium (DMEM) and Ham's F-12 medium, supplemented with

1% N_2, 20 µg/L basic fibroblast growth factor (bFGF), 2 mmol/L glutamine, 10,000 U/L penicillin, and 10 mg/L streptomycin. The cultures were kept in a standard humidified air incubator containing 5% CO_2 and maintained at 37°C. They were divided when the cells reached approximately 90% confluence. After passage, a portion of the single cell suspension was plated onto poly-L-lysine-coated glass cover slips or plastic culture dishes at a density of 10^5 cells/mL of medium. Twelve hours after plating, a portion of the cells was fixed in 4% paraformaldehyde for 20 min and washed with PBS three times. For immunocytochemistry, cover slips were washed in PBS and incubated in 1% H_2O_2 in PBS for 20 min. The cells were permeabilized and pre-incubated with blocking solution (containing 2% goat serum, 0.3% Triton X-100, and 0.1% BSA in PBS) for 30 min at room temperature. They were then incubated overnight with a primary antibody (nestin, 1:200, Millipore Bioscience Research Reagents, Temecula, CA, USA) diluted in the same blocking solution at 4°C, washed with PBS, and incubated with secondary antibodies diluted in the same blocking solutions for 30 min at 37°C. Then, the cells were observed with a light microscope (Leica, Solms, Germany). OECs were obtained from neonatal rat olfactory bulb and purified as described before [12]. After purification, a portion of the cultured OECs were fixed and processed for immunocytochemistry to detect the specific antigen rat anti-p75-NGFR (low-affinity nerve growth factor receptor, p75, 1:400, Abcam, Cambridge, UK), using a two-step method described previously [12].

Animals, surgical procedures, and transplantation
All protocols involving the use of animals were in compliance with the National Institutes of Health Guide for the Care and Use of Laboratory Animals, and were approved by the Animal Care and Use Committee, Sichuan University, Chengdu, China. Female Sprague-Dawley (SD) rats weighing about 200 ± 20 g were used in the study (Table 1). They were randomly assigned to five groups: a sham-operated group (rats with skull exposed but not subjected to weight impaction, and receiving saline injections instead of cultured cells); a TBI group (rats subjected to TBI and receiving saline treatment); an NSC group (rats subjected to TBI and receiving NSCs transplantation); an OEC group (rats subjected to TBI and receiving OECs transplantation); and a co-transplantation group (rats subjected to TBI and receiving co-transplantation of both NSCs and OECs).

For the TBI model, rats were anesthetized by intraperitoneal injection of 3.6% chloral hydrate (1 mL/100 g). The scalp was incised on the midline, exposing the skull. A 5 mm hole was drilled into the right parietal bone, not touching the dura mater. A 50 g-weight hammer was allowed to fall from a 30 cm height along guide stick to create a contusion brain injury model. At the end of the procedure, the exposed dura was covered with bone wax and the scalp sutured. The rats were placed in a warmed, oxygenated recovery chamber with free access to food and water under controlled temperature (24 ± 21°C) and humidity (55 ± 5%) as well as a 12/12 h light–dark cycle. Postoperative care included injections of penicillin to prevent infection.

Before transplantation, the cells from a third passage were trypsinized (0.125% trypsin, 5 min), and gently titrated into serum containing medium to inactivate the trypsin, then washed three times by gently pelleting the cells, followed by a low-speed centrifugation (900 g). They were resuspended in DMEM/F-12 to yield/reach a final concentration of 1×10^7 cells/mL. Trypan blue was used to assess their viability. The suspension was kept on ice and gently triturated before each injection to keep the suspension dispersed and free of cell clumps. NSCs and OECs were labeled with Hoechst 33342 and CM-Dil, and then engrafted into tissues around the injury site through the microinjection needle of a stereotaxic instrument. Four injections were made, each containing 5.0 μL of suspended cells, delivered at 1 μL/min. For the co-grafting group, 50% NSCs and 50% OECs were injected, suggesting that the total number of cells for each treatment was the same. Sham-operated animals and TBI control animals received only saline injections.

All transplant recipients received 10 mL of cyclosporine each, administered intraperitoneally, beginning 3 days before transplantation and continuing for 1 week.

Assessment of neurological function

Neurological function was evaluated by a modified neurological severity score (NSS) on the day before, and on days 7 and 14 after transplantation [17]. The evaluations consisted of motor (muscle status, abnormal movement), sensory (visual, tactile, proprioceptive), reflex, and balance tests; and were recorded on a scale of 0 to 18 (normal score, 0; maximal deficit score, 18). They were performed by blinded, trained observers. For the NSS, 1 point was scored for inability to perform the test or the lack of a tested reflex. Thus, a higher score would

point to a more severe injury. All rats were given enough time to become familiar with the testing environment before inflicting the brain injury. This was assessed by the rat's ability to perform all the tests, and then an NSS was assigned.

Tissue preparation

For assessment of terminal deoxynucleotidyl transferase-mediated dUTP nick end labeling (TUNEL) staining and reverse transcription-polymerase chain reaction (RT-PCR) 1 week after TBI, and for behavior immunohistochemistry 2 weeks after TBI, rats were anaesthetized and tissues further processed. For TUNEL and immunostaining, a total of 500 mL of 0.1 M/L PBS (pH 7.2 to 7.3, room temperature) was introduced into the left ventricle for 20 to 30 min, followed by 500 mL of 4% paraformaldehyde in 0.1 M/L PBS (pH 7.2 to 7.3, 4°C for 1 h). The brain was removed and immersed in the same fixative for 4°C for 24 hours, and then transferred to PBS containing 30% sucrose before cryosectioning. Serial sections of the brain tissues were sliced at a thickness of 30 μm using a cryotome (CM1900, Leica), and mounted on gelatin-pretreated slides. For RT-PCR, the brain tissues were directly harvested without perfusion, then frozen and kept at −80°C until used.

Survival and differentiation of grafted cells

Grafted cell survival was assessed by identifying fluorescent cells under fluorescence microscopy in brain sections. Three microscopic fields (400×) from each section of each rat in each group were acquired to perform subsequent statistical analysis. Differentiation of NSC-derived cells in the host brain was detected by fluorescence immunohistochemistry staining. The antibodies used included NeuN (for neuronal differentiation), GFAP (for astrocyte differentiation), and APC (for oligodendrocyte differentiation), respectively. In the above procedures, mouse anti-NeuN (1:1,000, Millipore Bioscience Research Reagents), rabbit anti-GFAP (1:200, Millipore Bioscience Research Reagents), and mouse anti-APC (1:200, Millipore Bioscience Research Reagents) were used, followed by routine immunoenzyme-linked immunocytochemistry.

Neuronal survival

To detect neuronal survival in brain, sections from tissue surrounding the injured brain were evaluated using routine immunofluorescence staining. The primary antibody was NeuN (1:1,000, Millipore Bioscience Research Reagents) and the second antibody was conjugated with Cy3 (red) fluorescent. For control, the primary antibody was omitted for all markers. Labeled cells and regenerating axons were examined with a fluorescence microscope.

Table 1 Animal numbers in each procedure

Group	Behavior test (7 and 14 days)	Apoptosis assessment (7 days)	Gene expression detection (7 days)
Sham	6	3	6
TBI	6	3	6
NSC	7	3	6
OEC	8	3	6
NSC + OEC	6	3	6

NSC, neural stem cell; OEC, olfactory en sheathing cell; TBI, traumatic brain injury.

TUNEL staining

TUNEL was used to detect apoptotic neurons in the host brain. For each rat, the brain tissues sectioned at 20 μm thickness were stained with TUNEL reagents according to the manufacturer's instructions. The sections were dried, rehydrated in PBS, and treated with proteinase K for 5 min at room temperature. After quenching the endogenous peroxidase activity with 3% H_2O_2 in methanol, the sections were successively treated with an equilibration buffer, working TdT enzyme for 4 h at 37°C and blocking buffer. Finally, the reaction was visualized by streptavidin-biotin-peroxidase complex and diaminobenzidine. Sections incubated without the enzyme were used as negative controls. There were two distinct patterns of TUNEL staining, as reported previously [18]. Some cells were densely labeled and showed clear apoptotic characteristics, such as perinuclear ring formation, patches, or an apoptotic body. Other cells were weakly labeled and considered to be necrotic cells. Only the densely labeled cells were counted as TUNEL-positive cells [19]. In order to compare the numbers of apoptotic cells, three fields (400×) from each section of each rat in each group were taken for statistical analysis.

RT-PCR

To explore the molecular mechanism underlying the restorative features observed in the host brain following transplantation, the expressions of IL-1, IL-6 (inflammatory factors), and BAD (apoptosis signal molecule) were determined. Total RNA from pericontusional tissues of each group was extracted using a commercially available kit (Fermentas, Burlington, ON, Canada). The procedure followed the manufacturer's instructions. In order to remove any contaminating genomic DNA, samples were incubated at 37°C for 40 min with DNase I, followed by DNase inactivation with a DNase inactivation reagent. For reverse transcription, 2.0 μg RNA per sample was reverse transcribed using a reverse transcription kit in a total volume of 50 μL according to the manufacturer's instructions. cDNA was diluted in TE buffer, aliquoted, and stored at –20°C. Primers for IL-6, BAD, and β-actin (as an internal control) were designed with the primer 5.0 software and then empirically tested. IL-1β (234 bp), forward GAGCTGAAAGCTCTCCACCT and reverse TTCCAT CTTCTTCTTTGGGT; IL-6 (378 bp), forward CTTG GGACTGATGTTGTTGA and reverse CTGGCTTTG TCTTTCTTGTTAT; and BAD (435 bp), forward CGA GTGAGCAGGAAGACGC and reverse AATTTCGAT CCCACCAGGAC. β-actin (227 bp), forward GTAAAG ACCTCTATGCCAACA and reverse GGACTCATCGT ACTCCTGCT. PCR semi-quantitative conditions were optimized by varying the amount of template and cycle number to determine a linear amplification range. Following PCR, the product was electrophoresed on a 1.5% agarose gel, post-stained with gold view, and identified by size. The optical density (OD) of each product band, including the objective gene and β-actin was obtained, and the OD ratio between investigated genes and β-actin were calculated to semi-quantify the objective gene level.

Statistical analysis

Statistical analysis was conducted using SPSS 16.0 software (SPSS Inc., Chicago, IL, USA). The measurement data are expressed as mean ± SD and were subjected to statistical analysis using one-way analysis of variance (ANOVA). When significant interactions were detected in any ANOVA paradigm, post-hoc Student-Newman-Keuls t-tests were used to demonstrate effects between individual groups. Values of $P < 0.05$ were considered statistically significant.

Results

Characterization of cultured cells

After 2 to 3 days of culture, cultured cells began to form neurospheres and showed increases in number and size by 5 days (Figure 1A). The cells stained with nestin were confirmed as NSCs (Figure 1B). These cells emitted blue fluorescence after Hoechst 33342 labeling under fluorescence microscopy (Figure 1C). OECs were successfully isolated and assumed a shuttle appearance (Figure 1D), and were identified by p75 immunostaining (Figure 1E) confirming that they were OECs. In order to track the transplanted OECs, CM-Dil was used to label OECs, as shown in Figure 1F.

Character of differentiation of NSCs

Immunocytochemistry staining was used to detect differentiation of NSCs into neurons (NeuN-positive), oligodendrocytes (APC-positive), and astrocytes (GFAP-positive) (Figure 2A, B, C, D). *In vitro*, NSCs exhibited the capacity to differentiate into neurons, astrocytes, and oligodendrocytes. NSC, neural stem cell.

NSS

Before TBI or sham operation, rats received a score of 0 and showed normal cerebral function. However, after TBI surgery, the rats showed impairment of locomotor functions and the NSS significantly increased when compared to the sham group ($P < 0.01$). In addition, separate or combined transplantation of NSCs and OECs resulted in prominent decreases in the NSS, suggesting a significant improvement of neurological function ($P < 0.05$; Figure 3).

Survival and integration of grafted cells in host tissues

Cells emitting blue fluorescence were found in pericontusional tissue, confirming these as transplanted NSCs (Figure 4A, B), while those emitting red fluorescence

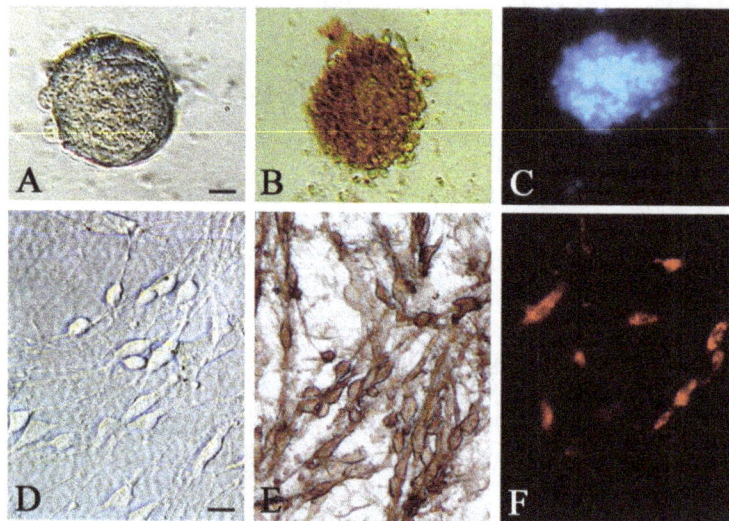

Figure 1 *In vitro* **characterization of NSCs and OECs.** Representative images of NSCs and OECs *in vitro*. **(A)** NSCs are tighter and larger 5 days after isolation from rat hippocampus, **(B)** nestin + neurosphere formation, and **(C)** neurons labeled with Hoechst 33342. **(D)** OECs present bipolar and multipolar cells with a three-dimensional, interlaced network after purified culture, **(E)** NGFR-p75+, and **(F)** labeled with CM-DiI. Scale bars are 30 μm in **(A)** and 50 μm in **(D)**. CM-DiI, chloromethyl-benzamidodialkyl carbocyanine; NSC, neural stem cell; OEC, olfactory en sheathing cell.

were identified as OECs (Figure 4C, D). This confirmed that grafted cells could survive and migrate around the injury site. Given that only half the number of NSCs were transplanted in the co-grafting group compared to the NSC group at the beginning of cell transplantation, it is clear that the number of surviving NSCs after co-grafting is 3.4-fold (68/20) higher compared with NSCs only transplantation into the brain. Moreover, compared with NSCs implanted alone, the number of surviving NSCs in the co-transplantation group is significantly

increased (P <0.05; Figure 4E). This finding demonstrates that OECs play an important role in enhancing the survival of NSCs.

Neuronal survival in host brain

In the sham-operated group, neurons presented a healthy and robust appearance (Figure 5A). After TBI, neurons surrounding the lesion site appeared shrunken and were significantly reduced in number when compared with the sham-operated group (Figure 5B). Notably, NSCs or OECs

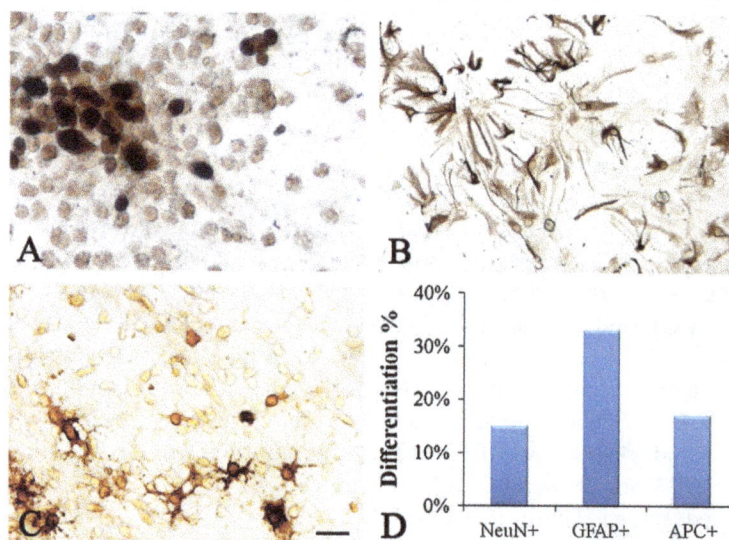

Figure 2 *In vitro* **characterization of NSC differentiation.** NSCs isolated from rats differentiate into neuron-like cells and glial cells, and express **(A)** NeuN (a neuron marker), **(B)** GFAP (an astrocyte marker), and **(C)** APC (an oligodendrocyte marker) as shown by immunocytochemical staining. **(D)** Quantitative differentiation (percent of NSCs). Scale bar = 100 μm, shown in **(C)**. NSC, neural stem cell.

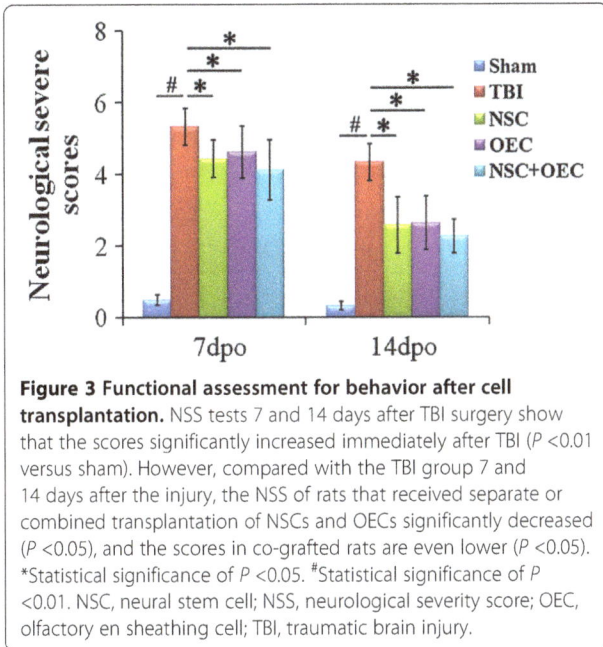

Figure 3 Functional assessment for behavior after cell transplantation. NSS tests 7 and 14 days after TBI surgery show that the scores significantly increased immediately after TBI (P <0.01 versus sham). However, compared with the TBI group 7 and 14 days after the injury, the NSS of rats that received separate or combined transplantation of NSCs and OECs significantly decreased (P <0.05), and the scores in co-grafted rats are even lower (P <0.05). *Statistical significance of P <0.05. #Statistical significance of P <0.01. NSC, neural stem cell; NSS, neurological severity score; OEC, olfactory en sheathing cell; TBI, traumatic brain injury.

grafting brought about a significant increase in the number of neurons (Figure 5C, D). Co-grafting of NSCs and OECs resulted in the largest number of surviving neurons (P <0.05 versus NSC group; P <0.05 versus OEC group; Figure 5E).

Neuronal apoptosis
TUNEL staining showed the presence of apoptotic cells with typical dark brown, rounded, or oval apoptotic bodies. Compared with the sham-operated group (Figure 6A), the number of apoptotic neurons in the brain significantly increased following TBI surgery (P <0.01). However, separate or combined transplantation treatment resulted in a significant decrease in the number of apoptotic cells (P <0.05 versus TBI; P <0.01 versus TBI; Figure 6B, C, D, E, F). Moreover, compared with separate transplantation of NSCs or OECs, the number of apoptotic cells decreased significantly in the co-grafted group (P <0.05; Figure 6C, D, E, F).

RT-PCR
To address the molecular mechanism for cell transplantation, the expressions of IL-1β, IL-6, and BAD genes were detected in the brain of rats subjected to TBI. Of note, although there is no statistical difference in expression of IL-1β following the different administrations, mRNA expression of IL-6 and BAD in the co-transplantation group exhibited a significant down-regulation in pericontusional regions at 7 days when compared with the OEC group (P <0.05; Figure 7A, B). Similarly, BAD gene expression was significantly reduced in the

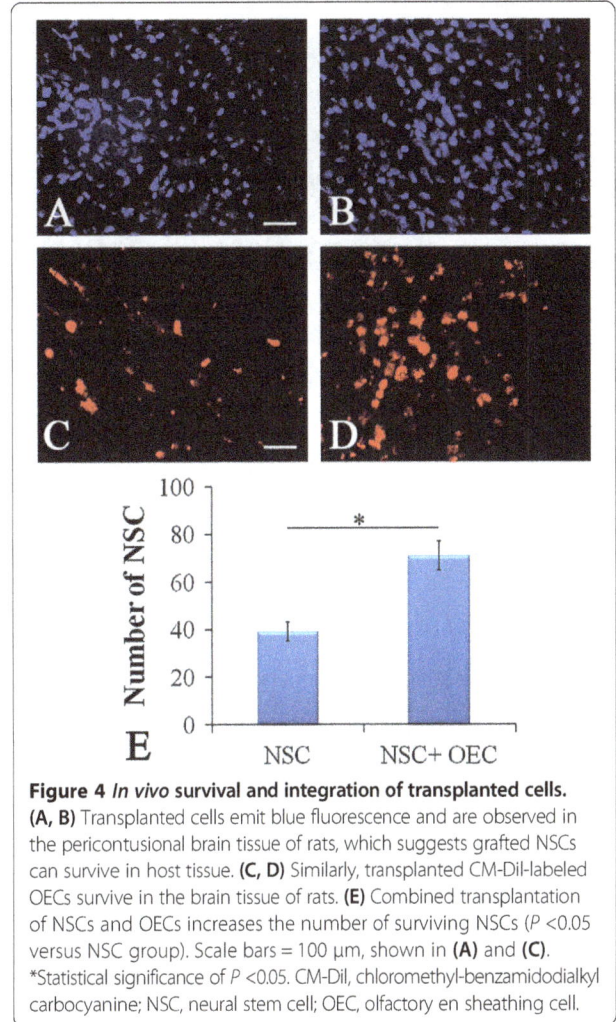

Figure 4 *In vivo* survival and integration of transplanted cells. (A, B) Transplanted cells emit blue fluorescence and are observed in the pericontusional brain tissue of rats, which suggests grafted NSCs can survive in host tissue. (C, D) Similarly, transplanted CM-Dil-labeled OECs survive in the brain tissue of rats. (E) Combined transplantation of NSCs and OECs increases the number of surviving NSCs (P <0.05 versus NSC group). Scale bars = 100 μm, shown in (A) and (C). *Statistical significance of P <0.05. CM-Dil, chloromethyl-benzamidodialkyl carbocyanine; NSC, neural stem cell; OEC, olfactory en sheathing cell.

NSC + OEC group compared with the TBI group or the NSC only group, (P <0.05; Figure 7A, B). This suggests that co-graft effects on behavior and anti-apoptosis may be linked to down-regulation of IL-6 and BAD.

Discussion
This study demonstrates that intracerebral implantation of NSCs and OECs after TBI effectively enhances survival of NSCs and improves neurological function. Moreover, co-grafting had the best results in attenuating posttraumatic neuronal apoptosis, compared with the single NSCs or OECs grafting. This could be associated with the observed down-regulation of IL-6 and BAD genes in the posttraumatic period.

Effects of grafts on behavior and morphology
NSCs transplanted into host tissue can produce neuro-active substances [20], which are important for neuronal survival and axonal growth [21,22]. However, in the injured milieu, survival of NSCs encounters challenges.

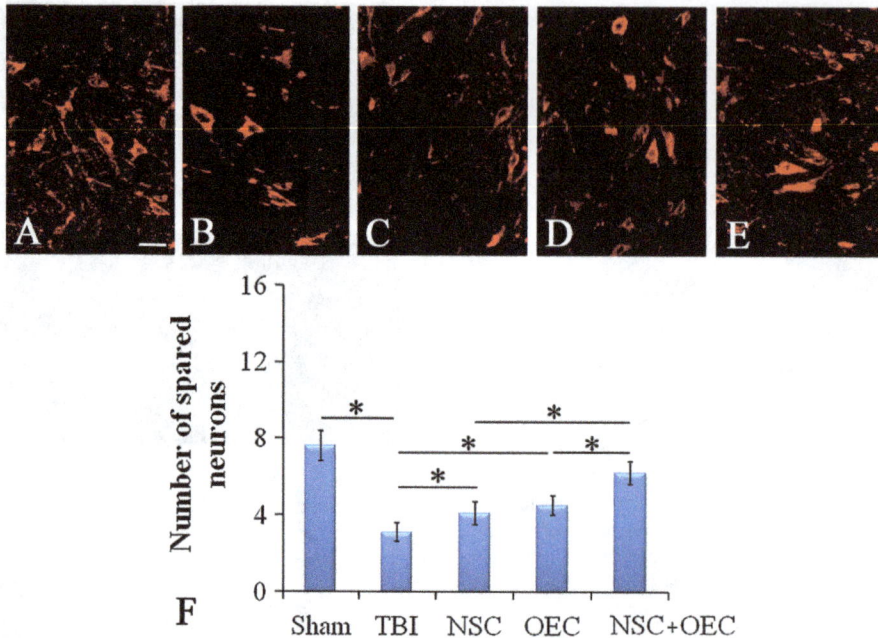

Figure 5 Neuronal survival in host brain. (A, B, F) The number of neurons labeled by NeuN in host brain significantly decreases following TBI when compared with sham (P <0.05). **(B, C, D, E, F)** However, separate or combined transplantation of NSCs and OECs increases neuronal number (P <0.05 versus TBI). **(C, D, E, F)** Furthermore, co-grafting group resulted in the highest number of surviving neurons; higher than the NSC only group or the OEC only group (P <0.05). Scale bars = 100 μm, shown in **(A)**. *Statistical significance of P <0.05. NSC, neural stem cell; OEC, olfactory en sheathing cell; TBI, traumatic brain injury.

As a result, additional supportive strategies to maintain NSCs survival are necessary. OECs, as a unique type of glial cell that arises from the neural crest, exhibit the ability to secrete several growth factors, and could therefore serve as support cells for NSCs survival. In our study, engrafted OECs survived and migrated together with NSCs in brain. They therefore may provide a favorable cellular substrate with molecules that could facilitate axonal binding and extension and neurotropic effects [23] for neuronal survival. In addition, OECs may

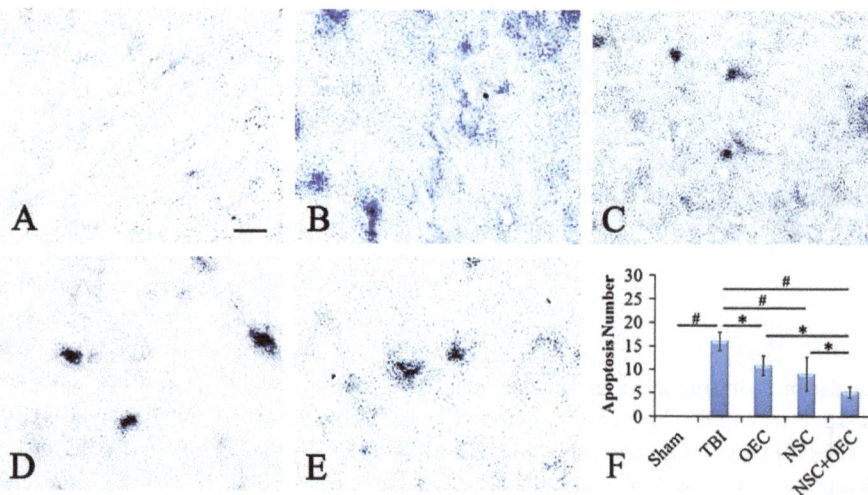

Figure 6 Neuronal apoptosis in host brain. (A, B, F) TUNEL staining shows that neuronal apoptosis increased significantly after TBI (P <0.01 versus sham group), **(B, C, D, E, F)** whereas separate or combined transplantation of NSCs and OECs has a reverse effect on neuronal apoptosis (P <0.05 versus TBI; P <0.01 versus TBI), and **(C, D, E, F)** results with co-grafting are the best (P <0.05 versus NSC; P <0.05 versus OEC). Bars = 100 μm, shown in **(A)**. *Statistical significance of P <0.05. #Statistical significance of P <0.01. NSC, neural stem cell; OEC, olfactory en sheathing cell; TBI, traumatic brain injury; TUNEL, terminal deoxynucleotidyl transferase-mediated dUTP nick end labeling.

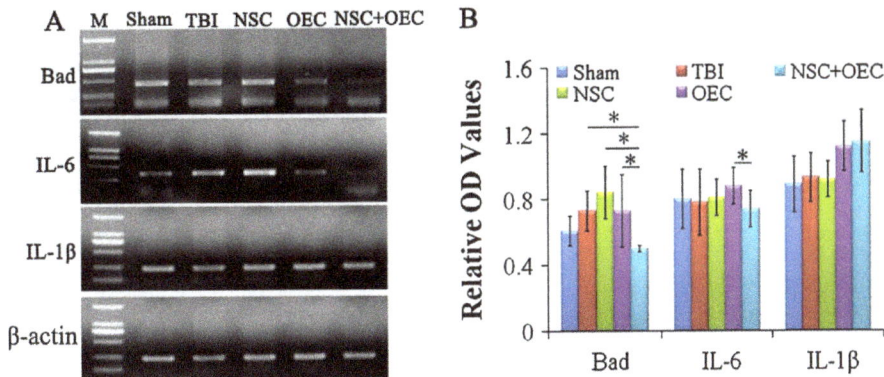

Figure 7 Changes of gene expression after cell transplantation. Gene expression of IL-1β, IL-6, and BAD in host brain were examined by **(A)** RT-PCR and **(B)** quantitative analysis. Although IL-1β gene expression is not statistically different after cell transplantation, IL-6 gene expression significantly decreased in the pericontusional regions of the co-transplantation group at 7 days compared with OEC only grafts (P <0.05). Moreover, BAD gene expression decreased significantly in the NSC + OEC group when compared with that of the TBI, NSC, and OEC groups (P <0.05). *Statistical significance of P <0.05. NSC, neural stem cell; OEC, olfactory en sheathing cell; TBI, traumatic brain injury.

be useful in myelin development or remyelination [24,25], and even in promoting axonal growth [21,23]. In this study, engrafted NSCs and OECs were well integrated into the host and enhanced structural and functional restoration in rats following TBI. Co-transplantation may be considered as a new strategy for the treatment of TBI.

Possible mechanism for structural restoration following co-grafting

The exact mechanism by which co-transplantation brings about functional restoration after TBI is unclear. An increase in neuronal survival may play an important role in this process. Other important events may include angiogenesis, formation of new synaptic junctions, and structural reorganization, as reported previously [15]. In our study, co-transplantation of NSCs and OECs exerted synergistic effects in amelioration of TBI, which may involve the following: 1) addition of OECs enhanced survival of NSCs, which is beneficial to structural restoration; 2) NSCs and OECs could secrete many types of growth factors that are useful for the formation of new synaptic junctions, and anti-apoptosis; 3) after TBI, lost neurons might be replaced by engrafted NSCs, while OECs could serve as 'bridges' to guide axonal elongation, or could promote myelination [24]; and 4) co-grafting may down regulate expression of cytokines, such as IL-6, and decrease BAD levels, so as to protect neurons from apoptosis via an anti-inflammatory mechanism.

Implications of down-regulation of IL-6 and BAD genes

In the investigation of mechanisms of cell death and survival, apoptosis genes and neurotrophic factors are commonly considered. However, the present study mainly shows that co-transplantation of NSCs and OECs can regulate expression of IL-6, in addition to BAD, a crucial

molecular signal involved in anti-inflammatory effects and apoptosis. IL-6 was originally identified as a major inducer of immune and inflammatory responses under injury conditions [26]. IL-6 *in vitro* enhances glutamate-mediated excitotoxicity in cerebellar granule cells, and can cause blood–brain barrier damage *in vivo* [27]. Transgenic mice overexpressing IL-6 display gliosis, neuronal cell loss, and learning disabilities with prominent neurodegeneration [28]. Hence, excessive IL-6-mediated inflammation is likely to play a fundamental role in the pathogenesis of the undesirable outcomes of TBI. In this study, we found that co-grafts could down regulate expressions of the inflammatory cytokine IL-6 but not IL-1β. This suggests that IL-6 may be a vital molecule in TBI following co-grafting. In addition, BAD, as a pro-apoptotic protein in the mitochondria-mediated apoptosis pathway [29,30], was also involved. The apoptotic activity of BAD is dependent on its phosphorylation status at Ser112, Ser136, and Ser155 [31]. When BAD is phosphorylated at these sites, it forms a complex with 14-3-3 proteins that cannot induce apoptosis [32]. In our study, BAD expression was greatly down regulated following co-transplantation. This could certainly lead to reduced apoptotic activity. Hence the prevention of cell apoptosis by the co-graft could be dependent on BAD regulation, a vital apoptosis signal molecule.

Conclusions

The present study provides new evidence to confirm the effects of co-grafting of NSCs and OECs in TBI rats, as demonstrated by restored structural integrity, attenuated neuronal apoptosis, promotion of host neuronal survival, and down-regulation of the expression of IL-6 and BAD genes in TBI rats. These findings could be useful in suggesting new strategies for treatment of TBI, and provide insight into potential underlying mechanisms.

Abbreviations
ANOVA: Analysis of variance; bFGF: Basic fibroblast growth factor; BSA: Bovine serum albumin; CM-DiI: Chloromethyl-benzamidodialkyl carbocyanine; CNS: Central nervous system; DMEM: Dulbecco's modified Eagle's medium; IL: Interleukin; NSC: Neural stem cell; NSS: Neurological severity score; OD: Optical density; OEC: Olfactory en sheathing cell; PBS: Phosphate-buffered saline; RT-PCR: Reverse transcription-polymerase chain reaction; SD: Sprague-Dawley; TBI: Traumatic brain injury; TUNEL: Terminal deoxynucleotidyl transferase-mediated dUTP nick end labeling.

Competing interests
The authors declare that they have no competing interests.

Authors' contributions
THW, QJX, and SJL designed the study. SJL, YZ, QJX, LYL, XZ, NL, and TYW performed the experiments. SJL, VB, and JM discussed the results and prepared the manuscript. All authors read and approved the final version of the manuscript.

Acknowledgment
This research was supported by a grant from the China National Science Foundation (number: 81271358, 81070991).

Author details
[1]Department of Histology, Embryology and Neurobiology, West China School of Preclinical and Forensic Medicine, Sichuan University, Chengdu, Sichuan 610041, China. [2]Institute of Neurological Disease, Translational Neuroscience Center, West China Hospital, Sichuan University, Chengdu, Sichuan 610041, China. [3]Department of Neurology, Johns Hopkins University School of Medicine, Baltimore, MD 21205, USA. [4]Institute of Neuroscience, Kunming Medical University, Kunming, Yunnan 650031, China.

References
1. Chauhan NB: Chronic neurodegenerative consequences of traumatic brain injury. *Restor Neurol Neurosci* 2014, 32:337–365.
2. Tran LV: Understanding the pathophysiology of traumatic brain injury and the mechanisms of action of neuroprotective interventions. *J Trauma Nurs* 2014, 21:30–35.
3. Wu X, Hu J, Zhuo L, Fu C, Hui G, Wang Y, Yang W, Teng L, Lu S, Xu G: Epidemiology of traumatic brain injury in eastern China, 2004: a prospective large case study. *J Trauma* 2008, 64:1313–1319.
4. Amaranath JE, Ramanan M, Reagh J, Saekang E, Prasad N, Chaseling R, Soundappan S: Epidemiology of traumatic head injury from a major paediatric trauma centre in New South Wales, Australia. *ANZ J Surg* 2014. doi: 10.1111/ans.12445.
5. Moppett IK: Traumatic brain injury: assessment, resuscitation and early management. *Br J Anaesth* 2007, 99:18–31.
6. Kumar A, Loane DJ: Neuroinflammation after traumatic brain injury: opportunities for therapeutic intervention. *Brain Behav Immun* 2012, 26:1191–1201.
7. Okano H: Neural stem cells and strategies for the regeneration of the central nervous system. *Proc Jpn Acad Ser B Phys Biol Sci* 2010, 86:438–450.
8. Skardelly M, Gaber K, Burdack S, Scheidt F, Hilbig H, Boltze J, Forschler A, Schwarz S, Schwarz J, Meixensberger J, Schuhmann MU: Long-term benefit of human fetal neuronal progenitor cell transplantation in a clinically adapted model after traumatic brain injury. *J Neurotrauma* 2011, 28:401–414.
9. Ma H, Yu B, Kong L, Zhang Y, Shi Y: Transplantation of neural stem cells enhances expression of synaptic protein and promotes functional recovery in a rat model of traumatic brain injury. *Mol Med Rep* 2011, 4:849–856.
10. Lang BC, Zhang Z, Lv LY, Liu J, Wang TY, Yang LH, Liao DQ, Zhang WS, Wang TH: OECs transplantation results in neuropathic pain associated with BDNF regulating ERK activity in rats following cord hemisection. *BMC Neurosci* 2013, 14:80.
11. Blumenthal J, Cohen-Matsliah SI, Levenberg S: Olfactory bulb-derived cells seeded on 3D scaffolds exhibit neurotrophic factor expression and pro-angiogenic properties. *Tissue Eng Part A* 2013, 19:2284–2291.
12. Wang YC, Li JL, Liu J, Zhao XM, Xia GN, Wang TH, Fu XM, Qi JG: Olfactory en sheathing cells transplantation promotes the recovery of neurological functions in rats with traumatic brain injury associated with down-regulation of Bad. *Cytotherapy* 2014, S1465–3249(13):00841–00844.
13. Oudega M: Schwann cell and olfactory en sheathing cell implantation for repair of the contused spinal cord. *Acta Physiol (Oxf)* 2007, 189:181–189.
14. Toft A, Tome M, Barnett SC, Riddell JS: A comparative study of glial and non-neural cell properties for transplant-mediated repair of the injured spinal cord. *Glia* 2013, 61:513–528.
15. Wang G, Ao Q, Gong K, Zuo H, Gong Y, Zhang X: Synergistic effect of neural stem cells and olfactory en sheathing cells on repair of adult rat spinal cord injury. *Cell Transplant* 2010, 19:1325–1337.
16. Abraham AB, Bronstein R, Reddy AS, Maletic-Savatic M, Aguirre A, Tsirka SE: Aberrant neural stem cell proliferation and increased adult neurogenesis in mice lacking chromatin protein HMGB2. *PLoS One* 2013, 8:e84838.
17. Hirjak D, Wolf RC, Stieltjes B, Hauser T, Seidl U, Thiemann U, Schroder J, Thomann PA: Neurological soft signs and brainstem morphology in first-episode schizophrenia. *Neuropsychobiology* 2013, 68:91–99.
18. Charriaut-Marlangue C, Ben-Ari Y: A cautionary note on the use of the TUNEL stain to determine apoptosis. *Neuroreport* 1995, 7:61–64.
19. Sobrado M, Lopez MG, Carceller F, Garcia AG, Roda JM: Combined nimodipine and citicoline reduce infarct size, attenuate apoptosis and increase bcl-2 expression after focal cerebral ischemia. *Neuroscience* 2003, 118:107–113.
20. Pituello F, Boudannaoui S, Foulquier F, Duprat AM: Are neuronal precursor cells committed to coexpress different neuroactive substances in early amphibian neurulae? *Cell Differ Dev* 1990, 32:71–81.
21. Lu P, Jones LL, Snyder EY, Tuszynski MH: Neural stem cells constitutively secrete neurotrophic factors and promote extensive host axonal growth after spinal cord injury. *Exp Neurol* 2003, 181:115–129.
22. Lepore AC, Fischer I: Lineage-restricted neural precursors survive, migrate, and differentiate following transplantation into the injured adult spinal cord. *Exp Neurol* 2005, 194:230–242.
23. Richter MW, Fletcher PA, Liu J, Tetzlaff W, Roskams AJ: Lamina propria and olfactory bulb en sheathing cells exhibit differential integration and migration and promote differential axon sprouting in the lesioned spinal cord. *J Neurosci* 2005, 25:10700–10711.
24. Sasaki M, Lankford KL, Radtke C, Honmou O, Kocsis JD: Remyelination after olfactory en sheathing cell transplantation into diverse demyelinating environments. *Exp Neurol* 2011, 229:88–98.
25. Wewetzer K, Radtke C, Kocsis J, Baumgartner W: Species-specific control of cellular proliferation and the impact of large animal models for the use of olfactory en sheathing cells and Schwann cells in spinal cord repair. *Exp Neurol* 2011, 229:80–87.
26. Wang H, Wang K, Zhong X, Dai Y, Qiu W, Wu A, Hu X: Notable increased cerebrospinal fluid levels of soluble interleukin-6 receptors in neuromyelitis optica. *Neuroimmunomodulation* 2012, 19:304–308.
27. Farkas G, Marton J, Nagy Z, Mandi Y, Takacs T, Deli MA, Abraham CS: Experimental acute pancreatitis results in increased blood–brain barrier permeability in the rat: a potential role for tumor necrosis factor and interleukin 6. *Neurosci Lett* 1998, 242:147–150.
28. Xie F, Fang C, Schnittke N, Schwob JE, Ding X: Mechanisms of permanent loss of olfactory receptor neurons induced by the herbicide 2,6-dichlorobenzonitrile: effects on stem cells and noninvolvement of acute induction of the inflammatory cytokine IL-6. *Toxicol Appl Pharmacol* 2013, 272:598–607.
29. Jia Y, Zuo D, Li Z, Liu H, Dai Z, Cai J, Pang L, Wu Y: Astragaloside IV inhibits doxorubicin-induced cardiomyocyte apoptosis mediated by mitochondrial apoptotic pathway via activating the PI3K/Akt pathway. *Chem Pharm Bull (Tokyo)* 2014, 62:45–53.
30. Lama D, Sankararamakrishnan R: Anti-apoptotic Bcl-XL protein in complex with BH3 peptides of pro-apoptotic Bak, Bad, and Bim proteins: comparative molecular dynamics simulations. *Proteins* 2008, 73:492–514.
31. Son D, Na YR, Hwang ES, Seok SH: PDGF-C induces anti-apoptotic effects on macrophages through Akt and Bad phosphorylation. *J Biol Chem* 2014. doi: 10.1074/jbc.M113.508994.
32. Quan JH, Cha GH, Zhou W, Chu JQ, Nishikawa Y, Lee YH: Involvement of PI 3 kinase/Akt-dependent Bad phosphorylation in Toxoplasma gondii-mediated inhibition of host cell apoptosis. *Exp Parasitol* 2013, 133:462–471.

15

Reduced acute neuroinflammation and improved functional recovery after traumatic brain injury by α-linolenic acid supplementation in mice

Abhishek Desai, Taeyeop Park, Jaquel Barnes, Karl Kevala, Huazhen Chen and Hee-Yong Kim[*] ⓘ

Abstract

Background: Adequate consumption of polyunsaturated fatty acids (PUFA) is vital for normal development and functioning of the central nervous system. The long-chain n-3 PUFAs docosahexaenoic acid (DHA) and eicosapentaenoic acid are anti-inflammatory and neuroprotective in the models of central nervous system injury including traumatic brain injury (TBI). In the present study, we tested whether a higher brain DHA status in a mouse model on an adequate dietary α-linolenic acid (ALA) leads to reduced neuroinflammation and improved spontaneous recovery after TBI in comparison to a moderately lowered brain DHA status that can occur in humans.

Methods: Mice reared on diets with differing ALA content were injured by a single cortical contusion impact. Change in the expression of inflammatory cytokines was measured, and cellular changes occurring after injury were analyzed by immunostaining for macrophage/microglia and astrocytes. Behavioral studies included rotarod and beam walk tests and contextual fear conditioning.

Results: Marginal supply (0.04 %) of ALA as the sole dietary source of n-3 PUFA from early gestation produced reduction of brain DHA by 35 % in adult offspring mice in comparison to the mice on adequate ALA diet (3.1 %). The DHA-depleted group showed significantly increased TBI-induced expression of pro-inflammatory cytokines TNF-α, IL-1β, and IL-6 in the brain as well as slower functional recovery from motor deficits compared to the adequate ALA group. Despite the reduction of pro-inflammatory cytokine expression, adequate ALA diet did not significantly alter either microglia/macrophage density around the contusion site or the relative M1/M2 phenotype. However, the glial fibrillary acidic protein immunoreactivity was reduced in the injured cerebral cortex of the mice on adequate ALA diet, indicating that astrocyte activation may have contributed to the observed differences in cellular and behavioral responses to TBI.

Conclusions: Increasing the brain DHA level even from a moderately DHA-depleted state can reduce neuroinflammation and improve functional recovery after TBI, suggesting possible improvement of functional outcome by increasing dietary n-3 PUFA in human TBI.

Keywords: Polyunsaturated fatty acids (PUFA), Docosahexaenoic acid (DHA), Alpha-linolenic acid (ALA), Traumatic brain injury (TBI), Inflammation, Diet, Nutrition

* Correspondence: hykim@nih.gov
Laboratory of Molecular Signaling, National Institute of Alcohol Abuse and Alcoholism, National Institutes of Health, 5625 Fishers Lane, Rm. 3N-07, Bethesda, MD 20892-9410, USA

Background

Modern dietary practice has resulted in an increased consumption of n-6 polyunsaturated fatty acids (PUFA) with a corresponding deficit in n-3 PUFA. This phenomenon has skewed the n-6 to n-3 PUFA ratio, which is about 15:1 in modern diets [1]. Neuronal membranes preferentially incorporate docosahexaenoic acid (DHA; 22:6n-3), and its deficiency leads to altered gene expression in the mouse brain [2]. As the brain tissue content of DHA depends on the amount of n-3 PUFA in the diet, decreased n-3 PUFA consumption would translate to DHA deficiency in the brain. DHA deficiency results in increased n-6 docosapentaenoic acid (DPAn-6; 22:5n-6) in the brain as a substitute for DHA. Mice reared on adequate n-3 PUFA diet have very low levels of DPAn-6 in the brain (with the approximate DPAn-6 to DHA ratio less than 0.01), which increases in mice on low n-3 PUFA diet with a corresponding decrease in DHA [3]. Therefore, the relative concentration of DPAn-6 in the neural membrane may be used as an index of DHA deficiency. Interestingly, significant amount of DPAn-6 has been detected in the human brain with the DPAn-6 to DHA ratio in the phospholipids of about 0.44 [4]. Assuming that the DHA/DPAn-6 proportion in mice extrapolates to humans, this indicates that modern human brains may not have the optimum DHA levels.

In addition to their role in development, n-3 PUFA, especially DHA and eicosapentaenoic acid (EPA; 20:5n-3), have been shown to regulate immunity [5]. Dysregulated inflammation is an important pathological factor in models of central nervous system injury. Inflammatory responses in the brain have been attributed to local cellular responses wherein glial cells, in particular, secrete proinflammatory cytokines and chemokines. Under the influence of chemokines, there is an influx of neutrophils and monocytes/macrophages into the brain tissue parenchyma facilitated by a state of non-selective permeability brought about by the disruption of the blood-brain barrier [6, 7]. The invading neutrophils, macrophages, and resident glial cells produce both pro- and anti-inflammatory cytokines such as interleukin (IL)-1β, tumor necrosis factor (TNF)-α, IL-6, and IL-10 [8].

Pre-treatment with n-3 PUFA confers resilience and protects against brain injury [9–11]. Administration of these fatty acids has also been reported to be neuroprotective after stroke [12] and reduce axonal damage after spinal cord injury [13, 14] and head injury [15]. We recently reported impaired recovery from traumatic brain injury (TBI) in mice that were severely depleted in brain DHA (~70 %) [16]. DHA deficiencies of this magnitude are not expected to be present in humans. However, brain DHA levels can be lower if the n-3 PUFA intake is insufficient, as in the case of infants fed with formula milk lacking n-3 PUFA showing lower levels of brain DHA than those on breast milk [17, 18]. In this study, we sought to generate higher DPAn-6 to DHA ratio in mouse brains similar to that in humans by providing low level of α-linolenic acid (ALA; 18:3n-3) in the diet for 4 months from late gestation. Their cellular and behavioral responses to TBI were compared to those of mice on adequate ALA diet which resulted in higher levels of brain DHA and only trace amount of DPAn-6.

Methods

A mouse model of low and adequate n-3 PUFA

Pregnant (E14) C57BL6/N mice purchased from Charles River were placed on a diet containing a low ALA content (0.04 %). The adequate n-3 PUFA group received a diet containing flaxseed oil as a source of ALA (3.1 % ALA) (Table 1). The fatty acid content of the diet is shown in Table 2. Male offspring were reared on the same low or adequate ALA diet till 4 months of age. The normal 12-h light period was maintained in the animal housing facility, and mice had free access to food and water.

TBI model

A single controlled cortical impact was delivered to the exposed brain as previously reported [16]. Mice were anesthetized with 5 % isoflurane and then maintained under anesthesia at 2.5–3 % isoflurane during surgery. The mouse head was fixed in a stereotaxic apparatus. A ~4 mm craniotomy was made with a drill over the left cerebral hemisphere between the bregma and lambda and the stereotaxic apparatus angled to make the plane of the dura perpendicular to the impact. The flat-tipped 3-mm-diameter pin of the precision TBI head impactor delivered a pneumatically controlled impact at 3.5 m/s velocity with 1.5 mm penetration. The injury site was covered with Surgicel and the craniotomy sealed with a plastic cap glued using cyanoacrylate. The incision was glued and a topical analgesic cream (EMLA) was applied for analgesia. Lidocaine jelly was instilled in the ears, and the mouse was placed in a cage over a hot water blanket at 37 °C.

Fatty acid analysis

The contralateral cerebral hemisphere of the brains from 5-month-old mice was homogenized in 1:1 volumes of methanol/butylated hydroxytoluene and Tris buffer (pH 7.4) for lipid extraction by the Bligh-Dyer method [19].

Table 1 Fatty acid sources in diets

Lipid source	Low ALA diet (g/kg)	Adequate ALA diet (g/kg)
Tocopherol-stripped safflower oil	19	17.7
Flaxseed oil	0	4.81
Hydrogenated coconut oil	81	77.49

Table 2 Fatty acid content of diets

Fatty acid	Low ALA diet (weight %)	Adequate ALA diet (weight %)
Lauric acid (12:0)	36.06 ± 0.80	35.29 ± 1.61
Myristic acid (14:0)	17.90 ± 0.17	16.64 ± 0.15
Palmitic acid (16:0)	11.35 ± 0.09	10.90 ± 0.19
Stearic acid (18:0)	12.06 ± 0.07	11.71 ± 0.20
Oleic acid (18:1n9)	3.85 ± 0.06	4.47 ± 0.16
Vaccenic acid (18:1n7)	0.26 ± 0.00	0.27 ± 0.01
Linoleic acid (18:2n6)	18.19 ± 0.47	17.19 ± 0.68
γ-Linolenic acid (18:3n6)	N.D.	0.07 ± 0.06
Arachidonic acid (20:4n6)	N.D.	N.D.
α-Linolenic acid (18:3n3)	0.04 ± 0.04	3.08 ± 0.15
Docosahexaenoic acid (22:6n3)	N.D.	N.D.

Data are expressed as mean ± SD ($n = 3$)

N.D. not detected

Chloroform and water were added to the homogenate to attain a chloroform to methanol to water ratio of 2:2:1.8. The homogenate was vortexed after displacing the air by nitrogen to prevent oxidation and centrifuged at 3000 rpm at 4 °C. The organic layers were collected, and the aqueous layer was treated for repeated extraction as above. The lipids were transmethylated at 100 °C for 2 h under nitrogen using borontrifluoride and methanol, and fatty acids were analyzed by gas chromatography [20].

qRT-PCR

At 4 h, 24 h, or 4 days after TBI, mice were deeply anesthetized with isoflurane and perfused quickly with chilled phosphate-buffered saline under continued anesthesia. The brain was removed, and the peri-contusional cortex was dissected and immediately immersed in RNAlater solution to preserve RNA integrity. The RNA was isolated using TRIzol and reverse transcribed using Applied Biosystems cDNA Reverse Transcription kit (Fisher Scientific, Waltham, MA, USA) and amplified using QuantiTect SYBR PCR kit (Qiagen, Valencia, CA, USA). Glyceraldehyde-3-phosphate dehydrogenase (GAPDH) was used as an internal control to normalize the gene expression levels. The gene expression changes are displayed relative to the respective control (sham) level.

Primer sequences were as follows:

TNF-α: forward 5′-CCCTCCAGAAAAGACACCAT G-3′, reverse 5′-GCCACAAGCAGGAATGAGAAG-3′

IL-1β: forward 5′-CCACCTTTTGACAGTGATGA-3′, reverse 5′-GAGATTTGAAGCTGGATGCT-3′

IL-6: forward 5′-GTCGGAGGCTTAATTACACA-3′, reverse 5′-TTTTCTGCAAGTGCATCATC-3′

IL-10: forward 5′-AGCCTTATCGGAAATGATCC-3′, reverse 5′-GGGAATTCAAATGCTCCTTG-3′

Chemokine (C–C motif) ligand 2 (CCL2): forward 5′-GGATCGGAACCAAATGAGAT-3′, reverse 5′-ATTT ACGGGTCAACTTCACA-3′

Cluster of differentiation (CD)-16: forward 5′-TTTGG ACACCCAGATGTTTCAG-3′, reverse 5′-GTCTTCCT TGAGCACCTGGATC-3′

CD-32: forward 5′-AATCCTGCCGTTCCTACTGAT C-3′, reverse 5′-GTGTCACCGTGTCTTCCTTGAG-3′

CD-206: forward 5′-CAAGGAAGGTTGGCATTTGT-3′, reverse 5′-CCTTTCAGTCCTTTGCAAGC-3′

Arg1: forward 5′-CTATGTGTCATTTGGGTGGA-3′, reverse 5′-TCTGGGAACTTTCCTTTCAG-3′

Ym1/2: forward 5′-CAGGGTAATGAGTGGGTTGG-3′, reverse 5′-CACGGCACCTCCTAAATTGT-3′

GAPDH: forward 5′-CCACTCACGGCAAATTCA AC-3′, reverse 5′-CTCCACGACATACTCAGCAC-3′

Protein expression

Mice were perfused with chilled phosphate-buffered saline (PBS) at 4 h, 24 h, and 4 days after TBI. The peri-contusional cortex was carefully dissected and homogenized in Tris-based lysis buffer containing protease inhibitors, sonicated and centrifuged at 4 °C at 12,000 rpm for 15 min. The supernatant was collected and stored at –80 °C until analysis. A commercial CCL2 ELISA kit (Raybiotech, Norcross, GA, USA), which is a colorimetry-based sandwich ELISA kit, was used to quantify the CCL2 protein expression according to the manufacturer's instructions. For the western blotting, samples were run in pre-formed 4–12 % gradient gels, transferred to polivinylidene difluoride membrane, and incubated with mouse anti-IL-1β antibody (Cell Signaling Technology, Danvers, MA, USA). Bands were visualized and quantified to assess the relative changes in expression of IL-1β using a Kodak Gel Logic 440 imaging system with ImageQuant 5.1 software (Molecular Dynamics, Sunnyvale, CA).

Immunofluorescence

At 3 days after TBI, the injured mice were perfused with chilled PBS and then with 4 % paraformaldehyde. The brains were immersed in paraformaldehyde for 24 h and subsequently dehydrated with ethanol and permeated/embedded with paraffin. Six-micrometer-thick sections were cut with a cryotome and mounted on charged slides. Four sections from the injury epicenter for each brain were later deparaffinized, subjected to antigen retrieval by boiling in citrate buffer for 20 min, and blocked with 5 % goat serum for 1 h at room temperature. They were then incubated overnight at 4 °C in anti-ionized calcium-binding adaptor molecule 1 (Iba-1) (catalog number 019-19741; Wako Chemicals, Richmond, Virginia, USA) or anti-glial fibrillary acidic protein (GFAP) antibody (catalog number G9269; Sigma-Aldrich, Saint Louis, MO, USA) solution followed by secondary antibody tagged with Alexa Fluor 488

(Thermo Fisher, Waltham, MA, USA). The fluorescence was visualized with a ×20 objective and quantified using the MetaMorph software (Molecular Devices Inc., Sunnyvale, CA, USA). Cells were counted in the peri-contusional cortex in three non-overlapping fields per section and the corresponding fields for the contralateral cortex.

Motor function tests

Motor deficits were assessed using the rotarod and beam walk tests. Mice were trained to balance on an accelerating rotarod (0 to 400 rpm) for 5 min. The training schedule began 4 days prior to the day of surgery and consisted of three trials each day for 3 days with the baseline performance recorded on the fourth day. The mice were tested daily for 6 days after surgery, and the average latency to fall over three trials on each day was recorded. The beam walk test consisted of walking across a 50-cm-long 0.7-cm-wide beam. The mice were trained for 2 days with three trials per day followed by recording the baseline performance on the day preceding surgery. The total hind limb steps and foot slips were counted on the day before surgery. The test was conducted daily after surgery for 7 days.

Fear conditioning

The fear conditioning experiment was performed over 3 days starting 3 weeks after injury with the first day serving as the day of habituation, the second as the day of fear conditioning, and the third as the day of testing the memory. Mice were individually placed inside the fear conditioning chamber (Freeze Monitor, San Diego Instruments, San Diego, CA, USA) on the first day and allowed to explore for 5 min. On the following day, mice were given two shocks at 120 and 150 s after being introduced into the fear conditioning chamber and were taken out of the chamber 60 s after the last shock. Each shock was 0.5 mA and lasted for 0.5 s. The mice were tested for fear memory 24 h after the fear conditioning session by placing them again in the fear conditioning chamber and assessing freezing for 5 min. Freezing in mice was defined as the absence of any movement except for breathing. Freezing was also monitored on the first day to ascertain baseline freezing.

Statistical analyses

The data for behavioral tests were analyzed using repeated measures two-way analysis of variance (ANOVA) with Prism 6 for Windows (GraphPad software Inc., La Jolla, CA, USA). Multiple comparisons between experimental groups were made using Fisher's least significant difference (LSD) test. Two-way ANOVA was also performed for cytokine expression and microglial phenotype analyses; Sidak's multiple comparisons test was used for comparing individual groups. Groups were compared for the fatty acid analysis and astroglia immunofluorescence by unpaired two-tailed Student's t test.

Results

Mice on adequate ALA diet have higher DHA levels in the brain

Higher levels of DHA, an endogenous product of ALA, were found in the brain of mice on the diet having 3.1 % ALA (Fig. 1) compared to those on the low ALA diet. The average value of DHA was 50 % higher in the mice on adequate ALA diet (14.23 ± 0.87 %) than in the mice on low ALA diet (9.29 ± 0.64 %) (a). The increase in DHA was mirrored by a corresponding decrease in n-6 PUFAs including arachidonic acid (AA; 20:4n-6) (8.54 ± 0.41 % vs 5.85 ± 0.45 %), n-6 docosatetraenoic acid (22:4n-6) (3.03 ± 0.14 % vs 1.53 ± 0.12 %), and DPAn-6. The DPAn-6 level decreased from 3.51 ± 0.3 % in the brain of low ALA diet mice to a nearly undetectable level in the mice on adequate ALA diet. As a consequence, the adequate ALA diet reduced the DPAn-6 to DHA ratio from $0.38 \pm$ to 0.05 to 0.01 ± 0.007 % (b) and the AA to DHA ratio from 0.92 ± 0.04 to 0.41 ± 0.02 % (c).

Mice with higher brain DHA show less neuroinflammation after TBI

The expression of pro-inflammatory cytokines TNF-α, IL-1β, IL-6, CCL2, and the anti-inflammatory cytokine IL-10 in the DHA-low and DHA-high brains was measured at 4 h, 24 h, and 4 days after TBI. TBI induced an increase in all pro-inflammatory cytokines examined. Two-way ANOVA revealed a significant elevation in the expression of TNF-α ($p < 0.0001$), IL-1β ($p < 0.0001$), IL-6 ($p < 0.0001$), and CCL2 ($p = 0.0008$) after TBI (Fig. 2). The TBI-induced production of these cytokines was affected by the brain DHA status. Sidak's multiple comparisons test revealed significantly lower expression of TNF-α (22.0 ± 1.8 vs 17.8 ± 2.4; $p = 0.007$) as well as IL-1β transcript levels (50.0 ± 9.2 standard deviation (SD) vs 30.9 ± 5.5; $p < 0.0001$) in the adequate ALA diet group at 4 h after TBI. Similar differences were present for IL-6 (46.7 ± 5.3 vs 15.7 ± 3.6; $p < 0.0001$) and CCL2 (44.6 ± 6.2 vs 19.7 ± 2.9; $p < 0.0001$) at 24 h after TBI. The expression of the anti-inflammatory cytokine IL-10, despite its elevation after TBI, was not significantly affected by diet for any of the time points considered in this study. To evaluate changes in protein expression, the CCL2 and IL-1β expression was assessed by ELISA and western blotting, respectively. CCL2 and IL-1β protein expression increased after TBI and remained elevated at all time points examined (Fig. 3). Two-way ANOVA showed significant effects for injury ($p < 0.001$) and diet ($p < 0.01$) for both the cytokines. Sidak's multiple comparisons test revealed a significant decrease in CCL2 expression at 24 h post-injury for mice on adequate

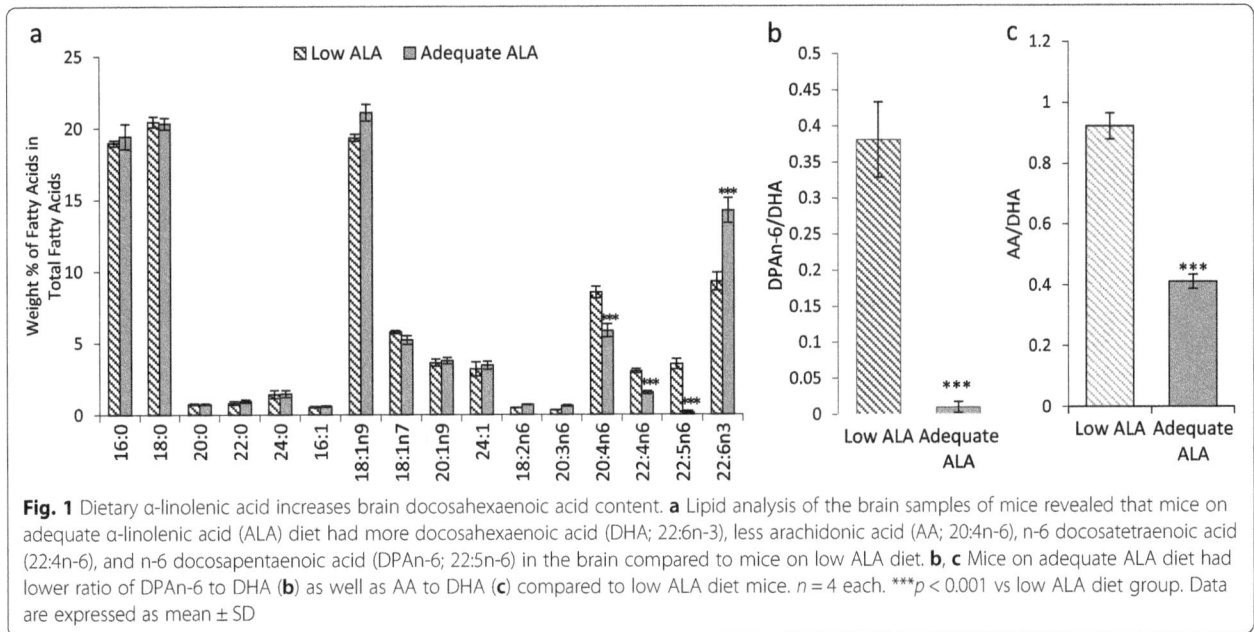

Fig. 1 Dietary α-linolenic acid increases brain docosahexaenoic acid content. **a** Lipid analysis of the brain samples of mice revealed that mice on adequate α-linolenic acid (ALA) diet had more docosahexaenoic acid (DHA; 22:6n-3), less arachidonic acid (AA; 20:4n-6), n-6 docosatetraenoic acid (22:4n-6), and n-6 docosapentaenoic acid (DPAn-6; 22:5n-6) in the brain compared to mice on low ALA diet. **b, c** Mice on adequate ALA diet had lower ratio of DPAn-6 to DHA (**b**) as well as AA to DHA (**c**) compared to low ALA diet mice. $n = 4$ each. ***$p < 0.001$ vs low ALA diet group. Data are expressed as mean ± SD

ALA diet compared to mice on low ALA diet ($p < 0.05$) (Fig. 3a). The expression of IL-1β protein was significantly lower at 4 days after injury for the adequate ALA diet mice compared to those on low ALA diet ($p < 0.05$) (Fig. 3b).

Acute post-injury astrogliosis is modulated by n-3 PUFA status without affecting microglial density

Iba-1 is expressed by microglia and macrophages. TBI resulted in a threefold increase in the number of Iba-1-positive cells around the contusion site compared to the

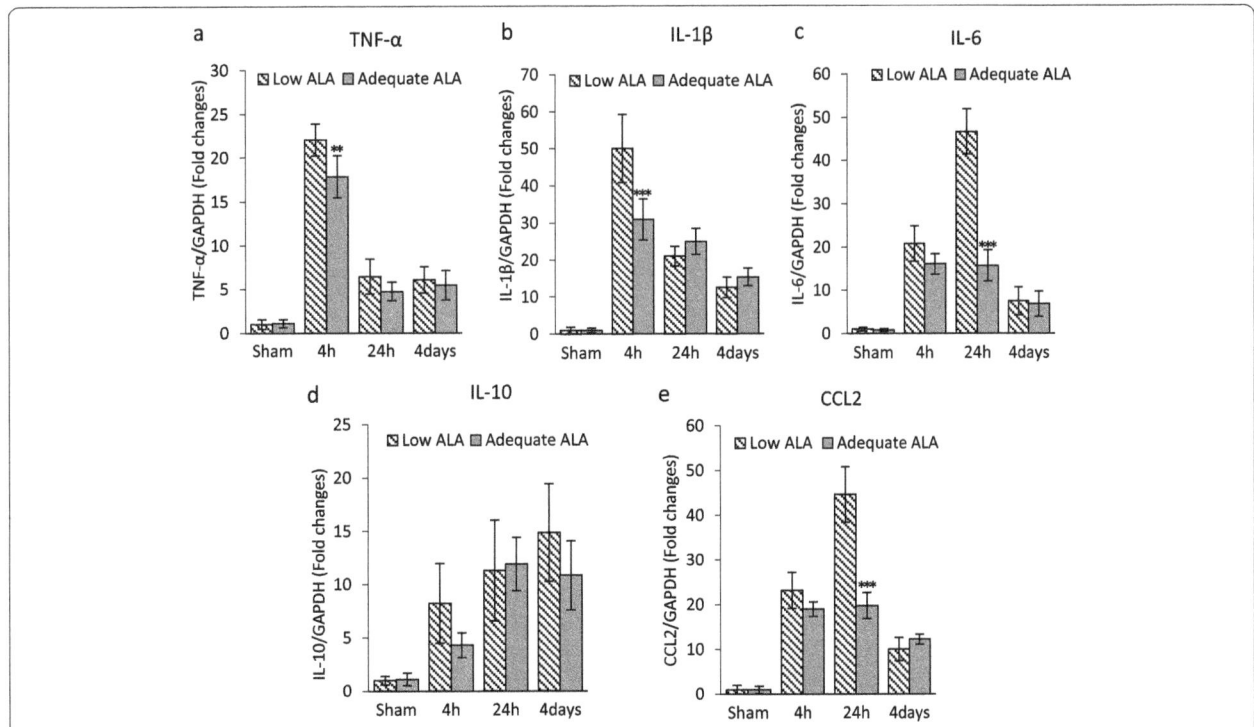

Fig. 2 a–e Suppression of TBI-induced acute inflammatory cytokine expression in mice with higher brain docosahexaenoic acid. TBI induced the gene expression of pro-inflammatory cytokines in the cerebral cortex. Adequate α-linolenic acid (ALA) diet resulted in lower expression of pro-inflammatory cytokines TNF-α, IL-1β, IL-6, and CCL2 after TBI as compared to the low ALA group. $n = 3$–4. ***$p < 0.001$, **$p < 0.01$ compared to the low ALA diet group for the respective time point. Data are expressed as mean ± SD

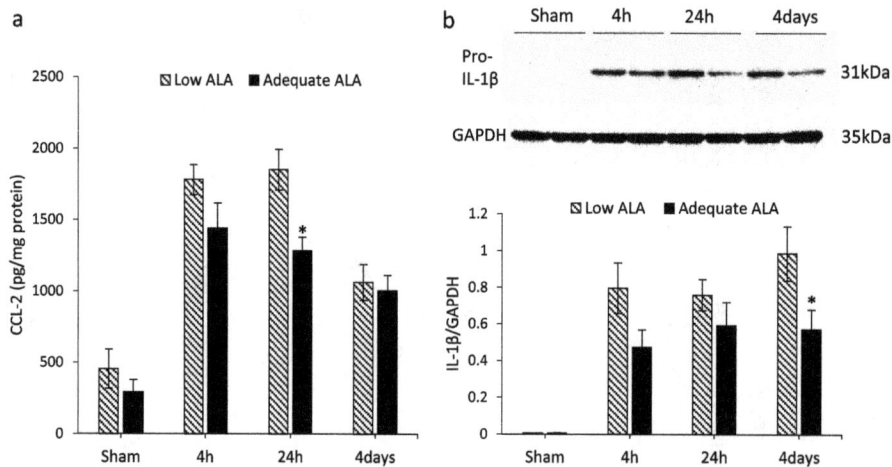

Fig. 3 a, b Suppression of traumatic brain injury-induced CCL2 and IL-1β protein expression in mice with higher brain docosahexaenoic acid. Traumatic brain injury caused induction of CCL2 and IL-1β protein expression in the cerebral cortex at the site of injury. The expression of both proteins was lower in mice on adequate α-linolenic acid (ALA) diet compared to the low ALA group. $N = 3$–4. $*p < 0.05$ compared to the low ALA diet group for the respective time points. Data are expressed as mean ± SEM

contralateral cortex (Fig. 4a). However, there was no significant difference in the number of Iba-1-positive cells between the diet groups. The mean Iba-1-positive cell count obtained from the contralateral cortex was 119.4 ± 2.0 and 129.1 ± 15.9 for the low ALA and adequate ALA diet group, respectively. In the injured mouse brains, mean counts of Iba-1-positive cells accumulated around the injury site were 349.3 ± 13.0 and 304.8 ± 17.7 for the low ALA and adequate ALA diet groups, respectively. GFAP immunoreactivity in the contralateral cortex was negligible (Fig. 4b). However, TBI induced a robust increase in GFAP immunofluorescence, indicating astrocyte activation. Mice with DHA deficiency showed higher GFAP immunofluorescence in the injured cortex ($p < 0.01$) compared to the mice that had greater DHA (2.6 ± 0.1 vs 2.1 ± 0.1, respectively).

Altering the brain n-3 PUFA has limited effect on microglial M1/M2 polarization

Since the microglial response to injury depends on their phenotype, we assessed the expression of CD-16 and CD-32 for M1 microglia and CD-206, arginase 1 (Arg-1), and Ym1/2 for M2 microglia. TBI induced distinct increases in the expression of all these markers, particularly from 24 h (Fig. 5). However, with the sole exception of CD-206, there was no statistically significant change in the relative expression of these M1/M2 markers due to n-3 PUFA differences. The expression of CD-206 was higher in the low ALA diet group ($p < 0.05$) (1.9 ± 0.1) at 24 h after TBI compared to the adequate ALA group (1.1 ± 0.2).

Mice with more brain DHA exhibit better motor recovery after TBI

TBI resulted in motor deficits observed in the rotarod as well as beam walk tests (Fig. 6). Repeated two-way ANOVA revealed a significant effect of diet on the latency to fall off the rotarod ($p < 0.01$). The motor performance of all mice recovered gradually with time. The mean time on the rotarod for the mice on low ALA diet, and thus with lower brain DHA, did not reach the pre-injury levels even on the sixth day after injury (248 s ± 14.5 standard error of mean (SEM) compared to the pre-injury time of 293 s ± 2 SEM) (Fig. 6a). However, the performance of the mice on adequate ALA diet that have more brain DHA was comparable to the pre-injury level (288.6 ± 5.1 SEM) by the fifth day (277.2 ± 7.6 SEM). In the beam walk test, the mean values for foot slips for the adequate ALA diet mice remained lower than those of the low ALA group throughout the test period as shown by the significant difference on day 2, 3, 4, and 6 after injury ($p < 0.05$) (Fig. 6b).

Contextual fear conditioning test was used to assess differences in fear memory after TBI. The mice on adequate ALA diet had significantly better memory 24 h after the fear conditioning for both sham ($p < 0.001$) and TBI animals ($p < 0.01$) compared to the low ALA group as indicated by more freezing (Fig. 6c). However, TBI by itself did not affect freezing.

Discussion

The present study investigated the effects of altering the brain DHA status on acute TBI outcome. The DHA level in mouse brains was modulated by differing levels

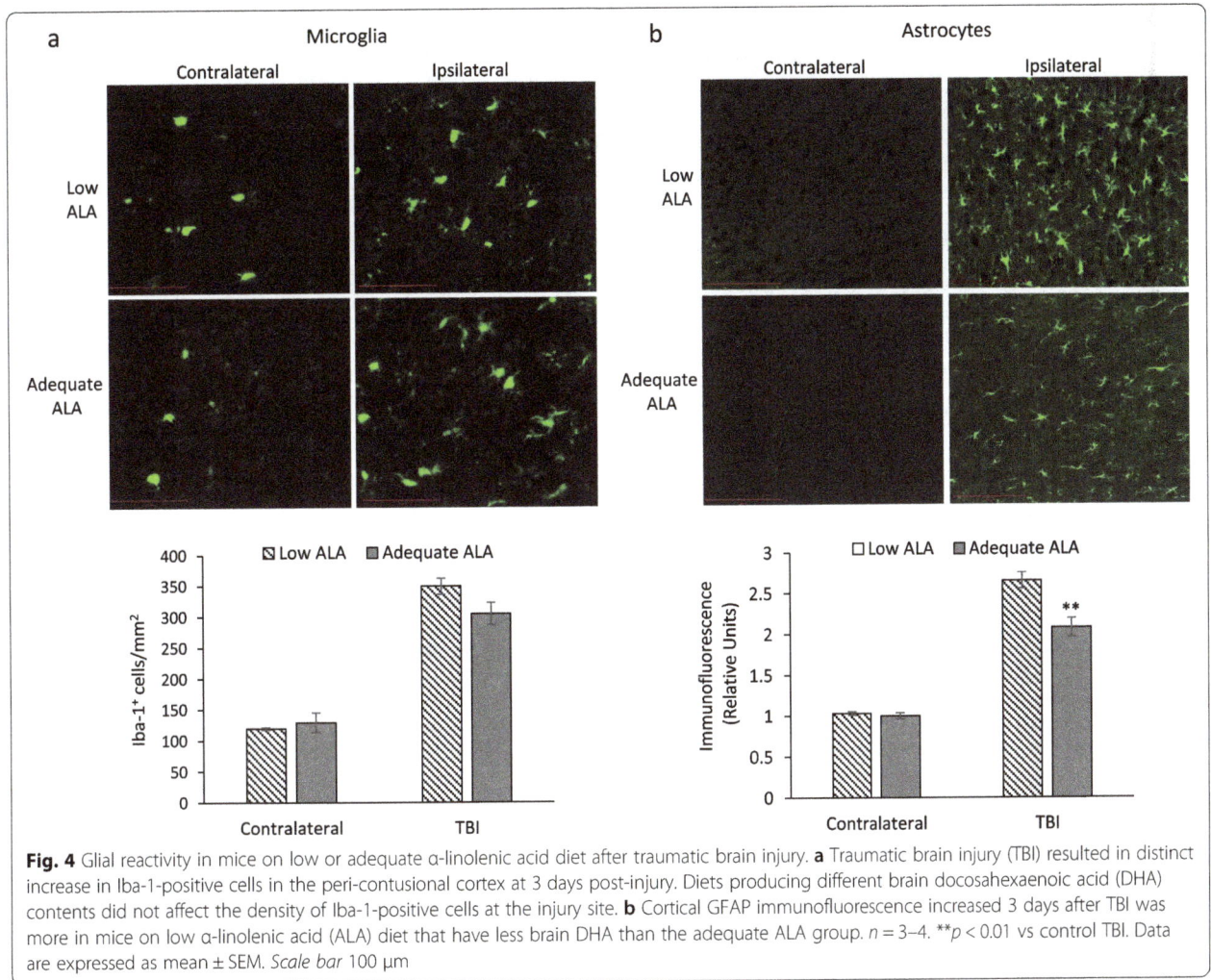

Fig. 4 Glial reactivity in mice on low or adequate α-linolenic acid diet after traumatic brain injury. **a** Traumatic brain injury (TBI) resulted in distinct increase in Iba-1-positive cells in the peri-contusional cortex at 3 days post-injury. Diets producing different brain docosahexaenoic acid (DHA) contents did not affect the density of Iba-1-positive cells at the injury site. **b** Cortical GFAP immunofluorescence increased 3 days after TBI was more in mice on low α-linolenic acid (ALA) diet that have less brain DHA than the adequate ALA group. $n = 3–4$. $**p < 0.01$ vs control TBI. Data are expressed as mean ± SEM. *Scale bar* 100 μm

of dietary ALA from late gestation to the adult stage. A moderately lower DHA level in the brain achieved by a diet lacking DHA and having low ALA was to model human brains with conspicuous presence of DPAn-6 [4]. With this diet, DPAn-6 was elevated in mouse brains with the DPAn-6 to DHA ratio of 0.38 (Fig. 1) which is similar to that observed in human brains (0.44) [4]. The brain DPA to DHA ratio below 0.01 that is normally observed in an n-3 PUFA-sufficient condition [3] was also achieved by providing 3.1 % ALA in diet.

Acute increase in inflammatory mediators is a part of fundamental tissue response to injury. Decrease in n-3 PUFA levels with a corresponding increase in the n-6 to n-3 PUFA ratio can lead to increase in inflammation [21]. Phospholipase A2 is activated after TBI [22], which elevates free fatty acid levels [23], leading to greater local availability of DHA and AA. While eicosanoids generated from AA can be neurotoxic under pathological conditions, docosanoids derived from DHA are often anti-inflammatory. Having higher DHA levels in the brain can lead to greater local free DHA levels after injury as

well as more anti-inflammatory DHA metabolites. These attributes likely decreased acute inflammatory cytokine expression after TBI in mice with higher brain DHA (Fig. 2). The transcription factor nuclear factor kappa light chain enhancer of activated B cells (NF-kB) that upregulates the expression of pro-inflammatory genes has been shown to be activated after TBI [24]. In contrast, DHA/EPA supplementation can reduce NF-kB activity and inflammation, as shown for neonatal hypoxia-ischemia [9] and LPS-stimulated macrophages [25]. In addition, increase in oxidative stress in the injured brain leads to generation of oxidation products of n-3 PUFA, and these products can inhibit NF-kB by activating peroxisome proliferator-activated receptor (PPAR)α [26]. Thus, it is likely that raising the brain DHA level reduced pro-inflammatory cytokines by affecting the activity of these transcription factors.

ALA-rich diet was reported to lower the production of IL-6, IL-1β, and TNF-α by peripheral blood mononuclear cells of hypercholesterolemic subjects compared to controls fed with either high linoleic acid diet or a typical

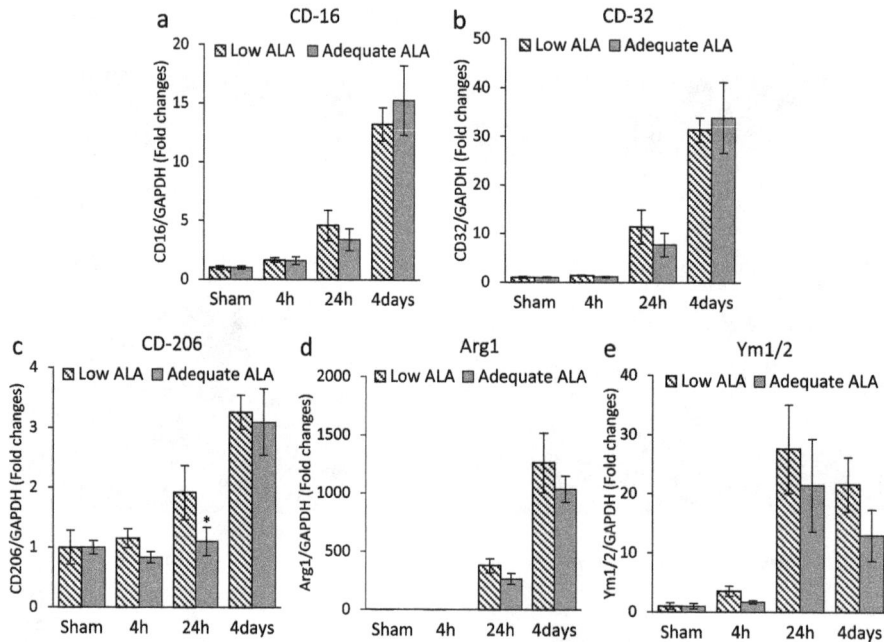

Fig. 5 Diets differing in α-linolenic acid content have limited effects on microglial polarization. The expression of M1 microglia/macrophage markers CD-16 and CD-32 (**a**, **b**) and M2 microglia/macrophage markers CD-206, Arg-1, and Ym1/2 (**c-e**) was increased in peri-contusional cortex after traumatic brain injury. Dietary α-linolenic acid (ALA) content showed no effect on the expression of these markers in general, with the exception of CD-206 at 24 h after TBI. $n = 3–4$. *$p < 0.05$ vs low ALA at the same time points. Data are expressed as mean ± SD

American diet [27]. These cytokines were also associated with injury-induced activation of not only macrophage/microglia but also astrocytes in the brain [28]. Pu et al. [11] have reported increase in pro-inflammatory cytokine expression along with an increase in microglia/macrophage count in n-3 PUFA-deficient mice after TBI. Our results are in agreement with the local increase in pro-inflammatory cytokines (Figs. 2 and 3). However, we did not find significant differences in the macrophage/microglial density around the injury site for the two diet groups (Fig. 4a). This may be a result of the differences in dietary n-3 PUFA used in the two studies. While we provided n-3 PUFA in the form of ALA in diet, Pu et al. [11] used fish oil (1.5 % DHA and EPA). This may change the blood levels of DHA/EPA that can impact the microglia activation after TBI. In addition, we had the mice on diet since

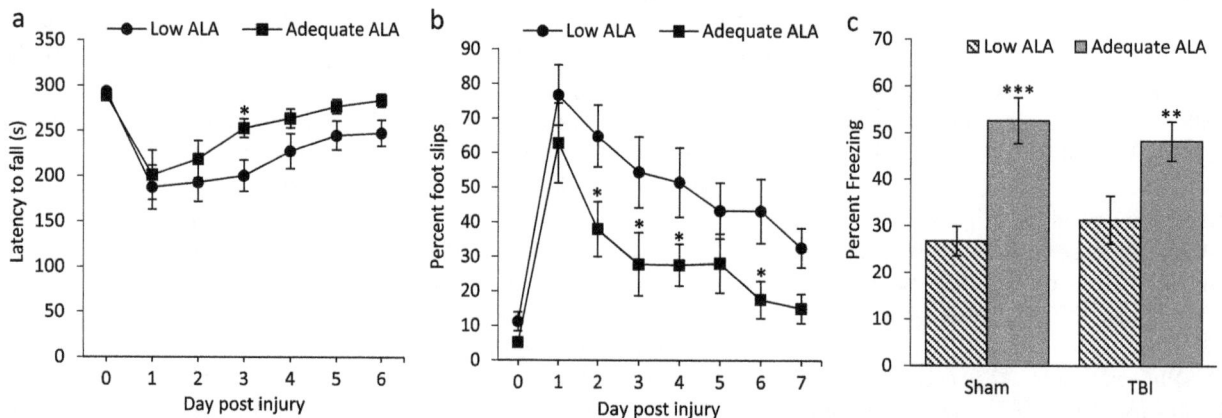

Fig. 6 Effect of low or adequate α-linolenic acid diet on motor and cognitive changes after TBI. **a**, **b** Impaired motor performance in the rotarod (**a**) and beam walk tests (**b**) due to TBI was recovered faster in mice on adequate α-linolenic acid (ALA) diet compared to those on the low ALA diet that had less brain DHA. **c** Mice on adequate ALA diet showed more freezing after contextual fear conditioning compared to the mice on low ALA diet for both sham and TBI mice. ***$p < 0.001$, **$p < 0.01$, *$p < 0.05$ compared to the respective low ALA diet group. Data are expressed as mean ± SEM. $n = 8–14$

late gestation, while in the study by Pu and colleagues, the mice were placed on diet at 3 weeks age. This is probably the reason for greater differences in brain DHA (about 35 % change) in our experiment as compared to the small but statistically significant changes of 10–15 % in the reported study. Furthermore, the DPAn-6 levels change dramatically with our dietary regiment but do not change in the case of Pu et al.'s study [11]. This is expected as the brain undergoes rapid accretion of DHA during early development when our dietary regimen was initiated while its levels recover at a slower rate after adolescence [3]. These factors may also account for the temporal differences in cytokine expression in these studies. Pu et al. assessed cytokine expression at 24 h post-injury and found significant differences between the two diet groups for TNF-α and IL-1β, while we found maximum expression and significant differences for these cytokines at 4 h in our time course analysis (Fig. 2). Nevertheless, we did observe changes in CCL2 and IL-1β protein expression at 24 h and 4 days, respectively (Fig. 3). Although we did not find a significant difference in the macrophage/microglial density near the injury site, there may also exist qualitative changes in these cells priming them toward a pro- or anti-inflammatory phenotype. The activated microglia/macrophages are categorized into a classical activated state or M1 and an alternate activated state or M2. M1 microglia/macrophages typically have a pro-inflammatory phenotype producing pro-inflammatory cytokines, having increased interaction with other immune cells, and contributing to oxidative/nitrosative stress [29]. On the other hand, M2 microglia/macrophages modulate phagocytosis and promote wound healing [29, 30]. We did not find any significant change in the M1/M2 phenotype marker expression for activated macrophage/microglia in the injured diet groups (Fig. 5). These findings suggest that the DHA-derived changes in inflammation may not be attributed to microglial activation at least in our experimental settings using ALA as the n-3 PUFA source.

Our data indicated increased induction of astrogliosis after TBI (Fig. 4b). Astrocyte activation is a complex process that can aid in limiting inflammation [31]. However, it can also lead to localized pro-inflammatory environment. For example, activation of astrocytes by TLR4 stimulation can lead to pro-inflammatory cytokine expression [32]. In contrast to microglial activation, astrogliosis was significantly increased in the DHA-depleted mouse brain. CCL2, which is mostly produced by astrocytes in the brain [33, 34], was significantly increased at 4 h after injury, indicating early activation of astrocytes. The brains from the mice on ALA adequate diet showed significantly reduced CCL2 at 24 h after injury compared to the low ALA diet group. It is possible that suppressed astrocyte activation with an increase in brain

DHA in the adequate ALA diet mice (Fig. 4b) may have contributed to the reduction in CCL2 at 24 h of injury. DHA inhibits endoplasmic reticulum stress in astrocytes in the in vitro ischemia model [35] and reduces endoplasmic reticulum stress after TBI [36]. Thus, reduction in endoplasmic reticulum stress in the mice on adequate ALA diet may have reduced astrocyte activation after TBI.

Severe DHA depletion in the brain brought about by multi-generational n-3 PUFA dietary restriction causes significant impairment in functional recovery after TBI [16]. Similarly, a relatively moderate lowering in brain DHA levels also impaired motor recovery from TBI (Fig. 6a, b). It is possible that neuroinflammation aggravated by DHA deficiency contributed to the worse recovery outcome, although causal relationship still needs to be established. The increase in brain DHA can be responsible for the increase in contextual fear learning/memory (Fig. 6c) as DHA/n-3 PUFA is known to improve cognition, although this parameter was not responsive to TBI.

Conclusions

Using a mouse model with brain DHA depletion, we demonstrate that increasing brain DHA can limit post-injury inflammation, reduce astrocyte activation, and improve functional recovery. This study suggests possible improvement of functional outcome by increasing brain DHA through diet in human TBI.

Abbreviations

ALA: α-linolenic acid; ANOVA: Analysis of variance; Arg-1: Arginase 1; CD: Cluster of differentiation; CCL2: Chemokine (C–C motif) ligand 2; DHA: Docosahexaenoic acid; DPAn-6: Docosapentaenoic acid; EPA: Eicosapentaenoic acid; GFAP: Glial fibrillary acidic protein; Iba-1: Ionized calcium-binding adaptor molecule 1; IL: Interleukin; LSD: Least significant difference; NF-kB: Nuclear factor kappa light chain enhancer of activated B cells; PPAR: Peroxisome proliferator-activated receptor; PUFA: Polyunsaturated fatty acid; SD: Standard deviation; SEM: Standard error of mean; TBI: Traumatic brain injury; TNF: Tumor necrosis factor

Acknowledgements

The authors acknowledge the Office of Laboratory Animal Science, National Institutes of Alcohol Abuse and Alcoholism for facilitating animal studies. This work was supported by the Defense Medical Research and Development Program (DMRDP) (W81XWH-11-2-0074) and Intramural Research Program of the National Institute of Alcohol Abuse and Alcoholism, National Institutes of Health.

Funding

This study was funded by the Henry M. Jackson Foundation and the Intramural Research Program of the National Institute of Alcohol Abuse and Alcoholism, National Institutes of Health. The funding agencies did not participate in planning the experiments, data analysis, or preparing the manuscript.

Authors' contributions

The experiments were designed by HYK and AD. The experiments were conducted by AD, TP, JB, KK, and HC. Analysis of data was done by AD and HYK. The manuscript was prepared by AD and HYK. All authors read and approved the final manuscript.

Competing interests

The authors declare that they have no competing interests.

Consent for publication

Not applicable.

References

1. Simopoulos AP. Evolutionary aspects of diet, the omega-6/omega-3 ratio and genetic variation: nutritional implications for chronic diseases. Biomed Pharmacother. 2006;60(9):502–7.
2. Sidhu VK, Huang BX, Desai A, Kevala K, Kim HY. Role of DHA in aging-related changes in mouse brain synaptic plasma membrane proteome. Neurobiol Aging. 2016;41:73–85.
3. Moriguchi T, Loewke J, Garrison M, Catalan JN, Salem N. Reversal of docosahexaenoic acid deficiency in the rat brain, retina, liver, and serum. J Lipid Res. 2001;42(3):419–27.
4. Hamazaki K, Choi KH, Kim HY. Phospholipid profile in the postmortem hippocampus of patients with schizophrenia and bipolar disorder: no changes in docosahexaenoic acid species. J Psychiatric Res. 2010;44(11):688–93.
5. Swanson D, Block R, Mousa SA. Omega-3 fatty acids EPA and DHA: health benefits throughout life. Adv Nutr. 2012;3(1):1–7.
6. Rossi D, Zlotnik A. The biology of chemokines and their receptors. Ann Rev Immunol. 2000;18(1):217–42.
7. Persidsky Y, Ramirez SH, Haorah J, Kanmogne GD. Blood–brain barrier: structural components and function under physiologic and pathologic conditions. J Neuroimmune Pharmacol. 2006;1(3):223–36.
8. Ziebell JM, Morganti-Kossmann MC. Involvement of pro-and anti-inflammatory cytokines and chemokines in the pathophysiology of traumatic brain injury. Neurotherapeutics. 2010;7(1):22–30.
9. Zhang W, Hu X, Yang W, Gao Y, Chen J. Omega-3 polyunsaturated fatty acid supplementation confers long-term neuroprotection against neonatal hypoxic–ischemic brain injury through anti-inflammatory actions. Stroke. 2010;41(10):2341–7.
10. Wu A, Ying Z, Gomez-Pinilla F. Dietary omega-3 fatty acids normalize BDNF levels, reduce oxidative damage, and counteract learning disability after traumatic brain injury in rats. J Neurotrauma. 2004;21(10):1457–67.
11. Pu H, Guo Y, Zhang W, Huang L, Wang G, Liou AK, Zhang J, Zhang P, Leak RK, Wang Y, Chen J, Gao Y. Omega-3 polyunsaturated fatty acid supplementation improves neurologic recovery and attenuates white matter injury after experimental traumatic brain injury. J Cereb Blood Flow Metab. 2013;33(9):1474–84.
12. Belayev L, Khoutorova L, Atkins KD, Bazan NG. Robust docosahexaenoic acid–mediated neuroprotection in a rat model of transient, focal cerebral ischemia. Stroke. 2009;40(9):3121–6.
13. King VR, Huang WL, Dyall SC, Curran OE, Priestley JV, Michael-Titus AT. Omega-3 fatty acids improve recovery, whereas omega-6 fatty acids worsen outcome, after spinal cord injury in the adult rat. J Neurosci. 2006;26(17): 4672–80.
14. Huang WL, King VR, Curran OE, Dyall SC, Ward RE, Lal N, Priestley JV, Michael-Titus AT. A combination of intravenous and dietary docosahexaenoic acid significantly improves outcome after spinal cord injury. Brain. 2007;130(11):3004–19.
15. Bailes JE, Mills JD. Docosahexaenoic acid reduces traumatic axonal injury in a rodent head injury model. J Neurotrauma. 2010;27(9):1617–24.
16. Desai A, Kevala K, Kim HY. Depletion of brain docosahexaenoic acid impairs recovery from traumatic brain injury. PLoS One. 2014;9(1), e86472.
17. Makrides M, Neumann MA, Byard RW, Simmer K, Gibson RA. Fatty acid composition of brain, retina, and erythrocytes in breast- and formula-fed infants. Am J Clin Nutr. 1994;60:189–94.
18. Jamieson EC, Farquharson J, Logan RW, Howatson AG, Patrick WJA, Weaver LT, Cockburn F. Infant cerebellar gray and white matter fatty acids in relation to age and diet. Lipids. 1999;34(10):1065–71.
19. Bligh EG, Dyer WJ. A rapid method of total lipid extraction and purification. Can J Biochem Physiol. 1959;37(8):911–7.
20. Wen Z, Kim HY. Alterations in hippocampal phospholipid profile by prenatal exposure to ethanol. J Neurochem. 2004;89(6):1368–77.
21. Liu HQ, Qiu Y, Mu Y, Zhang XJ, Liu L, Hou XH, Zhang L, Xu XN, Ji AL, Cao R, Yang RH, Wang F. A high ratio of dietary n-3/n-6 polyunsaturated fatty acids improves obesity-linked inflammation and insulin resistance through suppressing activation of TLR4 in SD rats. Nutr Res. 2013;33(10):849–58.
22. Shohami E, Shapira Y, Yadid G, Reisfeld N, Yedgar S. Brain phospholipase A$_2$ is activated after experimental closed head injury in the rat. J Neurochem. 1989;53:1541–6.
23. Dhillon HS, Dose JM, Scheff SW, Prasad MR. Time course of changes in lactate and free fatty acids after experimental brain injury and relationship to morphologic damage. Exp Neurol. 1997;146(1):240–9.
24. Ahmad A, Crupi R, Campolo M, Genovese T, Esposito E, Cuzzocrea S. Absence of TLR4 reduces neurovascular unit and secondary inflammatory process after traumatic brain injury in mice. PLoS One. 2013;8(3), e57208.
25. Mullen A, Loscher CE, Roche HM. Anti-inflammatory effects of EPA and DHA are dependent upon time and dose–response elements associated with LPS stimulation in THP-1-derived macrophages. J Nutr Biochem. 2010;21(5):444–50.
26. Mishra A, Chaudhary A, Sethi S. Oxidized omega-3 fatty acids inhibit NF-kB activation via a PPARα-dependent pathway. Arterioscler Thromb Vasc Biol. 2004;24(9):1621–7.
27. Zhao G, Etherton TD, Martin KR, Gillies PJ, West SG, Kris-Etherton PM. Dietary α-linolenic acid inhibits pro-inflammatory cytokine production by peripheral blood mononuclear cells in hypercholesterolemic subjects. Am J Clin Nutr. 2007;85(2):385–91.
28. Acarin L, González B, Castellano B. Neuronal, astroglial and microglial cytokine expression after an excitotoxic lesion in the immature rat brain. Eur J Neurosci. 2000;12(10):3505–20.
29. Cherry JD, Olschowka JA, O'Banion MK. Neuroinflammation and M2 microglia: the good, the bad, and the inflamed. J Neuroinflammation. 2014;11(1):98.
30. Fernandes A, Miller-Fleming L, Pais TF. Microglia and inflammation: conspiracy, controversy or control? Cell Mol Life Sci. 2014;71(20):3969–85.
31. Myer DJ, Gurkoff GG, Lee SM, Hovda DA, Sofroniew MV. Essential protective roles of reactive astrocytes in traumatic brain injury. Brain. 2006;129(10): 2761–72.
32. Gorina R, Font-Nieves M, Marquez-Kisinousky L, Santalucia T, Planas AM. Astrocyte TLR4 activation induces a pro-inflammatory environment through the interplay between MyD88-dependent NFkappaB signaling, MAPK, and Jak1/Stat1 pathways. Glia. 2011;59:242–55.
33. Berman JW, Guida MP, Warren J, Amat J, Brosnan CF. Localization of monocyte chemoattractant peptide-1 expression in the central nervous system in experimental autoimmune encephalomyelitis and trauma in the rat. J Immunol. 1996;156(8):3017–23.
34. Glabinski AR, Balasingam V, Tani M, Kunkel SL, Strieter RM, Yong VW, Ransohoff RM. Chemokine monocyte chemoattractant protein-1 is expressed by astrocytes after mechanical injury to the brain. J Immunol. 1996;156(11):4363–8.
35. Begum G, Kintner D, Liu Y, Cramer SW, Sun D. DHA inhibits ER Ca2+ release and ER stress in astrocytes following in vitro ischemia. J Neurochem. 2012; 120(4):622–30.
36. Begum G, Yan HQ, Li L, Singh A, Dixon CE, Sun D. Docosahexaenoic acid reduces ER stress and abnormal protein accumulation and improves neuronal function following traumatic brain injury. J Neurosci. 2014;34(10):3743–55.

Permissions

The contributors of this book come from diverse backgrounds, making this book a truly international effort. This book will bring forth new frontiers with its revolutionizing research information and detailed analysis of the nascent developments around the world.

We would like to thank all the contributing authors for lending their expertise to make the book truly unique. They have played a crucial role in the development of this book. Without their invaluable contributions this book wouldn't have been possible. They have made vital efforts to compile up to date information on the varied aspects of this subject to make this book a valuable addition to the collection of many professionals and students.

This book was conceptualized with the vision of imparting up-to-date information and advanced data in this field. To ensure the same, a matchless editorial board was set up. Every individual on the board went through rigorous rounds of assessment to prove their worth. After which they invested a large part of their time researching and compiling the most relevant data for our readers.

The editorial board has been involved in producing this book since its inception. They have spent rigorous hours researching and exploring the diverse topics which have resulted in the successful publishing of this book. They have passed on their knowledge of decades through this book. To expedite this challenging task, the publisher supported the team at every step. A small team of assistant editors was also appointed to further simplify the editing procedure and attain best results for the readers.

Apart from the editorial board, the designing team has also invested a significant amount of their time in understanding the subject and creating the most relevant covers. They scrutinized every image to scout for the most suitable representation of the subject and create an appropriate cover for the book.

The publishing team has been an ardent support to the editorial, designing and production team. Their endless efforts to recruit the best for this project, has resulted in the accomplishment of this book. They are a veteran in the field of academics and their pool of knowledge is as vast as their experience in printing. Their expertise and guidance has proved useful at every step. Their uncompromising quality standards have made this book an exceptional effort. Their encouragement from time to time has been an inspiration for everyone.

The publisher and the editorial board hope that this book will prove to be a valuable piece of knowledge for researchers, students, practitioners and scholars across the globe.

List of Contributors

Run Zhang, Yi Liu, Ke Yan, Xiang-Rong Chen, Peng Li, Fan-Fan Chen and Xiao-Dan Jiang
The National Key Clinic Specialty, The Neurosurgery Institute of Guangdong Province, Guangdong Provincial Key Laboratory on Brain Function Repair and Regeneration, Department of Neurosurgery, Zhujiang Hospital, Southern Medical University, Guangzhou 510282, China

Lei Chen
Department of Neurosurgery, Shenzhen Second People's Hospital, the First Affiliated Hospital of Shenzhen University, Shenzhen 518000, China

Kyria M. Webster, Mujun Sun, Terence J. O'Brien, Sandy R. Shultz and Bridgette D. Semple
Department of Medicine (The Royal Melbourne Hospital), The University of Melbourne, Kenneth Myer Building, Melbourne Brain Centre, Royal Parade, Parkville, VIC 3050, Australia

Peter Crack
Department of Pharmacology and Therapeutics, The University of Melbourne, Parkville, VIC 3050, Australia

Peter S Amenta, Jack I Jallo and Melanie B Elliott
Department of Neurological Surgery, Thomas Jefferson University Hospital, 1020 Locust Street, Thomas Jefferson University, Philadelphia, PA 19107, USA

Craig Hooper
Department of Cancer Biology, Thomas Jefferson University Hospital, 1020 Locust Street, Thomas Jefferson University, Philadelphia, PA 19107, USA

Ronald F Tuma
Department of Physiology, Temple University School of Medicine, 3500 N Broad St, Philadelphia, PA 19140, USA

Jian-Wei Pan, Hao Jiang, Feng Xiao and Ren-Ya Zhan
Department of Neurosurgery, The First Affiliated Hospital, School of Medicine, Zhejiang University, 79 Qingchun Road, Hangzhou 310003, People's Republic of China

Xiong-Wei Gao and Ya-Feng Li
Department of Neurosurgery, Sanmen People's Hospital, 171 Renmin Road, Sanmen 317100, People's Republic of China

Lara-Kirstie Riparip and Austin Chou
Brain and Spinal Injury Center, University of California, 1001 Potrero Ave, Bldg. 1, Room 101, San Francisco, CA 94110, USA

Josh M. Morganti and Susanna Rosi
Department of Physical Therapy and Rehabilitation Science, University of California, San Francisco, CA, USA
Neuroscience Graduate Program, University of California, San Francisco, CA, USA

Sharon Liu
Department of Neurological Surgery, University of California, San Francisco, CA, USA

Nalin Gupta
Department of Pediatrics, University of California, San Francisco, CA, USA

Hai-tao Zhu, Ji-chao Yuan, Wei-hua Chu, Xin Xiang, Fei Chen, Cheng-shi Wang, Hua Feng and Jiang-kai Lin
Department of Neurosurgery, Southwest Hospital, Third Military Medical University, 30 Gaotanyan Street, Chongqing 400038, China

Chen Bian
Department of Neurobiology, Third Military Medical University, 30 Gaotanyan Street, Chongqing 400038, China

Charu Garg, Joon Ho Seo, Jayalakshmi Ramachandran, Frances Calderon and Jorge E. Contreras
Department of Pharmacology, Physiology and Neurosciences, New Jersey Medical School, Rutgers University, 185 South Orange Ave, Newark, NJ 07103, USA

Donald G. Stein
Department of Emergency Medicine, Emory University, Atlanta, GA 30322, USA

Ji Meng Loh
Department of Mathematical Sciences, New Jersey Institute of Technology, University Heights, Newark, NJ 07102, USA

Kyria M. Webster, Mujun Sun, Bridgette D. Semple, Ezgi Ozturk, Terence J. O'Brien and Sandy R. Shultz
Department of Medicine, The Royal Melbourne Hospital, The University of Melbourne, Parkville, VIC 3050, Australia

David K. Wright
Anatomy and Neuroscience, The University of Melbourne, Parkville, VIC 3010, Australia
The Florey Institute of Neuroscience and Mental Health, Parkville, VIC 3052, Australia

Rachel K. Rowe and Jonathan Lifshitz
BARROW Neurological Institute at Phoenix Children's Hospital, Phoenix, AZ, USA
Department of Child Health, University of Arizona College of Medicine—Phoenix, Phoenix, AZ, USA
Phoenix Veteran Affairs Healthcare System, Phoenix, AZ, USA

Jordan L. Harrison
Basic Medical Sciences, University of Arizona College of Medicine—Phoenix, Phoenix, AZ, USA

Hongtao Zhang and Mark I. Greene
University of Pennsylvania Perelman School of Medicine, Philadelphia, PA, USA

Adam D. Bachstetter
Sanders-Brown Center on Aging, Spinal Cord and Brain Injury Research Center, and Department of Neuroscience, University of Kentucky, Lexington, KY, USA

Bruce F. O'Hara
Department of Biology, University of Kentucky, Lexington, KY, USA

Ingrid R Niesman, Jan M Schilling, Sarah E Kellerhals, Jacqueline A Bonds, Weihua Cui, April Voong, Sameh S Ali, David M Roth, Hemal H Patel, Piyush M Patel and Brian P Head
Veterans Affairs San Diego Healthcare System, 3350 La Jolla Village Drive, San Diego, CA 92161, USA
Department of Anesthesiology, University of California, San Diego, La Jolla, CA 92093, USA

Michela Campolo, Emanuela Esposito, Akbar Ahmad, Rosanna Di Paola, Irene Paterniti, Marika Cordaro and Giuseppe Bruschetta
Department of Biological and Environmental Sciences, University of Messina, Viale Ferdinando Stagno D'Alcontres, 31-98166 Messina, Italy

John L Wallace
Inflammation Research Network, University of Calgary, 3330 Hospital Drive NW, Calgary, Alberta T2N 4 N1, Canada

Salvatore Cuzzocrea
Manchester Biomedical Research Centre, Manchester Royal Infirmary, School of Medicine, University of Manchester, 29 Grafton Street Manchester, M13 9WU Manchester, UK

Lee A Shapiro
Neuroscience Research Institute, Scott & White Hospital, Central Texas Veterans Health System, Temple, TX, USA
Department of Surgery, Department of Neurosurgery, Department of Neuroscience and Experimental Therapeutics, College of Medicine, Texas A&M Health Science Center, Temple, TX, USA

Alexander M Kleschevnikov
Department of Neurosciences, University of California, San Diego, 9500 Gilman Drive, La Jolla, CA 92093, USA

Stan Krajewski
Sanford-Burnham Medical Research Institute, La Jolla, CA, USA

Weihua Cui
Department of Anesthesiology, Beijing Tiantan Hospital, Capital Medical University, Beijing, China

Sameh S Ali
Center for Aging and Associated Diseases, Helmy Institute of Medical Sciences, Zewail City of Science and Technology, Giza, Egypt

Charles Hudson and Paula C. Bickford
James A Haley Veterans Hospital, Research Service, Tampa, FL, USA

Niketa A. Patel and Denise R. Cooper
Department of Molecular Medicine, University of South Florida Morsani College of Medicine, 12901 Bruce B Downs Blvd, Tampa, FL 33612, USA

Lauren Daly Moss, Jea-Young Lee, Sandra Acosta and Paula C. Bickford
Department of Neurosurgery and Brain Repair, University of South Florida Morsani College of Medicine, Tampa, FL, USA

Naoki Tajiri
Department of Neurophysiology & Brain Science, Graduate School of Medical Sciences & Medical School, Nagoya City University, 1 Kawasumi, Mizuho-cho, Mizuho-ku, Nagoya, Aichi 467-8601, Japan

Cesario V. Borlongan
USF Health Center of Excellence for Aging and Brain Repair MDC-78, 12901 Bruce B Downs, Blvd, Tampa, FL 33612, USA

Maria N. Pavlova, Kristyn M. Ringgold, Paulien R. Barf, Amrita M. George, Mark R. Opp and Carmelina Gemma
Department of Anesthesiology and Pain Medicine, University of Washington, Seattle, WA 98001, USA

Hannah E. Thomasy
Neuroscience Graduate Program, University of Washington, Seattle, WA 98104, USA

Jenna N. Grillo
Department of Biology, University of Washington, Seattle, WA 98104, USA

Adam D. Bachstetter
Sanders-Brown Center on Aging, University of Kentucky, Lexington, KY 40536, USA

Jenny A. Garcia and Astrid E. Cardona
Department of Biology and South Texas Center for Emerging Infectious Diseases, University of Texas at San Antonio, San Antonio, TX 78249, USA

Heidi Y. Febinger
Interdepartmental Program in Neuroscience, University of Utah School of Medicine, Salt Lake City, Utah, USA

Su-Juan Liu, Xue Zhou and Ting-Hua Wang
Department of Histology, Embryology and Neurobiology, West China School of Preclinical and Forensic Medicine, Sichuan University, Chengdu, Sichuan 610041, China

Yu Zou, Qing-Jie Xia
Institute of Neurological Disease, Translational Neuroscience Center, West China Hospital, Sichuan University, Chengdu, Sichuan 610041, China

Visar Belegu and John W McDonald
Department of Neurology, Johns Hopkins University School of Medicine, Baltimore, MD 21205, USA

Long-Yun Lv, Na Lin, Ting-Yong Wang and Ting-Hua Wang
Institute of Neuroscience, Kunming Medical University, Kunming, Yunnan 650031, China

Abhishek Desai, Taeyeop Park, Jaquel Barnes, Karl Kevala, Huazhen Chen and Hee-Yong Kim
Laboratory of Molecular Signaling, National Institute of Alcohol Abuse and Alcoholism, National Institutes of Health, 5625 Fishers Lane, Rm. 3N-07, Bethesda, MD 20892-9410, USA

Index